Arthroplasty of the Upper Extremity

Graham J. W. King • Marco Rizzo
Editors

# Arthroplasty of the Upper Extremity

## A Clinical Guide from Elbow to Fingers

Springer

*Editors*
Graham J. W. King
Roth McFarlane Hand & Upper Limb Centre
St Joseph's Health Care
London, ON
Canada

Marco Rizzo
Department of Orthopedic Surgery
Mayo Clinic
Rochester, MN
USA

ISBN 978-3-030-68879-0 ISBN 978-3-030-68880-6 (eBook)
https://doi.org/10.1007/978-3-030-68880-6



This Springer imprint is published by the registered company Springer Nature Switzerland AG
The registered company address is: Gewerbestrasse 11, 6330 Cham, Switzerland

*I dedicate this book to my loving and supportive parents Ian and Ethelwynne; my beautiful wife and soul mate Denise; and my three amazing children Stephanie, Leanna, and Ian who provided me the opportunity, encouragement, and inspiration for this and many other projects that I have pursued during my "spare time." I am also grateful to my mentors Robert McMurtry, Cyril Frank, Bernard Morrey, and James Roth for their wisdom, guidance, and wise council.*

Graham J. W. King, MD, MSc, FRCSC
London, Ontario, Canada

*I would also dedicate this to my family: my wonderfully supportive and loving wife and daughter: Hope Marie and Hope Sol Rim without whom I would be lost. Thank you for encouraging and allowing me to pursue this work and the many others throughout my career. I remain indebted to your love, patience, and kindness. Special thanks also to my parents Nazario and Maria who've sacrificed so that I may have opportunities. Their love and example remain an inspiration. Thank you also to the mentors who've trained me: William Hardaker (1942–2015), teacher and mentor extraordinaire, who saw enough in me to give me a chance in orthopedics; James Urbaniak, for showing me the value and beauty of academic medicine; Richard Goldner, for demonstrating how dedicated, patient centered, and caring a surgeon can be; and Robert Beckenbaugh (1941–2020) for inspiring, teaching and nurturing my passion for arthroplasty.*

Marco Rizzo, MD
Rochester, Minnesota, United States of America

# Preface

Arthritis of the upper extremity often results in significant pain and disability. Arthroplasty of the arthritic elbow, wrist, and hand relieves pain, preserves motion, and improves function. While the experience in upper extremity arthroplasty is less extensive than those of the hip and knee, when successful, these procedures can be very rewarding for patients. The aim of this book is to guide practicing upper extremity surgeons, trainees, and therapists on the contemporary arthroplasty management of arthritis of the elbow, wrist, and hand.

The genesis of this book dates back to 2018. We were invited by the program chairs of The American Society for Surgery of the Hand Annual Meeting to co-chair a pre-course titled Arthroplasty: Elbow to Fingertips. We divided each joint into three parts: (1) design considerations, (2) primary arthroplasty, and (3) revision/failed arthroplasty. We invited national and international experts to participate and were delighted at their positive responses and enthusiasm for this endeavor.

The pre-course was a great success and sparked the interest of the representatives from Springer to create a book related to this subject matter. Given the success we experienced with the pre-course, it made sense to have the book mirror the same outline. Thankfully, most of the meeting presenters were able to contribute chapters. Countless hours of effort from the authors have been put into the making of this book. We are greatly indebted to them and sincerely appreciate their sacrificing time from family and work obligations to share their expertise and experience.

Having a book dedicated to arthroplasty of the elbow, wrist, and hand is unprecedented and should prove very useful to upper extremity surgeons. In addition, the structure of the chapters with sections for each anatomic region will be efficient for the reader. The design considerations chapters will reinforce the underlying pathology and provide a greater understanding of the thought processes related to rationale and development of implants. It is our hope that this will inspire further creativity and insights to advance the designs of current implants. The primary arthroplasty chapters will guide surgeons on the current indications, technique, and outcomes of primary joint arthroplasty. The revision/failed chapters should help guide the reader through the often difficult and challenging options associated with treating patients who have failed primary arthroplasty.

We sincerely appreciate the invitation from Springer to lead this effort and for their support throughout these past 2 years. We would like to especially thank Ms. Abha Krishnan for her steady support and stewardship through this entire process.

Finally, to our devoted families, who have quietly and lovingly supported us through this (and many) academic endeavors, we are eternally grateful. Your love and support inspire us and have made this possible.

London, ON, Canada Graham J. W. King
Rochester, MN, USA Marco Rizzo

# Acknowledgments

Arthroplasty of the upper extremity remains considerably less developed than that of the knee and hip due to the perceived lack of opportunities for manufacturers, limiting investment in research and development. Arthritis and disorders of the upper limb are very common and are major causes of disability and loss of function for daily activities, work, and sports. There have been significant advances in upper extremity joint arthroplasty in recent years; however, there continues to be an unmet need for patients who could benefit from reliable and durable implants. This project began as an idea to highlight the advances in arthroplasty of the upper limb and to serve as a basis for future work.

A total of 52 authors volunteered their time to contribute to this book. Each is an acknowledged expert in their area of subspecialty. We express our deepest appreciation to all the authors who provided their expertise. We would also like to thank the editors and the publisher for their support of this project, particularly during the height of the COVID-19 pandemic. It is our hope that this book will be useful for those interested in advancing the surgical treatment of patients requiring upper limb joint arthroplasty.

Graham J. W. King and Marco Rizzo

# Contents

# Contributors

**Brian Adams, MD** Department of Orthopedic Surgery, Baylor College of Medicine, Houston, TX, USA

**Julie Adams, MD** Department of Orthopaedic Surgery, University of Tennessee College of Medicine – Chattanooga, Erlanger Orthopaedic Institute, Chattanooga, TN, USA

**William R. Aibinder, MD** Shoulder & Elbow Surgery, SUNY Downstate Health Sciences University, Brooklyn, NY, USA

**Emilie J. Amaro, MD** Vanderbilt University Department of Orthopedics, Division of Hand Surgery, Nashville, TN, USA

**Douglas W. Bartels, MD** Department of Orthopedic Surgery, Mayo Clinic, Rochester, MN, USA

**Robert D. Beckenbaugh, MD** Department of Orthopedic Surgery, Mayo Clinic, Rochester, MN, USA

**Abhiram R. Bhashyam, MD PhD** Department of Orthopaedics and Sports Medicine, University of Washington, Seattle, WA, USA

**Chelsea Boe, MD** Department of Orthopaedics and Sports Medicine, University of Washington, Seattle, WA, USA

**Michel E. H. Boeckstyns, MD** Capio Private Hospital, Section for Hand Surgery, Hellerup, Denmark

Herlev-Gentofte University Hospital, Section for Hand Surgery, Hellerup, Denmark

**Anton Borgers, MD** Orthopedic Department, AZ Monica Hospital, Antwerp, Belgium

Orthopedic Department, AZ Turnhout Hospital, Turnhout, Belgium

**Samyd S. Bustos, MD** Division of Plastic and Reconstructive Surgery, Mayo Clinic, Rochester, MN, USA

**Logan W. Carr, MD** Department of Orthopedic Surgery, Baylor College of Medicine, Houston, TX, USA

**Joseph J. Crisco III, PhD** Bioengineering Laboratory, Department of Orthopaedics, The Warren Alpert Medical School of Brown University and Rhode Island Hospital, Providence, RI, USA

**Eric S. Dilbone, MD** Vanderbilt University Department of Orthopedics, Division of Hand Surgery, Nashville, TN, USA

**Kenneth J. Faber, MD MHPE FRCSC** Roth | McFarlane Hand and Upper Limb Centre, Western University, London, ON, Canada

**Giovanni Munz, MD** Hand Surgery and Reconstructive Microsurgery Unit, Azienda Ospedaliero-Universitaria Careggi, Florence, Italy

**Avi D. Goodman, MD** Department of Orthopaedics, Rhode Island Hospital/Brown University, Providence, RI, USA

Alpert Medical School of Brown University, Providence, RI, USA

**Amit Gupta, MD** Department of Orthopedic Surgery, University of Louisville, Louisville, KY, USA

**Doug Hanel, MD** Department of Orthopaedics and Sports Medicine, University of Washington, Seattle, WA, USA

**Daniel B. Herren, MD, MHA** Department of Hand Surgery, Schulthess Klinik, Zurich, Switzerland

**James P. Hovis, MD** Arizona Center for Hand Surgery, Phoenix, AZ, USA

**Mohammed S. Hussain, MD** University of Cincinnati, Department of Orthopaedic Surgery, Cincinnati, OH, USA

**James A. Johnson, PhD, PEng** Roth | McFarlane Hand & Upper Limb Centre, London, ON, Canada

St. Joseph's Health Care London, London, ON, Canada

Division of Orthopaedic Surgery, Western University, Schulich School of Medicine & Dentistry, London, ON, Canada

Mechanical and Materials Engineering, Department of Surgery, Western University, Faculty of Engineering, Schulich School of Medicine & Dentistry, London, ON, Canada

**Graham J. W. King, MD, MSc, FRCSC** Roth | McFarlane Hand & Upper Limb Centre, London, ON, Canada

St. Joseph's Health Care London, London, ON, Canada

Division of Orthopaedic Surgery, Western University, Schulich School of Medicine & Dentistry, London, ON, Canada

**Jerome Klawitter, PhD** Smith & Nephew, Austin, TX, USA

**Doga Kuruoglu, MD** Division of Plastic and Reconstructive Surgery, Mayo Clinic, Rochester, MN, USA

**Amy L. Ladd, MD** Chase Hand and Upper Limb Center, Department of Orthopaedic Surgery, Palo Alto, CA, USA

**Donald H. Lee, MD** Vanderbilt University Department of Orthopedics, Division of Hand Surgery, Nashville, TN, USA

**Massimo Ceruso, MD** Hand Surgery and Reconstructive Microsurgery Unit, Azienda Ospedaliero-Universitaria Careggi, Florence, Italy

**Yoshitaka Minamikawa, MD** Minamikawa Orthopaedic Surgery/Numba Hand Center, Naniwaku, Osaka, Japan

**Steven L. Moran, MD** Division of Plastic and Reconstructive Surgery, Mayo Clinic, Rochester, MN, USA

Department of Orthopedic Surgery, Mayo Clinic, Rochester, MN, USA

**Bernard F. Morrey, MD** Department of Orthopaedic Surgery, Mayo Clinic, Rochester, MN, USA

University of Texas Health Science Center, San Antonio, TX, USA

**Mark E. Morrey, MD** Department of Orthopaedic Surgery, Mayo Clinic, Rochester, MN, USA

**Sebastian A. Müller, MD, PD, FMH** Shoulder and Elbow Surgery, Division of Orthopaedic Surgery and Traumatology, University of Basel, Basel, Switzerland

**Peter M. Murray, MD** Department of Orthopedic Surgery, Mayo Clinic, Jacksonville, FL, USA

**Shawn W. O'Driscoll, MD, PhD** Department of Orthopedic Surgery, Mayo Clinic and Mayo Foundation, Rochester, MN, USA

**William F. Ogilvie, BS** Ensemble Orthopedics, LLC, Austin, TX, USA

**Marco Rizzo, MD** Department of Orthopedic Surgery, Division of Hand Surgery, Mayo Clinic, Rochester, MN, USA

**Susanne M. Roberts, MD** Division of Hand and Upper Extremity Surgery, Department of Orthopedic Surgery, Columbia University Medical Center, New York, NY, USA

**Phillip R. Ross, MD** University of Cincinnati, Department of Orthopaedic Surgery, Cincinnati, OH, USA

**Sandra Pfanner, MD** Hand Surgery and Reconstructive Microsurgery Unit, Azienda Ospedaliero-Universitaria Careggi, Florence, Italy

**Luis R. Scheker, MD** Kleinert Institute, Louisville, KY, USA

**Stephan F. Schindele, MD** Department of Hand Surgery, Schulthess Klinik, Zurich, Switzerland

**Scott P. Steinmann, MD** Department of Orthopaedic Surgery, University of Tennessee College of Medicine – Chattanooga, Erlanger Orthopaedic Institute, Chattanooga, TN, USA

Mayo Clinic, Rochester, MN, USA

**Peter J. Stern, MD** University of Cincinnati, Department of Orthopaedic Surgery, Cincinnati, OH, USA

**Ian A. Trail, MD, FRCS** Wrightington Hospital, Wigan, Lancashire, UK

**Matthias Vanhees, MD, PhD** Orthopedic Department, AZ Monica Hospital, Antwerp, Belgium

Orthopedic Department, Antwerp University Hospital, Edegem, Belgium

**Frederik Verstreken, MD** Orthopedic Department, AZ Monica Hospital, Antwerp, Belgium

Orthopedic Department, Antwerp University Hospital, Edegem, Belgium

**Arnold-Peter C. Weiss, MD** Department of Orthopaedics, Rhode Island Hospital/Brown University, Providence, RI, USA

Alpert Medical School of Brown University, Providence, RI, USA

**Scott W. Wolfe, MD** Hand and Upper Extremity Division, Hospital for Special Surgery, Department of Orthopedic Surgery, Weill Cornell Medicine, New York, NY, USA

**Maria Yan, MD** Division of Plastic and Reconstructive Surgery, Mayo Clinic, Rochester, MN, USA

**Nicole Zelenski, MD** Department of Orthopedic Surgery, Mayo Clinic, Rochester, MN, USA

# Part I

# Total Elbow Arthroplasty

# 1 Total Elbow Arthroplasty: Design Considerations

Sebastian A. Müller, Graham J. W. King, and James A. Johnson

## Introduction

The elbow is a complex tripartite joint, consisting of the ulnohumeral, the radiocapitellar, and the proximal radioulnar joints (PRUJ) [1] allowing for extension and flexion as well as forearm rotation. Compared to the joints of the lower limb, which are usually weight bearing, loading of the elbow is relatively low for many activities of daily living. However, forces transmitted across the elbow can be high for some activities exceeding three times body weight [2] and thereby challenging the longevity of total elbow arthroplasty (TEA). Several design considerations are necessary to restore the main motion of extension and flexion in the elbow as well as forearm rotation while respecting the high loading, which can occur. The overall goal of TEA is to achieve painless and stable motion for activities of daily living, vocations, and avocations [3]. The main indications for TEA include primary or posttraumatic osteoarthritis, rheumatoid arthritis, tumors, distal humeral fractures and nonunions, and dysfunctional instability. While the incidence of TEA continues to rise for acute trauma and posttraumatic sequelae, those for rheumatoid arthritis have decreased with the advent of more effective medical management [4–6]. TEA can be either linked transmitting higher forces along the implant or unlinked requiring intact ligaments and good bone stock. Convertible TEAs can be converted from an unlinked to a linked articula-

*Dr. King serves as a consultant and receives royalties from Wright Medical. Neither Dr. Johnson, Dr. Müller, nor any immediate family member has received anything of value from or has stock or stock options held in a commercial company or institution related directly or indirectly to the subject of this chapter.*

S. A. Müller
Shoulder and Elbow Surgery, Division of Orthopaedic Surgery and Traumatology, University of Basel, Basel, Switzerland

G. J. W. King
Roth | McFarlane Hand & Upper Limb Centre, London, ON, Canada

St. Joseph's Health Care London, London, ON, Canada

Division of Orthopaedic Surgery, Western University, Schulich School of Medicine & Dentistry, London, ON, Canada
e-mail: gking@uwo.ca

J. A. Johnson (✉)
Roth | McFarlane Hand & Upper Limb Centre, London, ON, Canada

St. Joseph's Health Care London, London, ON, Canada

Division of Orthopaedic Surgery, Western University, Schulich School of Medicine & Dentistry, London, ON, Canada

Mechanical and Materials Engineering, Department of Surgery, Western University, Faculty of Engineering, Schulich School of Medicine & Dentistry, London, ON, Canada
e-mail: jajohnso@uwo.ca


G. J. W. King, M. Rizzo (eds.), *Arthroplasty of the Upper Extremity*,
https://doi.org/10.1007/978-3-030-68880-6_1

tion if instability is problematic without having to revise the humeral or ulnar components [7–10]. They can also allow conversion from a distal humeral hemiarthroplasty to a TEA without removing the humeral stem.

Hemiarthroplasty of the distal humerus is an option for selected acute distal humeral fractures and nonunions, and likely require less weight restrictions than for TEA. However, the collateral ligaments must be repairable and a humeral component matched in size and shape to the native ulnar, and radial articulations are essential to reduce cartilage wear [11–13].

## Basic Biomechanics

### Kinematics of the Elbow

The primary function of the elbow is to position the hand in space for bimanual activities. The principal motions are flexion, extension, pronation, and supination. The flexion-extension motion has a full range of approximately 0–140 degrees, with an average 30–130 degrees needed for typical activities of daily living [3, 14, 15]. The flexion-extension axis passes through the center of curvature of the trochlear groove and the spherical center of the capitellum [16–20]. This axis varies slightly throughout the flexion-extension cycle, and hence the ulnohumeral articulation has been termed a "sloppy hinge" [16, 19]. This axis is approximately 3–5 degrees internally rotated from the medial and lateral epicondylar axis, and 4–8 degrees valgus relative to the humeral long axis [16, 17, 21]. An understanding of this relatively unique motion has led to the genesis of "loose hinge" TEA designs.

The carrying angle of the elbow, which differs from the aforementioned flexion axis, also has implications with respect to implant design [22]. The carrying angle is measured between the long axes of the humerus and ulna as measured in the coronal plane in full extension and supination. Carrying angles vary considerable among individuals, and are higher on average in women (10–15 degrees) than in men (7–12 degrees) [14]. Quite clearly, the establishment of this alignment is also important with regard to the design of the ulnohumeral articulation in implants.

Forearm rotation is governed primarily by the radiocapitellar joint, and proximal and distal radioulnar joints. The normal range is approximately 90 degrees of supination to 80 degrees of pronation, although 50 degrees in either direction is generally sufficient for most activities of daily living [3, 15]. The rotation axis runs from the center of the radial head to close to the fovea of the distal ulna [23, 24]. Reproducing the native forearm motion following implant reconstruction is primarily influenced by the shape and position of the radial head and capitellar surfaces for the total elbow replacement systems that replace both the ulnohumeral and radiohumeral articulations.

### Joint Loading of the Elbow

Muscle loading has a profound impact on articular biomechanics. The compressive forces generated across the articulations of the elbow have been shown to markedly increase joint stability [25–30]. Biomechanical cadaver-based studies have clearly demonstrated that active loading achieved by simulating contraction of the elbow flexors and extensors results in more consistent and repeatable flexion-extension motion pathways relative to passive control (where the arm is guided by the investigator) [29].

An understanding of the loads that occur at the elbow is very relevant with regard to total implant design and performance. To date, direct measurements using instrumented implants and wireless telemetry in patients have yet to be developed for the elbow, and thus an exact measurement of joint loading is not available. However, it is well established from a variety of studies that these magnitudes are far from trivial. The quantification of these loads currently relies on computational approaches. Both simplified two-dimensional models and more complex approaches that account for the numerous load-bearing structures that cross the joint (i.e., the articulation, ligaments, capsule, muscles, and tendons) have been employed [2, 31, 32]. At the radiocapitellar joint, up to three times body weight has been estimated [2]. The resultant force on the ulnohumeral joint can also approach three times body weight during weight-training activities. Push-up exercises can generate forces approximating 45% of body weight [33]. Also, the direction of the joint reaction force varies markedly throughout the flexion-extension cycle, and this of course has a strong influence on the axial and bending loads that must be accepted by the implant and interfaces with bone. With respect to the relative load distribution between the ulnar and radial sides, this is very dependent on the activity and position of the joint (both for flexion and forearm rotation). Experimental and analytical studies have reported variable results, with approximately a 60:40 ratio for the radio-capitellar and ulnohumeral sides [31, 34, 35]. In light of the foregoing, it is logical to postulate that elbow implants are subjected to a wide range of significant loads that vary markedly in magnitude and direction in patients during routine activities.

## Current Total Elbow Arthroplasty (TEA) Principals

The first implantation of a TEA was documented in 1942 [36], but TEA was not routinely used before the early 1970s. These constrained TEAs had a fixed hinge (Fig. 1.1) with reported loosening rates of 26–68% of one or both stems at the bone-cement interface within 3 years after insertion, which is why this concept was abandoned [37–43]. Semi-constrained linked and unlinked implants were introduced in the 1970s and have continued to evolve over the last 50 years [37, 44, 45].

Improvements in linked implant durability were achieved with the development of semi-constrained implants incorporating a sloppy hinge. These implants permit 7–10° of varus-valgus laxity and some internal-external rotational laxity like that present in the native elbow. With this concept some of the forces are absorbed by the soft tissues reducing loading to the cement interface and thus loosening [7, 46–48]. In general, overconstraint results in higher loads being transferred through the bone-implant interface [49], which can lead to mechanical loosening, while underconstraint results in elbow instability [50, 51].

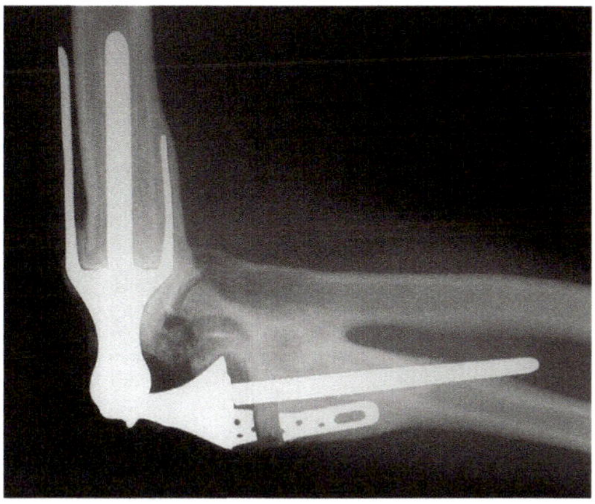

**Fig. 1.1** Custom-made linked TEA with anterior and posterior humeral flanges as well as a broken ulnar flange used for management of posttraumatic arthritis. The tip of the ulnar component has been implanted outside the intramedullary canal. A synostosis of the proximal ulna and radius is present. The olecranon is missing indicating poor triceps function

Unlinked implants transmit less force across the implant, which should theoretically reduce mechanical loosening. In the varus position, an unlinked TEA with intact ligaments transmits approximately half of the loads to the humeral stem when compared to a linked device [52]. This biomechanical advantage of unlinked TEA has yet to be confirmed with a reduction in wear and loosening in clinical studies [10, 30, 48, 53–55]. The stability of an unlinked device relies on secure ligament repair with strong healing, and good bone stock with no or little bony deformity [37, 44, 45, 53, 55–57] (Fig. 1.2). For an unlinked TEA, an intact or replaced radial head is important to improve stability [53, 58–60] (Fig. 1.3). If the aforementioned factors are lacking, a linked TEA is preferred [1, 46, 48, 52, 61–63]. However, forces on the implant increase for both linked and unlinked TEAs with insufficient ligaments in vitro, stressing the importance of ligament repair where possible for both design concepts [52] (Fig. 1.4).

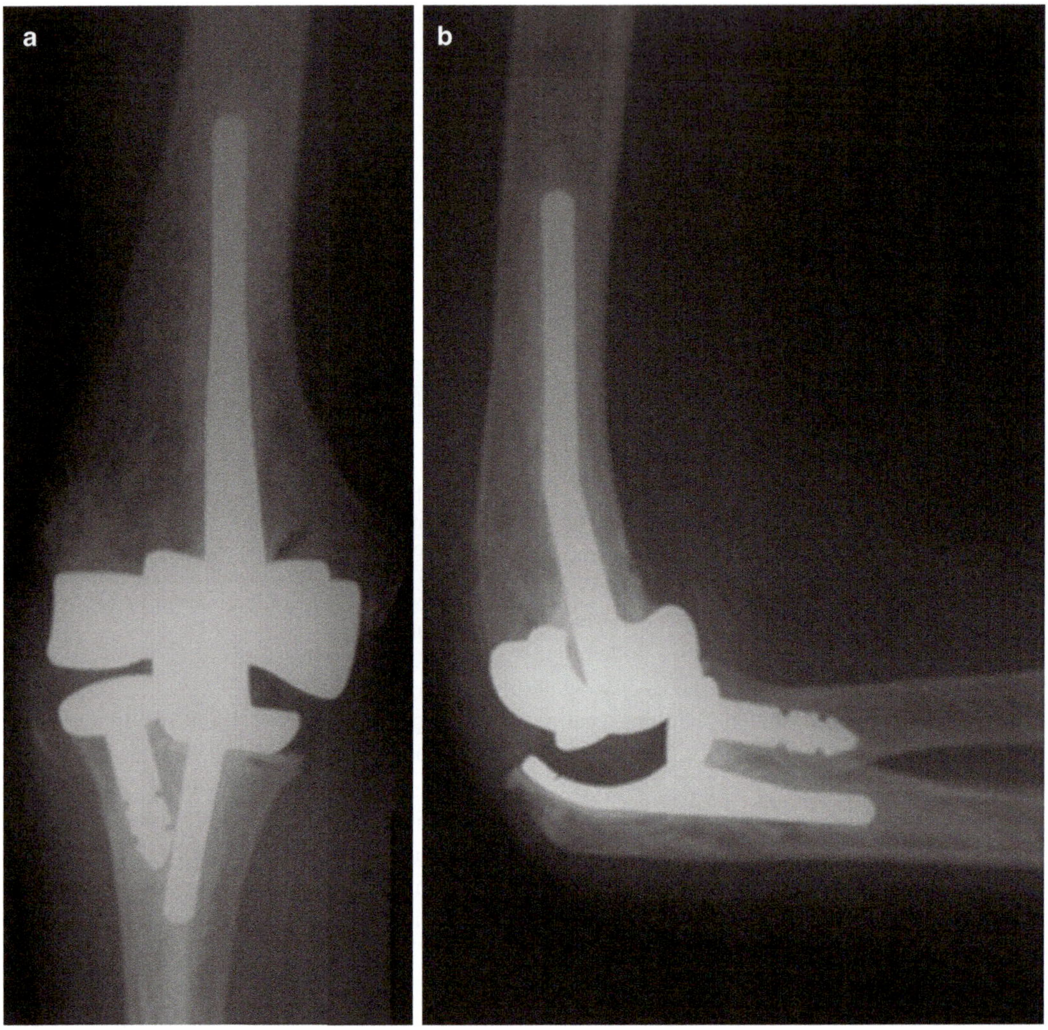


**Fig. 1.2** (**a**, **b**) Joint subluxation in an unstable TEA with a radial head replacement (Sorbie, Wright Medical)

Traditional TEA designs were either linked or unlinked. In case of revision from an unlinked to a linked TEA to address instability, often well-fixed stems had to be removed, which means major surgery (Fig. 1.3). Modern convertible TEA designs can more easily be converted from unlinked to linked in a short surgical procedure [8–10]. Moreover, conversion from a hemiarthroplasty to TEA is possible without removing the humeral stem [8, 9] (Fig. 1.5).

The 10-year survivorship of linked and unlinked TEA is 83–90% with better results in high-volume institutions and in lower-demand patients [64, 65]. Instability, loosening, and material wear continue to be the most common causes of TEA failure [64–66]. Therefore, design considerations include joint stability in unlinked TEA, wear reduction in linked TEA, and implant fixation in linked and unlinked TEA.

## Implant Fixation

Implants are usually fixed with acrylic bone cement into the distal humerus, proximal ulna, and proximal radius (if needed). Uncemented implants are not currently commercially avail-

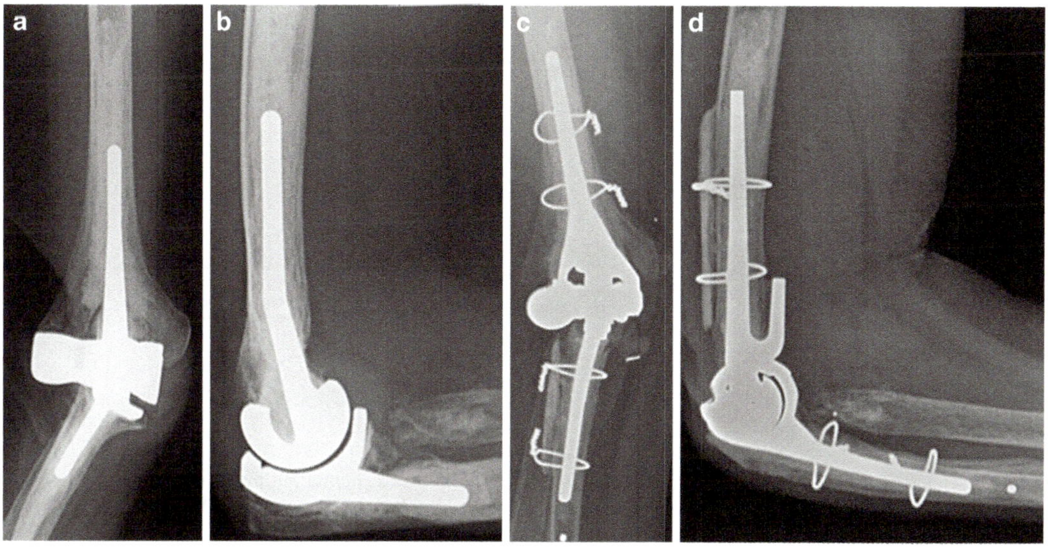


**Fig. 1.3** (**a**, **b**) Fifteen years following an unlinked TEA for osteoarthritis (Sorbie, Wright Medical), valgus instability developed due to attenuation of the medial collateral ligament. (**c**, **d**) Revision to a linked implant (Latitude, Wright Medical). The well-fixed stems were removed and humeral and ulnar shafts augmented with allograft struts

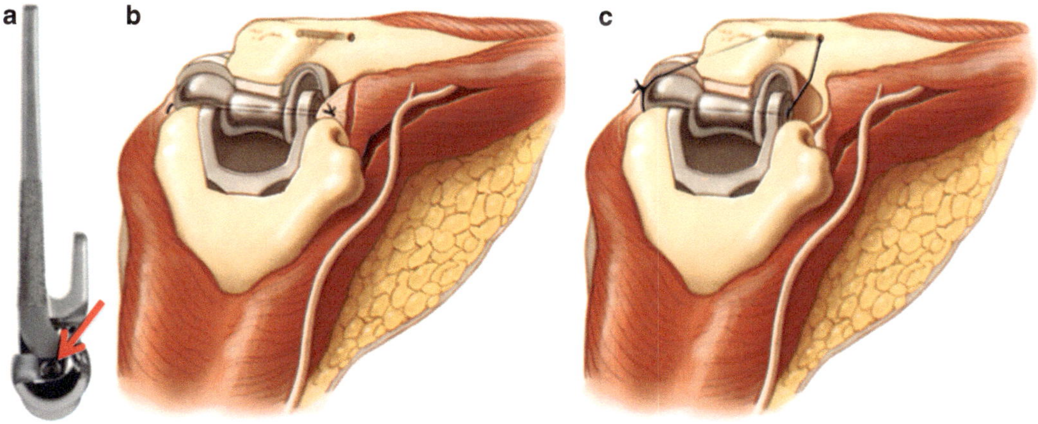


**Fig. 1.4** Convertible implant (Latitude EV, Wright Medical) with (**a**) a hole in the humeral spool (red arrow) for (**b**) reattachment of the collateral ligaments and the flexor and extensor muscles, respectively. (**c**) Additional stability can be achieved by placing a strong suture through the spool and a tunnel in the ulna protecting the reattached ligaments from varus-valgus, distraction, and rotational forces while healing. (From Wright Medical Group, N.V., Memphis, TN, USA; with permission)

able for TEA but have had some success for humeral component fixation [45, 67–69]. Secure fixation of the cement interfaces with implant and bone is required to accept the significant axial, bending, and torsional loads that can be generated at the articulation. The stem should be inserted carefully into the intramedullary canal to achieve an optimal cement mantle around the implant [70]. Modern cementing techniques using cement guns and cement restrictors have further improved stem fixation [71].

## Intramedullary Stem Design

Due to failures of early stemless or short-stem TEA designs (Fig. 1.6), intramedullary stem fixation has become standard in TEA [72, 73]. The

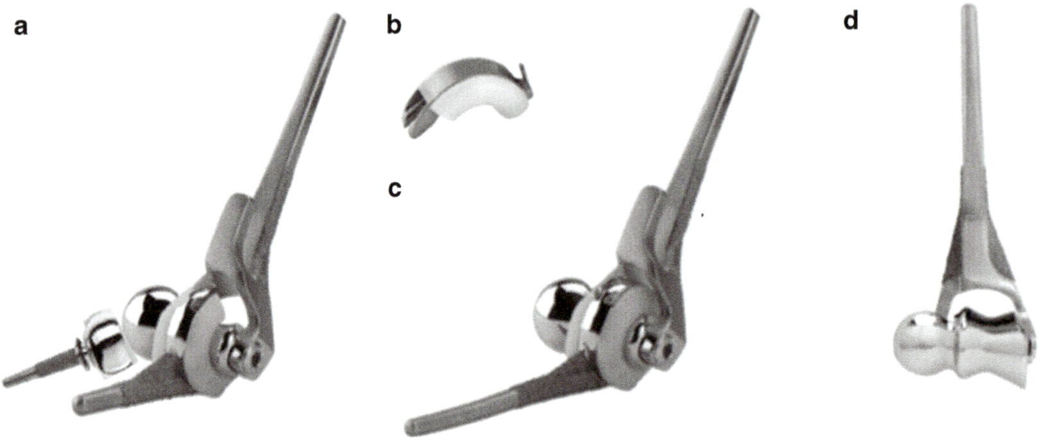


**Fig. 1.5** Convertible TEA (Latitude EV System, Wright Medical). (**a**) Unlinked TEA with radial head replacement, (**b**) ulnar cap to link system, (**c**) linked TEA without radial head, (**d**) hemiarthroplasty of distal humerus with anatomical humeral spool. (From Wright Medical Group, N.V., Memphis, TN, USA; with permission)

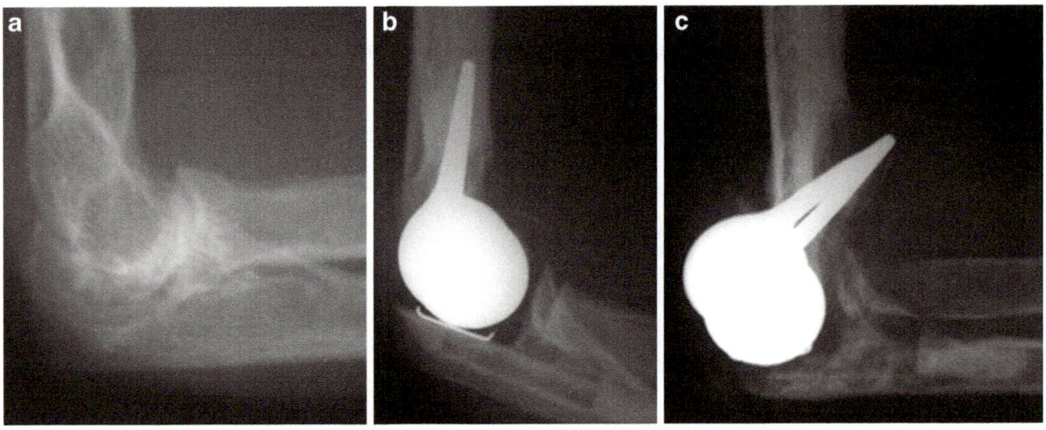


**Fig. 1.6** (**a**) Lateral radiograph of a patient with rheumatoid arthritis, (**b**) postoperative radiograph after a short stem TEA (Souter-Strathclyde, Stryker), (**c**) humeral loosening with implant failure at 5 years

optimal stem length is unknown and requires further study.

Adding an anterior flange to the humeral component permits the insertion of a bone graft on the anterior humerus, which may enhance the bony support at a point where the maximum stress has been found to occur with some implant designs. The idea is to reduce rotational and posterior-directed forces potentially causing loosening [2, 34, 72, 74, 75]. While the anterior flange seems to reduce the forces for some implants (GSB, Sulzer Medical [76]; Coonrad-Morrey, Zimmer [7]), this may not be the case for other implants. The anterior flange of the Latitude TEA, Wright Medical did not change the load distribution for axial or bending moments in an in vitro study [77]. The authors of this study suggested two possible reasons why an anterior flange may not be needed in this implant. First, the Latitude humeral component has medial and lateral fins on the distal portion increasing the cross-sectional area and thus the fixation within the cement (Fig. 1.5). Second, the Latitude implant is made of cobalt chrome, and as such the forces may not be transmitted to the distal humerus to the same extent as they are with less stiff titanium implants.

Finite element and in vitro studies [78, 79] have shown unequal load distribution with greatly

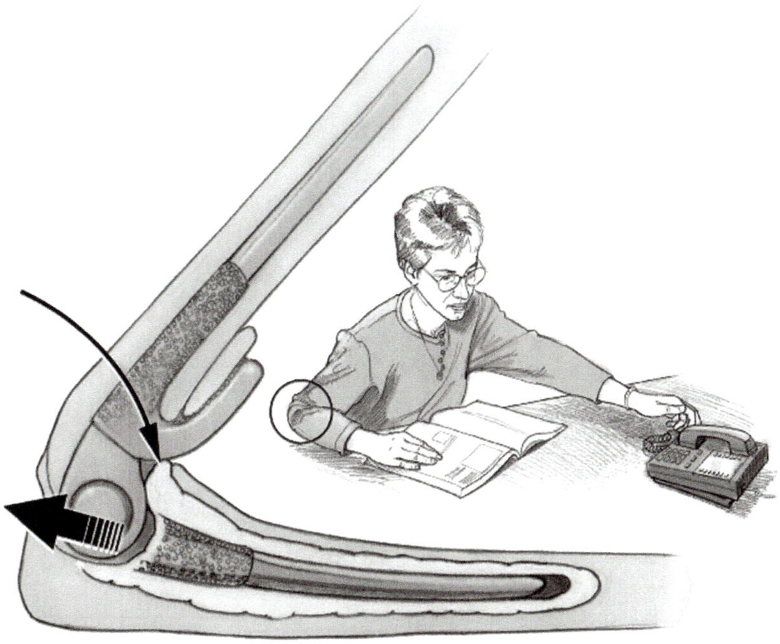

**Fig. 1.7** Schematic of a TEA illustrating anterior impingement of the coronoid process on the anterior flange resulting in pullout forces being applied to the ulnar component. (From Cheung and O'Driscoll [80]; with permission)

increased strain adjacent to the implant tip, but strain reduction relative to the epiphysis of humerus and ulna. This may lead to stress shielding, bone resorption, and fatigue failure, particularly in the ulna where there is no flange on the stem. The ideal stem shape, length, and materials with respect to improving the load distribution of elbow arthroplasty require further study.

Unlike the loaded joints of the lower limb, pullout forces, so-called pistoning, may cause ulnar stem loosening, particularly in linked TEA (Fig. 1.7). Impingement of the anterior humeral component flange with a prominent coronoid process or excessive cement must be avoided. Moreover, the ulnar stem should not be implanted too far distally [80]. Anterior flexion impingement should be reduced in future TEA designs allowing for high flexion angles regardless of the presence of an anterior flange.

Smooth stems favor debonding of the implant-cement interface and should be avoided in TEA. In vitro studies showed the highest axial load resistance was found for stems with rough surface treatment when compared to smooth stems. Titanium stems showed significantly higher load resistance compared to cobalt chrome stems for sintered beads, but similar results between materials with plasma spray coatings [81]. Shedding of sintered beads was of concern in these in vitro studies as well as the known weakening of the stem substrate in the course of their application (Fig. 1.8). Titanium plasma spray surface treatments are likely preferred for TEA.

In a laboratory setting, the ideal stem cross section was shown to be rectangular because it resisted the highest rotational forces when compared to triangular, oval, or round [82] (Fig. 1.9). Sharp rectangular stems, while providing the greatest resistance to torsion, should probably be avoided due to the concern about stress concentration in the cement mantle. To date, in vitro studies testing surface treatment and cross section have used straight stems with a constant cross section throughout the entire length, which does not reflect the anatomic situations with

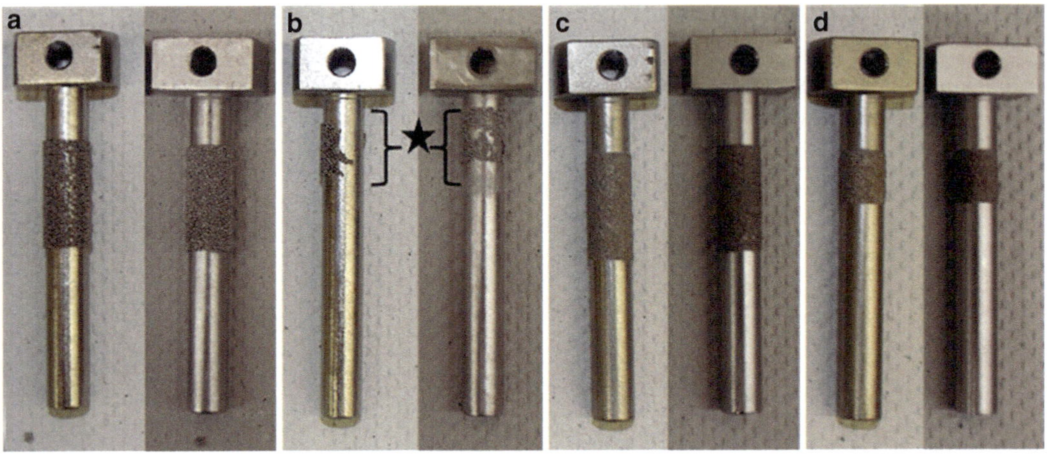


**Fig. 1.8** Titanium (left) and cobalt chrome (right) stems after in vitro testing. (**a**) 20 mm and (**b**) 10 mm beaded stems. (**c**) 20 mm and (**d**) 10 mm plasma spray-treated stems. Note debonding of the surface treatment in 10 mm beaded stems (star; B). (From Hosein et al. [81]; with permission)

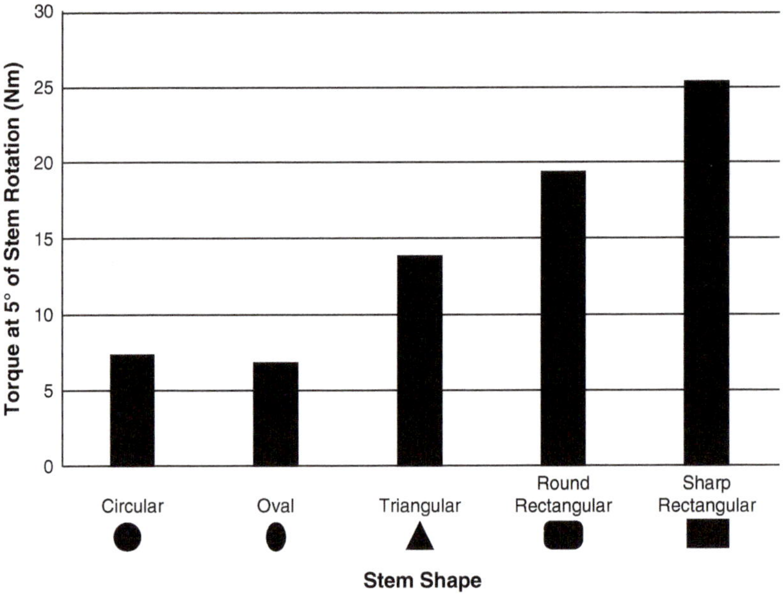


**Fig. 1.9** Resistance to rotational force in this in vitro study was found to differ depending on stem cross-sectional shape. The highest torque resistance was found for a rectangular cross section with sharp edges [82]

curved and tapered implants. Nevertheless, plasma spray-coated stems with a rectangular cross section are most likely favorable in vivo as well. Curved stems are more anatomic however; their removal is problematic relative to straight-tapered stems in the setting of infection. Further studies are needed to compare the durability of these two design concepts.

## Implant Positioning

Restoration of the extension and flexion axis is essential in TEA. Implant malpositioning alters ligament and capsular tension, muscle moment arms, and lines of action. This may increase wear of the articular surfaces and increase stresses in the implant-bone construct, possibly leading to component loosening or mechanical failure. It has been shown in an in vitro biomechanical study that the resultant load is significantly increased if the humeral component is positioned in anything but an anatomic location [83] (Fig. 1.10).

Correct positioning of the humeral stem relies on the accurate reproduction of the anatomic extension-flexion axis, which is determined by the vector through the centers of the capitellum and the trochlea. However, using visual cues to estimate the axis, alignment errors up to 10° in both directions occur even in the hands of subspecialty trained orthopedic surgeons [84] (Fig. 1.11). Improved surgical cutting guides or navigation systems may help to improve accuracy.

Among five methods for intraoperative determination of the extension-flexion axis from the proximal forearm, the most accurate is to use the ridge of the greater sigmoid notch in combination with the center of the radial head [85]. Modern TEA designs use surgical guides for joint axis determination and likely improve the accuracy of

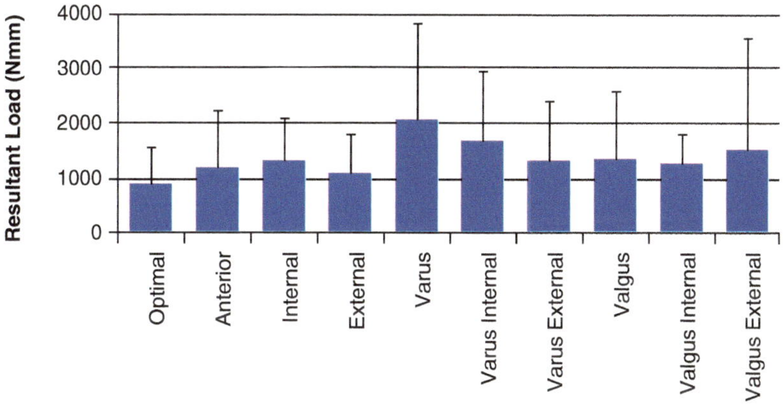


**Fig. 1.10** Mean bending load in the humeral stem of an instrumented TEA using a cadaver biomechanical model and an in vitro joint motion simulator. The resultant bending load (mean + SD) of the entire flexion range is shown. Malpositioning of the humeral component resulted in an increase in forces in the humeral stem. (From Brownhill et al. [83]; with permission)

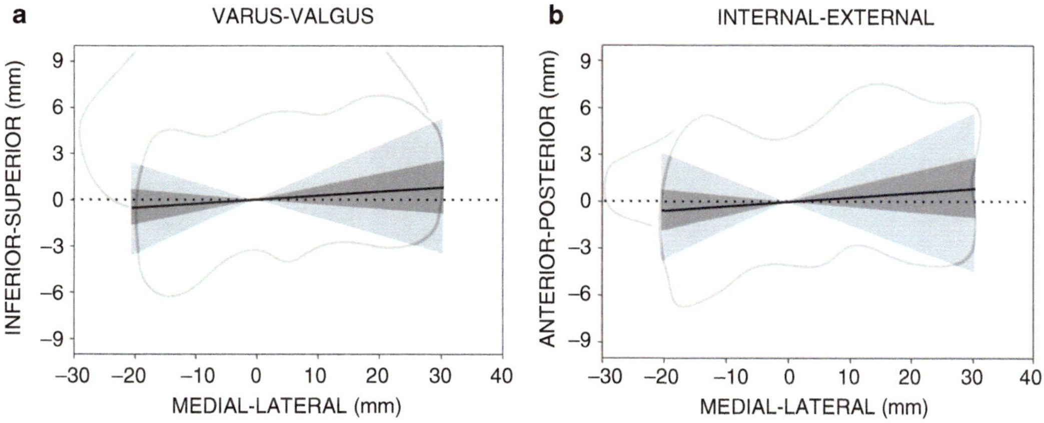


**Fig. 1.11** (**a**, **b**) Error in determination of extension-flexion axis of the elbow for varus-valgus and internal-external rotational alignment, respectively. The solid black line indicates the mean extension flexion axis. The dark gray area represents errors within one standard deviation of the mean line and the light gray area the remaining errors. (Adapted from Brownhill et al. [84]; with permission)

ulnar component positioning when the radial head is available.

More anatomic stem designs are required to improve alignment within the intramedullary canal as shown for the proximal ulna and distal humerus [86, 87]. Modular systems or custom-designed implants reverse engineered from CT imaging could be an option in cases of an altered intramedullary canal due to previous fractures, if long stems are needed [86], or to better accommodate the natural shape of the humerus and ulna, which varies between individuals [86, 87].

Computer navigation has been clinically used for spinal surgery as well as knee and hip arthroplasty but not for TEA so far. There are some in vitro studies evaluating navigation approaches using a laser scanner [88] also in combination with CT data from the diseased elbow [89] or CT data from the contralateral distal humerus [90], in order to define the correct implant position. Using this technology, commercially available humeral stems were found to impinge within the intramedullary canal in some cases causing alignment errors in rotation and translation. Impingement was not observed when shorter (more anatomic) stems were used. It was concluded that humeral stems with a fixed valgus angulation are difficult to implant correctly and more variability in varus-valgus stem angulations is needed to improve the accuracy of implant positioning [91]. Navigated implant placement was found to be superior to surgeon placement using standard mechanical instruments, particularly evident in the setting of distal humeral bone loss or deformity. Further work is needed to translate these in vitro findings into improved TEA designs and implantation techniques.

## Implant Wear

Wear of ultrahigh molecular weight polyethylene (UHMWPE) may induce osteolysis, which favors implant loosening [92–95]. Implant fatigue fractures may occur at the junction of a well-fixed and loose stem due to osteolysis (Fig. 1.12) as well as substrate weakening from the sintering of beaded surface treatments (Fig. 1.8) [96].

Whereas early TEA designs used metal on metal bearings, all current linked TEAs feature a

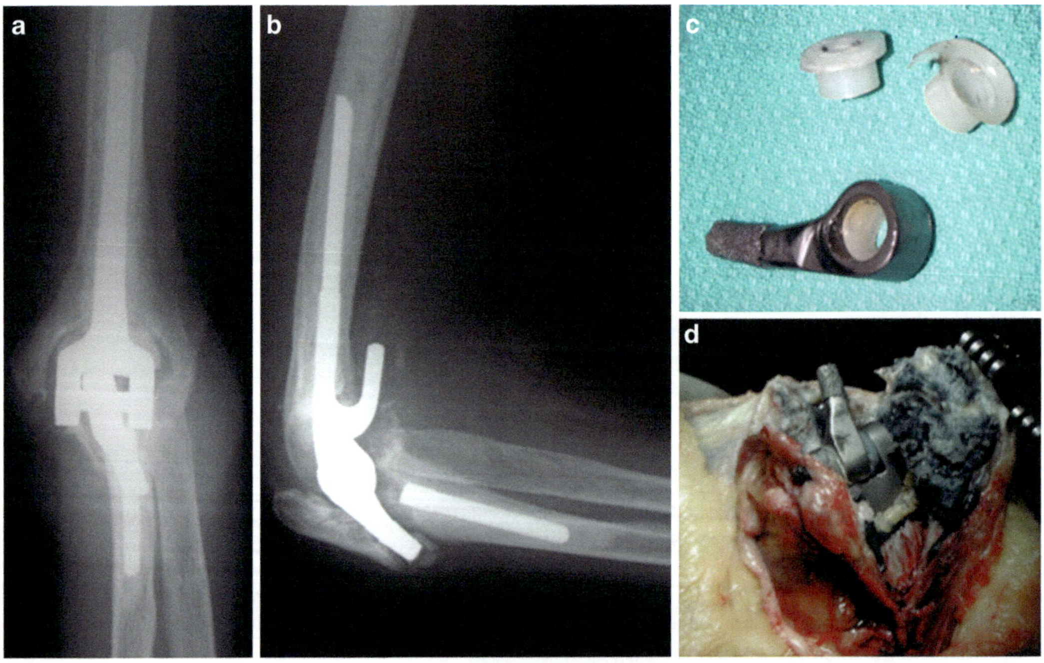


**Fig. 1.12** (**a**, **b**) Cantilever bending failure of the ulnar stem with periprosthetic fracture of the proximal ulna in a linked TEA (Coonrad-Morrey, Zimmer). (**c**, **d**) Bearing wear, osteolysis, and massive metallosis was noted at surgery

cobalt chrome surface that articulates against an UHMWPE bearing. Once the UHMWPE bearing surface is worn completely, the bushings need to be replaced to avoid metal on metal contact resulting in metallosis (Fig. 1.12). Some TEA designs use a "cylindrical" linking mechanism with a straight cobalt chrome pin [97–99]. Others use an "hourglass" or "concave cylinder" linkage designs with greater surface area of contact (Fig. 1.13). In a computational finite element analysis [51], the hourglass and concave cylinder linkages showed a significant decreased edge loading compared to a traditional cylindrical linkage design (Fig. 1.14). While edge loading

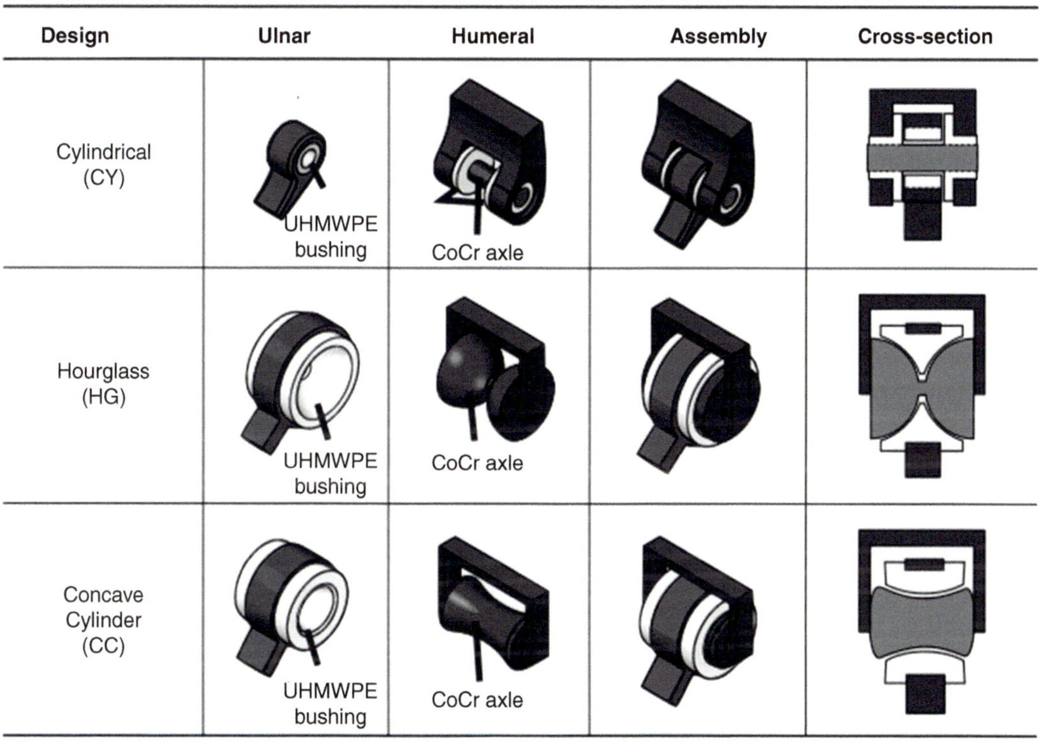


**Fig. 1.13** Schematic drawing of three different linkage mechanisms types. (From Willing et al. [51]; with permission)

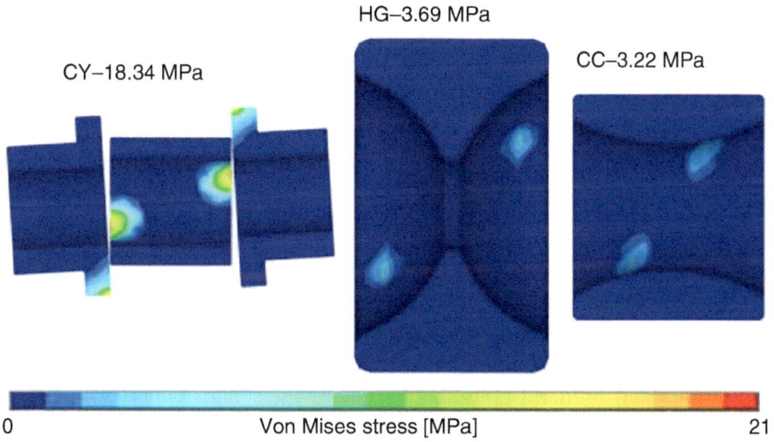


**Fig. 1.14** Significantly higher edge loading occurred for the cylindrical linkage design compared to hourglass and concave cylinder shapes. (From Willing et al. [51]; with permission)

was comparable for hourglass and concave cylinder designs, the concave cylinder design provided better varus-valgus stability and thus may be best suited for TEA with respect to reduction of wear, osteolysis, and implant failure [96].

## Design Considerations for Distal Humeral Hemiarthroplasty

### Overview

The first reported hemiarthroplasty of the distal humerus was implanted in 1925, which was made of aluminum and bronze with a protective rubber coating [100]. Other early implants composed of acrylic, nylon, or Vitallium were reported in case reports or small case series between 1947 and 1990 [101–105]. A series of ten elbows treated with a stemless stainless-steel or titanium hemiarthroplasty for posttraumatic conditions, rheumatoid arthritis, or ankylosis due to hemophilia was published in 1974. While elbows with posttraumatic conditions were stable, were painless, and had a functional range of motion in posttraumatic conditions, the results for inflammatory arthritis or hemophilia were unpredictable or poor [106].

The main treatment of distal humerus fractures remains ORIF in younger patients with reconstructable fractures and TEA for older patients with osteoporosis and unreconstructable fractures. There has been recent interest in distal humerus hemiarthroplasty for comminuted capitellar-trochlear and supracondylar fractures in patients too young for a TEA due to the lifelong activity restrictions required with these devices and concerns about implant longevity. The indications for distal humeral hemiarthroplasty also include failed ORIF, malunion or nonunion, and avascular necrosis of the capitellum or the trochlea [13, 107–110]. Some authors do not recommend distal humeral hemiarthroplasty in the younger population with distal humeral fractures due to a concern about long-term cartilage wear. These studies reported the outcome of nonanatomic distal humeral components where the contact with the native joint was likely suboptimal unlike newer anatomically shaped designs [11, 12].

The advantages of distal humeral hemiarthroplasty over TEA are the absence of polyethylene bearing wear and periarticular osteolysis from particulate debris. This may lower the risk of component loosening likely requiring less activity restrictions than for TEA [111]. With the introduction of commercially available, anatomical (Sorbie, Wright Medical; Latitude, Wright Medical) and nonanatomical (Kudo, Biomet) implants, outcome studies of hemiarthroplasties have increased over the last two decades [111]. The convertible Latitude EV system (Fig. 1.5) is the only available implant with a hemiarthroplasty option as most of the aforementioned implants are no longer marketed. It can be converted to a TEA by adding an ulnar stem and replacing the anatomical humeral spool with a differently shaped TEA spool. Hemiarthroplasty implants are currently not approved for use by the Food and Drug Administration for the United States but are available in many other countries.

Design considerations for distal humeral hemiarthroplasty stems are comparable to TEA. Stable soft tissue constraint is as important for a distal humeral hemiarthroplasty, similar to unlinked TEA. While a lack of polyethylene wear means osteolysis-mediated aseptic loosening is unlikely, cartilage degeneration of the proximal ulna and radial head is an important concern that requires further study.

### Joint Stability

Ligament repair and fixation of fractured epicondyles or condyles are necessary for joint stability, which can be challenging in the setting of comminution. An olecranon osteotomy surgical approach was commonly employed in early clinical series; it has fallen out of favor [108–110, 112, 113]. While allowing excellent exposure of the distal humeral articular surface and preservation of the collateral ligaments, nonunion, prominent hardware, and conversion to TEA were problematic [111]. Other approaches include triceps-splitting [114], triceps-reflecting (Bryan-Morrey)

[115, 116], medial or lateral epicondyle osteotomy [117, 118], and subperiosteal lateral collateral ligament release [107]. The authors prefer a triceps-preserving para-olecranon approach for acute fractures. It gives appropriate exposure, can be used for conversion to TEA as well, and does not require postoperative restrictions for the triceps repair with greater extension strength [119]. While comminuted parts of the joint surface need to be removed, fractured condyles and epicondyles with their attached collateral ligaments must be preserved for repair [111]. Determination of correct humeral component positioning may be challenging if both epicondyles are fractured, which may result in incorrect joint alignment and altered joint biomechanics. Using the superior aspect of the olecranon fossa to position the anterior flange and evaluating the tension of the soft tissues with a triceps-on approach are recommended to estimate the correct depth [111]. The humeral stem should be internally rotated 14° relative to the posterior humeral cortex [120].

Epicondyles can be fixed using sutures, K-wires, or small plates, and torn ligaments can be repaired with sutures through the hole in the humeral spool as for TEA (Fig. 1.4) [111]. A secure repair and healing of epicondyles and collateral ligaments is essential for joint stability, which is why strengthening should not be started before 8–12 weeks postoperatively [111]. Once the epicondyles are radiographically healed and the elbow is clinically stable, no specific weight restrictions such as recommended for TEA are required. However, the patient should be educated about the need to protect the hemiarthroplasty [111].

## Cartilage Wear Reduction

Nonanatomic TEA implants that have been used for hemiarthroplasty (Kudo; Biomet) lead to substantial cartilage attrition and are no longer on the market [12]. Degenerative radiographic changes have also been reported with anatomically shaped implants, more commonly for the Sorbie than for the Latitude; however, the clinical results have been favorable [13, 110].

An in vitro study found that the best joint congruity of the Latitude hemiarthroplasty with highest contact area was found if the humeral spool optimally fitted the greater sigmoid notch, followed by oversized implants. Undersized implants had the least congruity. Moreover, congruity was greater for active motion than passive motion indicating joint reduction due to muscle loading [121]. Compared to the native elbow, the mean contact area of an optimally sized implant decreased 44% for the ulnohumeral joint but only 4% for the radiocapitellar joint [122]. Altered varus and valgus angulations were found for optimally and undersized implants, whereas the oversized implants best reproduced native elbow kinematics. Based on this in vitro data, when choosing between two implant sizes, the larger one should be selected [111]. However, regardless of implant size, alterations in elbow biomechanics were found with abnormal articular contact, tracking, and loading and thus may result in cartilage degeneration over time [123]. Possible design modifications of the humeral spool could improve joint congruity and biomechanics. The stiffer nature of the metallic implant relative to the native cartilage of the distal humerus most likely wears the cartilage of ulna and radial head over time. Hence, future consideration should be given to more compliant implant materials, which should be more cartilage friendly. Long-term data regarding cartilage wear and distal humeral hemiarthroplasty durability is not yet available [111].

## Summary

TEA can be either unlinked or linked. Good bone stock, repaired ligaments, and an intact or replaced radial head are required for unlinked TEA. In cases of unstable unlinked TEA, convertible designs have the advantage to be converted to a linked status in a short surgery without the need of revising well-fixed stems. Wear and loosening is more often seen in linked TEA. Improvement of implant designs includes more anatomic stems with rectangular cross section and surface roughening. Modern concave cylinder-shaped UHMWPE linkage designs reduce wear and provide good stability. Precise surgical guidance for correct implant alignment and fixation is preferable.

Distal humeral hemiarthroplasty for nonreconstructable distal humeral fractures is a good option in selected patients with good short- to mid-term results. Likely less weight restrictions are required than for TEA. Repair of epicondyles, condyles, and collateral ligaments is essential. Joint stability and wear of the ulnar and radial joint surfaces remain challenging. More anatomic implants using more compliant articular materials may improve long-term results.

**Acknowledgment** The authors gratefully acknowledge Mr. Jakub Szmit for his assistance in the organization and presentation of this chapter.

## References

1. Pritchard RW. Total elbow joint arthroplasty in patients with rheumatoid arthritis. Semin Arthritis Rheum. 1991;21(1):24–9.
2. Amis AA, Dowson D, Wright V, Miller JH. The derivation of elbow joint forces, and their relation to prosthesis design. J Med Eng Technol. 1979;3(5):229–34.
3. Morrey BF, Askew LJ, Chao EY. A biomechanical study of normal functional elbow motion. J Bone Joint Surg Am. 1981;63(6):872–7.
4. Gay DM, Lyman S, Do H, Hotchkiss RN, Marx RG, Daluiski A. Indications and reoperation rates for total elbow arthroplasty: an analysis of trends in New York State. J Bone Joint Surg Am. 2012;94(2):110–7.
5. Triplet JJ, Kurowicki J, Momoh E, Law TY, Niedzielak T, Levy JC. Trends in total elbow arthroplasty in the Medicare population: a nationwide study of records from 2005 to 2012. J Shoulder Elb Surg. 2016;25(11):1848–53.
6. Rajaee SS, Lin CA, Moon CN. Primary total elbow arthroplasty for distal humeral fractures in elderly patients: a nationwide analysis. J Shoulder Elb Surg. 2016;25(11):1854–60.
7. Morrey BF. The elbow - master techniques in orthopaedic surgery. Wolters Kluwer. 2015.
8. Gramstad GD, King GJ, O'Driscoll SW, Yamaguchi K. Elbow arthroplasty using a convertible implant. Tech Hand Up Extrem Surg. 2005;9(3):153–63.
9. Leclerc A, King GJ. Unlinked and convertible total elbow arthroplasty. Hand Clin. 2011;27(2):215–27. vi
10. Strelzow JA, Frank T, Chan K, Athwal GS, Faber KJ, King GJW. Management of rheumatoid arthritis of the elbow with a convertible total elbow arthroplasty. J Shoulder Elb Surg. 2019;28(11):2205–14.
11. Adolfsson L, Hammer R. Elbow hemiarthroplasty for acute reconstruction of intraarticular distal humerus fractures: a preliminary report involving 4 patients. Acta Orthop. 2006;77(5):785–7.
12. Adolfsson L, Nestorson J. The Kudo humeral component as primary hemiarthroplasty in distal humeral fractures. J Shoulder Elb Surg. 2012;21(4):451–5.
13. Smith GC, Hughes JS. Unreconstructable acute distal humeral fractures and their sequelae treated with distal humeral hemiarthroplasty: a two-year to eleven-year follow-up. J Shoulder Elb Surg. 2013;22(12):1710–23.
14. Morrey BF. The elbow and its disorders. Philadelphia: WB Saunders; 2000.
15. Boone DC, Azen SP. Normal range of motion of joints in male subjects. J Bone Joint Surg Am. 1979;61(5):756–9.
16. Duck TR, Dunning CE, King GJ, Johnson JA. Variability and repeatability of the flexion axis at the ulnohumeral joint. J Orthop Res. 2003;21(3):399–404.
17. Bottlang M, Madey SM, Steyers CM, Marsh JL, Brown TD. Assessment of elbow joint kinematics in passive motion by electromagnetic motion tracking. J Orthop Res. 2000;18(2):195–202.
18. Stokdijk M, Meskers CG, Veeger HE, de Boer YA, Rozing PM. Determination of the optimal elbow axis for evaluation of placement of prostheses. Clin Biomech (Bristol, Avon). 1999;14(3):177–84.
19. Ericson A, Arndt A, Stark A, Wretenberg P, Lundberg A. Variation in the position and orientation of the elbow flexion axis. J Bone Joint Surg Br. 2003;85(4):538–44.
20. Morrey BF, Chao EY. Passive motion of the elbow joint. J Bone Joint Surg Am. 1976;58(4):501–8.
21. Duck TR, Dunning CE, Armstrong AD, Johnson JA, King GJ. Application of screw displacement axes to quantify elbow instability. Clin Biomech (Bristol, Avon). 2003;18(4):303–10.
22. An KN, Morrey BF, Chao EY. Carrying angle of the human elbow joint. J Orthop Res. 1984;1(4):369–78.
23. Carret JP, Fischer LP, Gonon GP, Dimnet J. Cinematic study of prosupination at the level of the radiocubital (radioulnar) articulations. Bull Assoc Anat (Nancy). 1976;60(169):279–95.
24. Kapandji A. Biomechanics of pronation and supination of the forearm. Hand Clin. 2001;17(1):111–22, vii
25. Armstrong AD, Dunning CE, Faber KJ, Duck TR, Johnson JA, King GJ. Rehabilitation of the medial collateral ligament-deficient elbow: an in vitro biomechanical study. J Hand Surg Am. 2000;25(6):1051–7.
26. Dunning CE, Zarzour ZD, Patterson SD, Johnson JA, King GJ. Muscle forces and pronation stabilize the lateral ligament deficient elbow. Clin Orthop Relat Res. 2001;388:118–24.
27. Dunning CE, Duck TR, King GJ, Johnson JA. Simulated active control produces repeatable motion pathways of the elbow in an in vitro testing system. J Biomech. 2001;34(8):1039–48.

28. Buchanan TS, Delp SL, Solbeck JA. Muscular resistance to varus and valgus loads at the elbow. J Biomech Eng. 1998;120(5):634–9.
29. Johnson JA, Rath DA, Dunning CE, Roth SE, King GJ. Simulation of elbow and forearm motion in vitro using a load controlled testing apparatus. J Biomech. 2000;33(5):635–9.
30. King GJ, Itoi E, Niebur GL, Morrey BF, An KN. Motion and laxity of the capitellocondylar total elbow prosthesis. J Bone Joint Surg Am. 1994;76(7):1000–8.
31. Amis AA, Dowson D, Wright V. Elbow joint force predictions for some strenuous isometric actions. J Biomech. 1980;13(9):765–75.
32. Chadwick EK, Nicol AC. Elbow and wrist joint contact forces during occupational pick and place activities. J Biomech. 2000;33(5):591–600.
33. An KN, Chao EY, Morrey BF, Donkers MJ. Intersegmental elbow joint load during pushup. Biomed Sci Instrum. 1992;28:69–74.
34. Halls AA, Travill A. Transmission of pressures across the elbow joint. Anat Rec. 1964;150:243–7.
35. Morrey BF, An KN, Stormont TJ. Force transmission through the radial head. J Bone Joint Surg Am. 1988;70(2):250–6.
36. Boerema I, de Waard DJ. Osteoplastische verankerung von metallprosthesen bei pseudarthrose und athroplastik. Acta Chir Scand. 1942;1942(86):511–24.
37. Lyall HA, Cohen B, Clatworthy M, Constant CR. Results of the Souter-Strathclyde total elbow arthroplasty in patients with rheumatoid arthritis. A preliminary report. J Arthroplast. 1994;9(3):279–84.
38. Dee R. Total replacement arthroplasty of the elbow for rheumatoid arthritis. J Bone Joint Surg Br. 1972;54(1):88–95.
39. Dee R. Total replacement of the elbow joint. Orthop Clin North Am. 1973;4(2):415–33.
40. Garrett JC, Ewald FC, Thomas WH, Sledge CB. Loosening associated with G.S.B. hinge total elbow replacement in patients with rheumatoid arthritis. Clin Orthop Relat Res. 1977;127:170–4.
41. Inglis AE, Pellicci PM. Total elbow replacement. J Bone Joint Surg Am. 1980;62(8):1252–8.
42. Soni RK, Cavendish ME. A review of the Liverpool elbow prosthesis from 1974 to 1982. J Bone Joint Surg Br. 1984;66(2):248–53.
43. Souter WA. Arthroplasty of the elbow with particular reference to metallic hinge arthroplasty in rheumatoid patients. Orthop Clin North Am. 1973;4(2):395–413.
44. Ewald FC, Jacobs MA. Total elbow arthroplasty. Clin Orthop Relat Res. 1984;182:137–42.
45. Kudo H, Iwano K, Watanabe S. Total replacement of the rheumatoid elbow with a hingeless prosthesis. J Bone Joint Surg Am. 1980;62(2):277–85.
46. Moro JK, King GJ. Total elbow arthroplasty in the treatment of posttraumatic conditions of the elbow. Clin Orthop Relat Res. 2000;370:102–14.
47. O'Driscoll SW, An KN, Korinek S, Morrey BF. Kinematics of semi-constrained total elbow arthroplasty. J Bone Joint Surg Br. 1992;74(2):297–9.
48. Ramsey ML, Adams RA, Morrey BF. Instability of the elbow treated with semiconstrained total elbow arthroplasty. J Bone Joint Surg Am. 1999;81(1):38–47.
49. Schuind F, O'Driscoll S, Korinek S, An KN, Morrey BF. Loose-hinge total elbow arthroplasty. An experimental study of the effects of implant alignment on three-dimensional elbow kinematics. J Arthroplast. 1995;10(5):670–8.
50. Szekeres M, King GJ. Total elbow arthroplasty. J Hand Ther. 2006;19(2):245–53.
51. Willing R, King GJ, Johnson JA. The effect of implant design of linked total elbow arthroplasty on stability and stress: a finite element analysis. Comput Methods Biomech Biomed Engin. 2014;17(11):1165–72.
52. Brownhill JR, Pollock JW, Ferreira LM, Johnson JA, King GJ. The effect of implant linking and ligament integrity on humeral loading of a convertible total elbow arthroplasty. Shoulder Elbow. 2019;11(1):45–52.
53. Inagaki K, O'Driscoll SW, Neale PG, Uchiyama E, Morrey BF, An KN. Importance of a radial head component in Sorbie unlinked total elbow arthroplasty. Clin Orthop Relat Res. 2002;400:123–31.
54. Kamineni S, O'Driscoll SW, Urban M, Garg A, Berglund LJ, Morrey BF, et al. Intrinsic constraint of unlinked total elbow replacements--the ulnotrochlear joint. J Bone Joint Surg Am. 2005;87(9):2019–27.
55. Schneeberger AG, King GJ, Song SW, O'Driscoll SW, Morrey BF, An KN. Kinematics and laxity of the Souter-Strathclyde total elbow prosthesis. J Shoulder Elb Surg. 2000;9(2):127–34.
56. Lowe LW, Miller AJ, Allum RL, Higginson DW. The development of an unconstrained elbow arthroplasty. A clinical review. J Bone Joint Surg Br. 1984;66(2):243–7.
57. Morrey BF, An KN. Articular and ligamentous contributions to the stability of the elbow joint. Am J Sports Med. 1983;11(5):315–9.
58. Trepman E, Vella IM, Ewald FC. Radial head replacement in capitellocondylar total elbow arthroplasty. 2- to 6-year follow-up evaluation in rheumatoid arthritis. J Arthroplast. 1991;6(1):67–77.
59. Duranthon LD, Augereau B, Alnot JY, Hardy P, Dreano T. GUEPAR total elbow prosthesis in rheumatoid arthritis. A multicentric retrospective study of 38 cases with an average 4-year follow-up. Rev Chir Orthop Reparatrice Appar Mot. 2001;87(5):437–42.
60. Ramsey M, Neale PG, Morrey BF, O'Driscoll SW, An KN. Kinematics and functional characteristics of the Pritchard ERS unlinked total elbow arthroplasty. J Shoulder Elb Surg. 2003;12(4):385–90.
61. Weiland AJ, Weiss AP, Wills RP, Moore JR. Capitellocondylar total elbow replacement. A long-term follow-up study. J Bone Joint Surg Am. 1989;71(2):217–22.
62. Morrey BF, Adams RA. Semiconstrained elbow replacement for distal humeral nonunion. J Bone Joint Surg Br. 1995;77(1):67–72.
63. Papagelopoulos PJ, Morrey BF. Treatment of nonunion of olecranon fractures. J Bone Joint Surg Br. 1994;76(4):627–35.

64. Jenkins PJ, Watts AC, Norwood T, Duckworth AD, Rymaszewski LA, McEachan JE. Total elbow replacement: outcome of 1,146 arthroplasties from the Scottish Arthroplasty Project. Acta Orthop. 2013;84(2):119–23.
65. Skytta ET, Eskelinen A, Paavolainen P, Ikavalko M, Remes V. Total elbow arthroplasty in rheumatoid arthritis: a population-based study from the Finnish Arthroplasty Register. Acta Orthop. 2009;80(4):472–7.
66. Welsink CL, Lambers KTA, van Deurzen DFP, Eygendaal D, van den Bekerom MPJ. Total elbow arthroplasty: a systematic review. JBJS Rev. 2017;5(7):e4.
67. van der Heide HJ, de Vos MJ, Brinkman JM, Eygendaal D, van den Hoogen FH, de Waal Malefijt MC. Survivorship of the KUDO total elbow prosthesis--comparative study of cemented and uncemented ulnar components: 89 cases followed for an average of 6 years. Acta Orthop. 2007;78(2):258–62.
68. Brinkman JM, de Vos MJ, Eygendaal D. Failure mechanisms in uncemented Kudo type 5 elbow prosthesis in patients with rheumatoid arthritis: 7 of 49 ulnar components revised because of loosening after 2–10 years. Acta Orthop. 2007;78(2):263–70.
69. Kleinlugtenbelt IV, Bakx PA, Huij J. Instrumented bone preserving elbow prosthesis in rheumatoid arthritis: 2–8 year follow-up. J Shoulder Elb Surg. 2010;19(6):923–8.
70. Chan KW, Ahmed AM, A. JJ. Joint replacement materials: Polymethylmethacrylate. Reconstructive Surgery of the Joints New York: Churchill Livingstone; 1996:p. 29–43.
71. Faber KJ, Cordy ME, Milne AD, Chess DG, King GJ, Johnson JA. Advanced cement technique improves fixation in elbow arthroplasty. Clin Orthop Relat Res. 1997;334:150–6.
72. Gschwend N. Present state-of-the-art in elbow arthroplasty. Acta Orthop Belg. 2002;68(2):100–17.
73. Morrey BF, Bryan RS. Complications of total elbow arthroplasty. Clin Orthop Relat Res. 1982;170:204–12.
74. Morrey BF. Total joint replacement. In: Morrey BF, editor. The elbow and its disorders WB. Philadelphia: Saunders; 1985. p. 546–69.
75. An KN, Hui FC, Morrey BF, Linscheid RL, Chao EY. Muscles across the elbow joint: a biomechanical analysis. J Biomech. 1981;14(10):659–69.
76. Herren DB, Ploeg H, Hertig D, Klabunde R. Modeling and finite element analysis of a new revision implant for the elbow. Clin Orthop Relat Res. 2004;420:292–7.
77. Quenneville CE, Austman RL, King GJ, Johnson JA, Dunning CE. Role of an anterior flange on cortical strains through the distal humerus after total elbow arthroplasty with a latitude implant. J Hand Surg Am. 2008;33(6):927–31.
78. Craik JD, Laffer CH, Richards SW, Walsh SP, Evans SL. Distal humerus cortical strains following total elbow arthroplasty. Proc Inst Mech Eng H. 2013;227(2):120–8.
79. Completo A, Pereira J, Fonseca F, Ramos A, Relvas C, Simoes J. Biomechanical analysis of total elbow replacement with unlinked iBP prosthesis: an in vitro and finite element analysis. Clin Biomech (Bristol, Avon). 2011;26(10):990–7.
80. Cheung EV, O'Driscoll SW. Total elbow prosthesis loosening caused by ulnar component pistoning. J Bone Joint Surg Am. 2007;89(6):1269–74.
81. Hosein YK, King GJ, Dunning CE. The effect of stem surface treatment and material on pistoning of ulnar components in linked cemented elbow prostheses. J Shoulder Elb Surg. 2013;22(9):1248–55.
82. Kedgley AE, Takaki SE, Lang P, Dunning CE. The effect of cross-sectional stem shape on the torsional stability of cemented implant components. J Biomech Eng. 2007;129(3):310–4.
83. Brownhill JR, Pollock JW, Ferreira LM, Johnson JA, King GJ. The effect of implant malalignment on joint loading in total elbow arthroplasty: an in vitro study. J Shoulder Elb Surg. 2012;21(8):1032–8.
84. Brownhill JR, Furukawa K, Faber KJ, Johnson JA, King GJ. Surgeon accuracy in the selection of the flexion-extension axis of the elbow: an in vitro study. J Shoulder Elb Surg. 2006;15(4):451–6.
85. Brownhill JR, Ferreira LM, Pichora JE, Johnson JA, King GJ. Defining the flexion-extension axis of the ulna: implications for intra-operative elbow alignment. J Biomech Eng. 2009;131(2):021005.
86. Brownhill JR, Mozzon JB, Ferreira LM, Johnson JA, King GJ. Morphologic analysis of the proximal ulna with special interest in elbow implant sizing and alignment. J Shoulder Elb Surg. 2009;18(1):27–32.
87. Brownhill JR, King GJ, Johnson JA. Morphologic analysis of the distal humerus with special interest in elbow implant sizing and alignment. J Shoulder Elb Surg. 2007;16(3 Suppl):S126–32.
88. McDonald CP, Brownhill JR, King GJ, Johnson JA, Peters TM. A comparison of registration techniques for computer- and image-assisted elbow surgery. Comput Aided Surg. 2007;12(4):208–14.
89. McDonald CP, Beaton BJ, King GJ, Peters TM, Johnson JA. The effect of anatomic landmark selection of the distal humerus on registration accuracy in computer-assisted elbow surgery. J Shoulder Elb Surg. 2008;17(5):833–43.
90. McDonald CP, Peters TM, King GJ, Johnson JA. Computer assisted surgery of the distal humerus can employ contralateral images for pre-operative planning, registration, and surgical intervention. J Shoulder Elb Surg. 2009;18(3):469–77.
91. McDonald CP, Peters TM, Johnson JA, King GJ. Stem abutment affects alignment of the humeral component in computer-assisted elbow arthroplasty. J Shoulder Elb Surg. 2011;20(6):891–8.
92. Cadambi A, Engh GA, Dwyer KA, Vinh TN. Osteolysis of the distal femur after total knee arthroplasty. J Arthroplast. 1994;9(6):579–94.
93. Peters PC Jr, Engh GA, Dwyer KA, Vinh TN. Osteolysis after total knee arthroplasty without cement. J Bone Joint Surg Am. 1992;74(6):864–76.

94. Revell PA, Weightman B, Freeman MA, Roberts BV. The production and biology of polyethylene wear debris. Arch Orthop Trauma Surg. 1978;91(3):167–81.
95. Schmalzried TP, Campbell P, Schmitt AK, Brown IC, Amstutz HC. Shapes and dimensional characteristics of polyethylene wear particles generated in vivo by total knee replacements compared to total hip replacements. J Biomed Mater Res. 1997;38(3):203–10.
96. Lee H, Vaichinger AM, O'Driscoll SW. Component fracture after total elbow arthroplasty. J Shoulder Elb Surg. 2019;28(8):1449–56.
97. Aldridge JM 3rd, Lightdale NR, Mallon WJ, Coonrad RW. Total elbow arthroplasty with the Coonrad/Coonrad-Morrey prosthesis. A 10- to 31-year survival analysis. J Bone Joint Surg Br. 2006;88(4):509–14.
98. Seitz WH Jr, Bismar H, Evans PJ. Failure of the hinge mechanism in total elbow arthroplasty. J Shoulder Elb Surg. 2010;19(3):368–75.
99. Wright TW, Hastings H. Total elbow arthroplasty failure due to overuse, C-ring failure, and/or bushing wear. J Shoulder Elb Surg. 2005;14(1):65–72.
100. Robnineau R. Contribution à l'étude de prothèses osseuses. Bull Mem Soc Nat Chir. 1927;53:886–96.
101. Mellen RH, Phalen GS. Arthroplasty of the elbow by replacement of the distal portion of the humerus with an acrylic prosthesis. J Bone Joint Surg Am. 1947;29(2):348–53.
102. Venable CS. An elbow and an elbow prosthesis; case of complete loss of the lower third of the humerus. Am J Surg. 1952;83(3):271–5.
103. Macausland WR. Replacement of the lower end of the humerus with a prosthesis; a report of four cases. West J Surg Obstet Gynecol. 1954;62(11):557–66.
104. Barr JS, Eaton RG. Elbow reconstruction with a new prosthesis to replace the distal end of the humerus. A case report. J Bone Joint Surg Am. 1965;47(7):1408–13.
105. Shifrin PG, Johnson DP. Elbow hemiarthroplasty with 20-year follow-up study. A case report and literature review. Clin Orthop Relat Res. 1990;254:128–33.
106. Street DM, Stevens PS. A humeral replacement prosthesis for the elbow: results in ten elbows. J Bone Joint Surg Am. 1974;56(6):1147–58.
107. Heijink A, Wagener ML, de Vos MJ, Eygendaal D. Distal humerus prosthetic hemiarthroplasty: midterm results. Strategies Trauma Limb Reconstr. 2015;10(2):101–8.
108. Lechasseur B, Laflamme M, Leclerc A, Bedard AM. Incipient malunion of an isolated humeral trochlea fracture treated with an elbow hemiarthroplasty: case report. J Hand Surg Am. 2015;40(2):271–5.
109. Schultzel M, Scheidt K, Klein CC, Narvy SJ, Lee BK, Itamura JM. Hemiarthroplasty for the treatment of distal humeral fractures: midterm clinical results. J Shoulder Elb Surg. 2017;26(3):389–93.
110. Smith GC, Bayne G, Page R, Hughes JS. The clinical outcome and activity levels of patients under 55 years treated with distal humeral hemiarthroplasty for distal humeral fractures: minimum 2-year follow-up. Shoulder Elbow. 2016;8(4):264–70.
111. Chang N, King GJW. Elbow hemiarthroplasty for the treatment of distal humerus fractures. Orthop Clin North Am. 2020;51(2):265–77.
112. Parsons M, O'Brien RJ, Hughes JS. Elbow hemiarthroplasty for acute and salvage reconstruction of intra-articular distal humerus fractures. Tech Shoulder Elbow Surg. 2005;6(2):82–97.
113. Argintar E, Berry M, Narvy SJ, Kramer J, Omid R, Itamura JM. Hemiarthroplasty for the treatment of distal humerus fractures: short-term clinical results. Orthopedics. 2012;35(12):1042–5.
114. Al-Hamdani A, Rasmussen JV, Sorensen AKB, Ovesen J, Holtz K, Brorson S, et al. Good outcome after elbow hemiarthroplasty in active patients with an acute intra-articular distal humeral fracture. J Shoulder Elb Surg. 2019;28(5):925–30.
115. Bryan RS, Morrey BF. Extensive posterior exposure of the elbow. A triceps-sparing approach. Clin Orthop Relat Res. 1982;166:188–92.
116. Burkhart KJ, Nijs S, Mattyasovszky SG, Wouters R, Gruszka D, Nowak TE, et al. Distal humerus hemiarthroplasty of the elbow for comminuted distal humeral fractures in the elderly patient. J Trauma. 2011;71(3):635–42.
117. Campbell WC. Incision for exposure of the elbow joint. Am J Surg. 1932;15(1):65–7.
118. de Vos MJ, Wagener ML, Verdonschot N, Eygendaal D. An extensive posterior approach of the elbow with osteotomy of the medial epicondyle. J Shoulder Elb Surg. 2014;23(3):313–7.
119. Studer A, Athwal GS, MacDermid JC, Faber KJ, King GJ. The lateral Para-olecranon approach for total elbow arthroplasty. J Hand Surg Am. 2013;38(11):2219–26. e3
120. Sabo MT, Athwal GS, King GJ. Landmarks for rotational alignment of the humeral component during elbow arthroplasty. J Bone Joint Surg Am. 2012;94(19):1794–800.
121. Desai SJ, Lalone E, Athwal GS, Ferreira LM, Johnson JA, King GJ. Hemiarthroplasty of the elbow: the effect of implant size on joint congruency. J Shoulder Elb Surg. 2016;25(2):297–303.
122. Lapner M, Willing R, Johnson JA, King GJ. The effect of distal humeral hemiarthroplasty on articular contact of the elbow. Clin Biomech (Bristol, Avon). 2014;29(5):537–44.
123. Desai SJ, Athwal GS, Ferreira LM, Lalone EA, Johnson JA, King GJ. Hemiarthroplasty of the elbow: the effect of implant size on kinematics and stability. J Shoulder Elb Surg. 2014;23(7):946–54.

# Primary Elbow Arthroplasty

# 2

William R. Aibinder and Kenneth J. Faber

## Introduction

Total elbow arthroplasty (TEA) is utilized to treat various degenerative, inflammatory, and traumatic pathologies involving the elbow joint [1–6]. The surgical goals include creating a painless and stable joint while maintaining or improving preoperative range of motion. Early designs yielded suboptimal clinical and functional outcomes [7–9]. Improved patient selection, recent advances in surgical approach and technique, as well as innovations in implant designs, have improved outcomes and implant survivorship [1–3, 10, 11]. Nonetheless, the durability of TEA remains inferior to the hip, knee, and shoulder. TEA is limited by a high rate of mechanical failure and loosening, although infection, triceps insufficiency, and ulnar neuropathy are also common [9, 12]. As such, a thorough understanding of TEA and appropriate patient selection is imperative to optimize outcomes. TEA should be reserved for low-demand patients, elderly patients, and those severely debilitated by elbow pain and/or instability who have failed other nonsurgical and surgical treatment options.

## Historical Perspective

In the early twentieth century, several custom implants were utilized; however, the success of these implants was limited [13]. Dee reported on 12 patients with rheumatoid arthritis treated using a linked prosthesis with good early outcomes [8]. The authors suggested that elbow arthroplasty should therefore be considered for other indications aside from rheumatoid arthritis. As a result, in the 1970s, there was an increasing interest in TEA design and use; however, high early complication rates were reported, up to 57% in one series [14–16]. The predominant failure mechanism was implant loosening that was attributed to a highly constrained articulation that transmitted excessive forces to the implant-bone interface. This led to the development of a "sloppy" hinge, often described as a semi-constrained prosthesis [17, 18].

In an effort to reduce loosening, several inventors developed unlinked prostheses that rely on the capsuloligamentous structures for stability [19–23]. Unlinked prostheses allow for their potential use in younger more active patients. More recently, convertible designs allow the surgeon to make intraoperative decisions on linking

W. R. Aibinder
Shoulder & Elbow Surgery, SUNY Downstate Health Sciences University, Brooklyn, NY, USA
e-mail: William.Aibinder@downstate.edu

K. J. Faber (✉)
Roth | McFarlane Hand and Upper Limb Centre, Western University, London, ON, Canada
e-mail: kjfaber@uwo.ca


G. J. W. King, M. Rizzo (eds.), *Arthroplasty of the Upper Extremity*,
https://doi.org/10.1007/978-3-030-68880-6_2

versus unlinking and have reported good early results [10, 11, 24–26].

Despite these design modifications, there has not been a significant increase in the utilization of TEA worldwide. Additionally, the indications for TEA have evolved over time. According to a New York State Department of Health database study, the number of TEA performed for rheumatoid arthritis decreased from 48% to 19% between 1997 and 2006 [6]. During the same time period, TEA performed for fracture increased from 43% to 69%. A recent study of the Australian registry demonstrated a similar trend with a substantial increase of TEA performed for trauma and a relatively low incidence of TEA performed for rheumatoid arthritis [1]. This is likely related to the development of effective disease-modifying antirheumatic drugs (DMARDs) and biologics used to treat early inflammatory arthropathy. Additionally, as indications for TEA expanded in the 1980s and 1990s, follow-up studies, particularly regarding younger active patients with post-traumatic etiology, have demonstrated a persistent high complication and reoperation rate [27–29]. As our understanding of elbow arthroplasty continues to evolve and progress, there is continued support for TEA in elderly low-demand patients in the treatment of inflammatory arthropathy, distal humerus fractures, and post-traumatic conditions that have failed other treatment options.

## Indications

As outlined above, the predominant indications for primary TEA include inflammatory arthropathy, acute comminuted unsalvageable distal humerus fractures in the elderly, post-traumatic elbow arthritis, tumors, and select cases of primary osteoarthritis [1–6, 10, 30–34].

### Rheumatoid Arthritis

Rheumatoid arthritis commonly affects the elbow. Larsen et al. described a classification for radiographic findings in patients with rheumatoid arthritis [35]. These findings are useful in identifying patients for TEA. Early stages are effectively treated with a combination of medications and synovectomy. More advanced stages such as grade 3 where there is loss of articular cartilage with bony resorption and grade 4 where there are severe bony destruction and gross instability are indications for TEA with good functional outcomes (Fig. 2.1).

Several key factors should be considered when performing a TEA on a patient with rheumatoid arthritis or other inflammatory arthropathy. First, given the systemic nature of the condition, assessment of other joints involved should be considered. Coordination with colleagues performing lower extremity arthroplasties and/or shoulder arthroplasties is imperative to optimize recovery and the ability to use gait aids. Additionally, an assessment of the patient's cervical spine is necessary for consideration of anesthetic requirements.

Second, a thorough history of the patient's current medications is necessary. Given the increased use of DMARDs and biologics, as well as steroids, consultation with the patient's rheumatologist is necessary. A discussion should be had with the patient regarding the increased risk of infection and wound complication associated with these medications. Some medications can be continued throughout the operative and perioperative periods, while others need to be suspended for a given period of time [36, 37]. Intraoperative stress-dose steroids are infrequently required and may depend on the patient's daily dosage.

### Distal Humerus Fracture

The expansion of indications for elbow arthroplasty to treat distal humerus fractures in the elderly was the result of poor outcomes and high complication rates with open reduction and internal fixation. Distal humerus fractures not amenable to fixation in elderly patients can be effectively treated with TEA [38–43] (Figs. 2.2 and 2.3). Several studies have demonstrated that in these cases, TEA leads to a faster return to function with decreased pain and stiffness

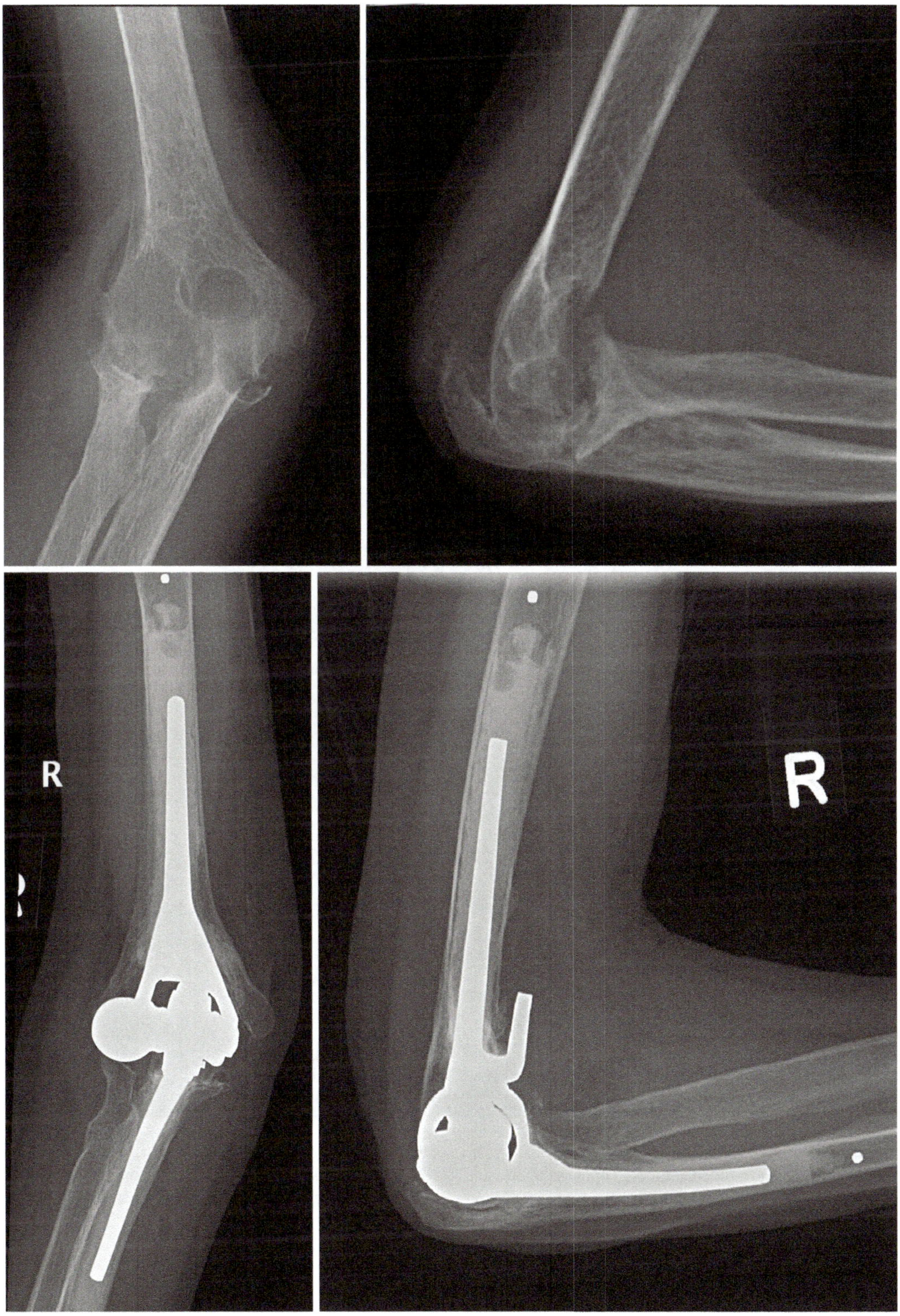


**Fig. 2.1** Pre- and postoperative radiographs of a 60-year-old female 4 years following linked total elbow arthroplasty for stage 4 rheumatoid arthritis

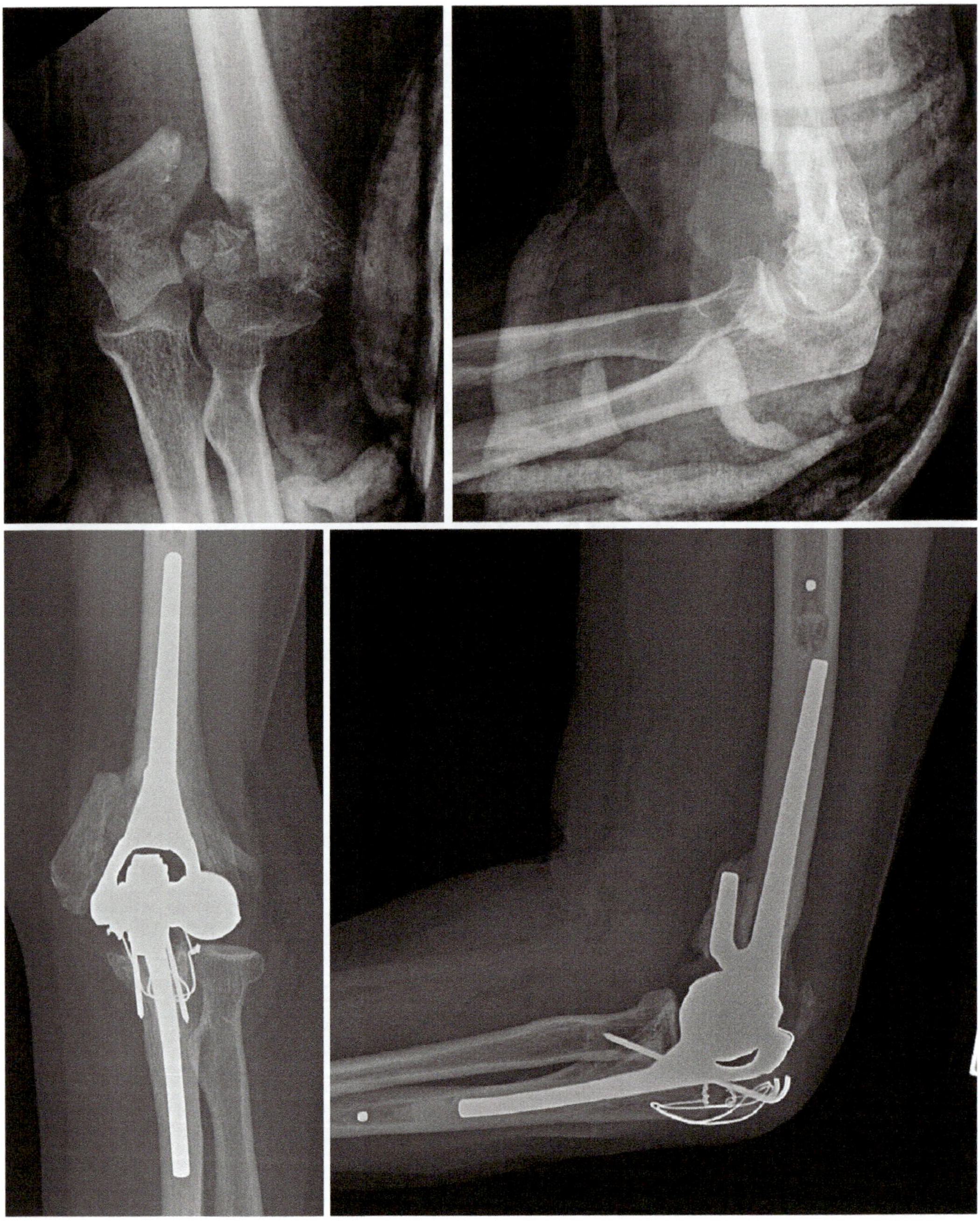

**Fig. 2.2** Pre- and postoperative radiographs of a 74-year-old female who had a failed attempt at open reduction and internal fixation of a distal humerus fracture. An olecranon osteotomy was used for exposure during the attempted fixation. An intraoperative conversion to a linked total elbow arthroplasty was performed in conjunction with a tension band repair of the olecranon osteotomy

compared to treating these fractures nonoperatively [44–46]. Elderly females with distal humerus fractures also tend to have better functional outcomes with a lower reoperation rate with TEA compared to open reduction and internal fixation [41, 47]. Nonetheless, when treating

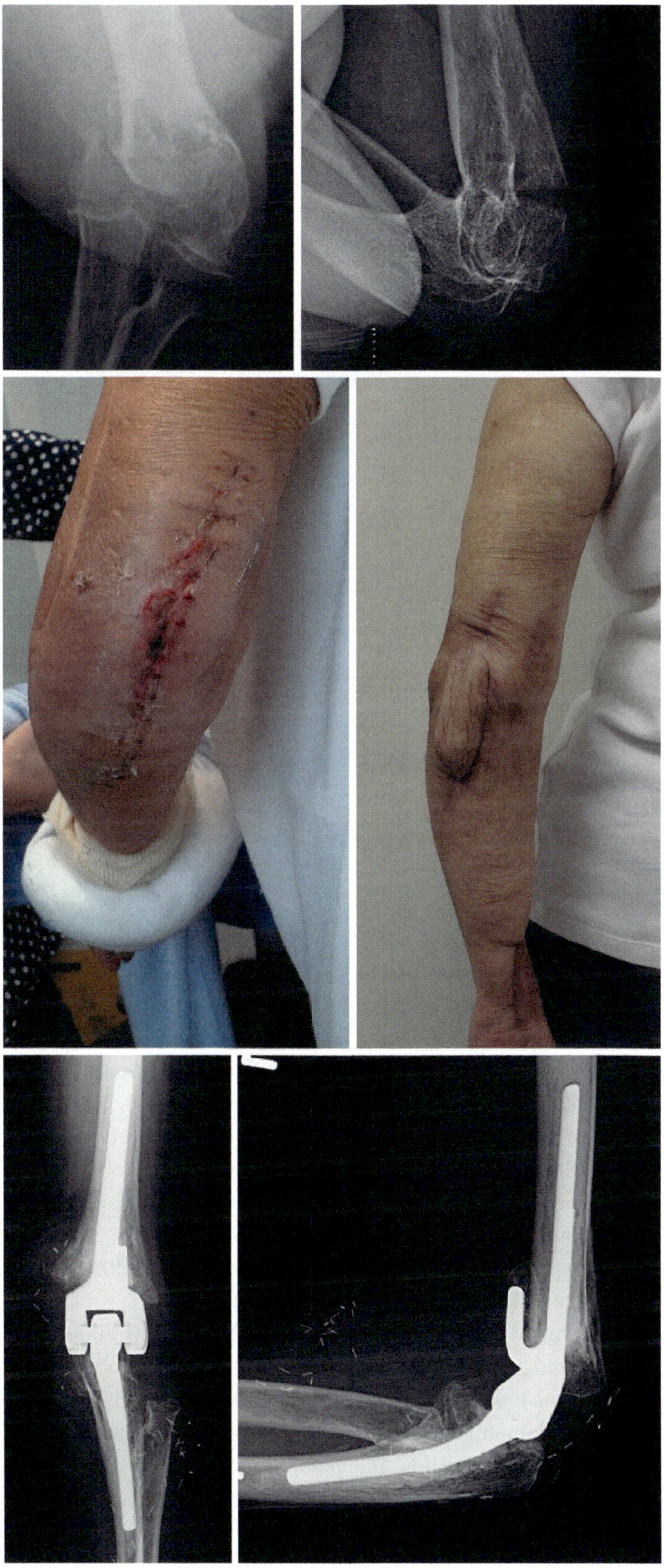

**Fig. 2.3** Pre- and 5-year postoperative radiographs of an 84-year-old female with a distal humerus fracture treated with total elbow arthroplasty. The postoperative course was complicated by a wound breakdown that was treated with a reversed radial forearm flap

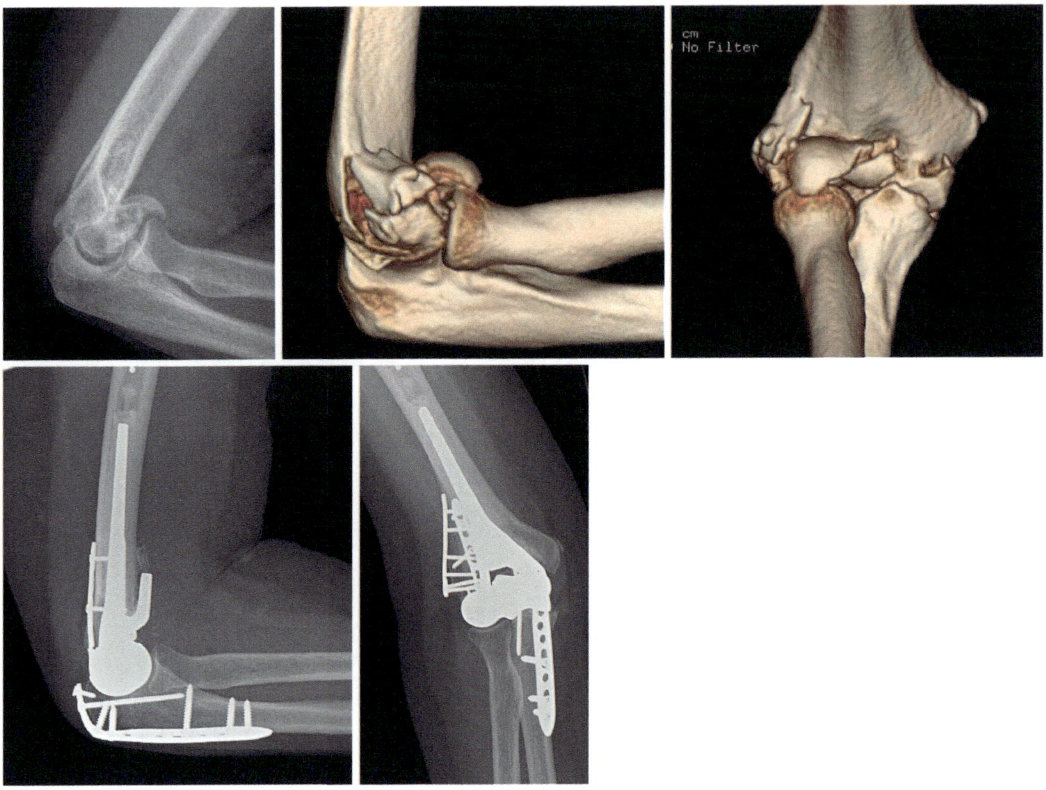


**Fig. 2.4** Radiographs and three-dimensional computed tomography of a 51-year-old female with a low transcondylar distal humerus fracture treated with an elbow hemiarthroplasty and open reduction and internal fixation of the lateral column. Exposure was obtained using an olecranon osteotomy

distal humerus fractures with TEA, careful evaluation of the proximal extent of the fracture is imperative to ensure that the humerus can support a conventional implant.

Elbow hemiarthroplasty is also a described treatment for nonconstructable distal humerus fractures (Fig. 2.4). Interest in this procedure spawned from concerns of premature ulnar component loosening in younger patients treated with total elbow replacements. The procedure involves replacement of the distal humerus with an anatomic prosthesis that articulates with the native ulna and radial head. This procedure requires collateral ligaments that are intact or that can be repaired in a manner that will ensure joint stability. A linked implant is required if stable condyles and competent ligaments that maintain stability cannot be achieved. Hemiarthroplasty is generally only indicated in younger patients with low transcondylar fractures that would be challenging to restore with stable fixation, particularly in patients who do not desire the lifelong restrictions of a total elbow prosthesis. Distal humeral hemiarthroplasty is less favorable in the elderly as it requires healing of the collateral ligaments leading to prolonged rehabilitation, higher rates of pain due to ulnar cartilage wear, and higher reoperation rates [48].

## Post-traumatic Arthritis

Following fracture, dislocation, or other injury about the elbow, there is often a development of post-traumatic degenerative changes or residual instability. Unlike inflammatory arthropathy and distal humerus fractures, TEA for post-traumatic arthritis of the elbow should not be sought as the initial treatment option given the comparatively worse clinical and functional outcomes [30]

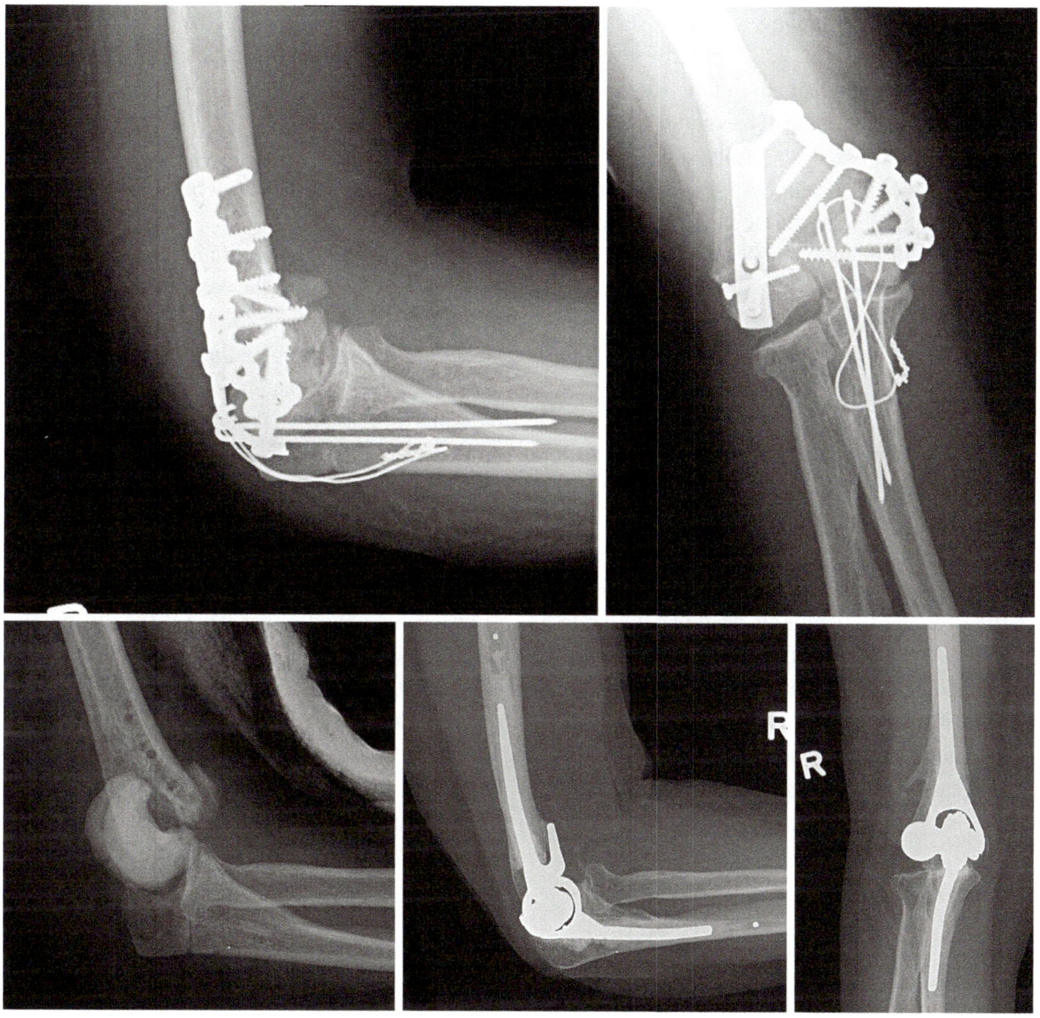


**Fig. 2.5** Radiographs of a 68-year-old female with a distal humerus fracture treated with open reduction and internal fixation. One month following surgery, joint culture was positive for *Staphylococcus epidermidis*, and a staged revision from an articulating spacer to a linked total elbow arthroplasty was performed

(Fig. 2.5). Despite the advances already described, survivability and durability of TEA in younger active patients are still uncertain. Surgeons and patients should exhaust all available nonoperative and operative treatment options including pain medication, corticosteroid injections, open and arthroscopic osteocapsular arthroplasty, and interposition arthroplasty. TEA should be reserved for when all these options fail and when patients have been counseled extensively on their activity restrictions following surgery.

Nonetheless, TEA is a reasonable option for post-traumatic arthritis with reasonable outcomes, particularly pain relief, reported in the literature [29, 40, 49]. There are specific factors to consider when performing a TEA in patients with post-traumatic arthritis. First, these patients tend to have prior skin incisions which need to be considered. Second, prior instrumentation may make implantation challenging, and careful preoperative planning is necessary. Third, as the majority of these patients are younger, surgeons may desire to use an unlinked prosthesis to limit mechanical failure; however, careful scrutiny of the ligament integrity is imperative pre- and intraoperatively. Fourth, the status of the ulnar nerve needs to be carefully evaluated preoperatively and addressed carefully, specifically in relation to medial osteophyte formation altering the cubital tunnel morphology and periarticular scarring about the nerve [50, 51].

### Tumors

Periarticular tumors involving the elbow have been treated with total elbow arthroplasty in certain situations. In a series of 47 patients treated at the Rizzoli institute, only 4% of patients developed an infection [32]. Similar findings were demonstrated by Athwal et al. with no infections in their series of 20 patients despite a high rate of radiation and/or chemotherapy in the cohort [34]. Both studies demonstrated a relatively high rate (25%) of nerve injury. Overall, the use of total elbow arthroplasty in the treatment of primary and metastatic tumors is a reasonable modality.

### Primary Osteoarthritis

Primary TEA is rarely indicated for primary osteoarthritis of the elbow [52] (Fig. 2.6).

The condition is commonly seen in the dominant extremity of males who are manual laborers and in their 40s and 50s [53]. The ulnohumeral cartilage is often spared in these patients, and the primary symptoms are pain at the end range of motion, stiffness, and mechanical symptoms. These symptoms are often effectively addressed with an elbow debridement, either open or arthroscopic. However, some patients have cartilage loss and develop pain at the mid-arc range of motion and may be candidates for TEA. Unlike patients with inflammatory arthropathy, these patients tend to have a high baseline level of function. A thorough preoperative discussion is necessary to ensure that patients are willing to abide by the activity restrictions of a primary TEA in exchange for the potential pain relief. Providers must discuss with the patients the risk of mechanical failure and the challenges with addressing these complications in the revision setting.

## Postoperative Rehabilitation

The postoperative rehabilitation plan should be structured to minimize the risk of early complications and to restore elbow function. The initial postoperative dressing includes significant protective padding and an anterior splint that avoids pressure on the surgical site and prevents elbow motion [54]. Motion exercises are initiated once satisfactory wound healing is established. The limits of motion are determined by the motion attained intraoperatively. Static progressive flexion and extension splinting is occasionally required for patients that have difficulty regaining functional arcs of motion. Resisted exercises are permitted once satisfactory motion has been restored in patients treated with a triceps-"on" approach. Resisted exercises are withheld for 3 months when a triceps-"off" approach is used. Triceps-"off" approaches include the Bryan-Morrey triceps-reflecting approach (Fig. 2.7) [55], the longitudinal triceps-splitting approach (Fig. 2.8) as described by Gschwend et al. [56], and triceps turndown approaches [57, 58]. The triceps-"on" approach includes the paratricipital approach as described by Alonso-Llames, which is limited by the ability to appropriately prepare the ulnar canal [59]. The lateral para-olecranon approach (Fig. 2.9) allows the ability to maintain the continuity of the extensor mechanism to accelerate rehabilitation while improving visualization and access to the ulnar canal for preparation [60]. This is the authors' preferred approach for TEA.

Most authors recommend a lifetime lifting limitation of 2.5 kg.

## Outcomes

Outcomes following primary TEA vary substantially depending on the indication as has been demonstrated through various published studies.

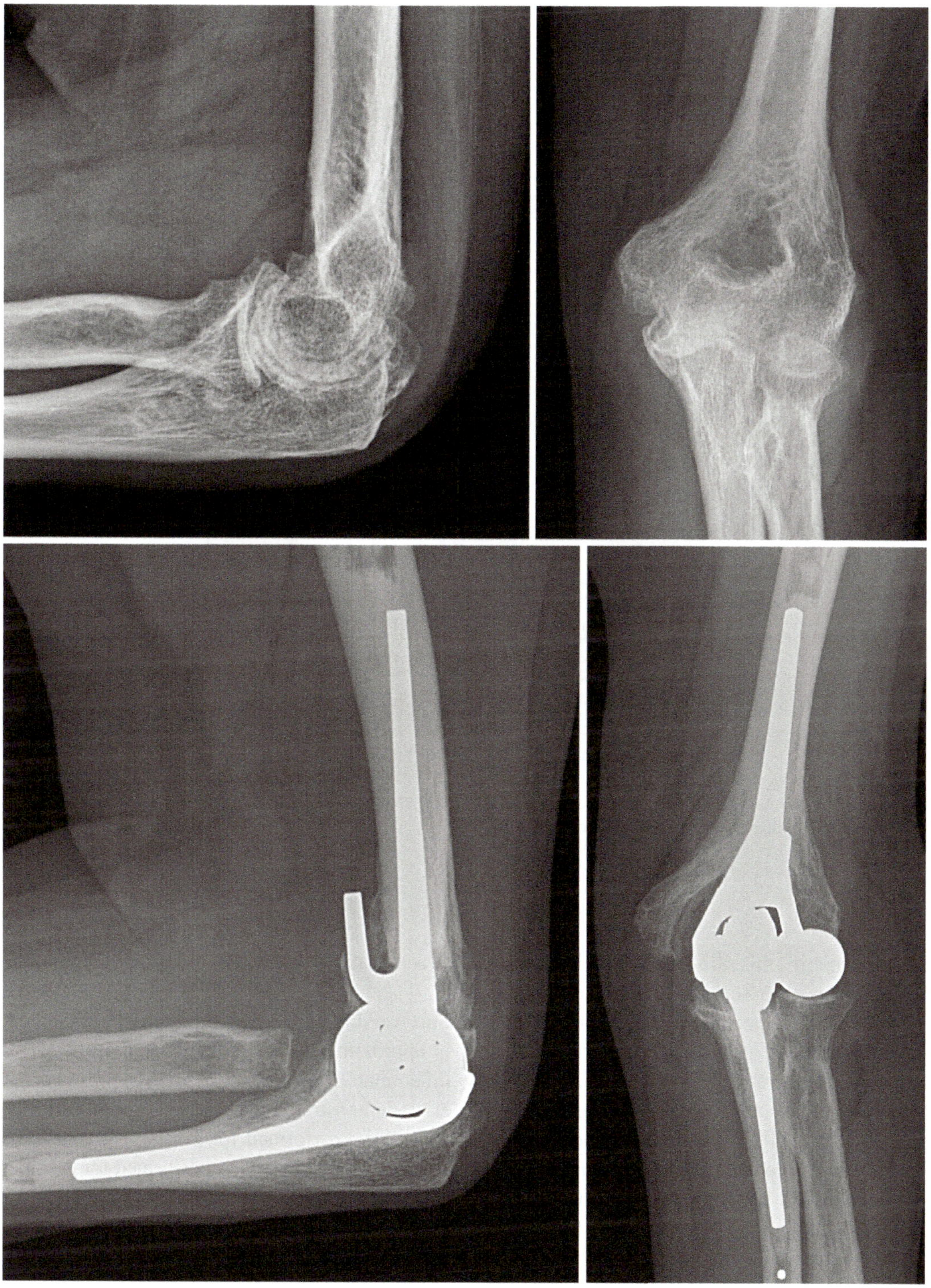

**Fig. 2.6** Preoperative and 2-year postoperative radiographs of a 60-year-old female with primary osteoarthritis treated with linked total elbow arthroplasty. (Courtesy Dr. G King)

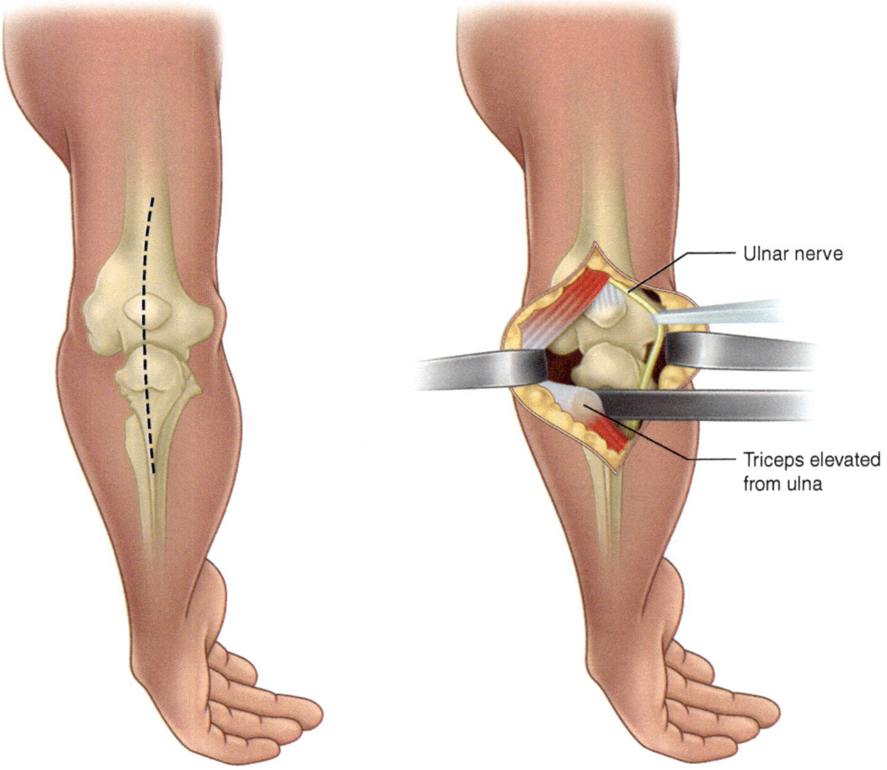


**Fig. 2.7** Bryan-Morrey triceps-reflecting approach. A posterior skin incision is used to expose the triceps. The ulna nerve is mobilized, and the triceps is elevated from the proximal ulna in a medial to lateral direction. The lateral triceps is kept in continuity with the anconeus

More recently, this difference has been highlighted through several systematic reviews demonstrating improved outcomes and decreased revision rates in primary TEA performed for inflammatory arthropathies and trauma compared to post-traumatic and degenerative conditions [1, 30, 31]. The difference in outcomes may be related directly to the etiology or indirectly to the lower activity demands of certain patients. Surgeon volume and experience likely also impact on outcomes. A report from the Scottish Joint Registry found that implant longevity was greater with experienced surgeons performing more than ten cases per year [3]. Nonetheless, it is prudent to evaluate the outcomes of primary TEA by indication.

## Rheumatoid Arthritis

Survivorship at 10 years following primary TEA is approximately 90% for cases performed for inflammatory arthropathy [1–5, 61–64]. Viveen et al. demonstrated that the revision rate for primary TEA performed for primary osteoarthritis was twice as high as TEA performed for rheumatoid arthritis [1].

In a study of the Finnish registry reviewing 1457 primary TEA performed for rheumatoid arthritis, the authors found a 10-year survival rate of 83%. The etiology for revision included aseptic loosening as the most common, followed by dislocation, periprosthetic fracture, infection, and fracture of the prosthesis [5]. A study from the

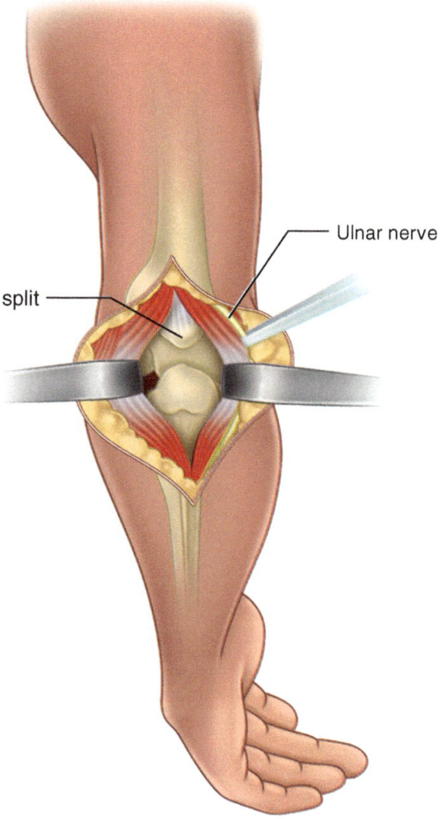


Fig. 2.8 Gschwend triceps-splitting approach. The ulna nerve is mobilized, and the triceps is split longitudinally and reflected from the ulna medially and laterally to expose the elbow joint

Mayo Clinic evaluating the Coonrad-Morrey "sloppy" hinge prosthesis at a minimum of 10-year follow-up in 78 elbows demonstrates only moderate or severe postoperative pain in 2 (2.6%) patients with a mean range of motion from 28° to 131° [61]. The mean Mayo Elbow Performance Score (MEPS) improved from 42 preoperatively to 87 at final follow-up.

Several studies have assessed the outcomes of unlinked TEA in the setting of rheumatoid arthritis with 10-year survivorship ranging between 70% and 93% [65–68]. The primary complication in most studies is aseptic loosening rather than instability.

More recently, outcomes regarding the use of a convertible TEA have been reported in the literature [10, 26]. In one study with a mean follow-up of 6 years, the authors linked 55 TEA, while 27 were unlinked [10]. The determination for linking was based on preoperative and intraoperative finding of collateral ligament integrity. There was no difference between the two groups with respect to complications, survivorship, revision rate, and reoperation rate. The overall complication rate was 32%. All instability complications occurred in the unlinked cohort, while aseptic ulnar component loosening occurred in the linked cohort. A convertible implant allows the treating surgeon to make an algorithmic intraoperative decision to optimize a patient's outcome while decreasing the postoperative complication risk. Nonetheless, multiple mid- and long-term studies have demonstrated successful outcomes of primary TEA in the setting of rheumatoid arthritis.

## Distal Humerus Fractures

In long-term studies, the survivorship of TEA for distal humerus fractures was between 76% and 90% at 10 years [38, 39]. Interestingly, in the series from the Mayo Clinic, if excluding patients with rheumatoid arthritis, the survivorship increased to 92% [38]. The mean range of motion was from 24° to 123° and a mean MEPS score 90.5. Still 11% of elbows underwent revision for infections, and 18% underwent revision for implant complications. Five other elbows sustained periprosthetic fractures.

In a prospective randomized trial, TEA and open reduction internal fixation yielded similar results at 2-year follow-up [47]. The reoperation rate in the TEA group was 12% compared to 26% in the ORIF group; however, this did not reach statistical significance. Furthermore, a recent study demonstrated no difference in outcome for TEA performed for acute distal humerus fractures or as a salvage for failed internal fixation [40]. The indications for TEA in the salvage group were nonunion, post-traumatic arthritis, hardware failure, intrinsic stiffness, fibrosis, instability, and malunion. It is important to note that the mean age in the salvage group was 60 years, compared to 74 years in the acute TEA group.

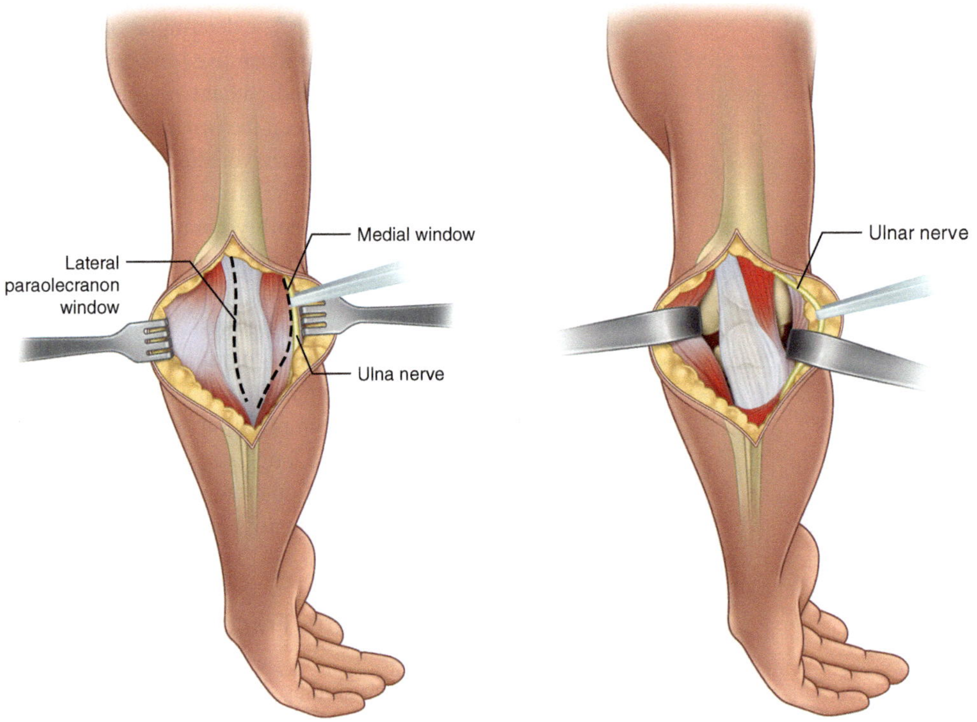


**Fig. 2.9** The lateral para-olecranon approach. The ulna nerve is mobilized, and two longitudinal arthrotomies are used to access the joint. The medial arthrotomy is established in the floor of the cubital tunnel and extends proximally along the medial edge of the triceps. The lateral arthrotomy involves splitting the lateral one third of the triceps from the medial two thirds. The lateral triceps is kept in continuity with the anconeus. The majority of the triceps tendon insertion is undisturbed on the olecranon

Thus, when determining the appropriate treatment option for elderly patients with comminuted distal humerus fractures, surgeons must be able to apply all the available data and individualize care with consideration for bone quality, fracture extension, patient activity level, life expectancy, and anticipated complications and need for revision. Nonetheless, primary TEA for unsalvageable distal humerus fractures yields reasonable functional outcomes in carefully selected low-demand patients. Surgeons need to be cognizant of the not insignificant rate of component revision, infection, and periprosthetic fracture that occurs with TEA in the treatment of distal humerus fractures [38, 39, 69]. In some instances, low-demand, medically unwell patients with distal humerus fractures may achieve satisfactory outcomes with nonoperative management as well [45].

An alternative in younger patients with an unsalvageable distal humerus fracture is a distal humerus hemiarthroplasty [70–74]. Several studies have demonstrated reasonable functional outcomes with hemiarthroplasty. In one study of 26 elbows, Smith et al. demonstrated a mean MEPS score of 90 but demonstrated a worse functional outcome in patients who had wear of the proximal ulna [71]. This is a common finding, occurring in up to 50% of the elbows studied [71, 73, 74]. Nestorson et al. demonstrated good outcomes in 42 patients at a mean of 34 months [72]. Five patients had wear of the olecranon with a mean MEPS of 90 and DASH of 20. No studies have demonstrated a high rate of instability; rather ulnar wear is the most common complication; however, in most patients it is asymptomatic.

## Post-traumatic Arthritis

In one study, implant survivorship at 15 years was 70% with increased failure associated with younger age at index arthroplasty [28]. Only 74% of patients were subjectively satisfied. Bushing wear was attributed as the main cause of intermediate-term failure. An earlier study demonstrated a 27% complication rate despite good functional outcome and resolution of pain [49]. These studies demonstrate that patients who are anticipating heavy use of their elbow need to be cautioned as to the expected outcomes with TEA for the treatment of post-traumatic arthritis.

A more recent study reviewed 14 patients at a mean follow-up of 46 months demonstrating good clinical and functional outcomes with only 3 experiencing complications [75]. Two of these had worsened ulnar neuropathy, and a third was complicated by a wound infection and periprosthetic humeral shaft fracture. Although a small and short follow-up series, the outcomes are more promising.

Still, patients need to be extensively counseled on the high rate of complications and activity limitations prior to proceeding with primary TEA.

Additionally, some authors have suggested that distal humeral hemiarthroplasty is an alternative to TEA for patients with post-traumatic arthritis [70]. Werthel et al. reported on 16 patients with a mean age of 45 years at a mean follow-up of 51 months [70]. The mean MEPS score was 72 with 1 poor and 5 fair outcomes. Fifty percent of patients experienced a complication and 31% required a revision, 2 of which were revised to a TEA. Further studies are required to demonstrate the efficacy and safety of this alternative option.

## Primary Osteoarthritis

Primary TEA for primary osteoarthritis is rarely performed or indicated. There are a few small series reported [52, 76, 77]. In one series, 20 elbows were treated for primary osteoarthritis over the course of 27 years, and followed for a mean of 9 years [52]. The authors noted reasonable outcomes, with a nearly 50% complication rate. However, only three elbows required a return to the operating room with only three experiencing mechanical failure. Espag et al. reported the outcomes of an unlinked TEA for the treatment of primary osteoarthritis with only one revision despite five components having radiographic loosening [77]. It is important to note that the majority of patients in these studies were over the age of 65 years, and thus TEA was reserved for older patients.

## Conclusion

As we advance into the twenty-first century, the indications for primary TEA are transitioning from rheumatoid arthritis to the treatment of acute trauma and post-traumatic conditions. The outcomes in inflammatory arthropathy and acute trauma continue to generally be favorable, particularly in older low-demand patients. The indications for TEA, particularly in the post-traumatic setting, are continuing to increase, and it is anticipated that the use of TEA in younger patients will result in higher complication rates and the need for reoperation. Advancements in technology, with novel convertible prosthetic designs and improved stem fixation may provide better outcomes in younger patients as the evidence in the literature continues to grow, specifically in challenging conditions including dysfunctional instability and periarticular tumors.

## References

1. Viveen J, van den Bekerom MPJ, Doornberg JN, Hatton A, Page R, Koenraadt KLM, et al. Use and outcome of 1,220 primary total elbow arthroplasties from the Australian Orthopaedic Association National Joint Arthroplasty Replacement Registry 2008-2018. Acta Orthop. 2019;90(6):511–6.
2. Krukhaug Y, Hallan G, Dybvik E, Lie SA, Furnes ON. A survivorship study of 838 total elbow replacements: a report from the Norwegian Arthroplasty Register 1994-2016. J Shoulder Elb Surg. 2018;27(2):260–9.

3. Jenkins PJ, Watts AC, Norwood T, Duckworth AD, Rymaszewski LA, McEachan JE. Total elbow replacement: outcome of 1,146 arthroplasties from the Scottish Arthroplasty Project. Acta Orthop. 2013;84(2):119–23.
4. Fevang BT, Lie SA, Havelin LI, Skredderstuen A, Furnes O. Results after 562 total elbow replacements: a report from the Norwegian Arthroplasty Register. J Shoulder Elb Surg. 2009;18(3):449–56.
5. Skytta ET, Eskelinen A, Paavolainen P, Ikavalko M, Remes V. Total elbow arthroplasty in rheumatoid arthritis: a population-based study from the Finnish Arthroplasty Register. Acta Orthop. 2009;80(4):472–7.
6. Gay DM, Lyman S, Do H, Hotchkiss RN, Marx RG, Daluiski A. Indications and reoperation rates for total elbow arthroplasty: an analysis of trends in New York State. J Bone Joint Surg Am. 2012;94(2):110–7.
7. Venable CS. An elbow and an elbow prosthesis; case of complete loss of the lower third of the humerus. Am J Surg. 1952;83(3):271–5.
8. Dee R. Total replacement arthroplasty of the elbow for rheumatoid arthritis. J Bone Joint Surg Br. 1972;54(1):88–95.
9. Voloshin I, Schippert DW, Kakar S, Kaye EK, Morrey BF. Complications of total elbow replacement: a systematic review. J Shoulder Elb Surg. 2011;20(1):158–68.
10. Strelzow JA, Frank T, Chan K, Athwal GS, Faber KJ, King GJW. Management of rheumatoid arthritis of the elbow with a convertible total elbow arthroplasty. J Shoulder Elb Surg. 2019;28(11):2205–14.
11. Wagener ML, de Vos MJ, Hannink G, van der Pluijm M, Verdonschot N, Eygendaal D. Mid-term clinical results of a modern convertible total elbow arthroplasty. Bone Joint J. 2015;97-B(5):681–8.
12. Kim JM, Mudgal CS, Konopka JF, Jupiter JB. Complications of total elbow arthroplasty. J Am Acad Orthop Surg. 2011;19(6):328–39.
13. Prkic A, van Bergen CJ, The B, Eygendaal D. Total elbow arthroplasty is moving forward: review on past, present and future. World J Orthop. 2016;7(1):44–9.
14. Morrey BF, Bryan RS, Dobyns JH, Linscheid RL. Total elbow arthroplasty. A five-year experience at the Mayo Clinic. J Bone Joint Surg Am. 1981;63(7):1050–63.
15. Garrett JC, Ewald FC, Thomas WH, Sledge CB. Loosening associated with G.S.B. hinge total elbow replacement in patients with rheumatoid arthritis. Clin Orthop Relat Res. 1977;127:170–4.
16. Soni RK, Cavendish ME. A review of the Liverpool elbow prosthesis from 1974 to 1982. J Bone Joint Surg Br. 1984;66(2):248–53.
17. Schuind F, O'Driscoll S, Korinek S, An KN, Morrey BF. Loose-hinge total elbow arthroplasty. An experimental study of the effects of implant alignment on three-dimensional elbow kinematics. J Arthroplast. 1995;10(5):670–8.
18. O'Driscoll SW, An KN, Korinek S, Morrey BF. Kinematics of semi-constrained total elbow arthroplasty. J Bone Joint Surg Br. 1992;74(2):297–9.
19. Kudo H. Non-constrained elbow arthroplasty for mutilans deformity in rheumatoid arthritis: a report of six cases. J Bone Joint Surg Br. 1998;80(2):234–9.
20. Schneeberger AG, King GJ, Song SW, O'Driscoll SW, Morrey BF, An KN. Kinematics and laxity of the Souter-Strathclyde total elbow prosthesis. J Shoulder Elb Surg. 2000;9(2):127–34.
21. King GJ, Itoi E, Niebur GL, Morrey BF, An KN. Motion and laxity of the capitellocondylar total elbow prosthesis. J Bone Joint Surg Am. 1994;76(7):1000–8.
22. Kamineni S, O'Driscoll SW, Urban M, Garg A, Berglund LJ, Morrey BF, et al. Intrinsic constraint of unlinked total elbow replacements--the ulnotrochlear joint. J Bone Joint Surg Am. 2005;87(9):2019–27.
23. Ramsey M, Neale PG, Morrey BF, O'Driscoll SW, An KN. Kinematics and functional characteristics of the Pritchard ERS unlinked total elbow arthroplasty. J Shoulder Elb Surg. 2003;12(4):385–90.
24. Brownhill JR, Pollock JW, Ferreira LM, Johnson JA, King GJ. The effect of implant linking and ligament integrity on humeral loading of a convertible total elbow arthroplasty. Shoulder Elbow. 2019;11(1):45–52.
25. Gramstad GD, King GJ, O'Driscoll SW, Yamaguchi K. Elbow arthroplasty using a convertible implant. Tech Hand Up Extrem Surg. 2005;9(3):153–63.
26. Cinats D, Bois AJ, Hildebrand KA. Clinical outcomes and complications following primary total elbow arthroplasty using the Latitude prosthesis. Shoulder Elbow. 2019;11(5):359–71.
27. Schoch B, Wong J, Abboud J, Lazarus M, Getz C, Ramsey M. Results of total elbow arthroplasty in patients less than 50 years old. J Hand Surg Am. 2017;42(10):797–802.
28. Throckmorton T, Zarkadas P, Sanchez-Sotelo J, Morrey B. Failure patterns after linked semiconstrained total elbow arthroplasty for posttraumatic arthritis. J Bone Joint Surg Am. 2010;92(6):1432–41.
29. Siala M, Laumonerie P, Hedjoudje A, Delclaux S, Bonnevialle N, Mansat P. Outcomes of semiconstrained total elbow arthroplasty performed for arthritis in patients under 55 years old. J Shoulder Elb Surg. 2020;29(4):859–66.
30. Wang JH, Ma HH, Chou TA, Tsai SW, Chen CF, Wu PK, et al. Outcomes following total elbow arthroplasty for rheumatoid arthritis versus post-traumatic conditions: a systematic review and meta-analysis. Bone Joint J. 2019;101-B(12):1489–97.
31. Samdanis V, Manoharan G, Jordan RW, Watts AC, Jenkins P, Kulkarni R, et al. Indications and outcome in total elbow arthroplasty: a systematic review. Shoulder & Elbow, 2020-10, Vol.12 (5), p.353–61.
32. Casadei R, De Paolis M, Drago G, Romagnoli C, Donati D. Total elbow arthroplasty for primary and metastatic tumor. Orthop Traumatol Surg Res. 2016;102(4):459–65.

33. Henrichs MP, Liem D, Gosheger G, Streitbuerger A, Nottrott M, Andreou D, et al. Megaprosthetic replacement of the distal humerus: still a challenge in limb salvage. J Shoulder Elb Surg. 2019;28(5):908–14.
34. Athwal GS, Chin PY, Adams RA, Morrey BF. Coonrad-Morrey total elbow arthroplasty for tumours of the distal humerus and elbow. J Bone Joint Surg Br. 2005;87(10):1369–74.
35. Larsen A, Dale K, Eek M. Radiographic evaluation of rheumatoid arthritis and related conditions by standard reference films. Acta Radiol Diagn (Stockh). 1977;18(4):481–91.
36. Goodman SM, Figgie M. Lower extremity arthroplasty in patients with inflammatory arthritis: preoperative and perioperative management. J Am Acad Orthop Surg. 2013;21(6):355–63.
37. Yeganeh MH, Kheir MM, Shahi A, Parvizi J. Rheumatoid arthritis, disease modifying agents, and periprosthetic joint infection: what does a joint surgeon need to know? J Arthroplast. 2018;33(4):1258–64.
38. Barco R, Streubel PN, Morrey BF, Sanchez-Sotelo J. Total elbow arthroplasty for distal humeral fractures: a ten-year-minimum follow-up study. J Bone Joint Surg Am. 2017;99(18):1524–31.
39. Prasad N, Ali A, Stanley D. Total elbow arthroplasty for non-rheumatoid patients with a fracture of the distal humerus: a minimum ten-year follow-up. Bone Joint J. 2016;98-B(3):381–6.
40. Logli AL, Shannon SF, Boe CC, Morrey ME, O'Driscoll SW, Sanchez-Sotelo J. Total elbow Arthroplasty for distal humerus fractures provided similar outcomes when performed as a primary procedure or after failed internal fixation. J Orthop Trauma. 2020;34(2):95–101.
41. Frankle MA, Herscovici D Jr, DiPasquale TG, Vasey MB, Sanders RW. A comparison of open reduction and internal fixation and primary total elbow arthroplasty in the treatment of intraarticular distal humerus fractures in women older than age 65. J Orthop Trauma. 2003;17(7):473–80.
42. Gambirasio R, Riand N, Stern R, Hoffmeyer P. Total elbow replacement for complex fractures of the distal humerus. An option for the elderly patient. J Bone Joint Surg Br. 2001;83(7):974–8.
43. Cobb TK, Morrey BF. Total elbow arthroplasty as primary treatment for distal humeral fractures in elderly patients. J Bone Joint Surg Am. 1997;79(6):826–32.
44. Aitken SA, Jenkins PJ, Rymaszewski L. Revisiting the 'bag of bones': functional outcome after the conservative management of a fracture of the distal humerus. Bone Joint J. 2015;97-B(8):1132–8.
45. Desloges W, Faber KJ, King GJ, Athwal GS. Functional outcomes of distal humeral fractures managed nonoperatively in medically unwell and lower-demand elderly patients. J Shoulder Elb Surg. 2015;24(8):1187–96.
46. Zagorski JB, Jennings JJ, Burkhalter WE, Uribe JW. Comminuted intraarticular fractures of the distal humeral condyles. Surgical vs nonsurgical treatment. Clin Orthop Relat Res. 1986;202:197–204.
47. McKee MD, Veillette CJ, Hall JA, Schemitsch EH, Wild LM, McCormack R, et al. A multicenter, prospective, randomized, controlled trial of open reduction--internal fixation versus total elbow arthroplasty for displaced intra-articular distal humeral fractures in elderly patients. J Shoulder Elb Surg. 2009;18(1):3–12.
48. Rangarajan R, Papandrea RF, Cil A. Distal humeral hemiarthroplasty versus total elbow arthroplasty for acute distal humeral fractures. Orthopedics. 2017;40(1):13–23.
49. Schneeberger AG, Adams R, Morrey BF. Semiconstrained total elbow replacement for the treatment of post-traumatic osteoarthrosis. J Bone Joint Surg Am. 1997;79(8):1211–22.
50. Kawanishi Y, Miyake J, Omori S, Murase T, Shimada K. The association between cubital tunnel morphology and ulnar neuropathy in patients with elbow osteoarthritis. J Shoulder Elb Surg. 2014;23(7):938–45.
51. Moro JK, King GJ. Total elbow arthroplasty in the treatment of posttraumatic conditions of the elbow. Clin Orthop Relat Res. 2000;370:102–14.
52. Schoch BS, Werthel JD, Sanchez-Sotelo J, Morrey BF, Morrey M. Total elbow arthroplasty for primary osteoarthritis. J Shoulder Elb Surg. 2017;26(8):1355–9.
53. Stanley D. Prevalence and etiology of symptomatic elbow osteoarthritis. J Shoulder Elb Surg. 1994;3(6):386–9.
54. Marsh JP, King GJW. Total elbow arthroplasty. Oper Tech Orthop. 2013;23(4):253–64.
55. Bryan RS, Morrey BF. Extensive posterior exposure of the elbow. A triceps-sparing approach. Clin Orthop Relat Res. 1982;166:188–92.
56. Gschwend N. Our operative approach to the elbow joint. Arch Orthop Trauma Surg. 1981;98(2):143–6.
57. Campbell WC. Arthroplasty of the elbow. Ann Surg. 1922;76(5):615–23.
58. Marinello PG, Peers S, Styron J, Pervaiz K, Evans PJ. Triceps fascial tongue exposure for total elbow arthroplasty: surgical technique and case series. Tech Hand Up Extrem Surg. 2015;19(2):60–3.
59. Alonso-Llames M. Bilaterotricipital approach to the elbow. Its application in the osteosynthesis of supracondylar fractures of the humerus in children. Acta Orthop Scand. 1972;43(6):479–90.
60. Studer A, Athwal GS, MacDermid JC, Faber KJ, King GJ. The lateral para-olecranon approach for total elbow arthroplasty. J Hand Surg Am. 2013;38(11):2219–26.e3
61. Gill DR, Morrey BF. The Coonrad-Morrey total elbow arthroplasty in patients who have rheumatoid arthritis. A ten to fifteen-year follow-up study. J Bone Joint Surg Am. 1998;80(9):1327–35.
62. Little CP, Graham AJ, Karatzas G, Woods DA, Carr AJ. Outcomes of total elbow arthroplasty for rheumatoid arthritis: comparative study of three implants. J Bone Joint Surg Am. 2005;87(11):2439–48.
63. Plaschke HC, Thillemann TM, Brorson S, Olsen BS. Implant survival after total elbow arthroplasty: a retrospective study of 324 procedures per-

formed from 1980 to 2008. J Shoulder Elb Surg. 2014;23(6):829–36.
64. Pham TT, Delclaux S, Huguet S, Wargny M, Bonnevialle N, Mansat P. Coonrad-Morrey total elbow arthroplasty for patients with rheumatoid arthritis: 54 prostheses reviewed at 7 years' average follow-up (maximum, 16 years). J Shoulder Elb Surg. 2018;27(3):398–403.
65. Tanaka N, Kudo H, Iwano K, Sakahashi H, Sato E, Ishii S. Kudo total elbow arthroplasty in patients with rheumatoid arthritis: a long-term follow-up study. J Bone Joint Surg Am. 2001;83(10):1506–13.
66. van der Lugt JC, Geskus RB, Rozing PM. Primary Souter-Strathclyde total elbow prosthesis in rheumatoid arthritis. J Bone Joint Surg Am. 2004;86(3):465–73.
67. Landor I, Vavrik P, Jahoda D, Guttler K, Sosna A. Total elbow replacement with the Souter-Strathclyde prosthesis in rheumatoid arthritis. Long-term follow-up. J Bone Joint Surg Br. 2006;88(11):1460–3.
68. Kodama A, Mizuseki T, Adachi N. Kudo type-5 total elbow arthroplasty for patients with rheumatoid arthritis: a minimum ten-year follow-up study. Bone Joint J. 2017;99-B(6):818–23.
69. Kamineni S, Morrey BF. Distal humeral fractures treated with noncustom total elbow replacement. J Bone Joint Surg Am. 2004;86(5):940–7.
70. Werthel JD, Schoch B, Adams J, Steinmann S. Outcomes after hemiarthroplasty of the elbow for the management of posttraumatic arthritis: minimum 2-year follow-up. J Am Acad Orthop Surg. 2019;27(19):727–35.
71. Smith GC, Bayne G, Page R, Hughes JS. The clinical outcome and activity levels of patients under 55 years treated with distal humeral hemiarthroplasty for distal humeral fractures: minimum 2-year follow-up. Shoulder Elbow. 2016;8(4):264–70.
72. Nestorson J, Ekholm C, Etzner M, Adolfsson L. Hemiarthroplasty for irreparable distal humeral fractures: medium-term follow-up of 42 patients. Bone Joint J. 2015;97-B(10):1377–84.
73. Heijink A, Wagener ML, de Vos MJ, Eygendaal D. Distal humerus prosthetic hemiarthroplasty: midterm results. Strategies Trauma Limb Reconstr. 2015;10(2):101–8.
74. Burkhart KJ, Nijs S, Mattyasovszky SG, Wouters R, Gruszka D, Nowak TE, et al. Distal humerus hemiarthroplasty of the elbow for comminuted distal humeral fractures in the elderly patient. J Trauma. 2011;71(3):635–42.
75. Giannicola G, Scacchi M, Polimanti D, Cinotti G. Discovery elbow system: 2- to 5-year results in distal humerus fractures and posttraumatic conditions: a prospective study on 24 patients. J Hand Surg Am. 2014;39(9):1746–56.
76. Naqui SZ, Rajpura A, Nuttall D, Prasad P, Trail IA. Early results of the Acclaim total elbow replacement in patients with primary osteoarthritis. J Bone Joint Surg Br. 2010;92(5):668–71.
77. Espag MP, Back DL, Clark DI, Lunn PG. Early results of the Souter-Strathclyde unlinked total elbow arthroplasty in patients with osteoarthritis. J Bone Joint Surg Br. 2003;85(3):351–3.

# Non-septic Revision Total Elbow Arthroplasty

3

Mark E. Morrey and Bernard F. Morrey

## Introduction, Scope, and Goal

The requirements to effectively manage the failed elbow replacement continue to evolve and expand. Various implant designs have unique revision features. Increased longevity often results in more extensive osteolysis. Expanded indications and implantation in younger patients cause an increased incidence of failure. Multiple factors result in the elbow being more prone to infection. In this chapter we will attempt to identify and describe the management of those conditions both that are most likely to be encountered and that can also be reliably managed with appropriate experience and execution (Table 3.1). It is recognized that options have evolved and that this is more than one way to manage many aseptic loosening problems. Treatment of the infected TEA is beyond the scope of this work [15].

M. E. Morrey
Department of Orthopaedic Surgery, Mayo Clinic, Rochester, MN, USA
e-mail: Morrey.mark@mayo.edu

B. F. Morrey (✉)
Department of Orthopaedic Surgery, Mayo Clinic, Rochester, MN, USA

University of Texas Health Science Center, San Antonio, TX, USA
e-mail: Morrey.bernard@mayo.edu

## Periprosthetic Fracture

Fractures associated with elbow replacement have been classified according to the location and whether implant fixation has been compromised [11] (Fig. 3.1). What has been learned over the years is that Type I, metaphyseal fractures typically occur due to osteolysis from disease, from a worn articulation, or from loosening of the stem. In general metaphyseal humeral fractures are best ignored. If they remain symptomatic, then resection is simple and effective. Olecranon fractures are a different matter as such fractures compromise extension strength. If displaced more than 1 cm, they should be fixed. However if not markedly displaced, a fibrous union often occurs with conservative management restoring function with MEPS similar to those with osseous union [9] (Fig. 3.2). In this chapter, we are more concerned with Type II fractures of either the ulna or humerus. In all instances we have found the use of strut grafts of great value. Of additional relevance is the reliable incorporation of the strut graft which has served as the platform to develop the allograft prosthetic options discussed below.

Theoretically, all that is necessary for a Type II or III fracture with a well-fixed stem is to fix the fracture, or less commonly treat nonoperatively. However, in our experience the Type II fracture rarely if ever occurs with a well-fixed


G. J. W. King, M. Rizzo (eds.), *Arthroplasty of the Upper Extremity*,
https://doi.org/10.1007/978-3-030-68880-6_3

**Table 3.1** Variety of revision circumstances and solutions

**Revision Procedures for Failed Total Elbow Arthroplasty***

**A. Non-replacement salvage surgery**

Triceps repair, reconstruction
Bushing exchange
Radial head removal
Periprosthetic Fracture —— **Cortical allograft strut graft**

**B. Stem revision with adequate residual osseous support**

Implant stem fracture
Short, small stem implant failure —— **Recement**

**C. Stem revision requiring osseous augmentation**

Bone quality issue, osteolysis —— **Impaction / Type 1 APC**
Length deficiency – bone absent —— **Type 11-111 APC**

*This chapter will cover those 5 conditions underlined

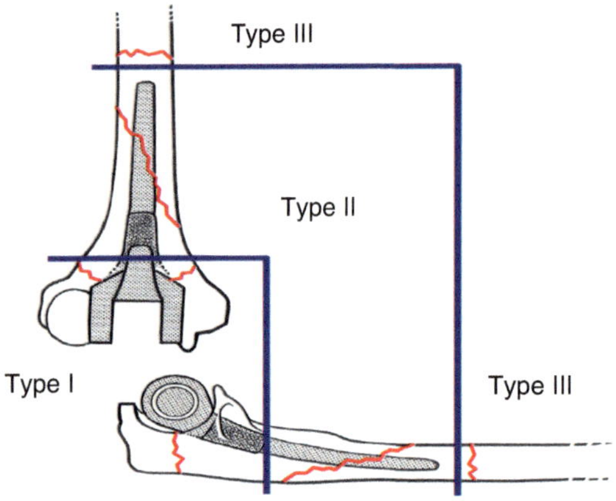


**Fig. 3.1** Periprosthetic fractures are classified by anatomic site: metaphysis, shaft involving the stem and beyond the tip of the stem. Management is based on the anatomic features as well as stability of fixation

implant since it is the loose stem that gives rise to [1] the osteolysis associated with these fractures. The effectiveness of strut grafting has been demonstrated to be approximately 90% in the Mayo experience [5, 13]. In reality strut grafting is used as an adjunct to other features of the revision that involve osseous augmentation as discussed later in this chapter. It may obviously also be used in conjunction with other fixation devices or strategies.

## Strut Graft Technique

The plan. Assess the needed graft length, taking into consideration a second strut which is often needed to better stabilize the fracture, but also to avoid cutting through the thin bone associated with this pathology with the cerclage wire fixation.

## The Strut

For the humerus we prefer a slightly curved strut graft harvested from the allograft so we can use the curvature of the graft to further strengthen the construct. A flat-surfaced graft is preferable for the ulna which is triangular in cross section providing a flat surface for incorporation of a flat graft.

## Application (Fig. 3.3)

1. The anterior strut is used to increase the length of the host bone if necessary. The extended flange provides an additional opportunity to address up to three additional cm of distal humeral bone loss.

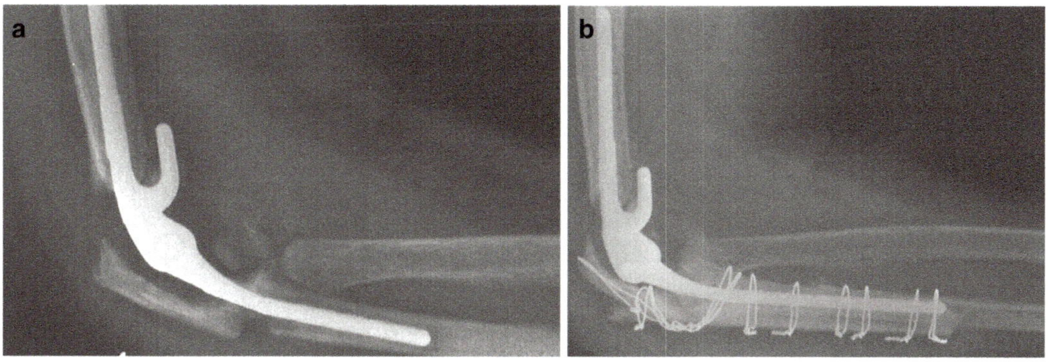


**Fig. 3.2** Olecranon periprosthetic fractures (**a**) should be stabilized if displaced to avoid extension weakness. The author prefers to avoid plates, and in this instance employed a supplemental strut allograft (**b**)

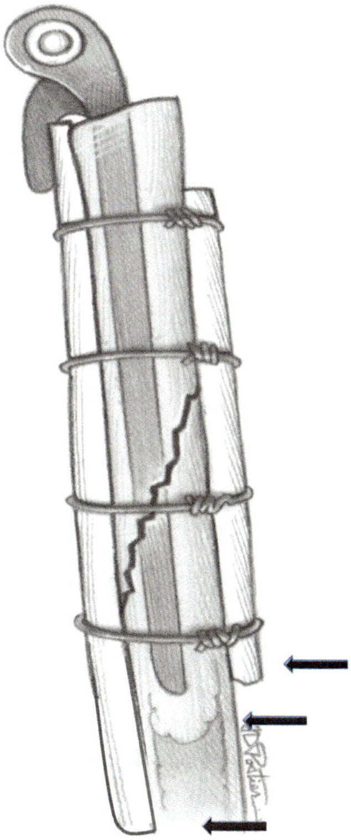

**Fig. 3.3** Allograft strut grafts are applied to the end at different locations (arrows) so as to avoid the stress riser effect from terminating at the same point. Authors use monofilament wire and avoid cables due to cost as well as tissue irritation at the end of the cable

2. The struts should not end at the same level and should bypass the fracture line by at least 2 diameters of the host bone, and the tip of the implant.
3. Avoid cables as they are expensive, the ends irritate the soft tissue, and they are unnecessary. We prefer looped Luque wires on the humerus and 14–16 gauge stainless steel wire for the ulna.
4. If necessary to avoid soft tissue irritation, taper the end of the graft with a burr.

## Revision with Adequate Residual Bone

Occurrence. Today most loose implants are associated with considerable bone compromise often with an associated periprosthetic fracture [1]. Failure of a short-stem primary device may offer the opportunity to reimplant into the native humerus or ulna without osseous augmentation [2]. Fracture of a prosthetic stem also affords the opportunity to recement into a well-fixed cement mantle.

Considerations. In the former instance, the evaluation is focused on the determination as to whether the osseous compromise can be addressed and a reimplantation is possible. This is most commonly accomplished with a longer stemmed implant. The revision stem should have a flange which is able to engage the anterior cortex. Alternatively, broken stems may occur because the distal stem is well fixed. In most instances a broken ulnar, most common, or humeral stem will require an osteotomy to remove the well-fixed stem(s).

## Technique: General Principles

As always the ulnar nerve is isolated and protected. If symptomatic it is decompressed and translocated. When possible the triceps is not detached from the ulna. The exposure must be adequate to effectively remove the implant and properly place the revised stem. Finally in all revision instances, the proper alignment, especially rotatory, of the stems must be meticulously achieved. With loss of column reference, the intermuscular septa may be used as a reference. But it is very important to perform a trial reduction with the ulnar component in place. With the elbow at 90 degrees of flexion, proper humeral axial rotation is defined with the thumb pointing to the shoulder. For ulnar bone loss, the trial reduction is employed to define the position whereby the ulnar component articulated without impingement at the humeral articulation. Recement into the host bone:

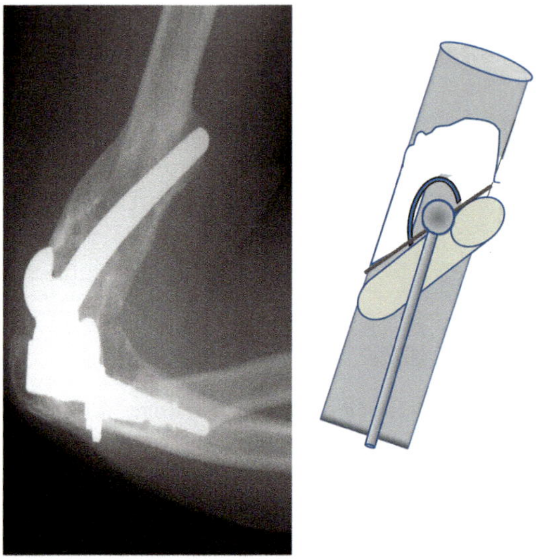

**Fig. 3.4** (**a**) When a loose implant is not centered in the canal, great care is required at revision to avoid following the cement mantel out the cortex. (**b**) If possible a defect should be made in the cement mantel as a pilot to align a drill bit that can drill into the host canal

1. *Exposing the normal canal.* The most important and difficult technical requirement is to bypass the involved bone and gain access to the normal canal. The medullary canal is identified by drilling past the cement plug. When the stem is not centered, extreme care must be taken to develop a pilot indentation in the cement allowing a drill bit to be directed in the proper orientation (Fig. 3.4). When revising the humeral component, the radial nerve should be exposed to avoid injury if the canal is breached. The surgeon should palpate the humerus as the drill is being advanced down the canal past the cement plug if present. In many instances this step is most safely done under fluoroscopic visualization. Alternatively, an arthroscope may be used to directly visualize the process.
2. *Canal preparation.* A guide wire is passed into the normal canal, and the well-fixed cement is serially removed to allow passage of the revision stem. If the guide pin is not centered through the residual cement, larger reamers may remove the cortex creating a stress riser.
3. *Cortex penetration.* Should the cortex be violated, depending on bone quality, consider placing an allograft strut over the cortical penetration.
4. *Cementation.* Once the canal has been adequately expanded, meticulous care is taken to remove any membrane that is adherent to the native bone. When the injection nozzle of the cement gun is too large to bypass the residual bone, every effort should be made to introduce sufficient cement to allow some fixation proximal to the revised implant. It is essential that the position of the humeral component allows the flange to engage the anterior cortex directly or with an interposed bone graft.

## Result

There is very little in the literature regarding the outcome of recementation without osseous augmentation [6]. The Mayo experience with 53 cases was reported in 2012 by Malone et al [8]. Using an objective bone quality rating scale, if bone quality was good, or deficiencies were addressed (bypassed by the stem), no loosening occurred in 78% of the ulnar stems and in 93% of the humeral components (Fig. 3.5). In three humeral and two ulnar components, the bone was inadequate and not addressed; all five subsequently loosened.

## Revising a Broken Stem

Ulna – the key is to obtain adequate exposure of the distal fragment:

1. The triceps is left attached to the olecranon. The location of the stem fracture is determined from the radiographs, and an osteotomy is performed which includes the triceps, olecranon, and proximal ulna (Fig. 3.6). We attempt to osteotomize in such a way as to allow firm grasping of the fractured stem and still have 2 cortical diameters of circumferential ulna intact to allow secure fixation of the revised ulnar component. If in doubt fluoroscopy may be used in this step.
2. A small "pencil" burr is employed to remove cement from around the fractured component.

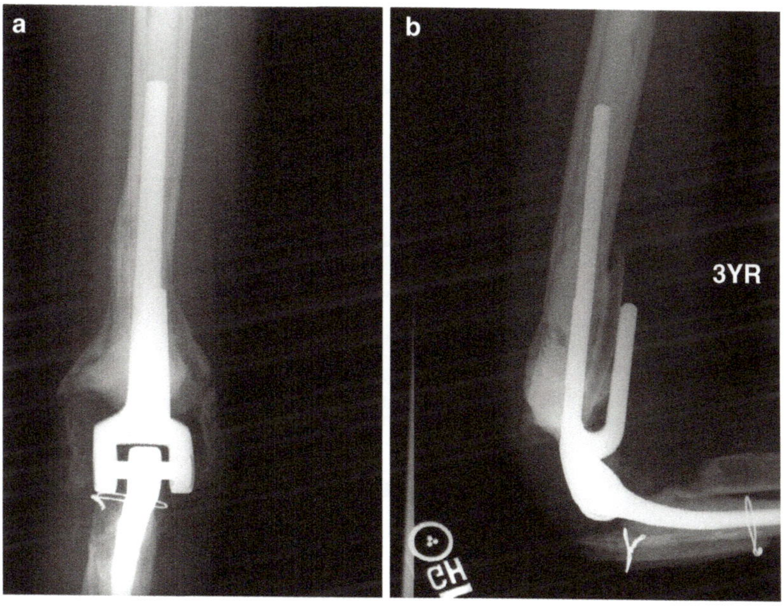


**Fig. 3.5** Serial expanding with flexible reamers allows the cement to be bypassed, in this instance with a recemented stem. (**a**) AP, (**b**) lateral stems centered in the canal bypassing the breached cortex

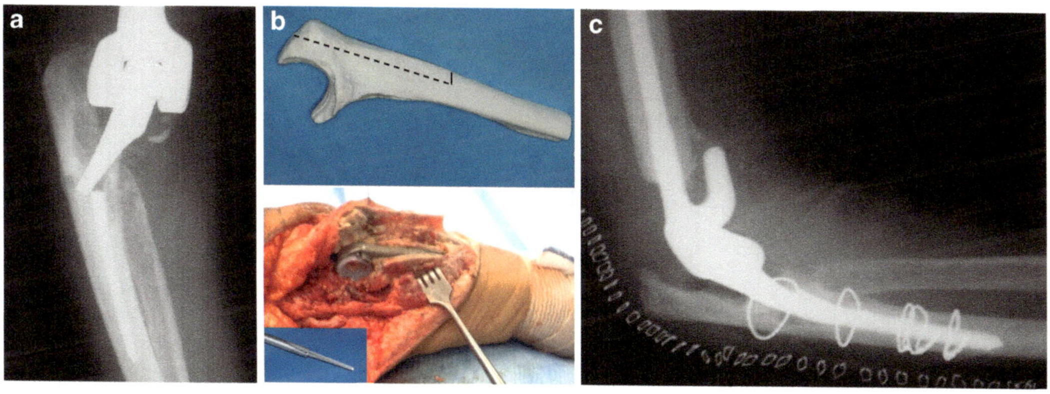


**Fig. 3.6** (**a**) A fractured well-fixed ulnar stem. (**b**) Model (top) and surgical exposure (bottom) with proximal ulnar osteotomy. (**c**) Lateral postoperative image of a reimplantated ulnar component

A needle-nosed vice grip is used to grasp the stem fragment, and it is removed with an attached impaction hammer.

3. The cement mantle is then expanded as described above sufficiently to introduce the same sized or a smaller implant if necessary. Note that if the canal is full of cement, we attempt to increase the length of the canal void by about a centimeter. A longer implant can then be adjusted in length using a metal-cutting blade to accommodate the length of the prepared canal.
4. The cortical window is replaced after the stem has been inserted with the cement still soft to avoid cement in the osteotomy interface and secured with cerclage wires. A strut graft is not typically needed.

Tip. As noted above it is critical to appreciate the position of the implant tip within the canal. It may not be necessary to increase the length of the implant as long as 2 cortical diameters of circumferential stem fixation is achieved (Fig. 3.7).

Humerus – The same considerations apply for the humeral stem fracture with a couple of additional features:

1. Care must be exerted to separate a well-incorporated flange from a distal humerus

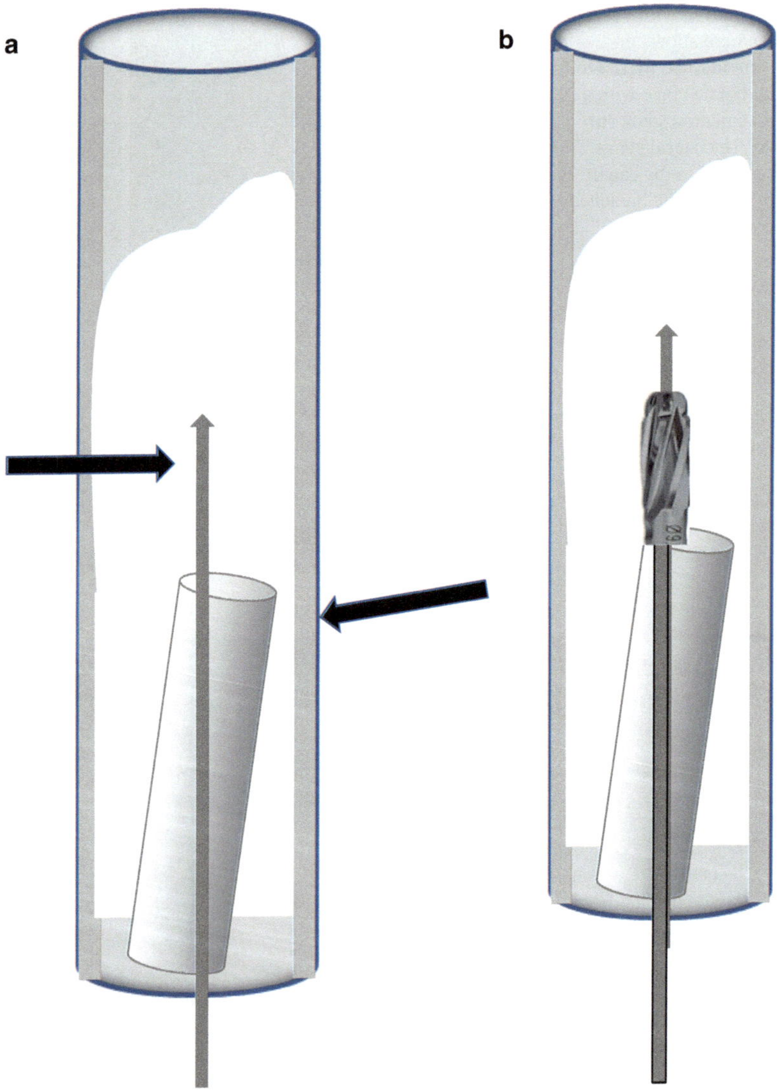

**Fig. 3.7** When a well-fixed excessive terminal cement does not allow ready removal, in some instances the canal may be "extended." (**a**) A drill bit is directed down the center of the cement plug, taking care to avoid breaching the cortex (lower arrow) (see Fig. 3.4b). A drill bit is carefully advanced as central as possible into the cement (top arrow). (**b**) The canal is the extended and expanded with serial reaming

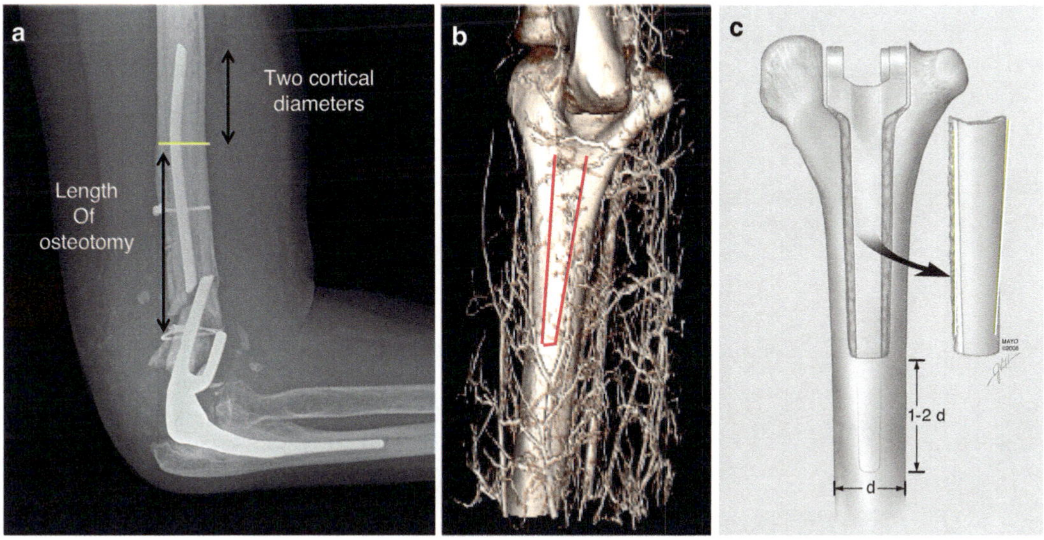


**Fig. 3.8** (**a**) A fractured well-fixed humeral stem. The length of the osteotomy should allow a 2-diameter circumferential fixation of the revision stem. (**b**) Avoid extensive soft tissue stripping to maintain as much vascularity as possible. (**c**) By designing a trapezoid, tapered window, a snug fit is attained when the window is replaced and secured with cerclage wire

fragment. An oscillating saw with a small blade is usually adequate.

2. The distal humeral osteotomy is in the form of a trapezoid and is removed from the posterior cortex. The length is, again, dictated by the location of the tip of the fractured stem (Fig. 3.8). The removed trapezoid bone is replaced after the stem has been inserted with the cement still soft to avoid cement in the osteotomy interface and secured with cerclage wires. A strut graft is not typically used.

## Expanded, Osteolytic Cortex: Impaction Grafting

Documentation of the efficacy of compressive impaction grafting to reconstruct lytic deficiency of both the acetabulum and proximal femur prompted the adaption of the concept to the elbow with similar problems [3, 4].

**Indications** This technique is used when osteolytic expansion of the cortex involves the length of a loose component. Ideally the expansion should be intact with no fracture, and the revision stem should be of adequate length to reach good host bone by about a 2-cortical diameter length.

**Contraindications** Fracture at the lytic/normal bone interface is a relative contraindication. Impaction grafting is still viable if a strut can be effectively used to treat the periprosthetic fracture and the revision stem enters normal host bone (Fig. 3.9). Note that if a long-stemmed device has become loose such that even a long-stemmed implant cannot reach the normal host canal, the interface can be reinforced with two struts, and a shorter stem can be used.

**Technique** This failure mode allows removal of the stem with cement, leaving only the poor-quality osteolytic shell. The membrane is carefully and completely removed – often this is a prolonged but necessary process. The unviolated portion of the host bone canal is entered and prepared to receive the revision stem. Cancellous allograft is placed through a bone mill. A plastic tube is inserted to the opening of the host canal. A second smaller tube that can slide through the larger tube is used to deliver PMMA and is inserted for a distance of about 2

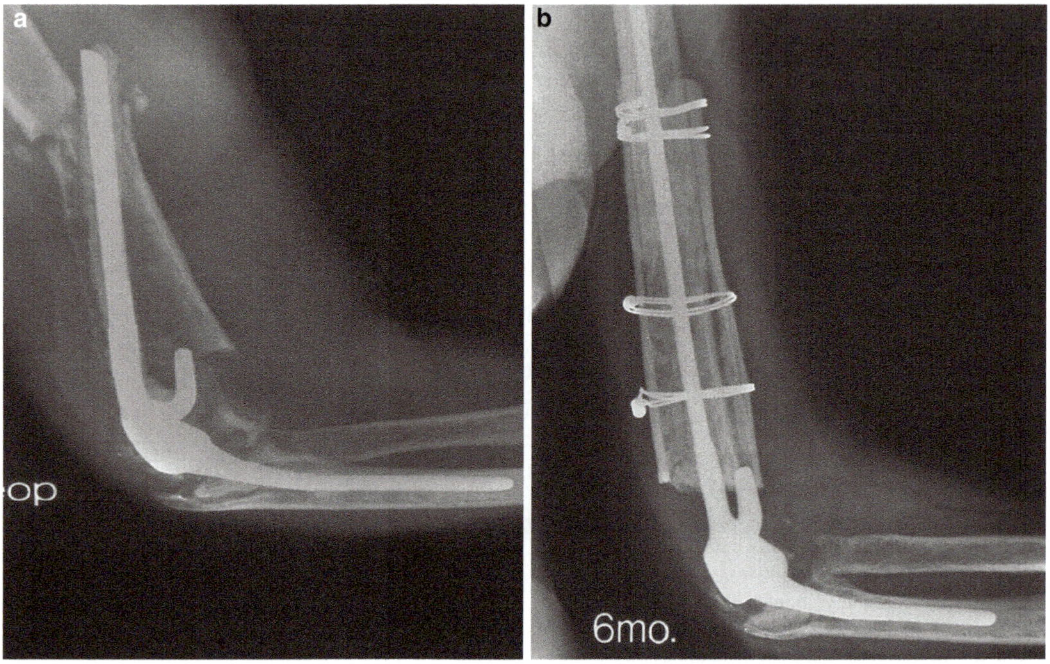


**Fig. 3.9** (**a**) Distal humeral osteolysis with anterior angulated fracture. (**b**) The fracture was anatomically reduced and stabilized with an allograft strut graft. This allowed an effective cancellous grafting technique to be executed

cortical diameters into the normal canal (Fig. 3.10). Cancellous chips 2–5 mm are then impacted around the larger, outer tube. Note that if the impacted bone should be so carefully and thoroughly inserted so as to allow the implant to be rigidly fixed in the bone when cemented.

**Cementation** Antibiotic cement is delivered with an injection system. The inner nozzle tube is cut so as to extend 2 cortical diameters past the large outer tube. The difference "d" in length between the two tubes is measured, and the cement is injected as the smaller inner tube is withdrawn for the predetermined length – "d" (Fig. 3.11). At the stage both tubes are withdrawn together to allow the cement to fill the new canal created by impacted bone around the created around the larger tube. The appropriate implant is then quickly but carefully inserted into the construct being especially careful not to disrupt the column of cancellous bone. Note that often the expansion allows direct contact with the implant flange. If this is not the case, then a bone graft is inserted to assure contact is established between the implant and host bone.

**Aftercare** The incorporation of impaction grafting occurs slowly. Great care is made to avoid torsion on the humerus if this is the replaced implant. A minimum of 3 months is felt to be needed to allow bone graft incorporation.

## Results

In 2004 Loebenberg et al. reported the Mayo experience with 12 of 14 satisfactory uses of this revision technique a mean of 4 years after surgery [4] (see Fig. 3.9). In 2013 Rhee et al. reported 15 of 16 successful procedures a mean of 7 years following surgery [12].

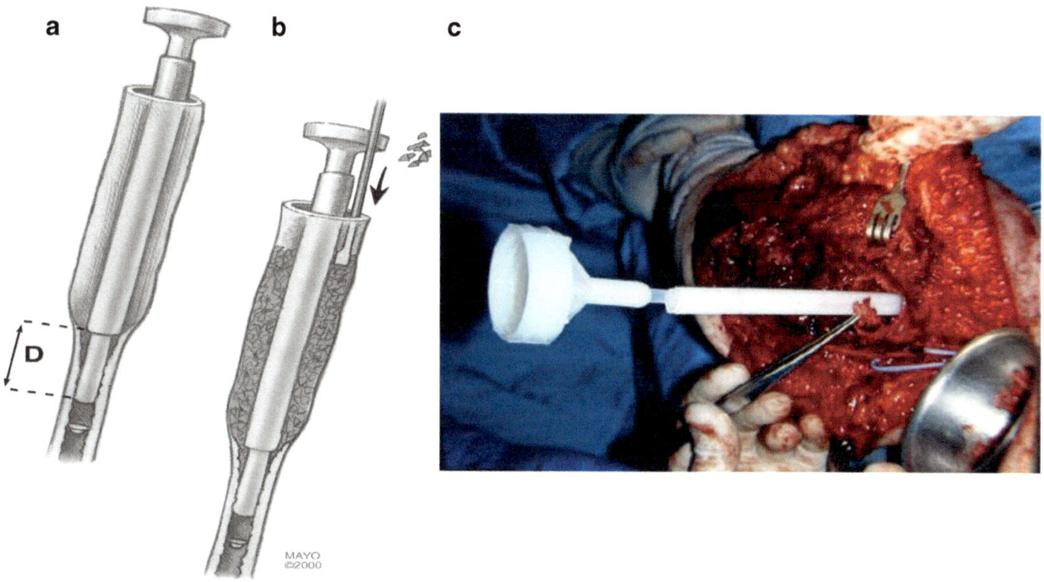


**Fig. 3.10** (**a**). The first step is to place the larger tube to the level of the expanded canal. The tube to be used for cement injection is measured to be ×2 diameters longer, "D," than the larger tube and is removed to facilitate bone grafting. (**b**, **c**) Cancellous chips are carefully and forcibly impacted around the tube

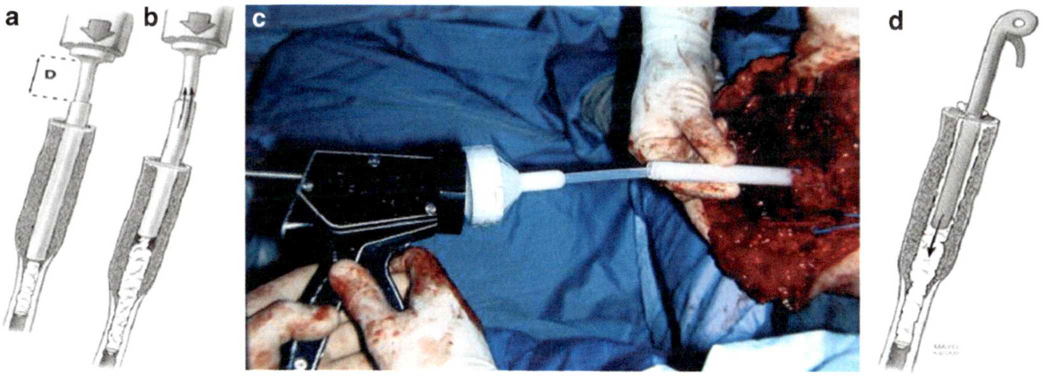


**Fig. 3.11** (**a**). The inner tube is inserted and fills the normal bone with cement by withdrawing injection to the previously determined depth, "D." (**b**, **c**) At this point the outer tube is withdrawn with the smaller tube as it injects the canal formed by the bone graft. (**d**) The implant is carefully inserted into the newly created and cemented canal

## Allograft Prosthetic Composite

Unfortunately, today many failures might be considered "catastrophic" due to extensive osseous violation both of the humerus and ulna. To address this problem, we have developed a system of allograft prosthetic composite (APC) revision strategies. Three types of deficiency can be so addressed: (1) Type I, expanded, lytic with minimal loss of longitudinal bone (Fig. 3.12a); (2) Type II, circumferential loss of bone, but implant stem can reach the native bone (Fig. 3.12b); and (3) Type III, massive loss of bone only addressed by custom stem length, or the Type III APC (Fig. 3.12c).

**Type I APC** *Indications:* Cortical expansion and thinning but minimal loss of bone length. *Contraindications:* Fracture of the expanded bone, especially if occurring at the interface with

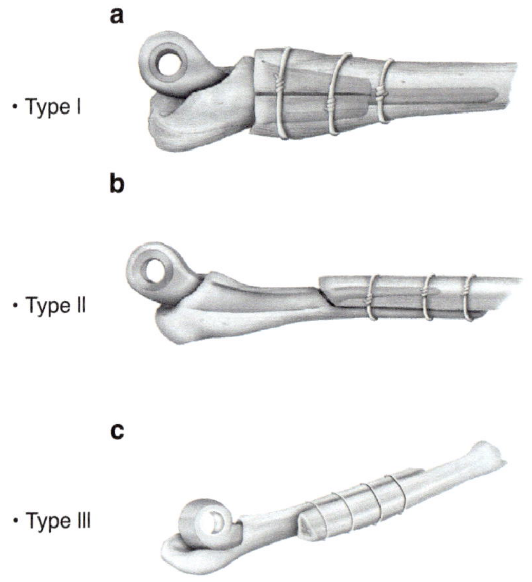


**Fig. 3.12** Three types of allograft prosthetic composite have been employed: (**a**) Type I – circumferential graft fixed to implant and inserted into circumferential osteolytic defect (**b**) Type II – length defect addressed with circumferential allograft, attached to host with extended cortical allograft strut. (**c**) If the implant cannot reach the host bone, the deficiency is replaced with an allograft replacement containing the prosthetic implant – "whole bone replacement"

normal host bone. Note: This employs a circumferential graft and is an alternative to the impaction graft option.

***Preoperative planning*** Carefully note the diameter of the expanded bone and assure a proper size of the allograft. Note: An oversized allograft can be trimmed to fit, but is very time-consuming; an undersized graft is at risk of non-incorporation. The host bone is sometimes longitudinally osteotomized to allow the expanded, lytic bone to collapse around the allograft. The complex is stabilized with monofilament cerclage wires.

**Technique**

1. Exposure. The principles described above are still respected. The ulnar and radial nerves are always identified and if necessary exposed and isolated/protected [14].
2. Preparation of host. The membrane is meticulously removed to enhance the likelihood of graft incorporation. The native normal medullary canal is exposed using the techniques described above. In the ideal situation, the implant stem bypasses the full length of the osteolytic bone, enters, and is cemented into the more normal host bone.
3. Fit and alignment. This is the most time-consuming and crucial technical step. (A) The first priority is to obtain a tight mechanical fit between the surfaces of the graft and host. This determines the position of the graft which is marked on host and graft bones. (B) The medullary canal of the allograft is then expanded with reamers to allow the stem to rotate sufficiently to achieve optimum rotational alignment. This is readily done as the thickness of the graft cortex is relatively unimportant.
4. Trial reduction. This step is critical to determine the sequence of implantation: graft to host to implant to graft/host complex, or implant to graft and then ACP to host. The determinants are the alignment and proper depth of insertion of the implant (Fig. 3.13).

**Type II APC** This composite includes a circumferential graft that provides fixation to the implant and addresses the linear deficiency. The graft then extends as a strut to provide reliable incorporation. In this composite the length of the implant is sufficient to bypass the deficiency and enter the host bone (Fig. 3.12b).

***Indications*** Loss of medullary fixation length of the humerus or ulna of about 2 or more cm (Fig. 3.14). Specific technical considerations:

1. Graft selection. Proximal half of an ulna allograft or either proximal or distal humeral allograft. The ulna allograft should also include the triceps tendon and be specific for the right or left side.
2. The graft that constitutes the strut and extends past the linear deficiency should be as robust as possible. Hence:
   (a) The allograft should be larger in diameter than the host to allow the central canal to

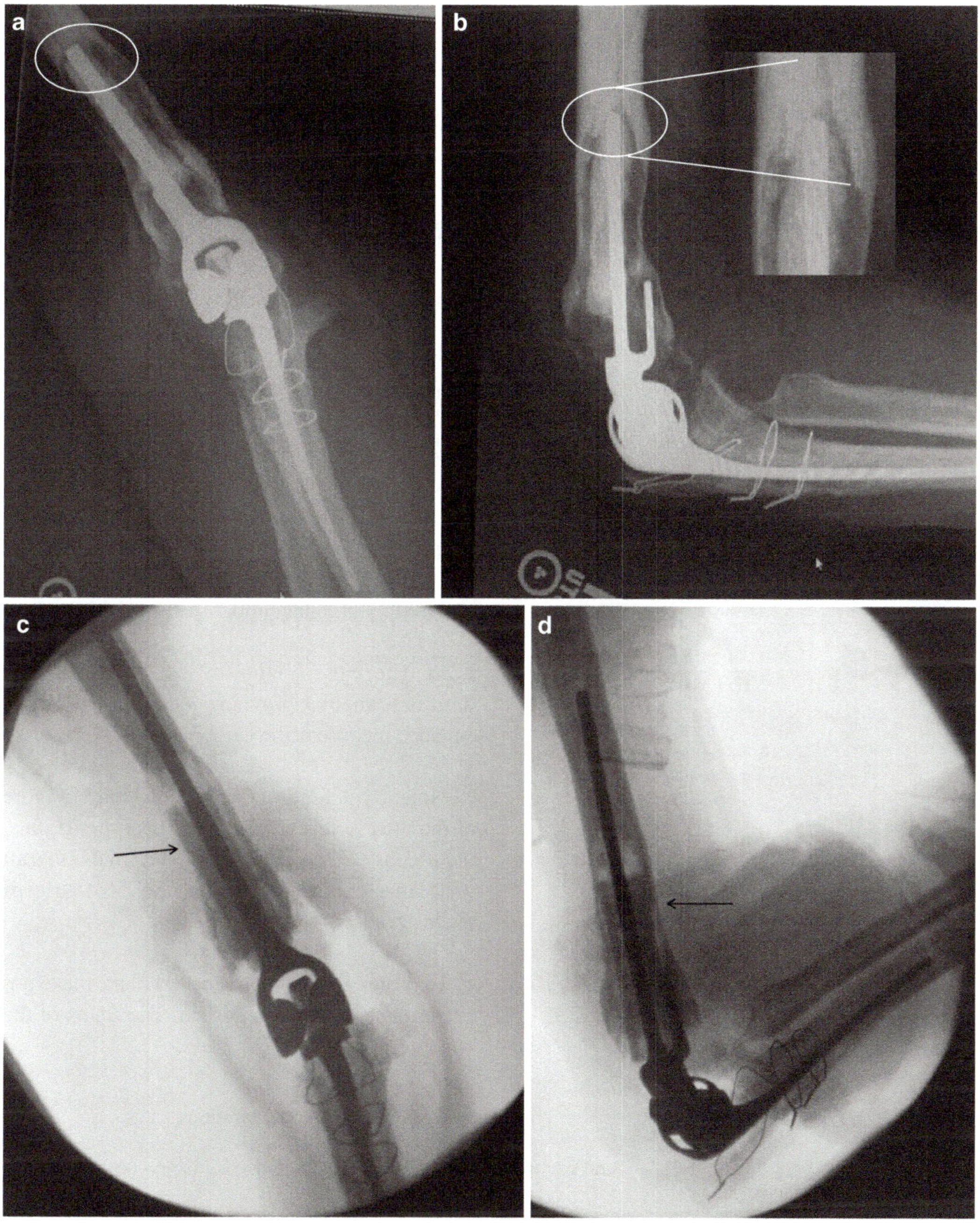


**Fig. 3.13** (**a**) An image of a typical osteolytic loosening involving the length of the humeral stem. Note thinning of the cortex and impending fracture. (**b**) Lateral view confirms fracture risk. Ovals. (**c**) AP after Type I APC construct showing stem bypassing the weakened area of humerus. The graft was extremely stable on the table and image (arrows) confirms favorable graft/host apposition, on both AP and lateral (**d**) views. The void between graft and host bone is filled with cement

align (Fig. 3.15). Note that in some instances, the stem of the implant must be slightly bent to negotiate the two canals.
(b) The strut should be as close to 50% of the circumference as possible.

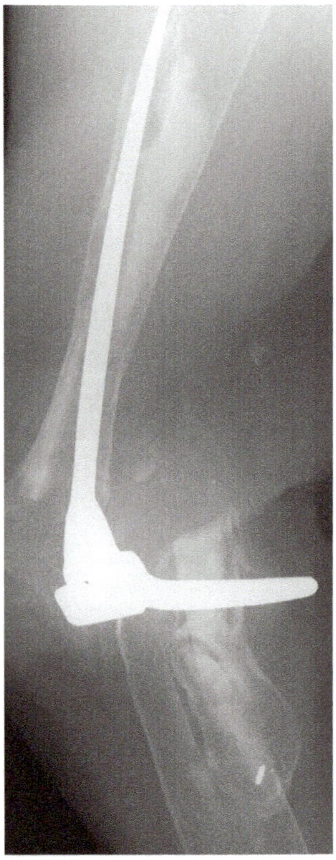

Fig. 3.14 Grossly loose device with destruction of both humerus and ulna

(c) The interface between the strut and circumferential graft should be "radiused" to avoid a stress riser (Fig. 3.16).
(d) Fixation to the host is with monofilament cerclage wires – these are perfectly adequate, less expensive, and less irritating than cable fixation.

3. The inner edge of the strut cortex should be removed to improve total host-graft contact and avoid the flat on curved effect (Fig. 3.17).
4. Prosthesis alignment remains critical, and similar considerations as mentioned for the Type I technique are applied for this composite.

***Type III APC*** This reconstruction effectively uses an intact allograft and simply replaces an absent bone. The implant need not be of an extra length since the host bone is too distant even for a long-stemmed device. The deficiency is replaced by an intact allograft (Fig. 3.12c).

***Ulna*** The cross section of the ulna in its mid third is triangular providing two flat surfaces to enhance incorporation (Fig. 3.18).

Note. By definition the proximal third or more of the ulna is absent. Hence in the Type III ulna, the triceps tendon is maintained on the allograft with the expectation of a possible triceps reconstruction.

1. Exposure. With the absence of bone, the exposure is easily accomplished. The status of the

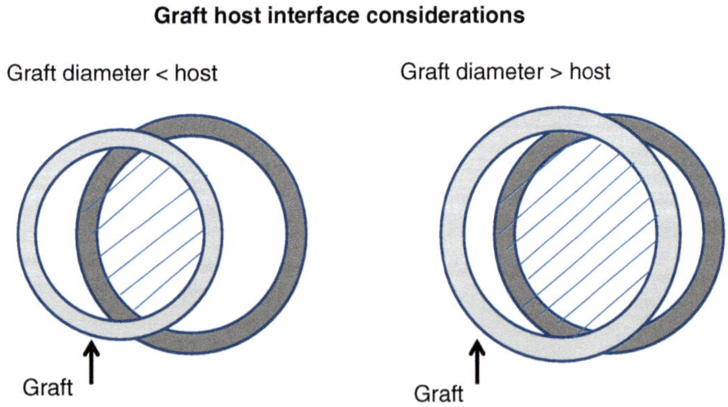


Fig. 3.15 The Type II strategy requires the donor bone to be larger than the host since the offset from the strut markedly lessens the ability of the stem to negotiate the host/graft interface

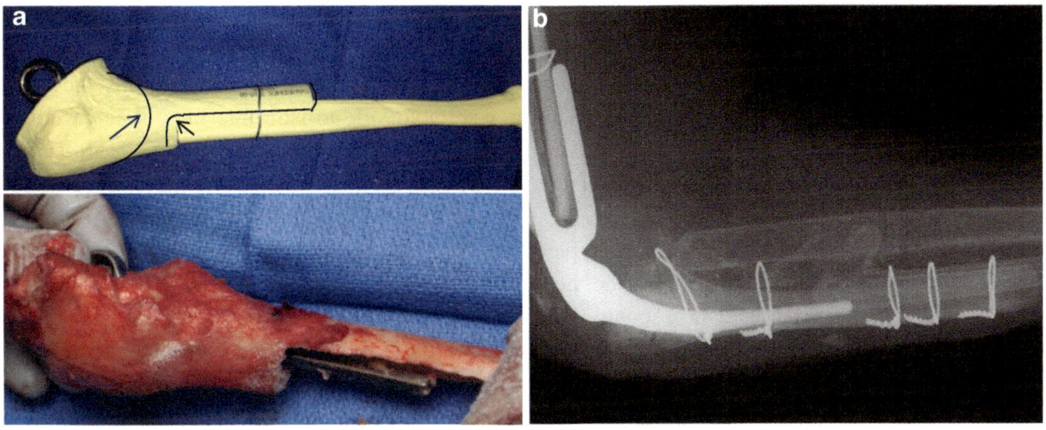


**Fig. 3.16** (**a**) Length deficiency is addressed by circumferential fixation of the implant and strut extension for reliable incorporation. Note the graft strut junction is "radiused" to avoid stress riser and potential fracture. (Top). (**b**) Lateral image of Type II APC

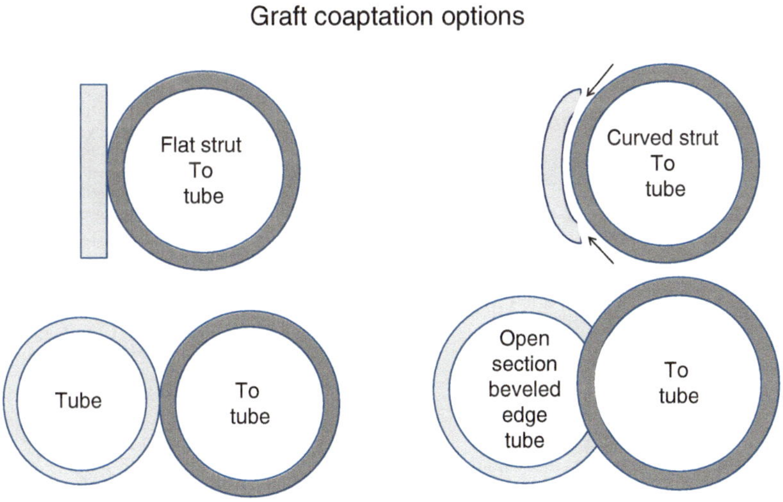


**Fig. 3.17** Top. For a strut graft, a curved-to-curved surface is much more effective than is a flat to curved construct. Bottom. So too with a whole bone interface, an open section coaptation is much more stable and likely to incorporate than a tube-to-tube interface

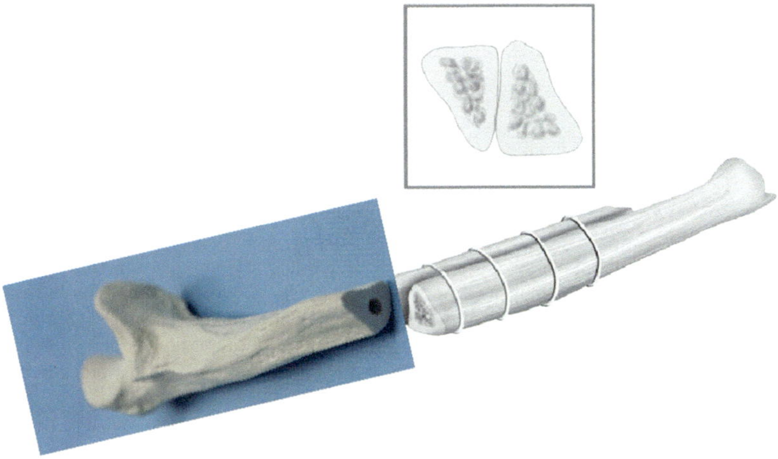

**Fig. 3.18** At the ulna, the triangular shaft allows for a natural flat to flat interface. The fibula, if used, allows for the identical surface coaptation

skin is carefully assessed to insure it can accommodate the increased bulk of the APC. Liberal consultation with a plastic surgeon characterizes the pre-procedure planning. The most important components of the dissection are identity and protection of the radial and ulnar nerves, as always.

2. Alignment of the implant. As with the Type I APC, the alignment is defined by the best coaptation of the graft and host bone. This relationship is first defined, and the allograft canal is expanded with reamers to allow flexibility to place the implant with proper axial rotation.
3. Graft preparation. At the humerus the most reliable side-to-side interface is achieved by creating an open section in the allograft for a length adequate to assure a high probability of union while still leaving adequate circumferential bone for stable implant fixation. The edges of the open section portion of the allograft are beveled or removed to enhance the amount of surface contact with the host bone (Fig. 3.19).

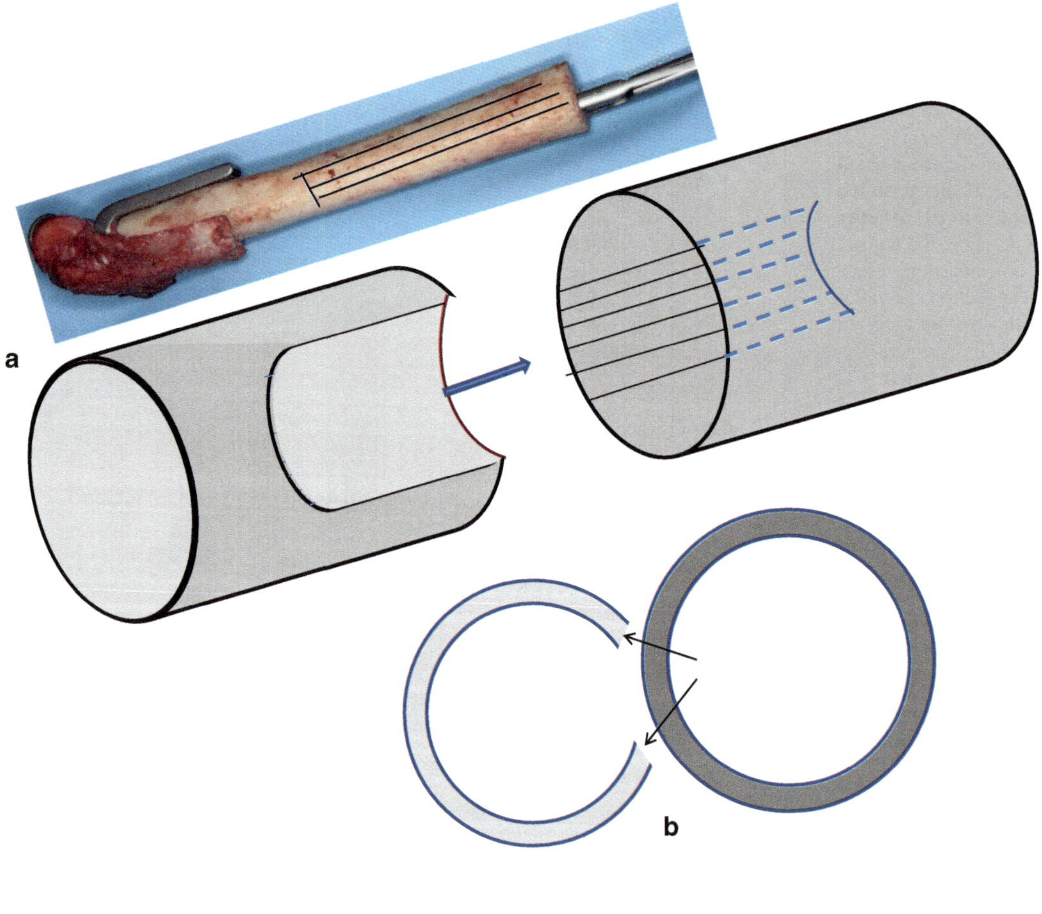


**Fig. 3.19** (**a**) At the humerus, the best interface for stability and healing creates an open section removing a strip of cortex comprising 25% or less of the circumference of the graft. (**b**) Improved contact is obtained by beveling the cut edge of the graft to conform to the surface of the host bone (arrows). (**c**) Radiograph of distal humeral fracture with proximal hardware that precludes access to the humeral canal. (**d**) Surgical photograph of a Type III allograph prosthetic composite fashioned as described above (**a**, **b**). (**e**) Post-procedure radiograph

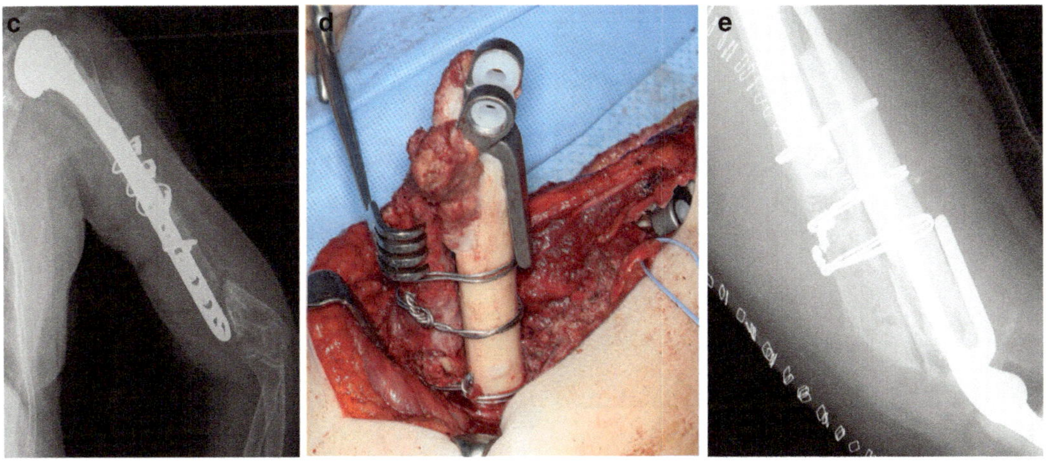


**Fig. 3.19** (continued)

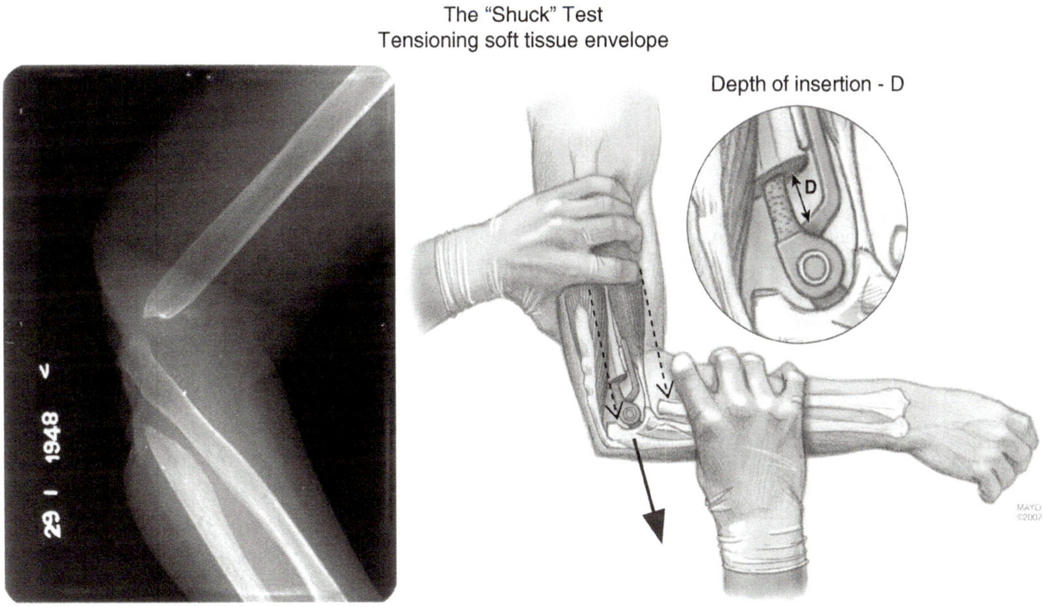


**Fig. 3.20** When extensive bone loss causes shortening, the proper depth of insertion is determined by the "shuck" test whereby the articulated trial is subjected to a downward force of the ulna. The amount of displacement "D" represents the depth of insertion to be observed of the humeral implant

4. Graft positioning. The axial relationships and balancing are very important in this reconstruction. We rely on the soft tissue tensioning test to determine the axial placement of the humeral graft (Fig. 3.20). For the ulna we avoid too distal placement by observing the tendency of the ulnar component to slide out of the ulna in flexion and adjusting distally as needed to avoid the tendency (Fig. 3.21). By definition the Type lll reconstruction is a "replace the bone" treatment. We employ the same landmarks as noted above for the Type I APC. However, in some ways rotation is a bit less critical due to the extensive nature of the bone loss, the APC defines, to some extent, a new kinematic axis for the elbow.

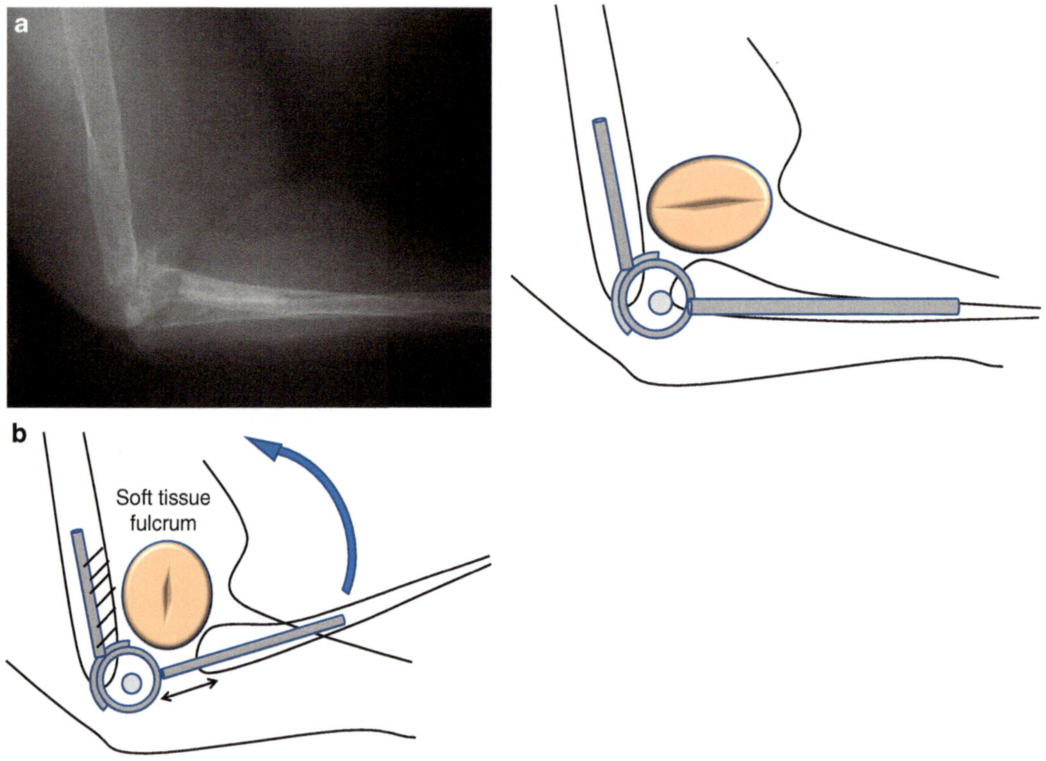


**Fig. 3.21** (**a**, left) Radiograph of an absent elbow joint with proximal migration of the ulna. Note soft tissue shadow of a large soft tissue envelope. (**a**, right) Simulation of an implanted prosthesis, whereby the humeral insertion is proximal as dictated by the level of resection. (**b**) With flexion the well-fixed humerus is stable, but the ulna component fails in shear due to the extracting shear forces caused by the soft tissue fulcrum of the anterior soft tissues occasioned by too proximal placement of the humeral component

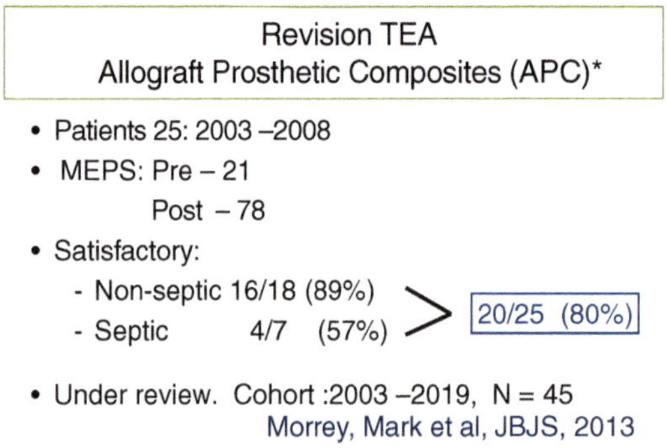


**Fig. 3.22** Original 5-year Mayo experience. The current cohort with >1-year surveillance is currently under an IRB-approved study

## Aftercare

The principle that governs postoperative activity is that success of the APC requires bone healing – 12 or more months. The Type I strategy is most vulnerable to ulnar loosening. Patients are especially advised to avoid internal and external rotation of the humerus with the elbow around 90 degrees of flexion. Radiographs are taken each month for the first 3 months, or until there is evidence of incorporation of the graft.

## Results

The Mayo experience is most extensive. Results of the first 25 procedures performed between 2003 and 2008 with a mean of 8 year surveillance were reported by Mansat et al. in [7]. Graft incorporation was 92% and the MEPS improved from 30 to 84. The most common causes of reoperation were infection (7 of 25 were infected revisions), fracture in 3, and loosening in 1 (Fig. 3.22). This experience now exceeds 45 patients and is under review [10].

## References


1. Foruria AM, Sanchez-Sotelo J, Oh LS, Adams RA, Morrey BF. The surgical treatment of periprosthetic elbow fractures around the ulnar stem following semiconstrained total elbow arthroplasty. J Bone Joint Surg Am. 2011;93(15):1399–407. PMID:21915545. https://doi.org/10.2106/JBJS.J.00102.
2. Ikävalko M, Belt EA, Kautiainen H, Lehto MU. Revisions for aseptic loosening in Souter-Strathclyde elbow arthroplasty: incidence of revisions of different components used in 522 consecutive cases. Acta Orthop Scand. 2002;73:257–63.
3. Lee DH. Impaction allograft bone-grafting for revision total elbow arthroplasty: a case report. J Bone Joint Surg Am. 1999;81-A:1008–12.
4. Loebenberg MI, Adams R, O'Driscoll SW, Morrey BF. Impaction grafting in revision total elbow arthroplasty. J Bone Joint Surg Am. 2005;87-A:99–106.
5. Kamineni S, Morrey BF. Proximal ulnar reconstruction with strut allograft in revision total elbow arthroplasty. J Bone Joint Surg Am. 2004;86-A(6):1223–9. PMID:15173296.
6. King GJ, Adams RA, Morrey BF. Total elbow arthroplasty: revision with use of a non-custom semiconstrained prosthesis. J Bone Joint Surg Am. 1997;79(3):394–400. PMID:9070529.
7. Mansat P, Adams RA, Morrey BF. Allograft-prosthesis composite for revision of catastrophic failure of total elbow arthroplasty. J Bone Joint Surg Am. 2004;86-A(4):724–35. PMID:15069136.
8. Malone AA, Sanchez JS, Adams R, Morrey B. Revision of total elbow replacement by exchange cementing. J Bone Joint Surg Br. 2012;94(1):80–5. PMID:22219252. https://doi.org/10.1302/0301-620X.94B1.26004.
9. Marra G, Morrey BF, Gallay SH, McKee MD, O'Driscoll S. Fracture and nonunion of the olecranon in total elbow arthroplasty. J Shoulder Elbow Surg. 2006;15(4):486–94. https://doi.org/10.1016/j.jse.2005.10.016. PMID: 16831655.
10. Morrey ME, Sanchez-Sotelo J, Abdel MP, Morrey BF. Allograft-prosthetic composite reconstruction for massive bone loss including catastrophic failure in total elbow arthroplasty. J Bone Joint Surg Am. 2013;95(12):1117–24. PMID:23783209. https://doi.org/10.2106/JBJS.L.00747.
11. Odriscoll S, Morrey BF. Periprosthetic fractures about the elbow. Orth Cl N Am. 1999;30:319.
12. Rhee YG, Cho NS, Parke CS. Impaction grafting in revision total elbow arthroplasty due to aseptic loosening and bone loss. JBJS Essent Surg Tech. 2013;3(3):e74.
13. Sanchez-Sotelo J, O'Driscoll S, Morrey BF. Periprosthetic humeral fractures after total elbow arthroplasty: treatment with implant revision and strut allograft augmentation. J Bone Joint Surg Am. 2002;84-A(9):1642–50. PMID:12208923.
14. Throckmorton TW, Zarkadas PC, Sanchez-Sotelo J, Morrey BF. Radial nerve palsy after humeral revision in total elbow arthroplasty. J Shoulder Elbow Surg. 2011;20(2):199–205. PMID:21106403. https://doi.org/10.1016/j.jse.2010.08.012.
15. Wee AT, Morrey BF, Sanchez-Sotelo J. The fate of elbows with unexpected positive intraoperative cultures during revision elbow arthroplasty. J Bone Joint Surg Am. 2013;95(2):109–16. PMID:23235940. https://doi.org/10.2106/JBJS.K.00121.

# Part II

# Radial Head Arthroplasty

# 4 Design Considerations in Radial Head Arthroplasty

Shawn W. O'Driscoll

## Outline

In this chapter, we will study three sets of issues that affect design considerations for radial head arthroplasty:

1. *Functional anatomy and biomechanics of the radial head*
2. *The prosthesis*
3. *Instruments and technique*

## Functional Anatomy and Biomechanics of the Radial Head

The radial head plays an important role in axial load bearing across the elbow as well as being an important constraint to valgus instability [1–5]. The radial head bears approximately 60% of the axial load across the elbow; however, the effect of forearm rotation has been controversial with different methods having found different results [1, 4].

Radial head excision shortens the moment arm resisting valgus torque on the elbow and therefore concentrates stressors on the lateral ulnohumeral joint and increases stress in the medial collateral ligament as shown in Fig. 4.1. This eventually leads to erosion of the bone in the lateral ulnohumeral joint as shown in Fig. 4.2. Multiple studies have shown that radial head excision substantially alters elbow kinematics, load bearing, and articular contact stressors [6–13]. Long-term studies after radial head excision document radiographic changes of arthritis, bone loss in the lateral ulnohumeral joint, and valgus drift (pseudolaxity) due to that bone loss [8]. Whether or not these long-term changes can be prevented by radial head replacement is not known yet, but biomechanical studies of radial head arthroplasty show that these disturbances in elbow kinematics, laxity, and load bearing can be corrected or prevented by prosthetic radial head replacement [7, 14, 15]. These biomechanical and clinical factors render a compelling argument in favor of radial head replacement, provided that the long-term safety and efficacy of this type of arthroplasty can be confirmed.

The three-dimensional shape and orientation of the radial head have a number of unique features. The radial head is elliptical in shape, not round, and is offset from the axis of rotation of the forearm such that there is a cam effect during rotation of the radial head. The radial head is also tilted (angulated) with respect to the neck of the radius. This is to accommodate a change in alignment of the long axis of the radius that occurs



S. W. O'Driscoll (✉)
Department of Orthopedic Surgery, Mayo Clinic and Mayo Foundation, Rochester, MN, USA
e-mail: odriscoll.shawn@mayo.edu


G. J. W. King, M. Rizzo (eds.), *Arthroplasty of the Upper Extremity*,
https://doi.org/10.1007/978-3-030-68880-6_4

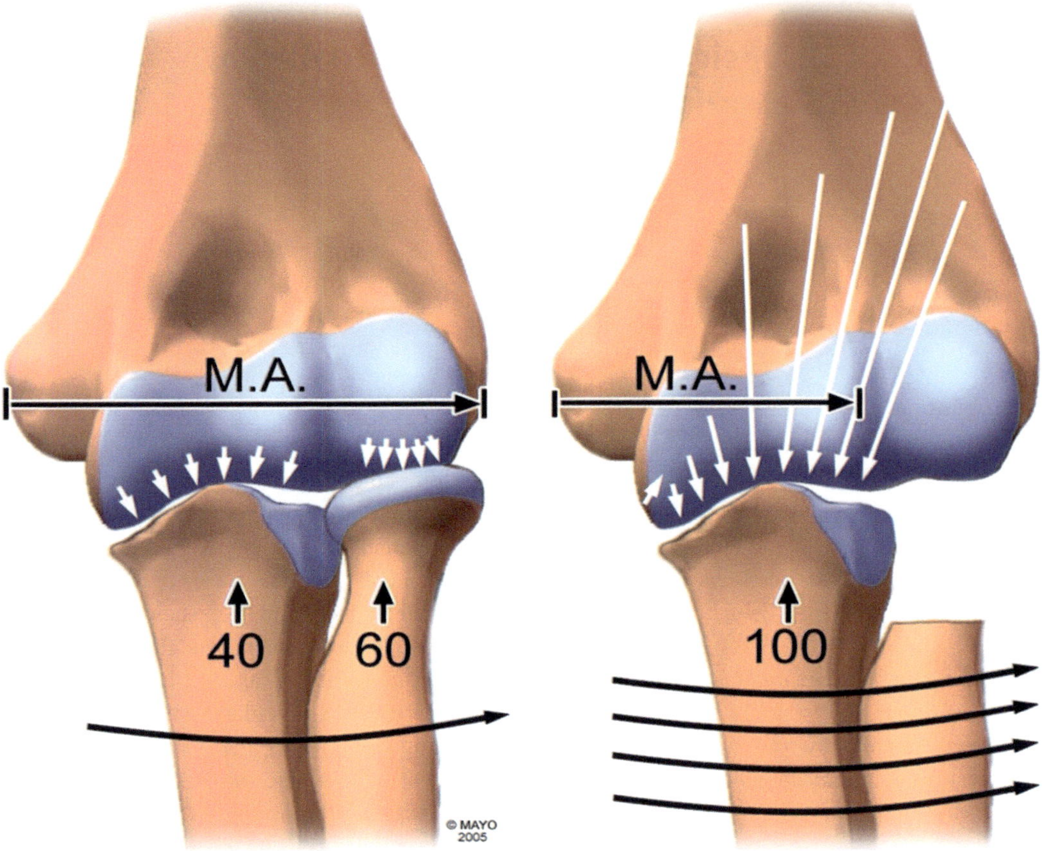


**Fig. 4.1** Radial head excision increases valgus torque on the elbow due to the shortened moment arm. This increases joint surface contact pressures in the lateral ulnohumeral joint and stress in the medial collateral ligament. (By permission of Mayo Foundation for Medical Education and Research (https://www.mayoclinic.org/copyright). All rights reserved)

during forearm rotation. As the distal radius crosses over the ulna at the wrist during pronation, the valgus alignment of the radius with respect to the humerus decreases. In other words, the radius does not rotate about its online axis, but rather about a long axis that passes through the radial head proximally and the ulna distally. The resulting crossover type of motion creates a windshield wiper motion of the radial head on the capitellum with forearm rotation.

As we consider these various anatomic, biomechanical, and functional aspects of the radial head, design specifications must take into consideration the needs for the radial head to [1] bear load, [2] articulate correctly, and/or [3] compensate for incorrect articulation. In theory, achievement of the first two design specifications would require a prosthetic radial head to be designed anatomically and positioned correctly by the surgeon. If this was thought not to be possible or feasible, then specification number 3 might be accomplished a number of different ways. For example, constraint within the prosthesis itself can be decreased through the use of a bipolar articulation. Constraint at the prosthetic-bone interface can be decreased with loose-fitting smooth stems. Finally, constraint at the prosthetic-joint surface interface can be reduced by altered shape (geometry) of the head itself.

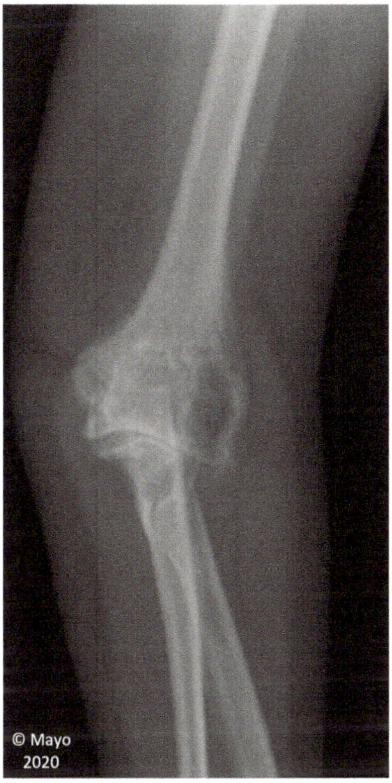


**Fig. 4.2** Increased valgus stress eventually leads to erosion of the bone in the lateral ulnohumeral joint. (By permission of Mayo Foundation for Medical Education and Research (https://www.mayoclinic.org/copyright). All rights reserved)

## Design Considerations of the Prosthesis

Design considerations relating to the prosthesis itself can be grouped into three categories:

- The head
- The stem
- The head-stem connection

### The Head

The head is the most obvious critical part of the prosthesis, since it articulates with the capitellum and ulna. Three features of the head are important or potentially important design considerations:

- Shape
- Position and orientation in 3-D space
- Material

#### Shape of the Radial Head

Since the prosthetic radial head will articulate with the capitellum, lateral trochlear ridge, and radial notch of the ulna, the ideal shape of the prosthetic head would either replicate native anatomy or be designed to compensate for any potential deleterious effects resulting from differences in shape. In this section we will focus on native radial head, which has been studied on cadaveric elbows, MRI images, and CT scans [16–19].

In the majority of native elbows, the outer surface of the radial head is asymmetrical in shape, representing an oval (or an ellipse) more than a circle (Fig. 4.3). King et al. measured cadaveric radial heads and found that the main difference between the maximum and minimum outer diameters (i.e., long axis vs. short axis) was 2 mm, ranging from 0 to 3 mm [16]. In other words, the radial head is not generally round, but it can be for those at one end of the spectrum.

The portion of the radial head that articulates with the capitellum is referred to as the "articular dish" (Fig. 4.3). The articular dish is generally round and symmetrical, but offset anterolaterally along the long axis of the radial head when the forearm is positioned in neutral rotation. This results in a cam effect such that the articular dish moves laterally and medially on the capitellum during forearm rotation [14]. The articular dish has an average depth of 2.3–2.4 mm, depending on the diameter of the head [16, 17]. The depth of a radial head prosthesis is a very important parameter, as it affects radiocapitellar contact area and peak stresses [20]. The depth of the prosthetic articular dish should probably be within 0.5 mm of that of the native radial head.

The radial head is also tilted (angulated) with respect to the neck of the radius. This is to accommodate a change in alignment of the long axis of the radius that occurs during the forearm rotation. As the distal radius crosses over the ulna at the wrist during pronation, the valgus alignment of

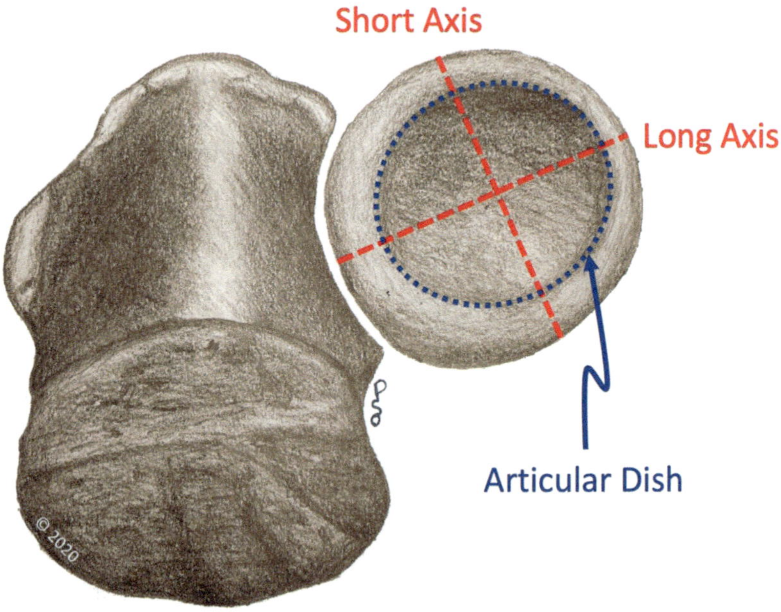


**Fig. 4.3** The native radial head is oval, with maximum and minimum outer diameters (i.e., long axis vs. short axis) that differ by about 2 mm. (By permission of Pierre S. O'Driscoll. All rights reserved)

the radius with respect to the humerus decreases. In other words, the radius does not rotate about its online access, but rather about a long axis that passes through the radial head proximally and the ulna distally. The resulting crossover type of motion creates a windshield wiper motion of the radial head on the capitellum.

To this point we have focused on geometric parameters describing the overall shape of the radial head (Fig. 4.4). There are several more aspects that relate to the surface contours specifically that are relevant to prosthetic design. We already described the fact that the articular dish is offset anterolaterally along the long axis of the radial head. A close look at the surface of the radial head will reveal two things about the rim, which forms the transition from the articular dish to the side of the radial head. First, it is broad posteromedially and narrow anterolaterally. The broad crescent-shaped rim posteromedially has a variable radius of curvature that articulates with the lateral trochlear ridge of the humerus and is an important load-bearing structure. In fact, load bearing in this region functions much like a "truss effect," the way a roof truss bears the load of a roof (Fig. 4.5). Radial head prostheses vary greatly in the extent to which they mimic this aspect of the articulation (Fig. 4.6) [14].

The second feature of the rim of the radial head to notice is that it is not generally in a single plane but undulates up and down (Fig. 4.7). These undulations are not symmetrical. This is quite noticeable during elbow arthroscopy while observing the rim calculating against the capitellum during pronation/supination. Although the functional importance of this feature has not yet been clarified, it likely confers some degree of optimization of either radiocapitellar contact or radiocapitellar stability, or a combination of the two.

## Position and Orientation of the Radial Head in 3-D Space

The radial head is offset from the axis of the intramedullary cavity of the radial neck as well as from the axis of rotation of the forearm such that there is a cam effect during rotation of the radial head. The radial head is also tilted (angulated) with respect to the neck of the radius. Replicating the position and orientation of the native radial head with a prosthetic radial head requires precisely defining the intramedullary axis of the neck (or proximal shaft in the case of a long-stem prosthesis) and the orientation and position of the head with respect to that axis. That could be done mechanically as illustrated

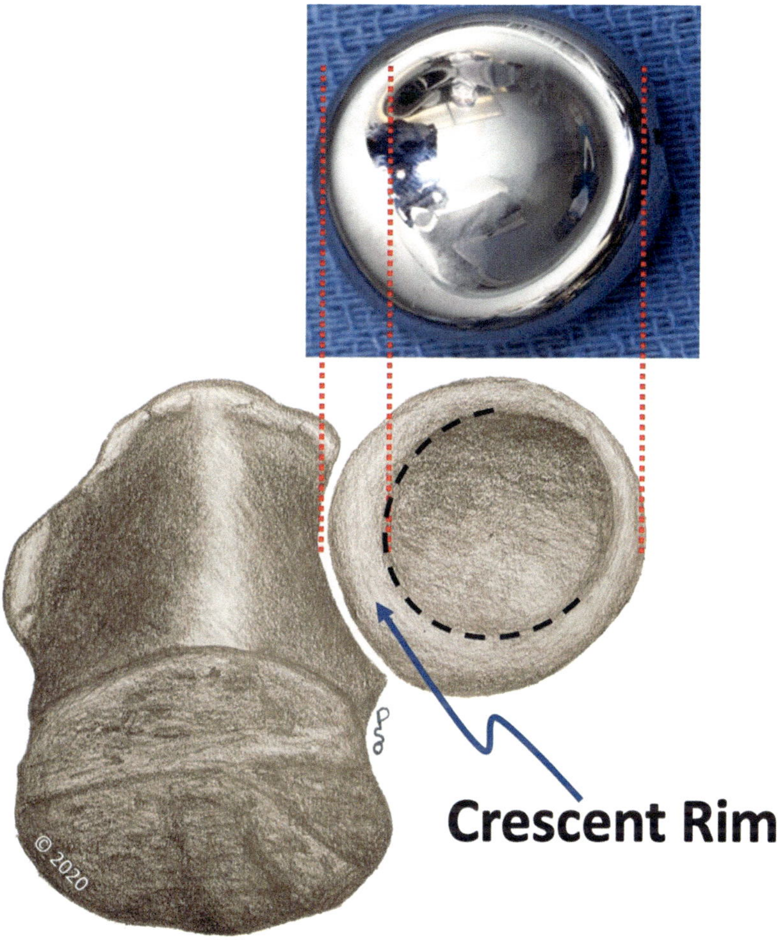


**Fig. 4.4** The articular dish is offset anterolaterally along the long axis of the radial head. The broad crescent-shaped rim posteromedially has a variable radius of curvature that articulates with the lateral trochlear ridge of the humerus and is an important load-bearing structure. (By permission of Pierre S. O'Driscoll. All rights reserved)

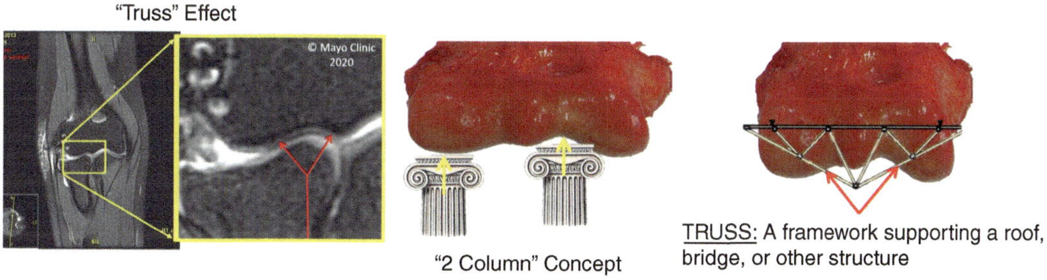


**Fig. 4.5** The load bearing in the broad crescent-shaped rim of the posteromedial radial head that articulates with the lateral trochlear ridge has a "truss" effect in the way it bears load – the way a roof truss bears the load of a roof. (By permission of Mayo Foundation for Medical Education and Research (https://www.mayoclinic.org/copyright). All rights reserved)

in Fig. 4.8, in which the intramedullary canal was reamed to determine its central axis. The angle between that intramedullary rod and a rigid plexiglass sheet fitted onto the rim of the head can be used to determine the head/neck angle. A long-stem prosthesis going into the radial shaft is more complex to design. For determining the spatial relationship between the

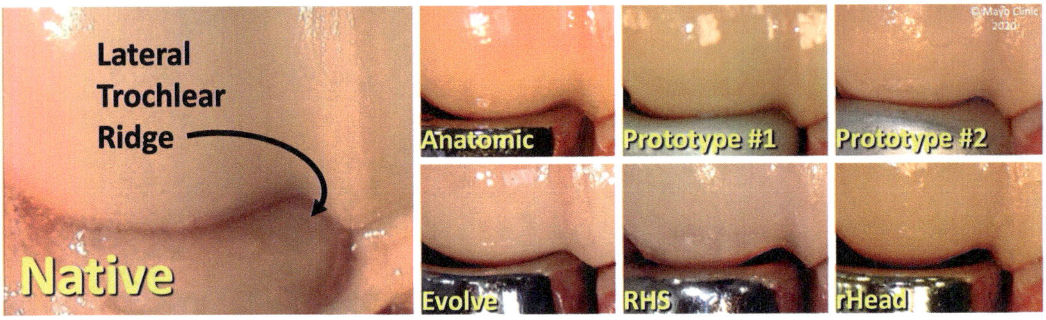


**Fig. 4.6** Radial head prostheses vary greatly in the extent to which they mimic the crescent rim that articulates with the lateral trochlear ridge (LTR). (By permission of Mayo Foundation for Medical Education and Research (https://www.mayoclinic.org/copyright). All rights reserved)

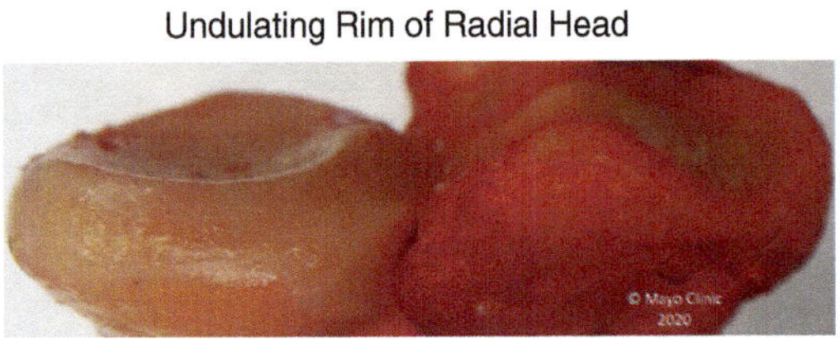


**Fig. 4.7** The rim of the radial head goes up and down, not lying in a single plane. (By permission of Mayo Foundation for Medical Education and Research (https://www.mayoclinic.org/copyright). All rights reserved)

head and intramedullary axis of the shaft of the radius, the engineering concept of a free body diagram is a valuable tool.

Getting the position and orientation of the head in 3-D space correct is important because incorrect placement will cause edge loading and therefore increased stress on the capitellar articular cartilage and subchondral bone. Additionally, increased or abnormal translational movement of the prosthesis across the capitellum will exacerbate any such wear.

## The Material

A discussion of the prosthetic material is included in the section related to the design of the head itself, although it is relevant to the stem as well. Various materials that have been employed in commercially available radial head prosthesis can be grouped according to whether they are nonmetallic or metallic. Nonmetallic materials have included silastic (silicone), PMMA (polymethyl methacrylate), and pyrocarbon. Metallic processes have been made of titanium, stainless steel, cobalt-chrome, or combination of titanium and cobalt-chrome.

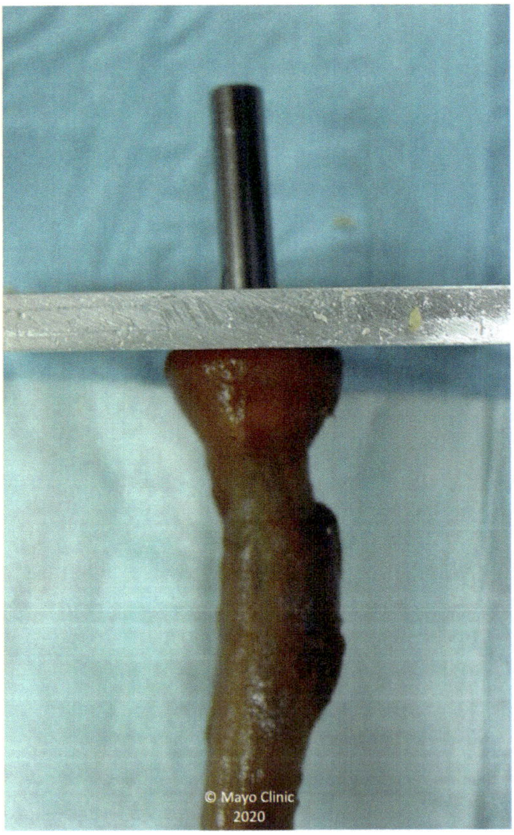


**Fig. 4.8** The radial head/neck junction is angulated in two planes. (By permission of Mayo Foundation for Medical Education and Research (https://www.mayoclinic.org/copyright). All rights reserved)

Silastic has fallen out of favor because of the potential for erosive destructive silicone synovitis that can occur over 2–3 decades as the soft silicone material breaks down and causes an inflammatory reaction in the synovium. PMMA use is not FDA approved for this use in the USA but has limited use in Europe. Pyrocarbon has lower hardness and stiffness compared to metal, which might confer a theoretical benefit with respect to decreasing cartilage wear on the distal humerus. That said, pyrocarbon is still orders of magnitude stiffer than native articular cartilage; any potential advantage of pyrocarbon over metal would almost certainly be less than the deleterious effects of poor radiocapitellar contact due to the shape or the orientation/position of the radial head. Marked increases in contact stresses that are known to be dangerous to articular cartilage and capable of eroding the subchondral bone can be expected with certain deviations from anatomic shape or orientation/position of the radial head.

Metallic radial heads currently in use generally have a cobalt-chrome head component. Solid titanium has been used in the past, but it has generally been realized that titanium is not a good bearing surface due to the possibility of developing titanium particulate debris and the associated osteolysis and soft tissue reaction.

## The Stem

The three main features related to the stem are:

- Fixed vs. loose-fitting (and cemented vs. uncemented if fixed)
- Length
- Shape

### Fixed Versus Loose-Fitting

Stems are either fixed or loose-fitting. Fixed stems can be either cemented or press-fitted for bone ingrowth. Fixed stems for bone ingrowth are made of titanium and have a porous surface that is plasma sprayed or grit-blasted, although other options may become available in the future such as coating with titanium beads, hydroxyapatite, or porous metal such as tantalum. Stems designed for cemented use are not porous coated although some surgeons prefer to cement noncemented stem designs, hoping to diminish problems of loosening.

Loose-fitting stems are generally undersized, with the hope that leaving a little bit of mobility of the stem inside the canal might compensate for any incorrect articulation of the head against the capitellum [21]. Loose-fitting stems are smooth, are polished, and made from cobalt-chrome or stainless steel, to diminish the shedding of metal particles that can cause metallosis and osteolysis. They should not be made from titanium, as titanium particles cause more biologic reaction than cobalt-chrome or stainless steel.

Each of these design concepts has advantages and disadvantages. Porous-coated stems that achieve bone ingrowth will likely remain stable over decades. However, failure of bone ingrowth with loosening and osteolysis is being reported much more commonly than I have experienced, and it is a very real clinical concern. The reasons for this are not yet completely clear. One factor is that bone ingrowth requires a very tight initial press fit with less than 100–200 microns of micromotion, which means that the radial canal must be carefully prepared and the prosthesis hammered into the bone [22]. Surgeons have concern about fracturing the radius, especially if the neck is comminuted, and therefore may be hesitant to insert a big enough stem. Fortunately, single, non-propagating hoop-stress fractures do not affect press-fit stability of porous titanium stems [23]. Nevertheless, fear of fracturing the radial neck does lead some surgeons to choose a suboptimal stem diameter, which may lead to loosening, pain, and osteolysis from titanium debris. Pain in the proximal radial forearm is pathognomonic for a loose prosthetic radial stem (Fig. 4.9).

To prevent loosening, some choose to cement the stem. If ingrowth does occur, stress shielding commonly occurs. Bone loss from stress shielding can be distinguished from that due to loosening, since stress shielding causes periosteal bone loss whereas loosening causes endosteal bone loss as seen in Fig. 4.10 [24]. One potential option to diminish stress shielding is to limit the porous texture to the proximal portion of the

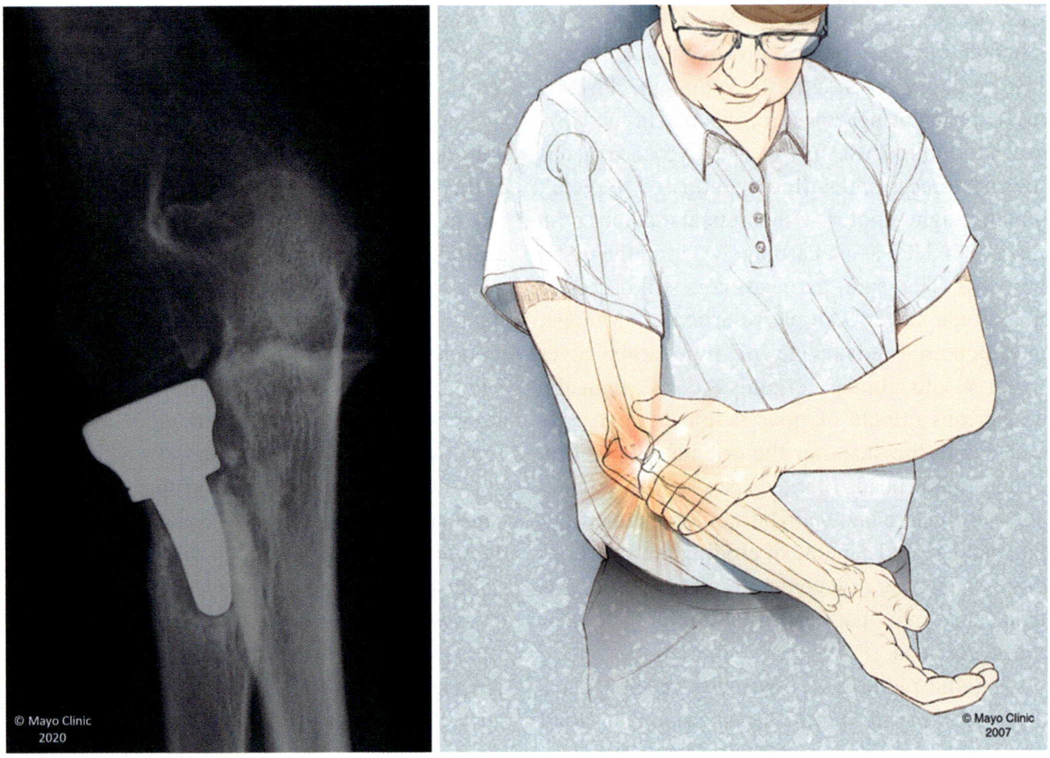


**Fig. 4.9** Pain in the proximal radial forearm is pathognomonic for a loose prosthetic radial stem. (By permission of Mayo Foundation for Medical Education and Research (https://www.mayoclinic.org/copyright). All rights reserved)

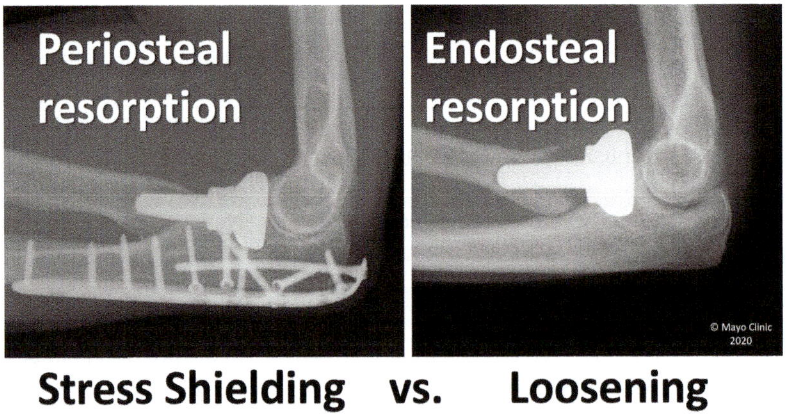


**Fig. 4.10** Bone loss from stress shielding causes periosteal bone loss, whereas loosening causes endosteal bone loss. (By permission of Mayo Foundation for Medical Education and Research (https://www.mayoclinic.org/copyright). All rights reserved)

stem. Doing so with grit-blasted stems does not seem to affect initial micromotion of the stem [25]. Future efforts to reduce stress shielding might focus on reducing the stiffness of the implant stem.

Ingrowth titanium stems are available in plasma spray and grit-blasted configurations. It would seem intuitive that a plasma spray surface would have a greater initial press-fit stability than a grit-blasted stem, but one biomechanical study showed no difference in micromotion between the two stem designs [26]. Whether or not there is a clinical difference in successful bone ingrowth is not known. However, removal of a well-fixed

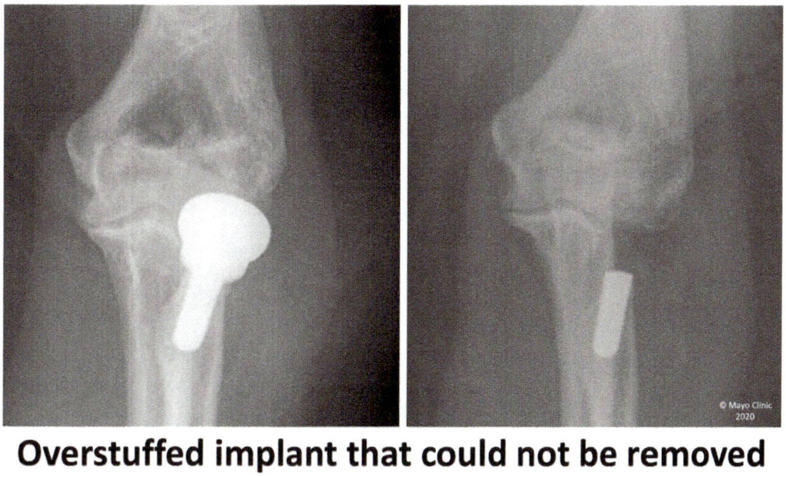


**Fig. 4.11** Removal of an ingrown plasma spray stem is difficult and sometimes impossible. In such circumstances, the stem may need to cut with a carbide burr. (By permission of Mayo Foundation for Medical Education and Research (https://www.mayoclinic.org/copyright). All rights reserved)

plasma spray stem is exceedingly difficult and sometimes impossible (Fig. 4.11), whereas ingrowth grit-blasted stems seem to be able to be hammered out of the bone with less difficulty.

Cemented long stems have been reported to have little tendency to loosen, but data for cemented short stems remains limited [27]. The main disadvantage of cemented stems is the possible need to remove the cement in the case of infection or malpositioning. This is very difficult in the proximal radius. Another concern is the potential for osteolysis if the stem loosens.

Loose-fitting stems have the advantage of simplicity of insertion and a theoretical capacity to accommodate for small imperfections in alignment (or shape) of the radial head with respect to the capitellum. The latter has not been proven. However, they have the disadvantage that the stem remains loose and may not be capable of providing the same load transfer to the capitellum as a well-fixed stem. Loose-fitting designs originated as temporary "spacers" implanted into unstable fracture dislocations of the elbow with the intention of removing them once soft tissue (and any other bony) healing had occurred [28, 29]. Due to the fact that removal of the spacer required subluxating the elbow, some surgeons stopped removing them, as they appeared to be well tolerated if left in place [28]. The loose fit is associated with a frequent occurrence of mild (sometimes moderate) proximal radial forearm pain ranging from 1 to 5/10, although removal is not often required. In fact, removal of press-fitted porous stems is reported more commonly than removal of loose-fitting smooth stems, since loose titanium ingrowth stems seem more likely to cause pain and osteolysis. Radiographic follow-up typically reveals endosteal lucencies and tilting of the stem (Fig. 4.12) [30–32].

Whether or not one stem interface with the bone will turn out to be superior to the others is not yet known. Stem fixation of prostheses in other joints has evolved toward a preference for non-cemented porous ingrowth stems. Loose-fitting stems in the hip, shoulder, and knee have essentially disappeared from clinical use.

## Stem Length

Stems can be separated into short and long, depending on whether or not the tip of the stem extends distally past the bicipital tuberosity into the shaft of the radius (Fig. 4.13). The reason that this distinction is so important is that the axis of the intramedullary canal of the radial neck does not line up with that of the shaft. Some prosthetic designs have an intermediate stem length. The problem with an intermediate stem length is that the long axis of the stem may not line up with either the intramedullary canal of the neck or the shaft, depending on how long the proximal radius is. Initial stability of a porous-coated, cementless titanium stem is related to the length of the stem

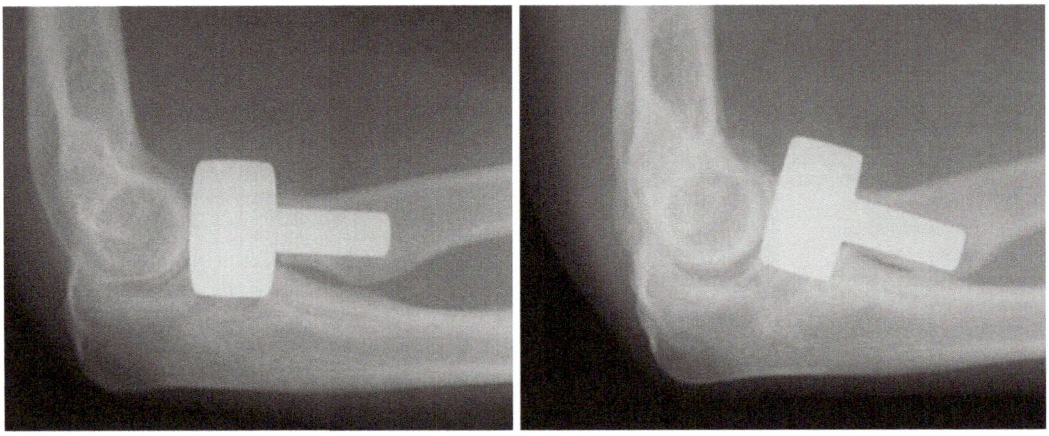

**Fig. 4.12** Radiographic lucencies are common with loose-fitting stems, which sometimes tilt in the canal. (Reprinted from O'Driscoll and Herald [45], Copyright 2011, with permission from Elsevier)

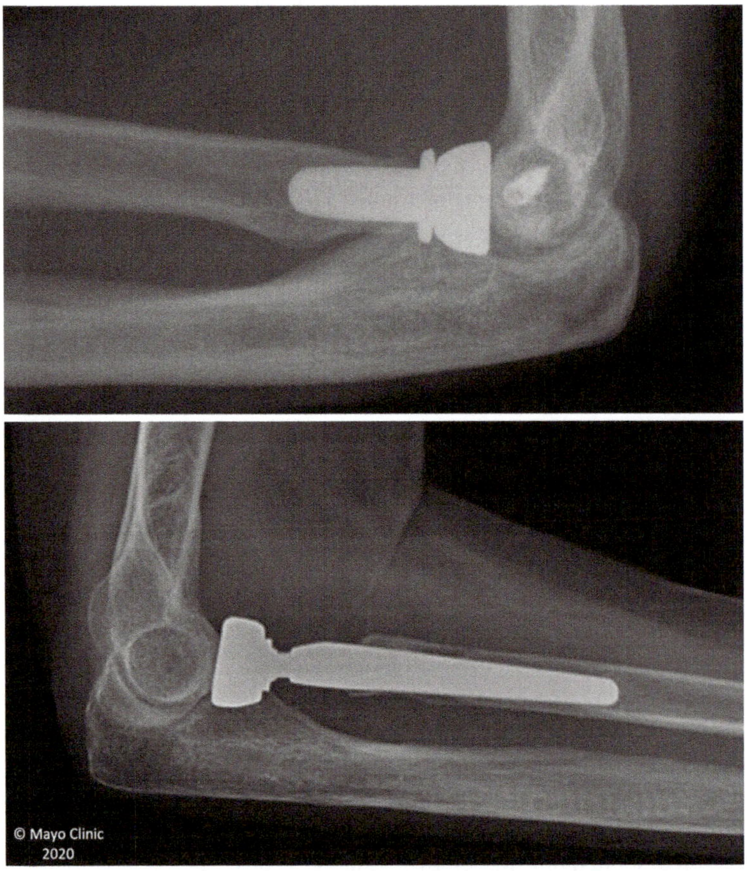


**Fig. 4.13** Stems can be short (top) or long (middle), depending on whether or not the tip of the stem extends distally past the bicipital tuberosity into the shaft of the radius. (By permission of Mayo Foundation for Medical Education and Research (https://www.mayoclinic.org/copyright). All rights reserved)

within the bone and the level of the cut (amount of radial neck resected) [33]. The cantilever quotient, defined as the ratio of combined head and neck length to total implant length, must be 0.4 or greater to ensure secure fixation (Fig. 4.14) [34]. As a generality, if the combined head and neck length is 15 mm or less, a short-stem design is appropriate. If the combined head and neck length is 18 mm or more, a long-stem design should be used.

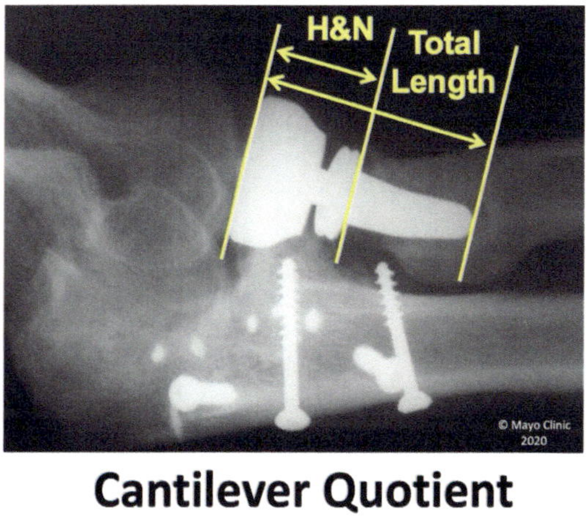


**Fig. 4.14** Stability, and therefore the likelihood of bone ingrowth, of a cementless stem is inversely related to cantilever quotient, defined as the ratio of combined head and neck length (*H&N*) to total implant length (*total length*). (By permission of Mayo Foundation for Medical Education and Research (https://www.mayoclinic.org/copyright). All rights reserved)

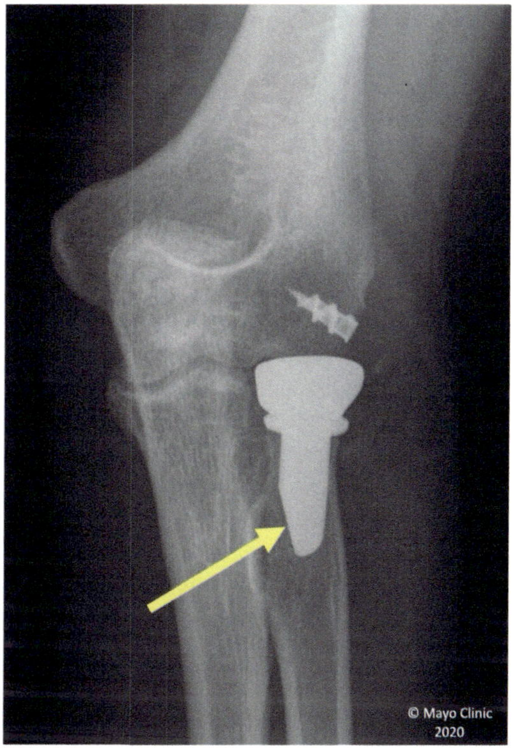


**Fig. 4.15** Example of a stem with a beveled tip (arrow), which has two theoretical benefits. (By permission of Mayo Foundation for Medical Education and Research (https://www.mayoclinic.org/copyright). All rights reserved)

## Stem Shape

As has been found with prosthetic stems in other joints, straight stems are preferable over curved stems. One of the problems with curved stems is that the preparation of the canal must perfectly match the shape and placement of the final component or there will be loosening. High loosening rates preceded withdrawal from the market of a radial head prosthesis which had a curved stem that also was relatively short (high cantilever quotient). No data yet exist to recommend whether the stem should be cylindrical or tapered. The exception would be a long-stem component going down into the shaft, because the intramedullary cavity of the proximal radius has a definite taper to it. Some stems have a bevel near the tip, which has two theoretical benefits (Fig. 4.15). One is that if the stem goes down past the bicipital tuberosity, the bevel might prevent bottoming out on the cortex distal to the tuberosity and fracturing the proximal radius. However, that does not seem to be a clinical problem reported with any stem design. The second theoretical advantage has to do with ease of insertion, but this is not a true advantage because once the non-beveled portion of the stem engages the intramedullary canal of the radial neck, it is mandatory that the stem be lined up with the long axis of the canal. It is not the first half of the stem that is difficult to insert correctly, but the final half of the stem, because it is during that phase when the head must clear the capitellum (assuming the head had been coupled onto the stem prior to insertion). By that point, it's no longer an option to have the stem angulated in the canal. Some designs try to get around this problem by having an in situ mechanism for coupling the head onto the stem, but each of these has its own potential problems as discussed below. Finally, the presence of a bevel might actually have some potential to compromise stem stability and therefore bone ingrowth. This is due to the fact that the broaches and reamers used to prepare the canal do not have a bevel, and therefore they leave a void between a portion of the stem and the bone.

## The Head-Stem Connection

Three aspects of the head-stem connection merit consideration:

1. Monopolar vs. bipolar
2. Coupling mechanism
3. Angle(s) and offset(s)

### Monopolar Versus Bipolar Connection

Bipolar connections have the theoretical advantage of compensating for any inaccuracies in alignment of the articulating head with the capitellum [35]. However, there are also some disadvantages. The primary disadvantage of a bipolar design is that any translation of the radial head with respect to the capitellum under axial load causes the bipolar component to tilt. As a result, the contribution of concavity compression to radiocapitellar stability is lost when the bipolar head tilts (Fig. 4.16) [36]. This also creates a tendency for the radial head to translate posteriorly with respect to the capitellum and therefore subluxate (Fig. 4.17). This can actually cause chronic attenuation of the lateral collateral ligament complex with tardy posterolateral rotatory instability (PLRI).

A bipolar radial head design has a UHMWPE bearing surface between the head and the stem and therefore has a potential for polyethylene particulate debris which can lead to osteolysis. Since radial head prostheses are generally implanted for trauma and post-traumatic conditions, rather than degenerative or inflammatory arthritis, the patients are often relatively young and high demand. Therefore, a radial head prosthesis should ideally have many decades of longevity. This is a concern for a polyethylene bearing surface.

Additionally, bipolar heads can partially or completely disengage. The mechanism for this disassembly is a force couple caused by an edge-loading compressive force on one side of the bipolar radial head and a distraction force on the other side caused by scar tissue surrounding the bipolar radial head. Complete dissociation requires reoperation. Partial disengagement can occur due to deformation or wear of the polyethylene. When this happens, the repeated partial coupling/uncoupling tends to cause further polyethylene wear and reactive synovitis (Fig. 4.18).

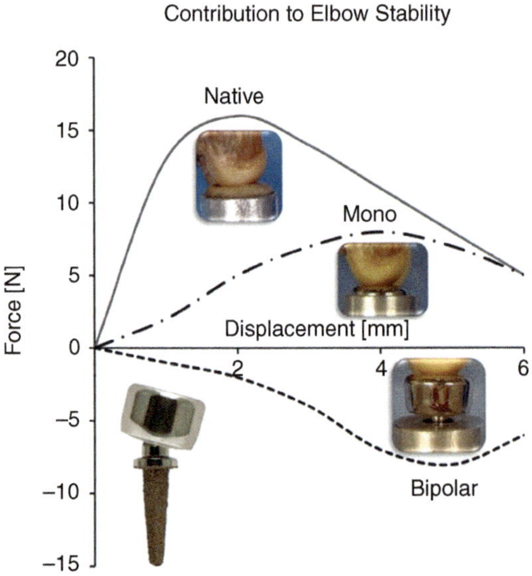


**Fig. 4.16** A bipolar radial head will tilt when subluxated, which diminishes the force resisting subluxation. If this same bipolar radial head is made to behave like a monoblock (Mono) prosthesis by locking it into place with a washer so it can no longer tilt, it is then able to resist subluxation in a manner similar to the native radial head. (By permission of Mayo Foundation for Medical Education and Research (https://www.mayoclinic.org/copyright). All rights reserved)

### Head-Stem Coupling Mechanism

The traditional Morse taper has functioned well in radial head arthroplasty, although it typically requires that the head and neck be coupled prior to insertion. This is not a problem in the acutely unstable elbow, which can be subluxated to get a straight shot down the canal and readily deliver the prosthesis over the capitellum. However, if the elbow is not unstable, or if the radial head prosthesis is being used for reconstruction in the post-traumatic setting, the lateral collateral ligament may need to be released in order to subluxate the elbow and insert the prosthesis. In situ couplers have been developed to secure the Morse taper, but these have proven bulky and difficult to use.

For this reason, a number of designs have attempted to permit coupling of the prosthesis in situ, typically with a slide on mechanism. The concept is valid, but two potential problems can occur (Figs. 4.19, 4.20, and 4.21). First, a coupling mechanism can come apart and dissociation can occur, requiring revision. Second, the

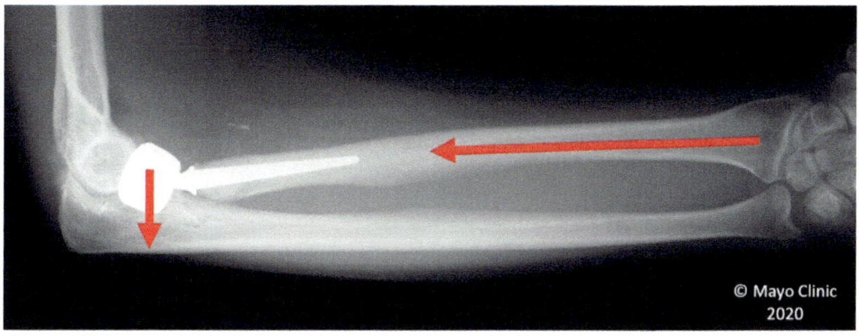


**Fig. 4.17** Bipolar radial heads have a tendency for the radial head to translate posteriorly with respect to the capitellum and therefore subluxate. This can actually cause chronic attenuation of the lateral collateral ligament complex with tardy posterolateral rotatory instability (PLRI). (By permission of Mayo Foundation for Medical Education and Research (https://www.mayoclinic.org/copyright). All rights reserved)

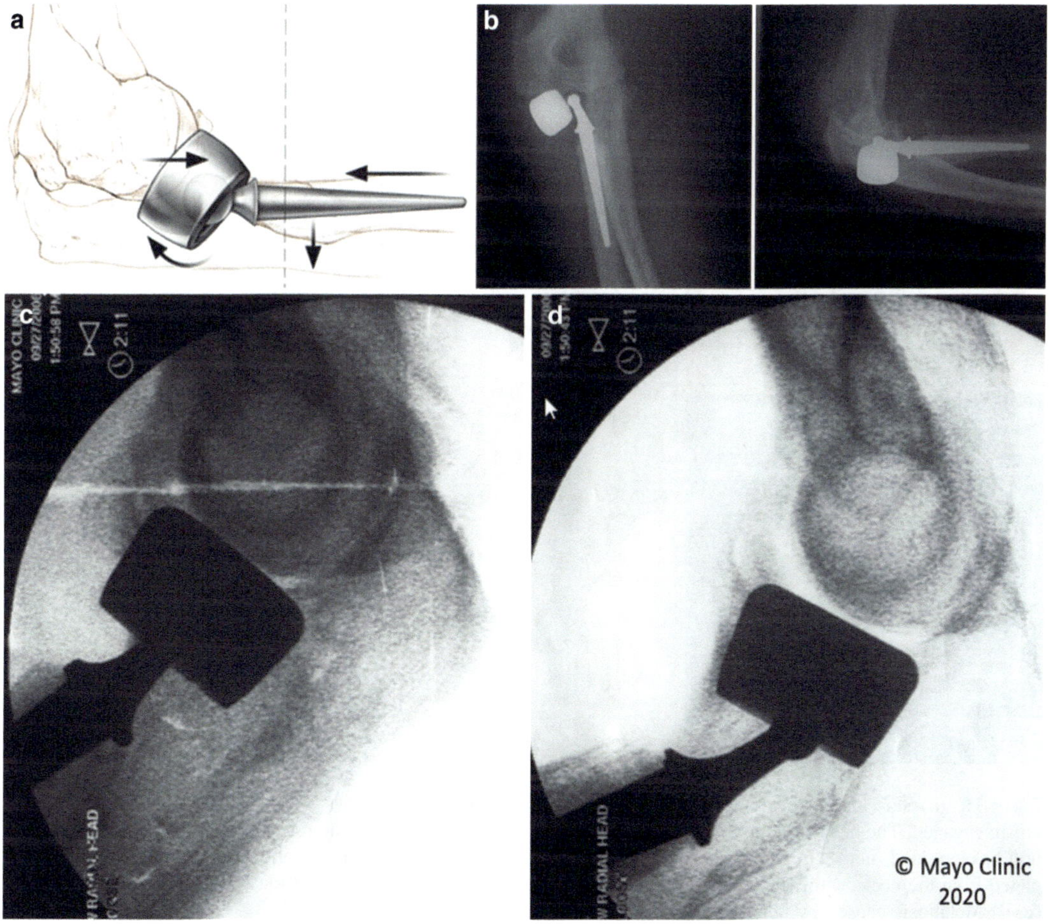


**Fig. 4.18** Bipolar heads can partially or completely disengage. The mechanism for this disassembly is a force couple caused by an edge-loading compressive force on one side of the bipolar radial head and a distraction force on the other side caused by scar tissue surrounding the bipolar radial head (**a**). Complete dissociation requires reoperation (**b**). Partial disengagement can occur due to deformation or wear of the polyethylene (**c**, **d**). When this happens, the repeated partial coupling/uncoupling tends to cause further polyethylene wear and reactive synovitis. (By permission of Mayo Foundation for Medical Education and Research (https://www.mayoclinic.org/copyright). All rights reserved)

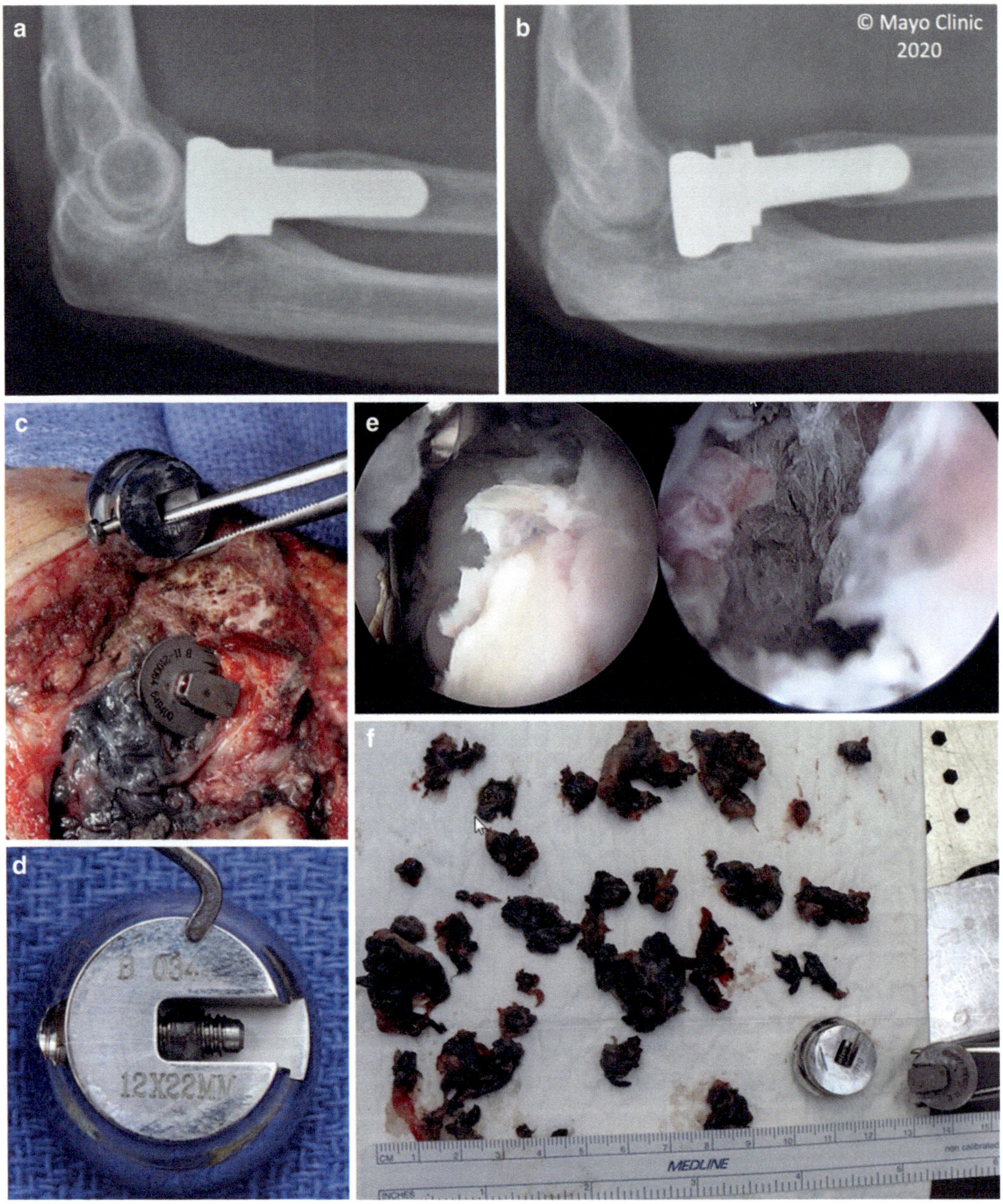


**Fig. 4.19** (**a**) Side-loading head with bolt locking mechanism engaged. The head lines up with the neck. (**b**) The bolt has loosened (not seen) and the head partially disengaged from the neck, with which it is no longer aligned. (**c**, **d**) Metallosis caused by abrasion of the head on the stem, as evidenced by worn laser markings. (**e**) Arthroscopic views showing titanium synovitis. (**f**) Metallosis due to the release of metal particles. (By permission of Mayo Foundation for Medical Education and Research (https://www.mayoclinic.org/copyright). All rights reserved)

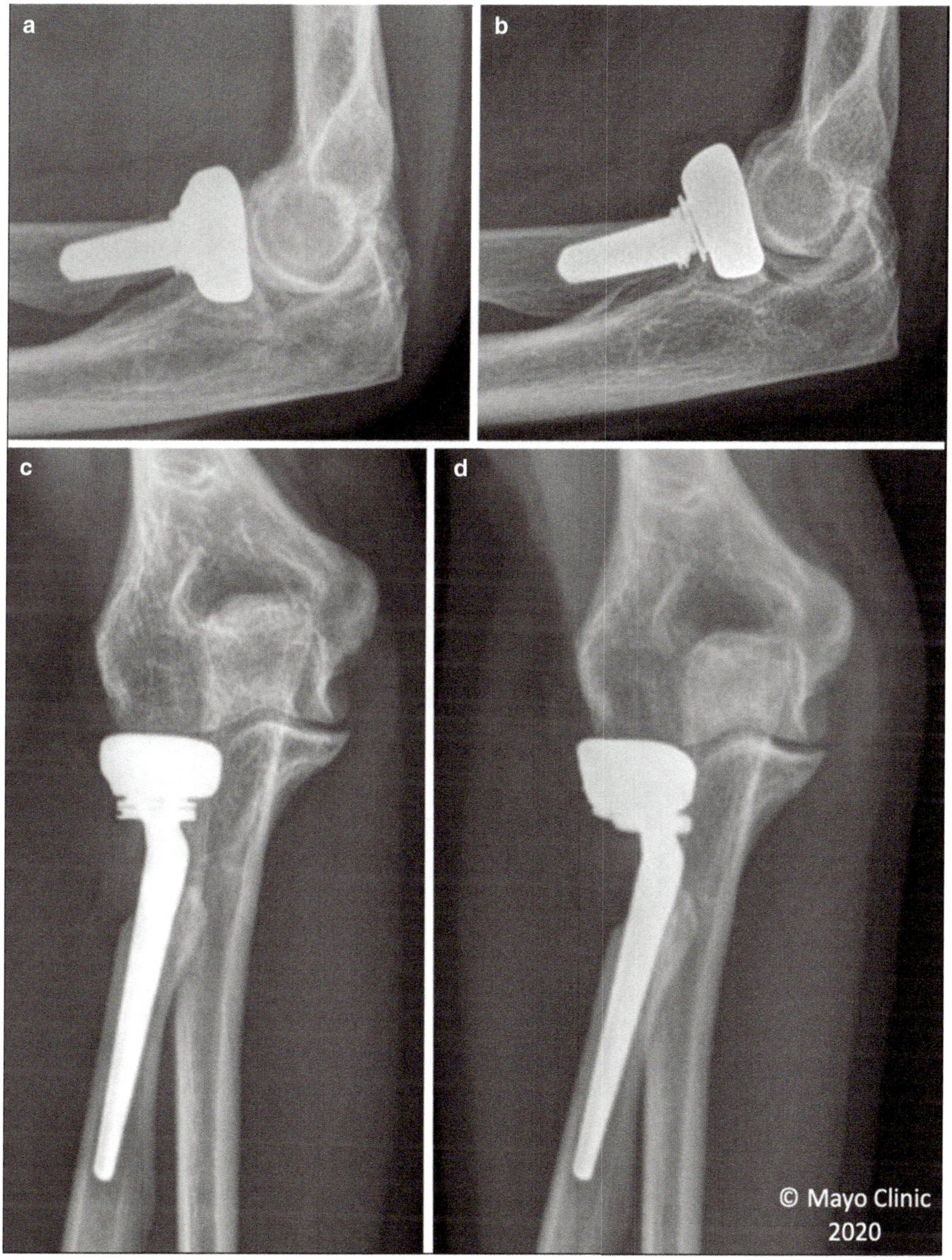


**Fig. 4.20** Examples of disengagement of a three-part Slide-Loc torsional locking mechanism. (**a** and **c**) Short and long stems assembled in situ. (**b** and **d**) The same prostheses disengaged, as evidenced by tilting (**b**) or translation (**d**) of the head/neck on the stem. (By permission of Mayo Foundation for Medical Education and Research (https://www.mayoclinic.org/copyright). All rights reserved)

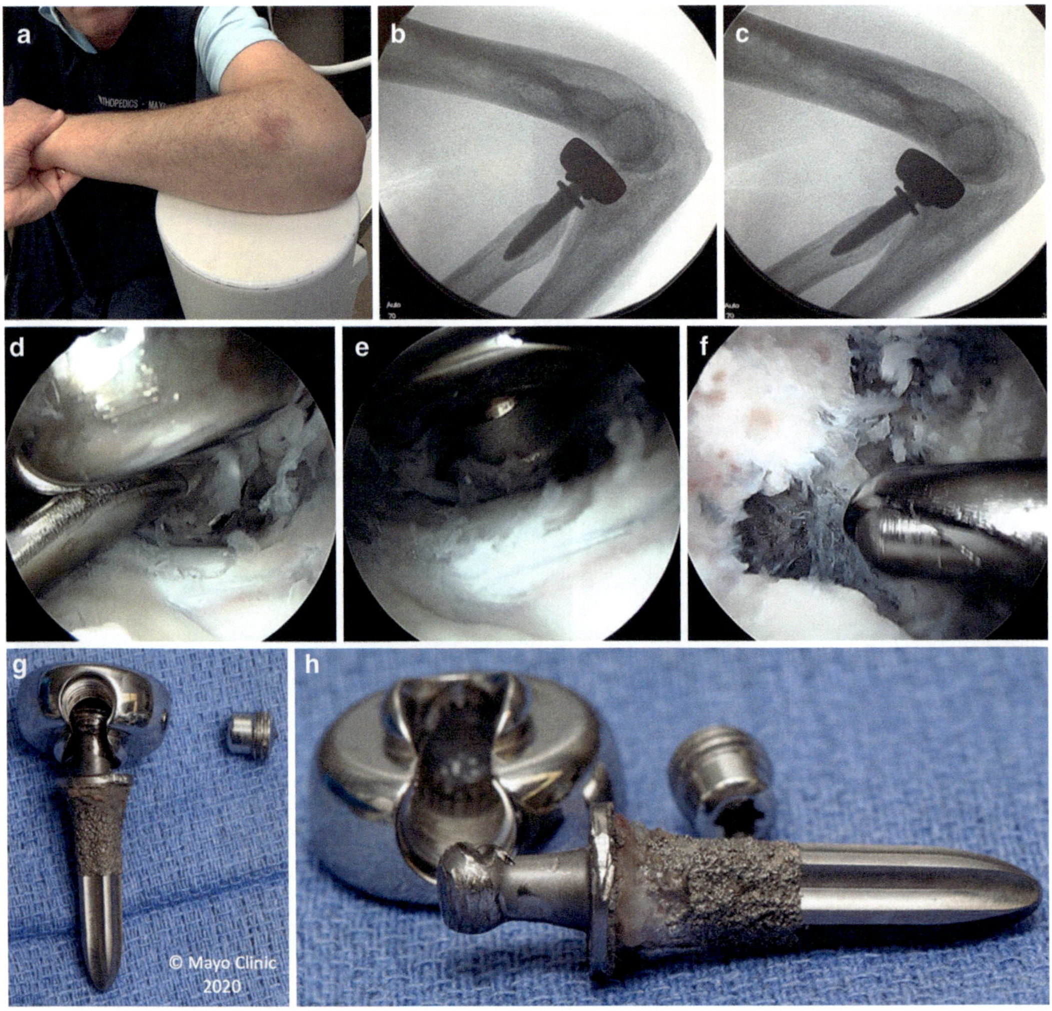


**Fig. 4.21** Example of disengagement of an adjustable angle locking mechanism using a bolt. (**a**) Positioning the elbow for comparison lateral X-rays in flexion and hyperflexion. (**b**) Lateral view in flexion. (**c**) Hyperflexion causes the head to tilt on the neck, indicating that the locking mechanism is no longer working, but causing metal-on-metal abrasion. (**d** and **e**) Arthroscopic reviews of the head/neck junction showing that it can be tilted. (**f**) Arthroscopic view showing synovitis. (**g** and **h**) Excoriations at the head/neck junction due to failed locking mechanism, explaining the surrounding titanium synovitis. (By permission of Mayo Foundation for Medical Education and Research (https://www.mayoclinic.org/copyright). All rights reserved)

locking mechanism can loosen and permit subclinical micromotion without apparent dissociation. This occurs regardless of whether the head is locked in place with a locking bolt or with a rotational torque. Micromotion at the head-stem interface causes abrasion and the release of metal particles that can lead to metallosis, synovitis, and osteolysis. It is not known at this point whether or not the types of problems that are seen with "trunnionosis" in the hip will be seen with these coupling mechanisms.

## Angle(s) and Offset(s)

The native radial head is angled in two planes with respect to the intramedullary canal of the radial neck. At the bicipital tuberosity, the intramedullary canal takes another change in direction such that there is angulation between the

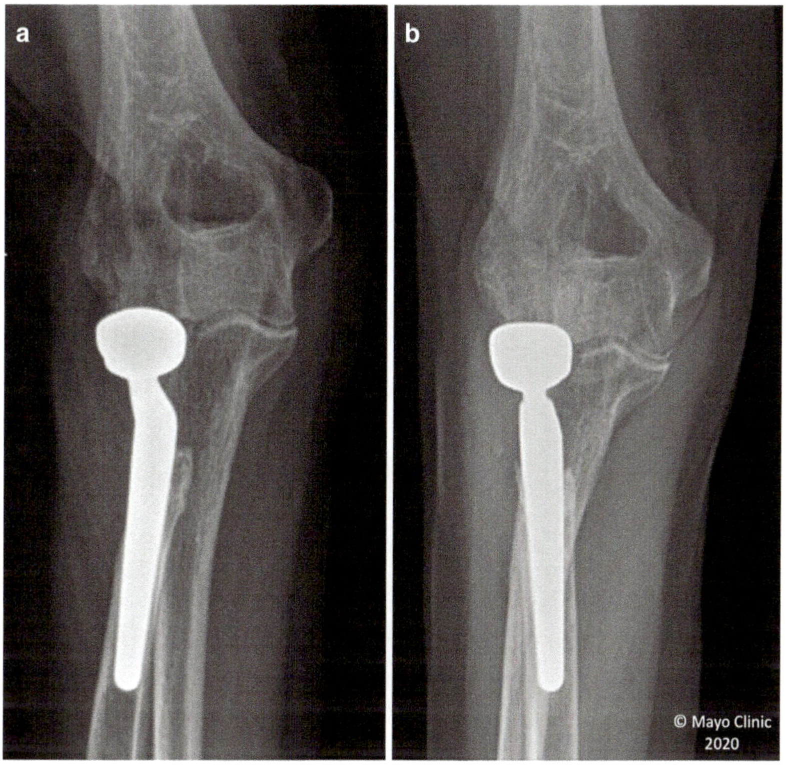


**Fig. 4.22** Long-stem prostheses need to take into consideration the angle between the neck and the proximal radial shaft (**a**). By mimicking the complex bi-planer, angulated anatomy of the radial head and proximal radius, adequately designed long-stem prosthesis can permit the biceps tendon and its insertion on the bicipital tuberosity to clear the ulna during pronation and supination (**b**). (By permission of Mayo Foundation for Medical Education and Research (https://www.mayoclinic.org/copyright). All rights reserved)

intramedullary axis of the radial neck and of the proximal radial shaft. This complex anatomy permits the biceps tendon and its insertion on the bicipital tuberosity to clear the ulna during pronation and supination (Fig. 4.22). In addition to the normal radial bow, this complex arrangement of head/neck and neck/shaft angles makes it possible for the radius to cross over the ulna during pronation. Standard stem length radial head prostheses need to take into consideration the angulation between the head and the neck. Long-stem prostheses also need to take into consideration the angle between the neck and the proximal radial shaft.

## Instruments and Technique

As with any prosthetic replacement, reliable precise instruments and reproducible technique are essential. Some aspects of the technique are more critical than others, but four key elements of radial head replacement merit discussion:

- Height (length)
- Stem diameter
- Head diameter
- Head rotation (for anatomic designs) and tilt

### Height (Combined Head and Neck Length)

Getting the height correct is one of the two most important technical variables [37–41]. Overstuffing is the term that has generally been used to mean lengthening of the radius by inserting a combined head and neck length that exceeds the bone and cartilage resected. Lengthening the radius by more than 2 mm causes increased radiocapitellar contact pressures resulting in cartilage necrosis and subchondral bone erosion (Fig. 4.23).

Instruments and a method for measuring the correct height of the radial head and neck are essential (Fig. 4.24). This is best done using a set of feeler gauges and an adjustable height gauge.

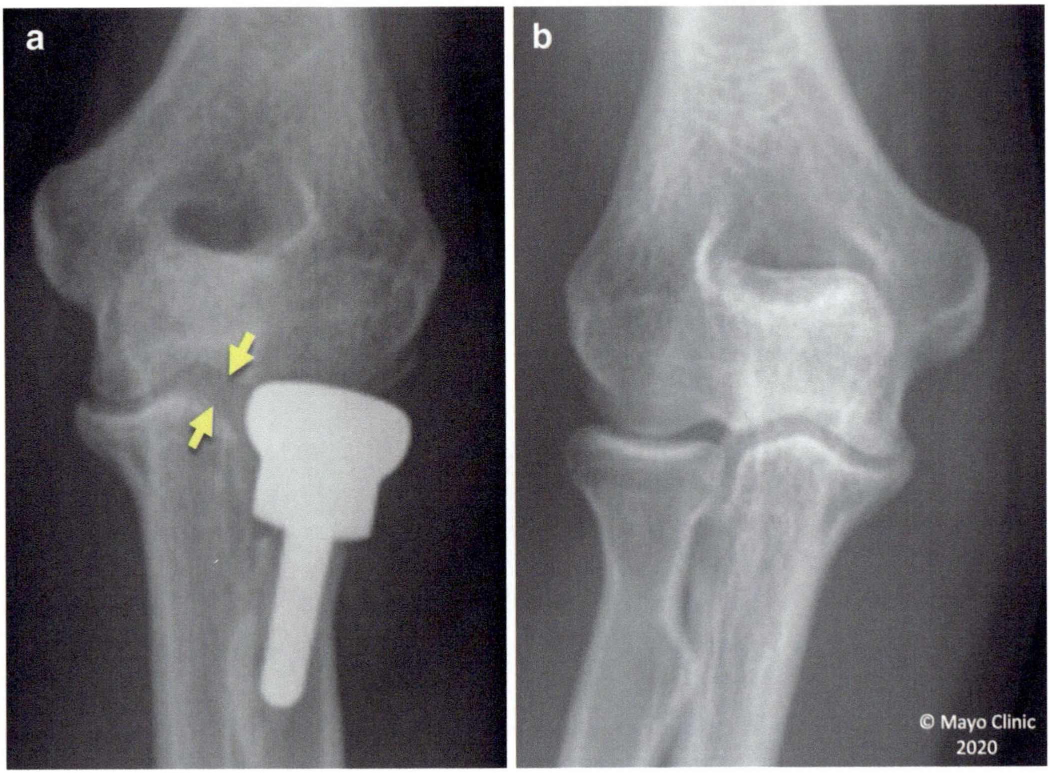


**Fig. 4.23** Lengthening the radius by more than 2 mm (overstuffing) causes increased radiocapitellar contact pressures resulting in cartilage necrosis and subchondral bone erosion. These radiographs show an increased ulnohumeral gapping (**a, arrows**) as compared to the contralateral elbow due to the radius being overlengthened/overstuffed (**b**). (By permission of Mayo Foundation for Medical Education and Research (https://www.mayoclinic.org/copyright). All rights reserved)

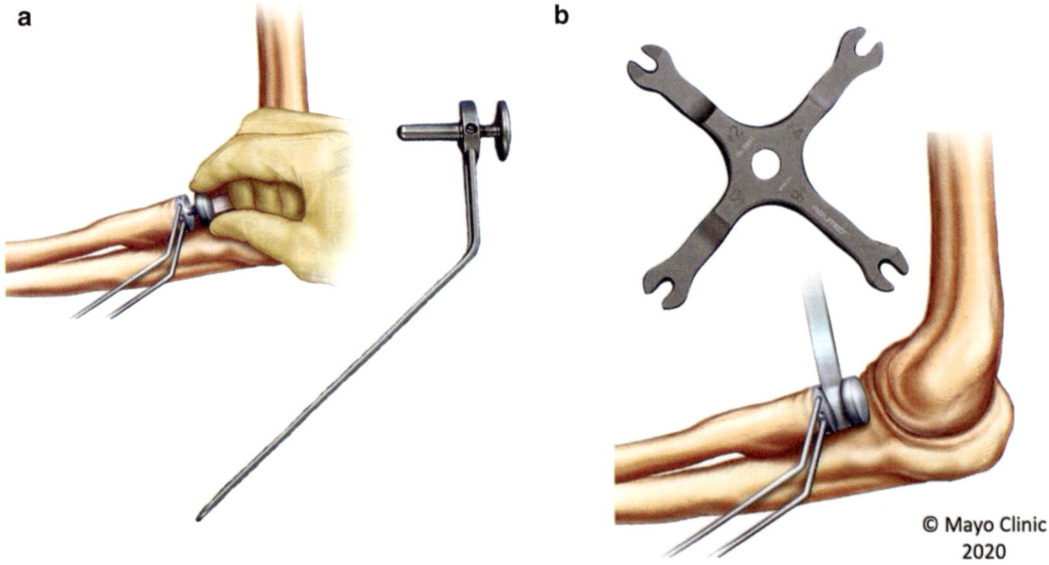


**Fig. 4.24** Instruments are required for measuring the correct height of the radial head and neck. Example of feeler gauges (**a**) and an adjustable height gauge (**b**). (By permission of Mayo Foundation for Medical Education and Research (https://www.mayoclinic.org/copyright). All rights reserved)

A critically important step in measuring height is to ensure that the ulnohumeral joint is reduced while performing the measurement. This can be done by placing the elbow at 90 degrees and applying a firm compressive force on the olecranon in line with the long axis of the humerus.

## Stem Diameter

Getting the stem direct diameter correct is essential to prevent loosening of a porous ingrowth stem. Some systems have broaches that are hammered in and others have reamers that are twisted. When using broaches, a "rule of thumb" is that if you can push it in with your thumb during surgery, you'll be able to pull it out with your finger and thumb at the time of revision. In other words it will not have adequate initial press-fit stability to permit bone ingrowth. Broaches and the final stem must be hammered into the canal to ensure reliable ingrowth [23].

## Head Diameter

The native radial head is asymmetrical and oval shaped, with a long axis that is generally about 2 mm longer than a short axis. Most systems rely on templating the excised radial head in a series of wells to determine head diameter. The excised head must fill the well tightly. If the well is bigger than the head, the prosthetic head will be bigger than the excised native head. If this happens, the next smaller size should be chosen. With some radial head systems, downsizing the implant by 2 mm further improves radiocapitellar contact [42–44]. A circular radial head should be sized according to the short axis, whereas an anatomic radial head should be sized according to the long axis.

## Head Rotation (For Anatomic Design) and Tilt

There is currently only one anatomic radial head implant design on the market. Head rotation is determined by lining up the laser marking on the head with a cautery mark on the lateral side of the radial neck placed at the midpoint of the neck with the forearm in neutral rotation. This also lines up with the Lister's tubercle at the wrist. No special instruments are needed.

The tilt is predetermined in all but one prosthesis on the market currently. That particular implant design requires the head to be locked onto the stem at the chosen tilt angle determined by the surgeon intraoperatively. There are no specific instruments provided to accomplish this.

## Summary and Future Considerations

The function and structure of the radial head is a much more complex than may be generally recognized. Prosthetic replacement design is still in the early stages and more scientific research is needed. As with replacement of other joints, the multiplicity of designs will likely diminish over time as clinical experience and scientific research shed light on which design features are the most important and successful. It is highly probable that certain features will have less tolerance for error than others. For example, a 3 mm (lengthening) error in radial height is almost certainly worse than a 3 mm error in rotational positioning of an asymmetric anatomic radial head. The former will have a deleterious effect on radiocapitellar contact pressures and lead to cartilage loss, whereas the latter represents a 15° malrotation, which studies in our laboratory show as well tolerated. The key priorities currently requiring attention include symptomatic loosening and osteolysis around ingrowth stems, cartilage and bone erosion due to nonanatomic radial head shapes on press-fitted stems, failure of head-stem coupling mechanisms, and the question of whether or not a loose-fitting stem in the canal truly functions as a prosthetic replacement and provides functional benefit over radial head excision in the long term.

**Acknowledgments** Pierre O'Driscoll created the anatomic illustration.

## References

1. Stormont TJ, An K-N, Morrey BF, Chao EY-S. Elbow joint contact study. Comparison of techniques. J Biomech. 1985;18:329–36.
2. Morrey BF, An K-N, Tanaka S. Valgus stability of the elbow. A definition of primary and secondary constraints. Clin Orthop. 1991;265:187–95.
3. Pomianowski S, Morrey BF, Neale PG, Park MJ, O'Driscoll SW, An KN. Contribution of monoblock and bipolar radial head prostheses to valgus stability of the elbow. J Bone Joint Surg Am. 2001;83-A(12):1829–34.
4. Hwang JT, Kim Y, Bachman DR, Shields MN, Berglund LJ, Fitzsimmons AT, et al. Axial load transmission through the elbow during forearm rotation. J Shoulder Elb Surg. 2018 Dec 28;27(3):530–7.
5. Hwang JT, Kim Y, Shields MN, Bachman DR, Berglund LJ, Fitzsimmons AT, et al. Effects of axial forearm instability on force transmission across the elbow. J Shoulder Elb Surg. 2019 Jan;28(1):170–7.
6. Jensen SL, Olsen BS, Sojbjerg JO. Elbow joint kinematics after excision of the radial head. J Shoulder Elb Surg. 1999;8(3):238–41.
7. Beingessner DM, Dunning CE, Gordon KD, Johnson JA, King GJ. The effect of radial head excision and arthroplasty on elbow kinematics and stability. J Bone Joint Surg Am. 2004 Aug;86-A(8):1730–9.
8. Antuna SA, Sanchez-Marquez JM, Barco R. Long-term results of radial head resection following isolated radial head fractures in patients younger than forty years old. J Bone Joint Surg Am. 2010 Mar;92(3):558–66.
9. Hall JA, McKee MD. Posterolateral rotatory instability of the elbow following radial head resection. J Bone Joint Surg Am. 2005 Jul;87(7):1571–9.
10. Schiffern A, Bettwieser SP, Porucznik CA, Crim JR, Tashjian RZ. Proximal radial drift following radial head resection. J Shoulder Elb Surg. 2011 Apr;20(3):426–33.
11. Morrey BF, Chao EY-S, Hui FC. Biomechanical study of the elbow following excision of the radial head. J Bone Joint Surg. 1979;61-A:63–8.
12. Ikeda M, Oka Y. Function after early radial head resection for fracture: a retrospective evaluation of 15 patients followed for 3-18 years. Acta Orthop Scand. 2000 Apr;71(2):191–4.
13. Herbertsson P, Josefsson PO, Hasserius R, Besjakov J, Nyqvist F, Karlsson MK. Fractures of the radial head and neck treated with radial head excision. J Bone Joint Surg Am. 2004 Sep;86-A(9):1925–30.
14. Bachman DR, Thaveepunsan S, Park S, Fitzsimmons JS, An KN, O'Driscoll SW. The effect of prosthetic radial head geometry on the distribution and magnitude of radiocapitellar joint contact pressures. J Hand Surg Am. 2015 Feb;40(2):281–8.
15. Johnson JA, Beingessner DM, Gordon KD, Dunning CE, Stacpoole RA, King GJ. Kinematics and stability of the fractured and implant-reconstructed radial head. J Shoulder Elbow Surg. 2005;14(1 Suppl S):195S–201S.
16. King GJ, Zarzour ZD, Patterson SD, Johnson JA. An anthropometric study of the radial head: implications in the design of a prosthesis. J Arthroplast. 2001;16(1):112–6.
17. van Riet RP, Van Glabbeek F, Neale PG, Bortier H, An KN, O'Driscoll SW. The noncircular shape of the radial head. J Hand Surg [Am]. 2003 Nov;28(6):972–8.
18. Swieszkowski W, Skalski K, Pomianowski S, Kedzior K. The anatomic features of the radial head and their implication for prosthesis design. Clin Biomech (Bristol, Avon). 2001;16(10):880–7.
19. Itamura J, Roidis N, Mirzayan R, Vaishnav S, Learch T, Shean C. Radial head fractures: MRI evaluation of associated injuries. J Shoulder Elb Surg. 2005 Jul-Aug;14(4):421–4.
20. Irish SE, Langohr GD, Willing R, King GJ, Johnson JA. Implications of radial head hemiarthroplasty dish depth on radiocapitellar contact mechanics. J Hand Surg Am. 2015 Apr;40(4):723–9.
21. Szmit J, King GJW, Johnson JA, Langohr GDG. The effect of stem fit on the radiocapitellar contact mechanics of a metallic axisymmetric radial head hemiarthroplasty: is loose fit better than rigidly fixed? J Shoulder Elb Surg. 2019 Dec;28(12):2394–9.
22. Moon JG, Berglund LJ, Domire Z, An KN, O'Driscoll SW. Stem diameter and micromotion of press fit radial head prosthesis: a biomechanical study. J Shoulder Elb Surg. 2009 Sep-Oct;18(5):785–90.
23. Chanlalit C, Shukla DR, Fitzsimmons JS, An KN, O'Driscoll SW. Effect of hoop-stress fracture on micromotion of textured ingrowth stems for radial head replacement. J Shoulder Elb Surg. 2011 Aug 9;21(7):949–54.
24. Chanlalit C, Shukla DR, Fitzsimmons JS, An KN, O'Driscoll SW. Stress shielding around radial head prostheses. J Hand Surg Am. 2012 Oct;37(10):2118–25.
25. Chanlalit C, Fitzsimmons JS, Moon JG, Berglund LJ, An KN, O'Driscoll SW. Radial head prosthesis micromotion characteristics: partial versus fully grit-blasted stems. J Shoulder Elb Surg. 2011 Oct 6;20(1):27–32.
26. Chanlalit C, Fitzsimmons JS, Shukla DR, An KN, O'Driscoll SW. Micromotion of plasma spray versus grit-blasted radial head prosthetic stem surfaces. J Shoulder Elb Surg. 2010 Feb 14;20(5):717–22.
27. Songy CE, Kennon JC, Barlow JD, Sanchez-Sotello J, O'Driscoll SW, Morrey ME. Radial head replacement for acute radial head fractures: outcome and survival of three implant designs with and without cement fixation. J Orthop Trauma. 2020;In Press.
28. Harrington IJ, Tountas AA. Replacement of the radial head in the treatment of unstable elbow fractures. Injury. 1981;12:405–12.
29. Knight DJ, Rymaszewski LA, Amis AA, Miller JH. Primary replacement of the fractured radial head with a metal prosthesis. J Bone Joint Surg. 1993;75-B:572–6.

30. Fehringer EV, Burns EM, Knierim A, Sun J, Apker KA, Berg RE. Radiolucencies surrounding a smooth-stemmed radial head component may not correlate with forearm pain or poor elbow function. J Shoulder Elb Surg. 2009 Mar-Apr;18(2):275–8.
31. Doornberg JN, Parisien R, van Duijn PJ, Ring D. Radial head arthroplasty with a modular metal spacer to treat acute traumatic elbow instability. J Bone Joint Surg Am. 2007 May;89(5):1075–80.
32. Shore BJ, Mozzon JB, MacDermid JC, Faber KJ, King GJ. Chronic posttraumatic elbow disorders treated with metallic radial head arthroplasty. J Bone Joint Surg Am. 2008 Feb;90(2):271–80.
33. Moon JG, Shukla DR, Fitzsimmons JS, An KN, O'Driscoll SW. Stem Length and Neck Resection on Fixation Strength of Press-Fit Radial Head Prosthesis: An In Vitro Model. J Hand Surg Am. 2019 Dec;44(12):1098 e1–8.
34. Shukla DR, Fitzsimmons JS, An KN, O'Driscoll SW. Effect of stem length on prosthetic radial head micromotion. J Shoulder Elb Surg. 2012;21(11):1559–64.
35. Judet T. Garreau de Loubresse C, Piriou P, Charnley G. a floating prosthesis for radial-head fractures. J Bone Joint Surg Br. 1996 Mar;78(2):244–9.
36. Moon JG, Berglund LJ, Zachary D, An KN, O'Driscoll SW. Radiocapitellar joint stability with bipolar versus monopolar radial head prostheses. J Shoulder Elb Surg. 2009 Sep-Oct;18(5):779–84.
37. Athwal GS, Rouleau DM, MacDermid JC, King GJ. Contralateral elbow radiographs can reliably diagnose radial head implant overlengthening. J Bone Joint Surg Am. 2011 Jul 20;93(14):1339–46.
38. Moon JG, Southgate RD, Fitzsimmons JS, O'Driscoll SW. Simple overlay device for determining radial head and neck height. Skelet Radiol. 2010 Mar 1;39(9):915–20.
39. Shukla DR, Vanhees MKD, Fitzsimmons JS, An KN, O'Driscoll SW. Validation of a Simple Overlay Device to Assess Radial Head Implant Length. J Hand Surg Am. 2018 Dec;43(12):1135 e1–8.
40. Ramazanian T, Müller-Lebschi JA, Yao Chuang M, Vaichinger AM, Fitzsimmons JS, O'Driscoll SW. Effect of incremental increase in radial neck height on coronoid and capitellar contact pressures. Shoulder & Elbow. 2019; In Press.
41. Berkmortel CJ, Gladwell MS, Ng J, Ferreira LM, Athwal GS, Johnson JA, et al. Effect of radial neck length on joint loading. J Shoulder Elb Arthroplasty. 2019;3
42. Bachman DR, Park SE, Thaveepunsan S, Fitzsimmons JS, An KN, O'Driscoll SW. Joint contact changes with under-sized prosthetic radial heads. J Orthop Trauma. 2018 Jul 30;32(11):e440–e4.
43. Lanting BA, Ferreira LM, Johnson JA, King GJ, Athwal GS. Radial head implant diameter: A biomechanical assessment of the forgotten dimension. Clin Biomech (Bristol, Avon). 2015;30(5):444–7.
44. Liew VS, Cooper IC, Ferreira LM, Johnson JA, King GJ. The effect of metallic radial head arthroplasty on radiocapitellar joint contact area. Clin Biomech (Bristol, Avon). 2003;18(2):115–8.
45. O'Driscoll SW, Herald JA. Forearm pain associated with loose radial head prostheses. J Shoulder Elbow Surg. 2011;21:92–7.

# Primary Radial Head Arthroplasty

5

Douglas W. Bartels, Julie Adams, and Scott P. Steinmann

## Introduction

Radial head arthroplasty has become a reliable treatment option for acute radial head fractures. There has also been expanded use in the setting of radial head malunion and nonunion, elbow instability, and arthritic conditions. Radial head fractures are relatively common with a reported incidence of 55 per 100,000 people in one population-based study [1], and they have been found to represent up to 33% of all fractures of the elbow [2]. A bimodal age distribution, mechanism of injury type, and sex distribution are present, with a subset of younger, typically male patients with high-energy trauma as well as a subset of older, typically female patients with low-energy trauma, often due to a fall from a ground level height [1]. With simple falls, the radial head is most often fractured with the arm in a pronated and partially flexed position which causes the radial head to transmit the force of the fall to the capitellum [3].

The most commonly utilized system for classification of radial head fractures was originally described by Mason [4] with a subsequent modification made by Johnston [5]. More recently, Hotchkiss [6] added a quantifiable value to the degree of displacement used to determine classification of radial head fracture. Mason type I injuries are nondisplaced or minimally displaced (<2 mm) injuries to the radial head or neck with no mechanical block to motion; type II injuries are fractures displaced greater than 2 mm without comminution; type III injuries are comminuted and displaced injuries; and type IV injuries are radial head fractures in the setting of concomitant ulnohumeral dislocation [Fig. 5.1] [3, 7]. Further modification of the Mason classification system was made by van Riet and Morrey [8] to quantify associated lesions about the elbow such as medial ligament injury, lateral ligament injury, and associated fractures to the humerus and ulna.

A number of treatment options exist based on the fracture classification and associated bony and soft tissue injuries. Simple, nondisplaced injuries can often be managed nonoperatively with a short period of immobilization for comfort, typically in a sling, followed by progressive

D. W. Bartels
Department of Orthopedic Surgery, Mayo Clinic, Rochester, MN, USA
e-mail: bartels.douglas@mayo.edu

J. Adams
Department of Orthopaedic Surgery, University of Tennessee College of Medicine – Chattanooga, Erlanger Orthopaedic Institute, Chattanooga, TN, USA

S. P. Steinmann (✉)
Department of Orthopaedic Surgery, University of Tennessee College of Medicine – Chattanooga, Erlanger Orthopaedic Institute, Chattanooga, TN, USA

Mayo Clinic, Rochester, MN, USA
e-mail: steinmann.scott@mayo.edu; scott.steinmann@erlanger.org


G. J. W. King, M. Rizzo (eds.), *Arthroplasty of the Upper Extremity*,
https://doi.org/10.1007/978-3-030-68880-6_5

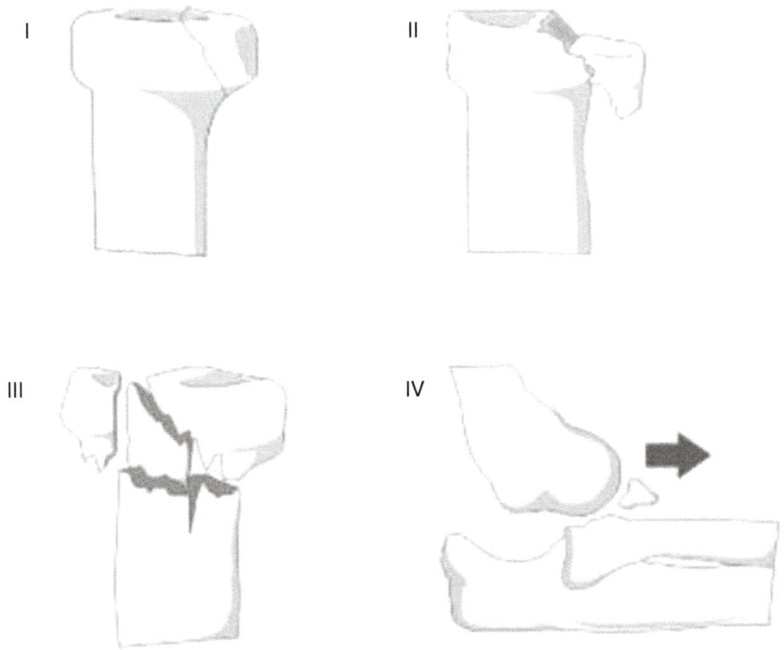


**Fig. 5.1** Mason-Johnston classification of radial head fractures. Type I, nondisplaced or minimally displaced; type II, displaced and angulated; type III, comminuted and displaced; and type IV, concomitant ulnohumeral dislocation. Originally published in Pires et al. [7]. (This is an open-access article distributed under the terms of the Creative Commons CC BY license, which permits unrestricted use, distribution, and reproduction in any medium, provided the original work is properly cited)

elbow range of motion. The examiner should assure that the elbow is not hindered by a bony block to motion, and the patient is encouraged to engage in early active motion, as the biggest risk of this injury is stiffness. Management of more complex fractures is highly variable, and options may include nonoperative care, fragment excision or radial head excision, open reduction internal fixation, and radial head arthroplasty. Radial head arthroplasty has become a reliable option for management of non-reconstructable fractures, nonunions, malunions, and, in some cases, primary radiocapitellar arthritis. Recent improvements in our understanding of the nature of these injuries, appropriate technical considerations, and treatment of associated injuries, as well as in some cases implant improvements, have advanced use of this procedure and made it a reliable and commonly used procedure.

## Anatomy and Biomechanics

The radial head is an eccentric concave structure that articulates with the convex capitellum. The outer portion of the radial head articulates with the lesser sigmoid notch of the ulna, and this portion is identified by thick articular cartilage. The radial head is elliptical rather than truly circular. Functionally, the elliptical nature of the radial head acts to produce a cam effect which translates the radial shaft radially during pronation [9]. The radial head is angled from the radial shaft on average 16.8°, but this is highly variable ranging from 6° to 28° [10].

Biomechanically, the radial head plays a role in load transmission, as well stability both of the elbow and axial stability of the forearm.

It has been shown that up to 60% of the load experienced by the forearm is transferred to the humerus through the radiocapitellar joint [11]. The elliptical nature of the radial head also plays a role in how load is experienced by the proximal radius. Load transmission is highly variable, based on position of the elbow in flexion versus extension, position of pronation and supination, and whether the elbow experiences a varus or valgus stress. Studies have shown that there is as much as a 10% decrease in load transmission through the radiocapitellar joint with a varus stress [12, 13]. While load transmission through the radiocapitellar joint decreases with varus stress, distraction forces with the elbow in varus are common [14]. This is important to consider in the post-operative setting.

A number of factors play an important role in maintaining appropriate elbow stability including the radiocapitellar and ulnohumeral articulations, their surrounding ligamentous structures, the coronoid, and the interosseous membrane [Fig. 5.2] [15]. The role of the anterior band of the medial collateral ligament as a primary stabilizer of the elbow to valgus stress is well documented [16, 17] with the radial head functioning as a secondary stabilizer. Both ligamentous and proximal radial structural integrity (either with native radial head or radial head arthroplasty) are necessary to confer elbow stability against valgus stress at time zero. This has been demonstrated in a number of studies that showed that radial head arthroplasty eliminated valgus instability in the ligamentously intact elbow; however, radial head arthroplasty could not fully eliminate valgus instability when the medial collateral ligament was compromised [18–21]. Coronoid fractures have also been found to play a role in valgus stability given that the anterior band of the medial collateral ligament inserts on the sublime tubercle at the base of the coronoid.

Posterolateral stability of the elbow is complex and relies on the integrity of both ligamentous and osseous structures to ensure proper stability. The primary stabilizer against posterolateral elbow instability has been shown to be the lateral ulnar collateral ligament (LUCL) [22, 23]. As with valgus stability of the elbow, the radial head plays a significant role as a secondary stabilizer against posterolateral instability at the elbow. The so-called "terrible triad" injury of the elbow consisting of elbow dislocation, radial head fracture, and coronoid fracture has significant implications on the posterolateral rotatory stability of the elbow. Not only does elbow dislocation often frequently result in disruption of the LUCL, but coronoid fracture leads to further instability. This is well demonstrated by the fact that both radial head arthroplasty and coronoid fracture fixation (in fractures of at least 50% of the coronoid) were necessary to fully restore elbow stability [24].

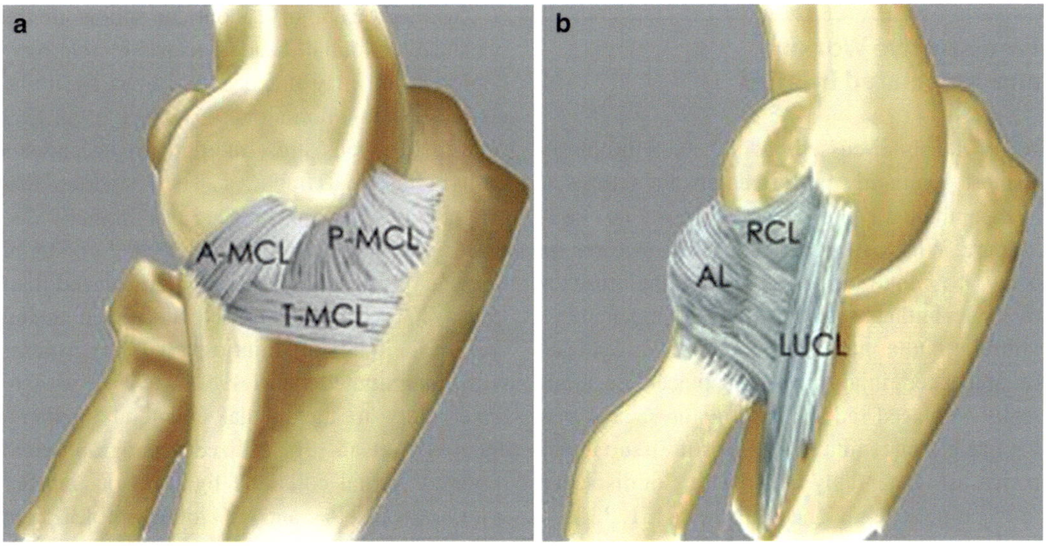


**Fig. 5.2** Illustrative representation of the medial (**a**) and lateral (**b**) ligamentous complexes of the elbow. A-MCL anterior band of the medial collateral ligament, P-MCL posterior band of the medial collateral ligament, T-MCL transverse band of the medial collateral ligament, AL annular ligament, RCL radial collateral ligament, LUCL lateral ulnar collateral ligament. Originally published in Acosta Batlle et al. [15]. (This is an open-access article distributed under the terms of the Creative Commons CC BY license, which permits unrestricted use, distribution, and reproduction in any medium, provided the original work is properly cited)

Finally, axial forearm stability is important to consider when discussing the status of the radial head and radial head arthroplasty. The radial head is crucially important to maintaining axial stability of the radius. Radial head fracture, especially severely comminuted fractures, has been shown to significantly affect axial radial stability [25]. Several studies have demonstrated the importance of additional structures in the forearm and wrist in maintaining axial radial stability, especially the interosseous membrane of the forearm and triangular fibrocartilage complex (TFCC) [26–28]. The interosseous membrane is a fibrous tissue complex running obliquely from the radius to the ulna which transmits forces between the radius and ulna and contributes to axial stability to the forearm [29]. The TFCC at the ulnar side of the wrist plays a significant role in maintaining not only normal wrist biomechanics but also forearm and elbow biomechanics [30].

Given the complex interplay of osseous and ligamentous structures in the elbow in conferring stability, it is important to consider the status of these structures during consideration of radial head arthroplasty.

## Preoperative Workup and Associated Injuries

As previously discussed, radial head arthroplasty is most commonly performed in the setting of a comminuted unreconstructable radial head fracture. While isolated radial head fractures do occur, it is important to be alert to the presence of concomitant fractures and/or ligamentous injuries. Studies have shown a relatively low rate of associated injury in nondisplaced or minimally displaced radial head fractures; however, the rate of concomitant bony or soft tissue injury increases substantially in the setting of displaced or comminuted radial head fractures [31, 32].

Osseous and cartilaginous injuries about the elbow are common in the setting of radial head fractures. Chondral or osteochondral injuries to the capitellum can occur in the presence of radial head fractures and may be underappreciated. One study noted that around a half of capitellar injuries were found to have associated radial head injuries, but only 2% of radial head fractures were found to have associated capitellar injury [33]. A variant of the Monteggia fracture has been identified in which a proximal ulna fracture is found to be associated with radial head fracture, rather than with just radial head dislocation alone. The presence of this injury pattern has been shown to result in poorer clinical outcomes when compared to traditional Monteggia-type injuries with radial head dislocation alone [34]. In 15% of patients with radial head fractures, a concomitant coronoid fracture has been documented [32]. Smaller coronoid fragments less commonly result in elbow instability but can be easily missed on plain radiographs. Larger fracture fragments are more easily recognized on basic imaging and clinically often result in substantial elbow instability, especially when associated with radial head fracture [35]. The rate of ulnohumeral elbow dislocation associated with radial head fracture has been reported to be between 10 and 15% [32]. Combined radial head fracture, elbow dislocation, and coronoid fracture have been term the "terrible triad" injury.

Ligamentous injury about the elbow in the presence of radial head fracture is relatively common and may not be recognized by initial clinical examination alone. Davidson et al. [31] performed valgus stress radiographs on patients with radial head fractures. They reported that no patients with nondisplaced or minimally displaced injuries had associated medial collateral ligament injuries. In patients with displaced fractures, 71% were found to have associated medial collateral ligament injuries, and in patients with comminuted injuries, 91% were found to have injury to the medial collateral ligament. Johansson et al. [36] utilized arthrography and reported medial collateral ligament or capsular injury in 4%, 21%, and 85% of Mason I, II, and III injuries, respectively. Finally, Itamura et al. [37] performed MRI on a series of 24 patients with Mason II or III fractures. They reported disruption of the medial collateral ligament in 54%, disruption of the lateral ulnar collateral ligament in 80%, disruption of both ligaments in 50%, capitellar osteochondral defects in 29%, capitellar bone bruises in 96%, and loose bodies in 92%.

The presence of a radial head fracture should prompt evaluation for concomitant ipsilateral upper limb injuries. About 6% of patients with radial head fractures were found to have concomitant ipsilateral hand or wrist fracture [32, 38]. The Essex-Lopresti injury is a radial head fracture with associated injury to the interosseous membrane of the forearm which results in longitudinal instability at the distal radioulnar joint [Fig. 5.3]. This injury pattern is often missed in the acute setting and more often presents as a chronic injury [39–41]. Regardless, missing this diagnosis can result in pain, stiffness, and weakness; thus, early recognition is of crucial importance. In addition to standard plain radiographs of the elbow, forearm, and wrist, obtaining bilateral anteroposterior grip views of both wrists in pronation in the more chronic setting has proven to be useful in comparing the degree of ulnar-positive variance which can suggest a possible disruption of the interosseous membrane [42]. Advanced imaging in the form of MRI and ultrasound has been suggested to have greater than 80% sensitivity in diagnosing interosseous membrane disruption in Essex-Lopresti injuries [43]. Intraoperatively, axial stability can be assessed by performing a "shuck" test by placing axial stress to the radius and assessing motion compared to the ulna [44] or by the radial pull test [45].

Evaluation of a radial head fracture includes plain film radiographs of the injured elbow, examination of the "joint above and joint below" including clinical palpation and history with imaging as indicated, and palpation for tenderness at the forearm, wrist, and medial

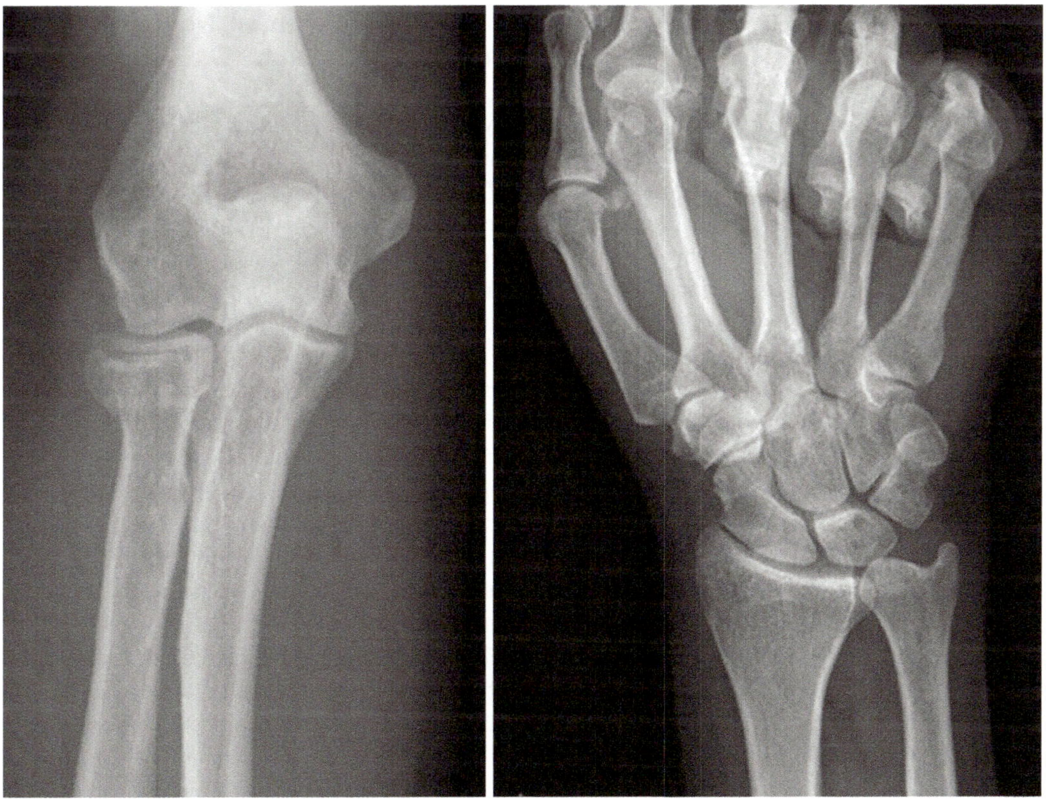

Fig. 5.3 AP elbow and wrist radiographs demonstrating a radial head fracture (left) and longitudinal instability resulting in ulnar-positive variance as seen in Essex-Lopresti injuries

and lateral elbow. Computed tomography (CT) scans may be very helpful to determine the source of bony fragments as plain film radiographs may be difficult to interpret, as well as presence or absence of associated injuries, the amount of comminution and number of fracture fragments. Three-dimensional reconstructions with joint subtraction views, may be particularly helpful.

## Indications for Radial Head Arthroplasty

### Acute Radial Head Fracture

Many radial head fractures (Mason I and many Mason II fractures) are amenable to nonoperative care. However, in the setting of some Mason II injuries, particularly those with a block to motion, open reduction internal fixation (ORIF) is generally the preferred treatment of reconstructable radial head fractures. Most Mason III fractures are best treated by radial head excision or arthroplasty. Ring et al. [46] found that all 15 patients with non-comminuted Mason-type II fractures had satisfactory results from ORIF. In contrast, 13 of 14 patients with Mason-type III comminuted fractures with more than 3 articular fragments had unsatisfactory results following ORIF. Additionally, many Mason III fractures are accompanied by concomitant injuries which may render the elbow unstable. For this reason, the preferred treatment for fractures deemed not reconstructable (i.e., more than three fragments or significant comminution) is often but not always radial head arthroplasty [47–50]. It is important to recognize patient factors will influence this as well as surgeon factors. Young active patients may have better bone quality to work with, and better healing capacity, and given the implications of a radial head arthroplasty in a young patient with a long expected lifespan, if the radial head can be repaired, this is often favored. Radial head arthroplasty is technically easier than fixation of comminuted multifragmentary fractures, so the element of surgeon skill and facility with repair plays a factor.

### Radial Head Fractures with Instability

When medial or lateral collateral ligament injury is discovered in the presence of radial head fracture, the elbow can remain unstable even in the setting of successful closed reduction of an elbow dislocation. Ashwood et al. [51] have demonstrated good outcomes in patients who underwent radial head arthroplasty for fractures not deemed reconstructable in the setting of elbow instability with ligament damage. Medial collateral ligament insufficiency and distal radioulnar joint injury have become well-recognized indications for radial head repair or arthroplasty [44]. Terrible triad injuries have proven to be a definite indication for radial head arthroplasty (when the head is not reconstructable) with lateral ulnar collateral ligament repair and with or without fixation of the coronoid [44, 49].

### Radial Head Malunion, Nonunion, or Previous Excision

Symptomatic radial head malunion and nonunion are potentially problematic complications of failed fracture fixation or failure of the nonoperatively managed fracture. Residual articular depression of 2 mm or angulation of 30° can result in a loss of up to 80% of stability at the radiocapitellar joint [52]. While published outcomes are somewhat limited, early data has demonstrated that radial head arthroplasty can be used as a salvage operation in the setting of radial head malunion or nonunion as long as the capitellum is not damaged [53]. Finally, radial head arthroplasty is an option for revision surgery in selected patients who previously underwent radial head excision and have subsequently failed due to proximal migration of the radius with distal radioulnar joint pain, pain from impingement of the radial neck on the capitellum, or valgus instability. When considering radial head arthroplasty in the setting of malunion, it is important to consider whether bony morphology of the radial neck and shaft is amenable to supporting an implant. Significant radial neck angulation and poor residual bone stock are factors to consider as they make radial head arthroplasty more technically challenging. One must also consider the status of the capitellar cartilage. In some settings the capitellar cartilage may be thinned or injured, and may not tolerate the interface of a metallic radial head on this imperfect cartilage, leading to pain.

## Essex-Lopresti Injury

Radial head replacement is often done in the setting of concern for axial instability of the forearm, or Essex-Lopresti injury. Essex-Lopresti injuries continue to be a challenge for appropriate diagnosis and treatment. In the acute setting, these are associated with an injury to the lateral side of the elbow, typically a radial head fracture, injury to the interosseous membrane of the forearm, and the TFCC. If the radial head is excised and the true extent of forearm instability is unrecognized, patients may present with ulnar impaction, forearm instability and pain, and impingement at the capitellum-radial neck junction. The management of these injuries is a subject of controversy both in the acute setting and the chronic setting. In the acute setting, typically radial head replacement is a component of the treatment; for patients identified in the chronic setting, radial head replacement may or may not be an appropriate option, as the presence of a metallic implant articulating with a worn capitellar cartilage may not restore forearm stability and may become a source of pain [54]. Current thought in the management of Essex-Lopresti injury is that concomitant TFCC and/or interosseous membrane injury should be treated with repair or reconstruction in order to restore load sharing between the radius and ulna [55].

## Contraindications for Radial Head Arthroplasty

Absolute contraindications to radial head arthroplasty are rare and include presence of active infection in the elbow. When radial head fracture is felt to be amenable to open reduction internal fixation, this treatment modality should be pursued as the first option. Capitellar arthrosis is a relative contraindication to radial head arthroplasty. As discussed previously, capitellar articular damage is common in the setting of radial head fracture [37]. Despite this, a subset of patients may have satisfactory outcomes in spite of some degree of capitellar arthrosis. Finally, alternatives to radial head arthroplasty should be considered if there is concern about the ability of the proximal radius to support an implant whether that is due to significant malalignment, surgical absence, or fracture propagation along the neck/shaft or bone resorption.

## Surgical Approaches

The patient is positioned supine on a standard operative table. A small bump can be utilized under the scapula of the operative extremity in order to more easily position the arm across the patient's chest. The operative table can be slightly tilted away from the surgeon to further assist with visualization and arm positioning. A sterile or nonsterile tourniquet is applied to the upper arm. The extremity is prepped and draped in the usual sterile fashion.

Although, in the past, a posterior incision was favored as a "utilitarian" approach, the authors favor an incision directly laterally to easily access the radial head with advantages of a smaller incision and less chance of seroma formation. If there is a need to address medial-sided pathology, a separate medial incision may easily be made [56, 57]. A laterally based incision typically runs from just proximal to the lateral epicondyle extending toward the supinator crest of the ulna. Following skin incision, full-thickness skin flaps are created [Fig. 5.4].

Access to the radial head can be achieved through either a Kocher approach between the ECU and the anconeus interval or alternatively a split of the extensor digitorum communis (EDC) tendon. In patients with instability from damage to the LCL, a Kocher approach is preferred as this facilitates ligament repair intraoperatively. In the setting of acute radial head fracture, the LCL and

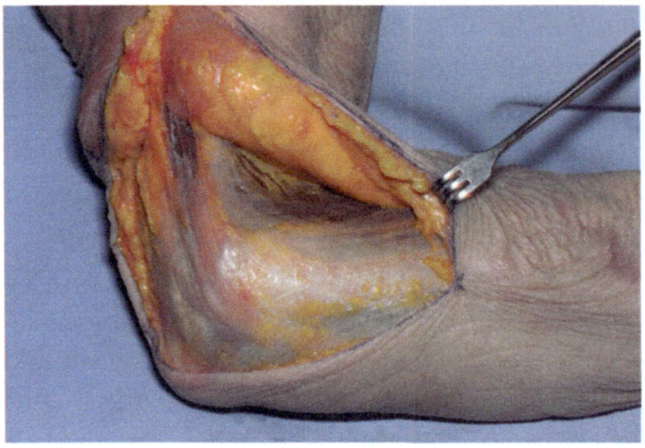

**Fig. 5.4** Posterior skin incision utilized and brought down to the antebrachial fascia on the lateral elbow. (Permissions obtained from Wolters Kluwer)

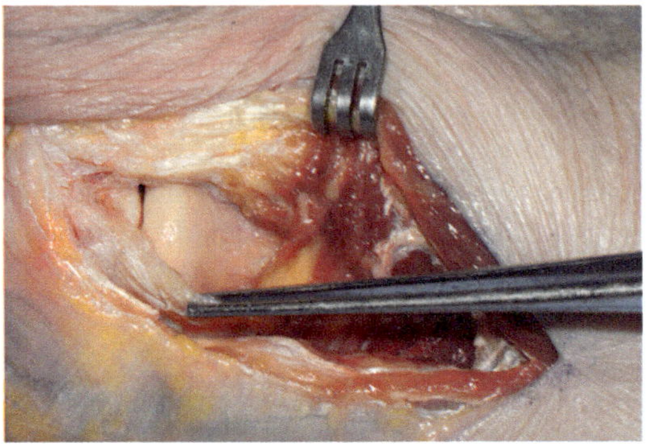

**Fig. 5.6** Capsular incision at the anterior border of LUCL to reveal the radial head. (Permissions obtained from Wolters Kluwer)

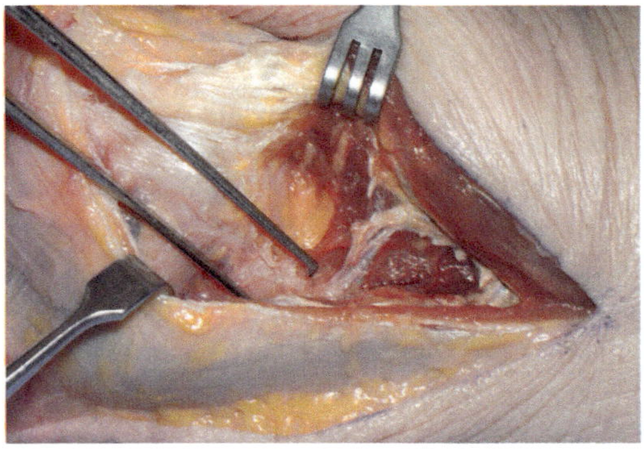

**Fig. 5.5** Identification of the LUCL in Kocher's interval. The common extensor tendon of the LCL has been elevated to demonstrate this anatomic structure

extensor muscle origin are frequently avulsed from the lateral epicondyle, thus providing a window for the surgeon to utilize to gain exposure to the radial head. In this setting, the surgeon can gently palpate the lateral side of the elbow to identify the disrupted interval and exploit this for exposure, thus "using the approach the patient gives you." When no instability is present, care must be taken by the surgeon to avoid iatrogenic injury to the LUCL if the Kocher interval is used. The interval between the ECU and anconeus can often be found by identifying a fat stripe under the fascia between these two muscles. The fascia is incised from the lateral epicondyle distally taking care to elevate the ECU anteriorly and anconeus posteriorly. The LCL is split centrally protecting the posterior portion of this complex containing the LUCL [Fig. 5.5], and the capsule is incised along the anterior border of the ligament, approximately 1 cm above the crista supinatoris. The extensor origin is carefully freed from the LUCL and retracted anteriorly with the radial collateral ligament [Fig. 5.6], taking care not to damage the LUCL as this will iatrogenically cause posterolateral rotatory instability. Care should also be taken to protect the posterior interosseous nerve by maintaining the forearm in pronation especially when retracting anterior structures. Retractors used anteriorly around the radial neck should be used with caution to avoid compression or injury to the posterior interosseous nerve.

In patients with an intact LCL, we highly favor an alternative approach which utilizes an EDC tendon origin split. With this approach, the EDC tendon and underlying radial collateral and annular ligaments are split longitudinally at or just above the mid-aspect or "equator" of the radial head. Care should be taken to avoid making the split too posterior as this can potentially damage the LUCL. The forearm should be maintained in pronation during the approach to avoid injury to the posterior interosseous nerve. Anatomic studies have shown that the posterior interosseous nerve can typically be found at the radial neck around 4 cm from the proximal margin of the radial head; the margin of safety may be increased by pronating the forearm [58]. A recent cadaveric series investigated the "3-finger method of Henry," providing recommendations to the surgeon regarding the "safe" locations of the elbow before one becomes worried about encountering the PIN or the radial nerve distally or proximally [59]. They suggest a safe zone of two fingerbreadths from the radiocapitellar joint to the midpoint of the axis of the radius with the forearm in pronation before the PIN is encountered.

## Surgical Technique and Tips

After gaining appropriate exposure to the radial head, the radial head is inspected to determine what treatment is appropriate (excision of fragments, ORIF, or radial head replacement). If radial head arthroplasty is chosen, any free osseous fragments are removed from the wound and preserved on the back table to act as a template for sizing purposes and to ensure that all of the radial head has been excised [Fig. 5.7]. If the radial head has been previously excised or is healed in a malunited state, templating for the diameter of the implant can be done using plain radiographs of the contralateral elbow.

A micro sagittal saw can be utilized to excise a small amount of radial neck to make a more uniform surface for eventual seating of the radial head implant if required. When performing resection of residual head, forearm rotation should be assessed to ensure that resection is performed perpendicular to the radial neck and that the resection is level on all sides.

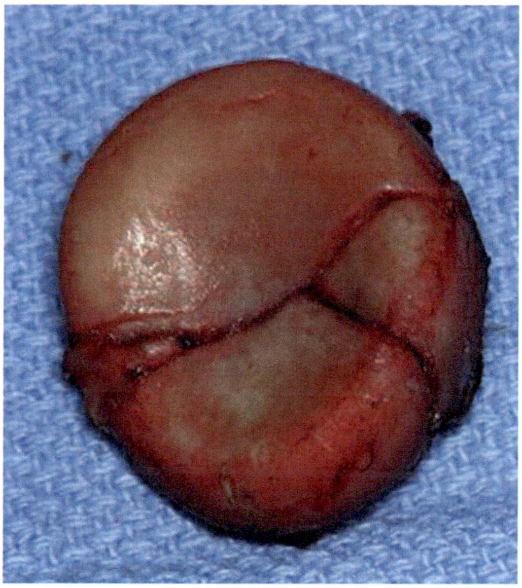

Fig. 5.7 Excised radial head that has been reconstituted in order to act as a template for implant

Following radial head excision, a "pull test" should be performed to evaluate for longitudinal instability of the forearm [45, 60]. To perform this test, a bone-reduction tenaculum is used to grasp the residual proximal radius. Then, a longitudinal pull of approximately 20 lb is applied in line with the radius. Fluoroscopy can then be used to quantify the amount of proximal migration of the radius. Greater than 3 mm of proximal radial migration with the "pull test" suggests disruption of the interosseous membrane [45].

The longitudinal height of the implant should be judged based on the reconstructed radial head. CT-based anatomic studies have proven useful in determining appropriate radial head height as well. Doornberg et al. [61] demonstrated that the native radial head lies on average 0.9 mm distal to the proximal margin of the less sigmoid notch. Thus, landmarks such as the lateral aspect of the coronoid at the lesser sigmoid notch can be used to determine the appropriate implant height. Care should be taken not to use an implant that is too long as this has been found to result in capitellar destruction and pain [62, 63]. Unfortunately, "overstuffing" of the joint is a common error, particularly in the setting of an elbow with LCL insufficiency. Radiocapitellar gapping has not been found to be a reliable measure of radial height as the LCL is often lax in patients undergoing radial head arthroplasty. Direct visualization of ulnohumeral gapping is a reliable indicator of overstuffing of the radiocapitellar joint; however, fluoroscopy was not found to reliably detect overstuffing [64].

Similarly, radial head diameter should be determined based on the reconstituted radial head that was previously removed from the wound. It has been suggested that the diameter of the implant be slightly undersized compared to the true diameter of the native radial head [50]. Typically the inner "dish" diameter, not the outer "dish" diameter of the native radial head, represents the size of implant that one should choose.

An implant with a diameter that is too large will load on the outer margins of the lesser sigmoid notch, whereas an implant with a diameter that is too small will point load on the central portion of the lesser sigmoid notch [18].

The radial neck is then reamed by hand removing cancellous bone until cortical bone is encountered. Exposure to the radial neck for reaming and implant seating can be facilitated with the use of leverage-based retractors [Fig. 5.8], again taking care to avoid excessive retraction anteriorly to avoid injury to the PIN. These can be placed around the radial neck, taking care to protect the posterior interosseous nerve, to deliver it laterally out of the wound. A variety of stem fixation is available, including press fit, cemented, or intentionally loose stems. We favor intentionally loose stem, smooth stem placement, based upon long-term favorable outcome studies [65]. For these implants, a trial stem one size smaller than the final reamer is selected, and an appropriately sized trial head is attached to the stem. The use of a stem size smaller than the final reamer allows for movement of the stem in the intramedullary canal. This is crucial as the implant functionally acts as a spacer with motion of the radial head being driven by the annular ligament and the articulations of the implant with the capitellum and lesser sigmoid notch. If the implant is found to track improperly through range of motion, it may be necessary to downsize the stem as this would allow for proper rotation of the stem in the medullary canal. It has been shown that movement of the stem in the medullary canal is well-tolerated and radiographic lucencies are not correlated with patient-reported symptoms [53, 66–68]. Intraoperative fluoroscopy can also be utilized to confirm appropriate implant thickness by ensuring that the medial ulnohumeral joint space is parallel on anteroposterior imaging. Additionally, imaging of the wrist may be considered to ensure that ulnar variance is equal bilaterally.

Once fit is found to be satisfactory, the real radial head implant is placed [Fig. 5.9], and the elbow is assessed for range of motion as well as stability. A valgus stress to the elbow should be applied, and if the medial joint space demonstrates opening, then medial collateral ligament injury should be suspected. If instability on the lateral side (LCL) is present, ligament repair should be performed. This often can be done by creating bone tunnels or suture anchors to repair the LCL to the epicondylar origin with the elbow in approximately 30° of flexion and the arm in pronation [18].

Elbow range of motion should be formally assessed prior to wound closure. Cadaveric studies have shown that the radiocapitellar space is reduced with the elbow in flexion when compared to the elbow in extension [69]. Thus, oversizing of the radial head component has the potential to reduce post-operative flexion as a large implant can impinge in the radial fossa of the distal humerus prior to achieving full flexion.

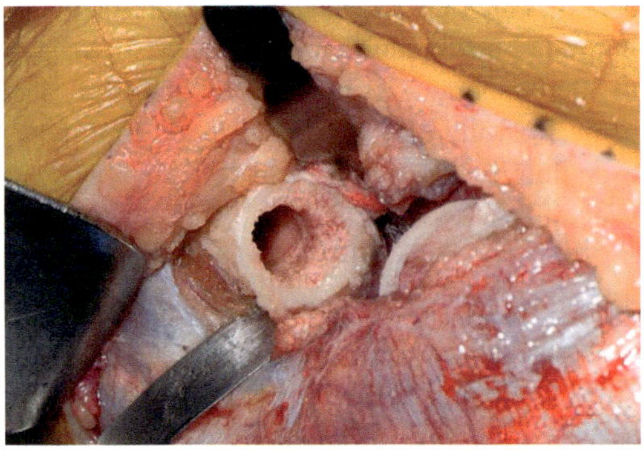

**Fig. 5.8** Radial canal delivered laterally for ease with reaming and implant placement. Care should be taken when placing the anterior retractor to avoid damage to the PIN

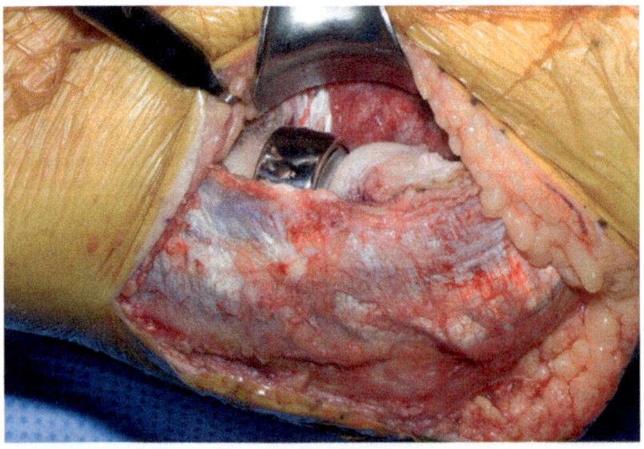

**Fig. 5.9** Picture demonstrating an implanted radial head replacement through and EDC split approach with appropriate joint reduction

## Post-Operative Management Following Primary Radial Head Arthroplasty

The post-operative management depends largely upon the presence and extent of any concomitant ligament or osseous injuries.

Generally following surgery, the operative extremity should be splinted at approximately 90 degrees, elevated, and rested for several days in order to minimize swelling and reduce the risk of wound dehiscence. Range of motion may begin as early as day one or two following surgery. Patients who have instability on the lateral side are typically immobilized in a position of pronation and flexion; forearm rotation is permitted with the elbow in full flexion only. Gradually the elbow is extended, again depending upon the stability achieved at the time of surgery and the confidence in the repair. Nighttime extension splinting should be utilized to regain terminal extension, beginning around 6 weeks following surgery [50, 70]. Outside of regaining early appropriate range of motion, specific post-operative rehabilitation programs are largely dictated by the presence of concomitant injury and the stability of any additional osseous or ligament repair. Of note, several studies have demonstrated the utility of overhead motion protocols in patients with suspected elbow instability [71–73]. This rehabilitation protocol is designed to convert gravity from a distracting to a stabilizing force in order to maintain congruency at the elbow.

Heterotopic ossification prophylaxis is commonly used following radial head arthroplasty. Heterotopic ossification has been found to occur in up to 43% of patients who experienced fracture dislocations of the elbow [74]; however, little to no data exists on the rate of heterotopic ossification following radial head arthroplasty. Indomethacin has been proposed as the medication of choice to act as prophylaxis against heterotopic ossification and also provide some post-operative pain control [50]. Nevertheless, there remains a paucity of data regarding the efficacy of indomethacin in preventing heterotopic ossification in the elbow, and there is no uniform agreement on the duration, dosage, and timing of this medication. Some patients tolerate indomethacin well, while others find GI upset problematic; thus, routine use of a proton pump inhibitor should be considered. Additionally, while radiotherapy is frequently employed as prophylaxis against heterotopic ossification in other locations about the body [75], there is little support for its use in protecting against heterotopic ossification in the elbow [76].

Post-operatively, plain radiographs consisting of a true anteroposterior and lateral of the elbow can be obtained to ensure appropriate implant position and to act as a baseline for comparison with future radiographs [Fig. 5.10].

## Complications

Complications following radial head arthroplasty are not infrequent, but most are minor with little functional consequence. Elbow and forearm stiffness is common following radial head arthroplasty; however, with appropriate rehabilitation a functional range of motion is achieved in most patients. Morrey et al. [77] evaluated 47 consecutive elbows that underwent radial head arthroplasty and subsequently required revision surgery. Revision surgery was indicated for stiffness in 18 elbows. As previously discussed, nerve injury is possible with radial head replacement. This may range from cutaneous nerve injury to major peripheral nerve injury [56]. Maintaining the forearm in pronation and ensuring safe retractor placement are intraoperative techniques that should be utilized to reduce the risk of posterior interosseous nerve injury. Finally, general complications such as infection, weakness, and complex regional pain syndrome are possible following radial head replacement.

## Prognostic Factors and Outcomes Following Primary Radial Head Arthroplasty

Implant design has been the focus of much of the outcomes data regarding radial head arthroplasty. This has been well-discussed in the previous chapter. Additionally, given that much of the data

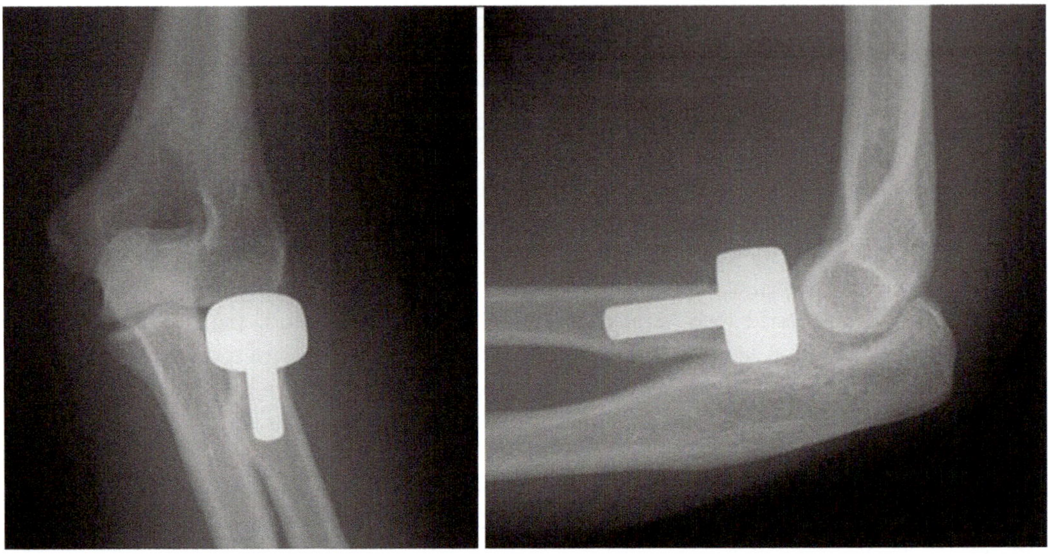

**Fig. 5.10** Post-operative AP (left) and lateral (right) radiographs of the elbow. These images demonstrate a parallel medial ulnohumeral joint and an implant well aligned with the capitellum

on outcomes is relatively heterogeneous with regard to implant characteristics, it is difficult to determine if certain patient-specific factors affect outcomes data. Nevertheless, data seem to suggest that there are certain patients or situational factors that exist for predicting outcomes following radial head arthroplasty.

## Acute Versus Delayed Presentation

One of the most important prognostic factors for outcomes following radial head arthroplasty is injury chronicity. A recent systematic review by Fowler et al. [78] identified 19 studies looking at outcomes following radial head arthroplasty and calculated a composite mean for Mayo Elbow Performance Score (MEPS) for each included study. They showed higher MEPS (90) for patients treated with radial head arthroplasty acutely when compared to those patients treated in a delayed setting [81]. This is further supported by data compiled by Morrey [44] who cites 92% patient satisfaction when undergoing radial head arthroplasty in the setting of acute fracture versus 48% patient satisfaction in patients who had delayed radial head arthroplasty as a reconstructive technique.

## Injury Pattern

Fowler et al. [78] showed no significant difference in pooled MEPS following radial head replacement performed in the setting of isolated radial head injury (89) versus complex injury pattern (87) as long as the concomitant pathology was appropriately addressed intraoperatively. This speaks to the importance of ensuring appropriate preoperative workup as well as performing comprehensive intraoperative assessment of elbow stability [Fig. 5.11].

## Return to Prior Level of Activity

Radial head replacement has proven to be a reliable treatment option for a number of surgical indications and has been found to successfully restore functional range of motion and grip strength over time [79]. Dunn et al. [80] sought to evaluate post-operative outcomes in more

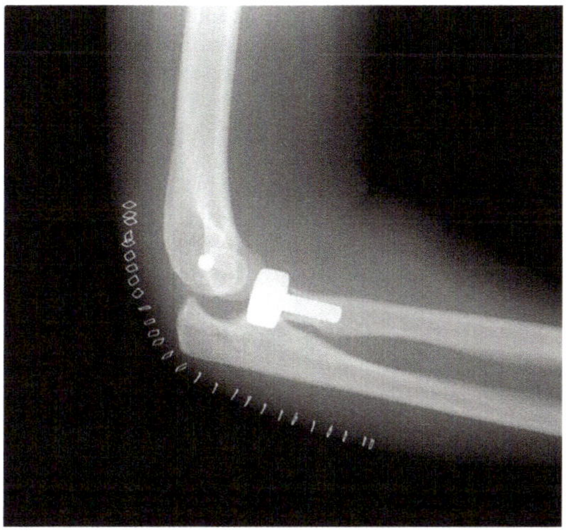

**Fig. 5.11** Persistent joint instability on radiograph despite radial head arthroplasty

high-demand patients and thus retrospectively reviewed all active duty military members who underwent radial head replacement following radial head fracture. They found that 77% of patients were able to return to active duty military service or sport; however, only half of those patients that did return reported that they were able to return to their preinjury level of function. Jung et al. [81] evaluated 57 recreational athletes who underwent radial head arthroplasty in the setting of radial head fracture and reported a relatively low return to sport rate of only 53% demonstrating that it may be difficult for the average patient to return to high level of activity following radial head replacement.

## Summary

Radial head arthroplasty has demonstrated good outcomes and is an appropriate treatment option for acute radial head fractures, elbow instability, and failed fracture reconstruction. Crucial to a successful outcome following radial head arthroplasty are appropriate preoperative workup, knowledge of surgical anatomy, technique of implantation, and rehabilitation. Further research is necessary to improve implant designs to best optimize patient outcomes.

## References

1. Duckworth AD, Clement ND, Jenkins PJ, Aitken SA, Court-Brown CM, McQueen MM. The Epidemiology of Radial Head and Neck Fractures. J Hand Surg. 2012;37(1):112–9.
2. Harrington IJ, Tountas AA. Replacement of the radial head in the treatment of unstable elbow fractures. Injury. 1981;12(5):405–12. Epub 1981/03/01.
3. Antuña S, Tabeayo Alvarez ED, Barco R, Morrey BF. 37 – Radial Head Fracture: General Considerations, Conservative Treatment, and Radial Head Resection. In: Morrey BF, Sanchez-Sotelo J, Morrey ME, editors. Morrey's the elbow and its disorders. 5th ed. Philadelphia: Elsevier; 2018. p. 375–87.
4. Mason ML. Some observations on fractures of the head of the radius with a review of one hundred cases. Br J Surg. 1954;42(172):123–32. Epub 1954/09/01.
5. Johnston GW. A follow-up of one hundred cases of fracture of the head of the radius with a review of the literature. Ulster Med J. 1962;31:51–6. Epub 1962/06/01.
6. Hotchkiss RN. Displaced fractures of the radial head: internal fixation or excision? J Am Acad Orthop Surg. 1997;5(1):1–10. Epub 1997/01/01.
7. Pires RES, Rezende FL, Mendes EC, Carvahlo AER, Filho IAA, Reis FB, et al. Radial head fractures: Mason Johnston's classification reproducibility. Malays Orthop J. 2011;5(2):6–10.
8. van Riet RP, Morrey BF. Documentation of associated injuries occurring with radial head fracture. Clin Orthop Relat Res. 2008;466(1):130–4. Epub 2008/01/16.
9. Forthman C, Henket M, Ring DC. Elbow dislocation with intra-articular fracture: the results of operative treatment without repair of the medial collateral ligament. J Hand Surg Am. 2007;32(8):1200–9. Epub 2007/10/10.
10. Van Riet RP, Van Glabbeek F, Neale PG, Bimmel R, Bortier H, Morrey BF, et al. Anatomical considerations of the radius. Clinical anatomy. 2004;17(7):564–9. Epub 2004/09/18.
11. Halls AA, Travill A. Transmission of Pressures across the elbow joint. Anat Rec. 1964;150:243–7. Epub 1964/11/01.
12. van Riet RP, Van Glabbeek F, Baumfeld JA, Neale PG, Morrey BF, O'Driscoll SW, et al. The effect of the orientation of the radial head on the kinematics of the ulnohumeral joint and force transmission through the radiocapitellar joint. Clin Biomech. 2006;21(6):554–9. Epub 2006/03/15.
13. Markolf KL, Lamey D, Yang S, Meals R, Hotchkiss R. Radioulnar load-sharing in the forearm. A study in cadavera. J Bone Joint Surg Am. 1998;80(6):879–88. Epub 1998/07/09.
14. Berkmortel CJ, Gladwell MS, Ng J, Ferreira LM, Athwal GS, Johnson JA, et al. Effect of radial neck length on joint loading. J Shoulder Elbow Arthroplasty. 2019;3:2471549219829964.

15. Acosta Batlle J, Cerezal L, López Parra MD, Alba B, Resano S, Blázquez SJ. The elbow: review of anatomy and common collateral ligament complex pathology using MRI. Insights Imaging. 2019;10(1):43.
16. Hotchkiss RN, Weiland AJ. Valgus stability of the elbow. J Orthop Res. 1987;5(3):372–7. Epub 1987/01/01.
17. Morrey BF, Tanaka S, An KN. Valgus stability of the elbow. A definition of primary and secondary constraints. Clin Orthop Relat Res. 1991;265:187–95. Epub 1991/04/01.
18. King GJ, Zarzour ZD, Rath DA, Dunning CE, Patterson SD, Johnson JA. Metallic radial head arthroplasty improves valgus stability of the elbow. Clin Orthop Relat Res. 1999;368:114–25. Epub 1999/12/29.
19. Beingessner DM, Dunning CE, Gordon KD, Johnson JA, King GJ. The effect of radial head excision and arthroplasty on elbow kinematics and stability. J Bone Joint Surg Am. 2004;86(8):1730–9. Epub 2004/08/05.
20. Sabo MT, Shannon H, De Luce S, Lalone E, Ferreira LM, Johnson JA, et al. Elbow kinematics after radiocapitellar arthroplasty. J Hand Surg Am. 2012;37(5):1024–32. Epub 2012/04/07.
21. An K, Morrey B. Biomechanics of the elbow. In: Morrey B, editor. The elbow and its disorders. 2nd ed. Philadelphia: W.B Saunders; 1993. p. 61–72.
22. O'Driscoll SW, Bell DF, Morrey BF. Posterolateral rotatory instability of the elbow. J Bone Joint Surg Am. 1991;73(3):440–6. Epub 1991/03/01.
23. Fedorka CJ, Oh LS. Posterolateral rotatory instability of the elbow. Curr Rev Musculoskelet Med. 2016;9(2):240–6. Epub 2016/05/20.
24. Schneeberger AG, Sadowski MM, Jacob HA. Coronoid process and radial head as posterolateral rotatory stabilizers of the elbow. J Bone Joint Surg Am. 2004;86(5):975–82. Epub 2004/05/01.
25. Lapner M, King GJ. Radial head fractures. Instr Course Lect. 2014;63:3–13. Epub 2014/04/12.
26. Werner FW, LeVasseur MR, Harley BJ, Anderson A. Role of the Interosseous membrane in preventing distal radioulnar gapping. J Wrist Surg. 2017;6(2):97–101. Epub 2017/04/22.
27. Adams JE, Osterman MN, Osterman AL. Interosseous membrane reconstruction for forearm longitudinal instability. Tech Hand Up Extrem Surg. 2010;14(4):222–5. Epub 2010/11/26.
28. Huang YX, Teng YJ, Yi XH, Pan J. A biomechanical study on the interosseous membrane and radial head in cadaveric forearms. Acta Orthop Traumatol Turc. 2013;47(2):122–6. Epub 2013/04/27.
29. McGinley JC, Kozin SH. Interosseous membrane anatomy and functional mechanics. Clin Orthop Relat Res. 2001;383:108–22. Epub 2001/02/24.
30. Skalski MR, White EA, Patel DB, Schein AJ, RiveraMelo H, Matcuk GR Jr. The traumatized TFCC: an illustrated review of the anatomy and injury patterns of the triangular fibrocartilage complex. Curr Probl Diagn Radiol. 2016;45(1):39–50. Epub 2015/06/29.
31. Davidson PA, Moseley JB Jr, Tullos HS. Radial head fracture. A potentially complex injury. Clin Orthop Relat Res. 1993;297:224–30. Epub 1993/12/01.
32. van Riet RP, Morrey BF, O'Driscoll SW, Van Glabbeek F. Associated injuries complicating radial head fractures: a demographic study. Clin Orthop Relat Res. 2005;441:351–5. Epub 2005/12/07.
33. Ward WG, Nunley JA. Concomitant fractures of the capitellum and radial head. J Orthop Trauma. 1988;2(2):110–6. Epub 1988/01/01.
34. Givon U, Pritsch M, Levy O, Yosepovich A, Amit Y, Horoszowski H. Monteggia and equivalent lesions. A study of 41 cases. Clin Orthop Relat Res. 1997;337:208–15. Epub 1997/04/01.
35. Regan W, Morrey B. Fractures of the coronoid process of the ulna. J Bone Joint Surg Am. 1989;71(9):1348–54. Epub 1989/10/01.
36. Johansson O. Capsular and ligament injuries of the elbow joint. A clinical and arthrographic study. Acta chir Scand Suppl. 1962;Suppl 287:1–159. Epub 1962/01/01.
37. Itamura J, Roidis N, Mirzayan R, Vaishnav S, Learch T, Shean C. Radial head fractures: MRI evaluation of associated injuries. J Shoulder Elb Surg. 2005;14(4):421–4. Epub 2005/07/15.
38. Wildin CJ, Bhowal B, Dias JJ. The incidence of simultaneous fractures of the scaphoid and radial head. J Hand Surg. 2001;26(1):25–7. Epub 2001/02/13.
39. Adams JE, Culp RW, Osterman AL. Interosseous membrane reconstruction for the Essex-Lopresti injury. J Hand Surg Am. 2010;35(1):129–36. Epub 2010/02/02.
40. Trousdale RT, Amadio PC, Cooney WP, Morrey BF. Radio-ulnar dissociation. A review of twenty cases. J Bone Joint Surg Am. 1992;74(10):1486–97. Epub 1992/12/01.
41. Artiaco S, Fusini F, Colzani G, Massè A, Battiston B. Chronic Essex-Lopresti injury: a systematic review of current treatment options. Int Orthop. 2019;43(6):1413–20.
42. Tomaino MM. The importance of the pronated grip x-ray view in evaluating ulnar variance. J Hand Surg Am. 2000;25(2):352–7. Epub 2000/03/21.
43. Loeffler BJ, Green JB, Zelouf DS. Forearm instability. J Hand Surg Am. 2014;39(1):156–67. Epub 2013/12/10.
44. Morrey BF. 39 - Prosthetic Radial Head Replacement. In: Morrey BF, Sanchez-Sotelo J, Morrey ME, editors. Morrey's the Elbow and its Disorders. 5th ed. Philadelphia: Elsevier; 2018. p. 395–402.
45. Smith AM, Urbanosky LR, Castle JA, Rushing JT, Ruch DS. Radius pull test: predictor of longitudinal forearm instability. J Bone Joint Surg Am. 2002;84(11):1970–6. Epub 2002/11/14.
46. Ring D, Quintero J, Jupiter JB. Open reduction and internal fixation of fractures of the radial head. J Bone Joint Surg Am. 2002;84(10):1811–5. Epub 2002/10/16.
47. Fowler JR, Goitz RJ. Radial head fractures: indications and outcomes for radial head arthroplasty.

Orthop Clin North Am. 2013;44(3):425–31, x. Epub 2013/07/06.
48. Madsen JE, Flugsrud G. Radial head fractures: indications and technique for primary arthroplasty. Eur J Trauma Emerg Surg. 2008;34(2):105–12. Epub 2008/04/01.
49. Acevedo DC, Paxton ES, Kukelyansky I, Abboud J, Ramsey M. Radial head arthroplasty: state of the art. J Am Acad Orthop Surg. 2014;22(10):633–42. Epub 2014/10/05.
50. King GJW. Fractures of the Head of the Radius. In: Wolfe SW, Pederson WC, Cozin SH, Cohen MS, editors. Green's operative hand surgery. 7th ed. Philadelphia: Elsevier; 2017.
51. Ashwood N, Bain GI, Unni R. Management of Mason type-III radial head fractures with a titanium prosthesis, ligament repair, and early mobilization. J Bone Joint Surg Am. 2004;86(2):274–80. Epub 2004/02/13.
52. Shukla DR, Fitzsimmons JS, An KN, O'Driscoll SW. Effect of radial head malunion on radiocapitellar stability. J Shoulder Elb Surg. 2012;21(6):789–94. Epub 2012/04/24.
53. Shore BJ, Mozzon JB, MacDermid JC, Faber KJ, King GJ. Chronic posttraumatic elbow disorders treated with metallic radial head arthroplasty. J Bone Joint Surg Am. 2008;90(2):271–80. Epub 2008/02/05.
54. Edwards GS Jr, Jupiter JB. Radial head fractures with acute distal radioulnar dislocation. Essex-Lopresti revisited. Clin Orthop Relat Res. 1988;234:61–9. Epub 1988/09/01.
55. Hutchinson S, Faber KJ, Gan BS. The Essex-Lopresti injury: more than just a pain in the wrist. Can J Plast Surg. 2006;14(4):215–8.
56. Dowdy PA, Bain GI, King GJ, Patterson SD. The midline posterior elbow incision. An anatomical appraisal. J Bone Joint Surg. 1995;77(5):696–9. Epub 1995/09/01.
57. Patterson SD, Bain GI, Mehta JA. Surgical approaches to the elbow. Clin Orthop Relat Res. 2000;370:19–33. Epub 2000/02/08.
58. Tornetta P 3rd, Hochwald N, Bono C, Grossman M. Anatomy of the posterior interosseous nerve in relation to fixation of the radial head. Clin Orthop Relat Res. 1997;345:215–8. Epub 1998/01/07.
59. Simone JP, Streubel PN, Sanchez-Sotelo J, Steinmann SP, Adams JE. Fingerbreadths rule in determining the safe zone of the radial nerve and posterior interosseous nerve for a lateral elbow approach: an anatomic study. J Am Acad Orthop Surg Glob Res Rev. 2019;3(2):e005. Epub 2019/07/25.
60. Kachooei AR, Rivlin M, Shojaie B, van Dijk CN, Mudgal C. Intraoperative Technique for Evaluation of the Interosseous Ligament of the Forearm. J Hand Surg. 2015;40(12):2372–6.e1. Epub 2015/11/09.
61. Doornberg JN, Linzel DS, Zurakowski D, Ring D. Reference points for radial head prosthesis size. J Hand Surg Am. 2006;31(1):53–7. Epub 2006/01/31.
62. Van Glabbeek F, Van Riet RP, Baumfeld JA, Neale PG, O'Driscoll SW, Morrey BF, et al. Detrimental effects of overstuffing or understuffing with a radial head replacement in the medial collateral-ligament deficient elbow. J Bone Joint Surg Am. 2004;86(12):2629–35. Epub 2004/12/14.
63. Van Riet RP, Van Glabbeek F, Verborgt O, Gielen J. Capitellar erosion caused by a metal radial head prosthesis. A case report. J Bone Joint Surg Am. 2004;86(5):1061–4. Epub 2004/05/01.
64. Athwal GS, Frank SG, Grewal R, Faber KJ, Johnson J, King GJ. Determination of correct implant size in radial head arthroplasty to avoid overlengthening: surgical technique. J Bone Joint Surg Am. 2010;92(Suppl 1 Pt 2):250–7. Epub 2010/09/25.
65. Marsh JP, Grewal R, Faber KJ, Drosdowech DS, Athwal GS, King GJ. Radial head fractures treated with modular metallic radial head replacement: outcomes at a mean follow-up of eight years. J Bone Joint Surg Am. 2016;98(7):527–35. Epub 2016/04/08.
66. Doornberg JN, Parisien R, van Duijn PJ, Ring D. Radial head arthroplasty with a modular metal spacer to treat acute traumatic elbow instability. J Bone Joint Surg Am. 2007;89(5):1075–80. Epub 2007/05/03.
67. Grewal R, MacDermid JC, Faber KJ, Drosdowech DS, King GJ. Comminuted radial head fractures treated with a modular metallic radial head arthroplasty. Study of outcomes. J Bone Joint Surg Am. 2006;88(10):2192–200. Epub 2006/10/04.
68. Moro JK, Werier J, MacDermid JC, Patterson SD, King GJ. Arthroplasty with a metal radial head for unreconstructible fractures of the radial head. J Bone Joint Surg Am. 2001;83(8):1201–11. Epub 2001/08/17.
69. Birkedal JP, Deal DN, Ruch DS. Loss of flexion after radial head replacement. J Shoulder Elb Surg. 2004;13(2):208–13. Epub 2004/03/05.
70. Calfee R, Madom I, Weiss AP. Radial head arthroplasty. J Hand Surg Am. 2006;31(2):314–21. Epub 2006/02/14.
71. Wolff AL, Hotchkiss RN. Lateral elbow instability: nonoperative, operative, and postoperative management. J Hand Ther. 2006;19(2):238–44.
72. Lee AT, Schrumpf MA, Choi D, Meyers KN, Patel R, Wright TM, et al. The influence of gravity on the unstable elbow. J Shoulder Elbow Surg. 2013;22(1):81–7.
73. Schreiber JJ, Paul S, Hotchkiss RN, Daluiski A. Conservative management of elbow dislocations with an overhead motion protocol. J Hand Surg. 2015;40(3):515–9.
74. Shukla DR, Pillai G, McAnany S, Hausman M, Parsons BO. Heterotopic ossification formation after fracture-dislocations of the elbow. J Shoulder Elb Surg. 2015;24(3):333–8. Epub 2015/01/21.
75. Popovic M, Agarwal A, Zhang L, Yip C, Kreder HJ, Nousiainen MT, et al. Radiotherapy for the prophylaxis of heterotopic ossification: a systematic review and meta-analysis of published data. Radiother Oncol. 2014;113(1):10–7. Epub 2014/09/16.
76. Ploumis A, Belbasis L, Ntzani E, Tsekeris P, Xenakis T. Radiotherapy for prevention of heterotopic ossification of the elbow: a systematic review of the literature. J Shoulder Elb Surg. 2013;22(11):1580–8. Epub 2013/10/22.

77. van Riet RP, Sanchez-Sotelo J, Morrey BF. Failure of metal radial head replacement. J Bone Joint Surg. 2010;92(5):661–7. Epub 2010/05/04.
78. Fowler JR, Henry SE, Xu P, Goitz RJ. Outcomes following radial head Arthroplasty. Orthopedics. 2016;39(3):153–60. Epub 2016/04/06.
79. Kaur MN, MacDermid JC, Grewal RR, Stratford PW, Woodhouse LJ. Functional outcomes post-radial head arthroplasty: a systematic review of literature. Shoulder Elbow. 2014;6(2):108–18. Epub 2014/04/01.
80. Dunn JC, Kusnezov NA, Koehler LR, Eisenstein ED, Kilcoyne KG, Orr JD, et al. Radial head arthroplasty in the active duty military service member with minimum 2-year follow-up. J Hand Surg. 2017;42(8):660.e1–7. Epub 2017/05/28.
81. Jung M, Groetzner-Schmidt C, Porschke F, Grutzner PA, Guehring T, Schnetzke M. Low return-to-sports rate after elbow injury and treatment with radial head arthroplasty. J Shoulder Elb Surg. 2019;28(8):1441–8. Epub 2019/06/23.

# Revision/Failed Radial Head Arthroplasty

6

Emilie J. Amaro, Eric S. Dilbone, James P. Hovis, and Donald H. Lee

## Introduction

The radial head confers significant stability to the elbow joint while also allowing for multiplanar range of motion. Radial head fractures are common, accounting for 1.5–4% of all fractures, and occur in approximately one third of elbow fractures [1, 2]. The radial head is a key stabilizer to valgus, axial, and posterolateral stress, and therefore appropriate clinical management is paramount in order to restore elbow function. The management of radial head fractures is dependent on fracture morphology, comminution, displacement, articular involvement, ligamentous stability, and associated injuries of the elbow [3].

Several classification systems exist to help guide the clinical management of radial head fractures. Mason first classified radial head fractures in 1954, and a modified classification has been created based on the degree of comminution and displacement. A Mason-type I injury describes a nondisplaced or minimally displaced fracture, a Mason-type II injury describes a displaced fracture, while a Mason-type III injury describes a comminuted and displaced fracture of the radial head [1]. In 1962, Johnston described a fourth type which involves a radial head fracture as well as an ulnohumeral joint dislocation [4]. These classifications were later modified by Broberg, Morrey, and Hotchkiss [5, 6].

There is a general consensus that Mason I and Mason II radial head fractures without mechanical blocks to motion can be managed with a short period of immobilization followed by early range of motion. Several studies have demonstrated that long-term outcomes are largely favorable with nondisplaced or minimally displaced radial head fractures treated with nonoperative management [7, 8]. Mason II fractures with displacement that interfere with motion are frequently treated via open reduction internal fixation (ORIF) with countersunk screws, headless compression screws, or plate fixation. However, Mason III fractures with significant comminution are challenging injuries to manage, and debate remains over the standard treatment. Surgical options include ORIF, radial head excision, and radial head arthroplasty [6]. Ring et al. performed a retrospective study on 56 patients and demonstrated that Mason II and Mason III fractures with 3 or less articular fragments have favorable outcomes with ORIF [9]. However, fractures with more than three articular fragments had poor outcomes defined as early failure or nonunion, decreased range of motion, or a fair or poor rating using the Broberg and Morrey rating system[9]. Thus,

E. J. Amaro · E. S. Dilbone · D. H. Lee (✉)
Vanderbilt University Department of Orthopedics, Division of Hand Surgery, Nashville, TN, USA
e-mail: emilie.j.amaro.1@vumc.org; eric.dilbone@vumc.org; donald.h.lee@vanderbilt.edu

J. P. Hovis
Arizona Center for Hand Surgery, Phoenix, AZ, USA



G. J. W. King, M. Rizzo (eds.), *Arthroplasty of the Upper Extremity*, https://doi.org/10.1007/978-3-030-68880-6_6

ORIF is effective for fractures with a few articular fragments, whereas fractures with significant comminution are better managed with radial head excision or prosthetic replacement.

Radial head excision is a reasonable surgical option in patients with a comminuted radial head fracture with stable elbow and forearm ligaments. Herbertsson et al. reviewed 61 patients with Mason II and Mason III fractures treated with radial head excision and found that patients had a good or fair functional outcome with minimal change in range of motion at 18 years following surgery [10]. However, radial head resection leads to altered elbow and wrist kinematics contributing to several anatomic complications. The radial head acts as a restraint to axial load by maintaining the anatomic length of the forearm, and is also an important secondary stabilizer to valgus stress, particularly in a ligamentous deficient elbow with a concomitant medial collateral ligamentous injury [11]. While displaced and comminuted radial head fractures may occur in isolation, they are commonly associated with concurrent ligamentous and bony injury about the elbow. An anatomic study performed by Beingessner revealed that radial head resection led to impaired rotational kinematics and elbow laxity to varus and valgus stress in a ligamentous deficient elbow [12]. Thus, radial head resection is contraindicated in radial head fractures with associated elbow instability, particularly with a deficient medial collateral ligament. Furthermore, proximal migration of the residual radius following radial head resection often leads to ulnar-positive variance and chronic wrist pain [13]. Radial head resections are therefore contraindicated in Essex-Lopresti fractures, defined as radial head or neck fractures with associated injury to the DRUJ and interosseous membrane. Subsequent resection in this situation would destabilize the forearm.

The advent and further advances of radial head prostheses have vastly impacted the way complex elbow trauma is treated. Radial head arthroplasty remains the treatment of choice in complex, comminuted radial head fractures with concomitant ligamentous or bony injury [14, 15]. Radial head prostheses restore elbow stability and range of motion. In 2001, Moro et al. studied 25 patients with unsalvageable radial head fractures and found that 17 patients had excellent/good outcomes and only 3 had poor outcomes using the Mayo Elbow Performance Index following radial head arthroplasty [15]. All patients reported high subjective markers and satisfaction with the procedure. Furthermore, several studies have demonstrated better outcomes with arthroplasty when compared to ORIF in the treatment of Mason III fractures. Ruan et al. demonstrated that when using the Broberg and Morrey functional elbow assessment, 92% of patients treated with arthroplasty had a good or excellent result, while only 12.5% of patients treated with ORIF demonstrated good or excellent results [16]. Chen et al. demonstrated that radial head arthroplasty was associated with fewer complications compared to ORIF when treating comminuted radial head fractures [17].

Radial head prosthetics have also been used in chronic conditions affecting the radiocapitellar joint including malunion, nonunion, and post-traumatic arthritis. However, radial head arthroplasty is not without complication. Complications requiring reoperation are cited in up to 45% of cases [18]. Implant loosening, technical failure, stiffness, radiocapitellar arthritis, and infection are all known complications of radial head arthroplasty.

## Current Concepts in Reconstruction

The first reported radial head arthroplasty was performed in 1941 by Speed using a ferrule cap [19, 20]. Following initial experimentation, silastic radial head implants became popular in the 1960s with a design developed by Alfred Swanson [21]. Initial reports demonstrated favorable clinical outcomes, which were thought to be secondary to maintaining radial length and radiocapitellar contact [21]. However, long-term data published in the early 1980s demonstrated that silastic particles lead to a reactive synovitis [22]. Furthermore, the silastic material was too deformable leading to high rates of implant fracture and residual elbow instability [23]. Silicone implants have poor biomechanical properties and therefore are now seldom used in practice. After silastic implants fell out of favor in the early 1980s, radial head implants have undergone innovations in design and presently most are manufactured using cobalt-chrome, titanium, or pyrolytic carbon [19, 24].

Currently, there are two major designs used in radial head replacements, unipolar and bipolar prosthetics [25]. Unipolar constructs are generally noncemented stem designs that are fit loosely within the radial canal or are secured to the proximal radial canal with press-fit insertion. With the smooth designs, the stem component is intentionally left loose to allow for radiocapitellar congruence with forearm range of motion [26]. Due to the loose fit, there is a lucency surrounding the implant stem seen on radiographs that is expected, although the long-term clinical relevance of this lucency is unknown [27]. Press-fit designs have a stem coating to allow for stem bony ingrowth. Immense care must be taken in press-fit designs as microfractures are common when inserting the stem [28]. Bipolar stems have a constrained joint at the radial head-neck junction to reapproximate the native joint [27]. Bipolar prosthetics are typically cemented or press fit into the radial canal to limit the degrees of freedom built into the implant. Bipolar designs are thought to decrease stress while increasing congruity at the radiocapitellar joint although this remains unproven. Both unipolar and bipolar implants are typically modular in design, i.e., have separate radial stem and head components, that allow for various combinations of head and stem sizes.

## Outcomes

Outcomes with radial head arthroplasty to treat complex elbow trauma appear satisfactory [17, 29]. A review performed by Bonnevialle et al. demonstrated that satisfactory clinical outcomes were seen in 60–80% of cases [30]. However, many of the studies evaluated short-term outcomes with long-term outcomes being largely unknown [31]. Laumonerie performed a large literature review demonstrating that reported rates of reoperation following radial head replacement range from 0 to 45% [18]. Furthermore, Duckworth et al. reviewed 105 patients who underwent radial head replacement following elbow trauma and found that 28% of patients required a reoperation within 6.7 years [32]. This was further validated by Cristofaro et al. who found a 25% rate of reoperation in patients who underwent a radial head replacement with an 8-year follow-up period [33]. Both younger age and silastic implants were independent and significant risk factors for further surgery [32].

However, Harrington et al. provided contradictory outcomes demonstrating that metal radial head prosthetics provide elbow stability with a few complications in patients with a mean follow-up of 12 years [14]. Furthermore, Reinhardt et al. performed a study evaluating the rate of reoperation and cost of treating radial head fractures with ORIF compared to radial head arthroplasty. The results demonstrated that following ORIF, patients were more likely to undergo a reoperation and had a higher total cost of care when compared to patients who underwent a radial head arthroplasty [34]. These results held true through a subgroup analysis evaluating patients both with and without a concurrent elbow dislocation [34]. Thus, radial head arthroplasty remains both a cost-effective and clinically successful treatment method for radial head fractures. However, radial head arthroplasty is not without complications. Commonly reported complications include aseptic loosening, stiffness, technical and implant failure, radiocapitellar arthritis, and infection [35].

## Aseptic Loosening

A recent systematic review regarding failure modes of radial head arthroplasty cited symptomatic, aseptic loosening as the most common mode of failure (Fig. 6.1a–c) [35]. Based on post hoc analyses, 30% of implants failed due to aseptic loosening, with an average time to failure of 34 months [35]. Aseptic loosening is seen among all methods of fixation including press-fit,

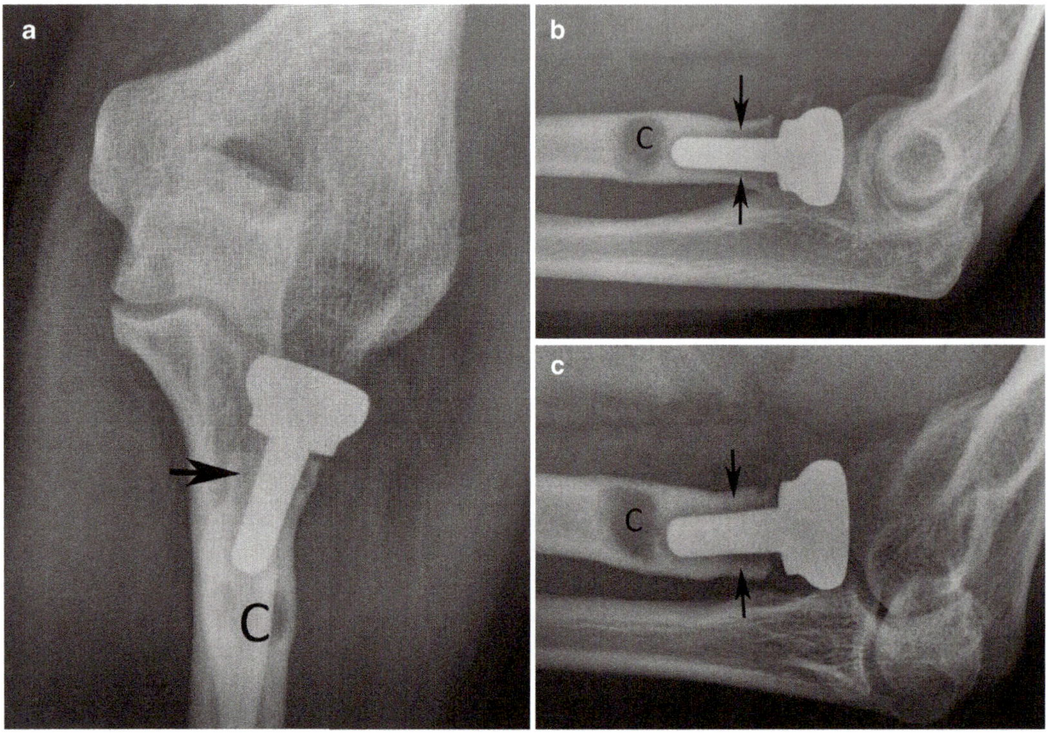


**Fig. 6.1** (**a**–**c**) Anteroposterior (**a**), lateral (**b**), and oblique (**c**) radiographs of the elbow with loosening of a press-fit radial head implant. Note the area of lucency around the stem (arrows) and cyst formation (C) distal to the tip of the implant

cemented, loose fitting, and expandable stems. As discussed, unipolar designs can be placed with a loose fit within the intramedullary canal to allow for radiocapitellar congruence with forearm range of motion. This can be seen radiographically as a lucency surrounding the implant. However, progression of the radiolucency radiographically can be associated with clinical pain and loosening of the implant.

One study found a lower incidence of aseptic loosening among bipolar designs compared to unipolar designs and hypothesized that this is secondary to lower stress transmission at the bone-implant interface [31]. Studies have demonstrated that bipolar prosthetics indeed have less micromotion and reduced stress at the bone-implant interface [36]. Furthermore, cemented bipolar arthroplasties and loose-fitting smooth unipolar implants are associated with less loosening than press-fit designs [37–39]. This suggests that poor bony ingrowth onto the stem leads to increased micromotion, which facilitates loosening of press-fit designs. Further advances in press-fit stem designs are needed, and surgeon preference and familiarity with the implant should factor into the choice of implant design used. As aseptic loosening remains the most commonly cited mode of failure in patients with radial head arthroplasty, patients should have close and long-term radiographic follow-up.

Treatment of aseptic loosening of a radial head implant includes implant revision, with or without cement and a longer stem implant, or implant removal [40]. Preoperative serologic studies and intraoperative cultures should be obtained. The choice of implant (unipolar vs. bipolar) and fixation technique (cemented vs. uncemented) will vary with the implant design and intraoperative factors such as anatomy of proximal radius at the time of revision. Other potential options could include total elbow arthroplasty (in cases of ulnohumeral arthritis) and radiocapitellar prosthesis (not currently available) (Algorithm 6.1) [35].

## Stiffness

Stiffness is a common complication following elbow trauma or reconstruction and can be secondary to multiple etiologies including soft tissue contractures, heterotopic ossification (HO), extra- and intra-articular malunions, nonunions, and loss of articular cartilage [41, 42]. In the setting of radial head arthroplasty, stiffness is caused by oversizing the radial head implant, implant loosening and migration, heterotopic ossification, or soft tissue contractures. Stiffness following radial head arthroplasty is common and has been cited as the mode of failure in 20% of all cases [35]. In one meta-analysis of patients with failed radial head arthroplasty undergoing revision surgery for stiffness, loose-fitting prostheses were revised 7 times more frequently when compared to press-fit prosthetics (20 of 53 loose-fit prostheses versus 3 of 47 press-fit prostheses; $p < 0.01$) [35]. Among the 20 intentionally loose-fit prostheses, unipolar designs were revised for stiffness more often than bipolar designs.

Heterotopic ossification (HO), an abnormal formation of bone, has a predilection for the elbow joint and is the leading cause of extrinsic elbow contracture leading to clinical stiffness (Fig. 6.2a,

**Algorithm 6.1** Treatment algorithm for failure due to aseptic loosening

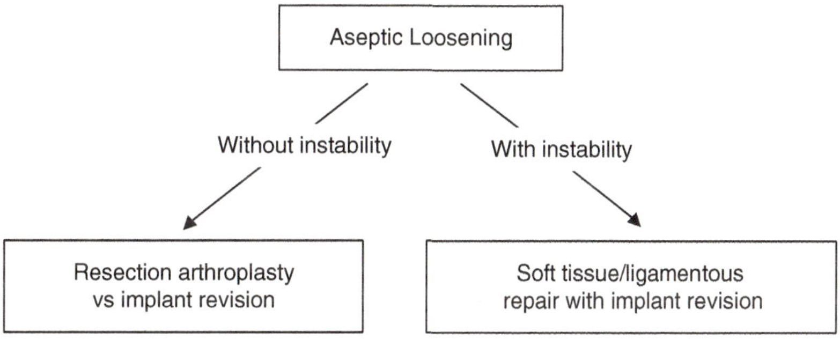


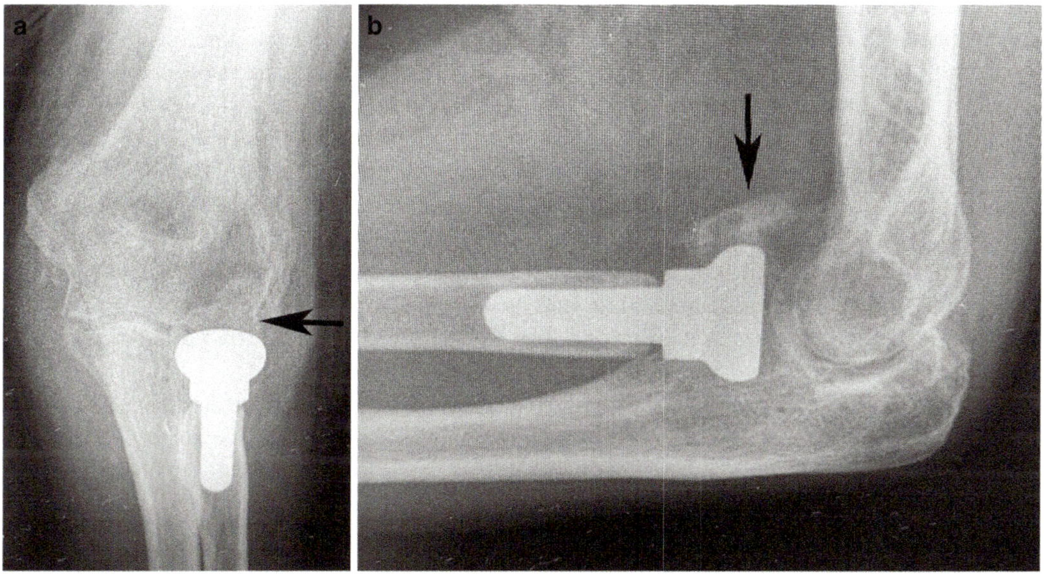

**Fig. 6.2** (**a–b**) Anteroposterior (**a**) and lateral (**b**) radiographs of non-bridging heterotopic ossification (arrow) following a radial head replacement

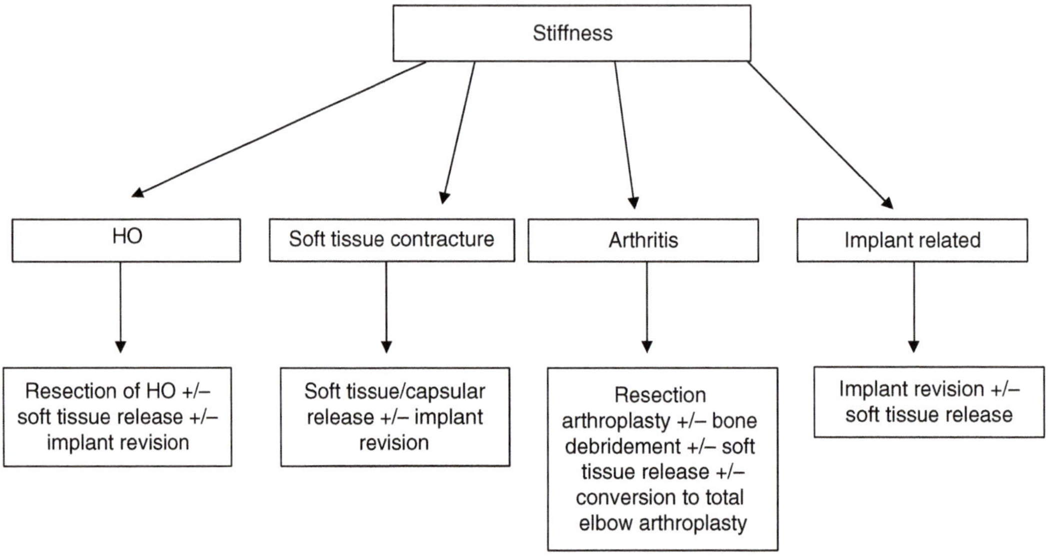


**Algorithm 6.2** Treatment algorithm for failure due to stiffness

b) [43]. The rate of HO following elbow trauma has been reported to be as high as 89% [44]. HO is a frequent complication following radial head arthroplasty. Moro et al. found a 30% rate of HO following radial head replacement, while Ha et al. reported that 38% of all patients showed signs of HO [15, 27]. Furthermore, 53% of these patients required removal or revision of implants due to heterotopic ossification [27]. As HO can impair functional outcomes, many studies have been performed on mechanisms to prevent abnormal bone formation. Currently, NSAIDs and radiotherapy are the two therapies used to prevent HO. However, their efficacy is not well established and these therapies are not without risk. NSAIDs have been shown on the molecular level to impair bone formation, while radiotherapy is associated with skin breakdown and poor wound healing. Therefore, the decision to prophylactically treat patients following a radial head replacement secondary to elbow trauma is very provider specific and varies significantly throughout the literature [45].

The indication and type of operative treatment of elbow contractures following a radial head replacement is dependent on the degree of elbow stiffness, functional impairment, and the etiology of the stiffness (soft tissue, heterotopic ossification, arthritis, implant-related problems). Soft tissue contractures without arthritis, heterotopic ossification, and implant-related problems (loosening, improper sizing) can be treated with capsular release. In elbows with mild to moderate arthritis or heterotopic ossification, limited bone debridement may be used to augment soft tissue release. Severe arthritis, however, would require some form of arthroplasty (fascial interposition or total elbow arthroplasty). In cases of radial head implant-related elbow stiffness (loose implant, improper sizing, implant-related arthritis), options include implant revision, with or without cement and a longer stem implant, and implant excision (Algorithm 6.2).

## Technical and Implant Failure

While radial head replacement appears to be a reproducible and systematic surgical procedure, there are several technical considerations that must be made. In particular, maintaining the anatomic length of the radius has been found to significantly impact elbow kinematics and load transfer at the ulnohumeral joint with direct clinical repercussions. Glabbeek et al. studied the

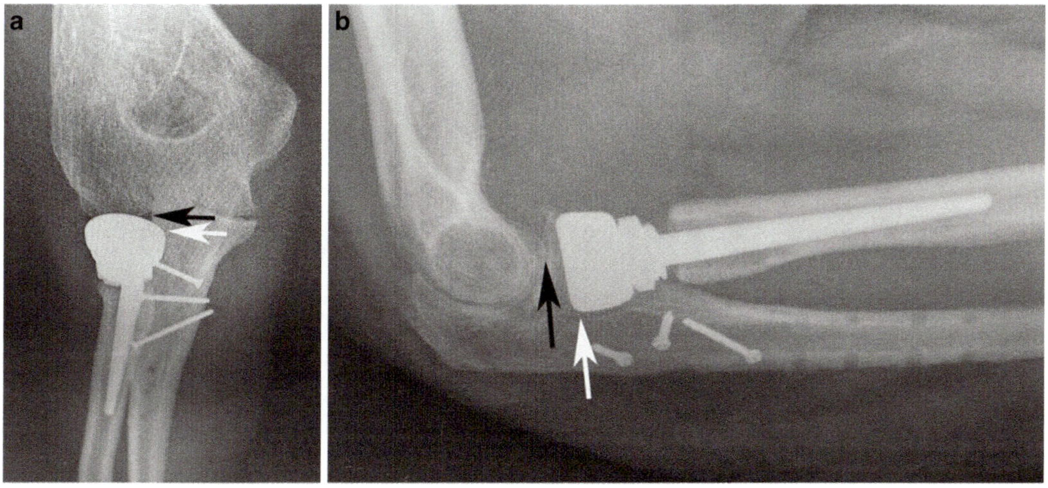


**Fig. 6.3** (**a–b**) Anteroposterior (**a**) and lateral (**b**) radiographs of a shortened radial head implant (white arrow) placed shorter than the proximal margin of the lateral coronoid facet (black arrow)

kinematics and forces at the elbow in cadaveric elbows with resected radial heads that were artificially lengthened or shortened [46]. Their data suggest that lengthening or shortening the radius by as little as 2.5 mm affected the varus/valgus stability at the elbow as well as contact pressures at the radiohumeral and ulnohumeral joints. Shortening the radius led to valgus laxity at the elbow with the ulna maintaining an internally rotated position (Fig. 6.3a, b). Overlengthening the radius, or overstuffing, led to a varus deformity of the elbow, which was most pronounced at 30 degrees of elbow flexion. Lengthening the radius by 5 mm led to such a profound overstuffing of the joint that the sensors became irreversibly deformed, distorting further data collection. Furthermore, Cohn et al. performed a cadaveric study and found that only 2 mm of radial lengthening could be tolerated without significant overloading of the radiocapitellar joint [47]. These studies clearly demonstrate that small deviations from the anatomic length of the radius can lead to significant changes in joint stability and forces across the elbow.

Overlengthening is a relatively frequent complication of radial head arthroplasty (Fig. 6.4a, b). Burkhart et al. followed 19 patients following a bipolar radial head prosthetic and found that 2 cases of dislocation and 1 case of bony erosion were attributable to overlengthening [29]. Overstuffing the joint is thought to lead to pain, early onset of radiocapitellar arthritis, and stiffness. As cadaveric studies have demonstrated that small changes in radial length lead to large biomechanical changes, it is difficult to ascertain an exact percentage of cases that fail directly due to overstuffing. However, appropriately sizing both the radial head diameter and length is paramount to a satisfactory outcome in radial head replacement.

Radial head implant sizing is typically templated by the size of the explanted radial head as well as by the fracture fragment sizes. Radiographic findings that indicate overstuffing mainly rely on joint symmetry. The proximal aspect of the radial head should be at the level of the most proximal extent of the lesser sigmoid notch or the lateral edge of the coronoid (Fig. 6.5). At the time of surgery, the radial head implant under fluoroscopy can appear up to 2 mm proximal to the most proximal margin of the lesser sigmoid notch due to the thick cartilage in this location [48]. Additionally there should be no widening of the lateral aspect of the ulnohumeral joint relative to the contralateral elbow, and the medial ulnohumeral joint space should be parallel [49].

Other technical failures include the failure to repair ligamentous injury following repair of the radial head in a ligamentous deficient elbow. As

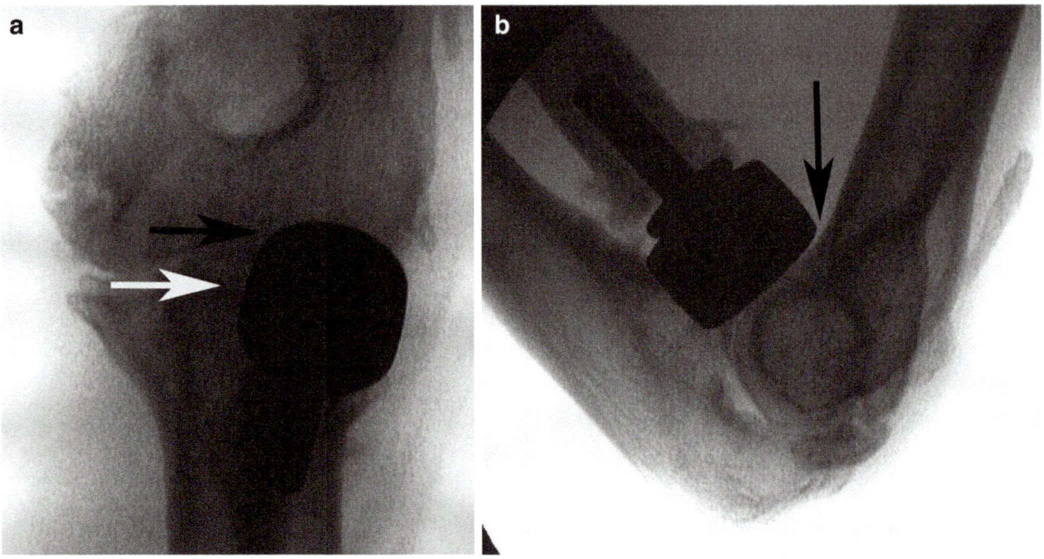


**Fig. 6.4** (**a**–**b**) Anteroposterior (**a**) and lateral (**b**) radiographs showing a large radial head implant that overstuffs the radiocapitellar joint. Note that the proximal margin of the radial head implant (black arrow) is too proximal to the proximal margin of the lateral coronoid facet (white arrow) (**a**). The implant also blocks elbow flexion (black arrow) (**b**)

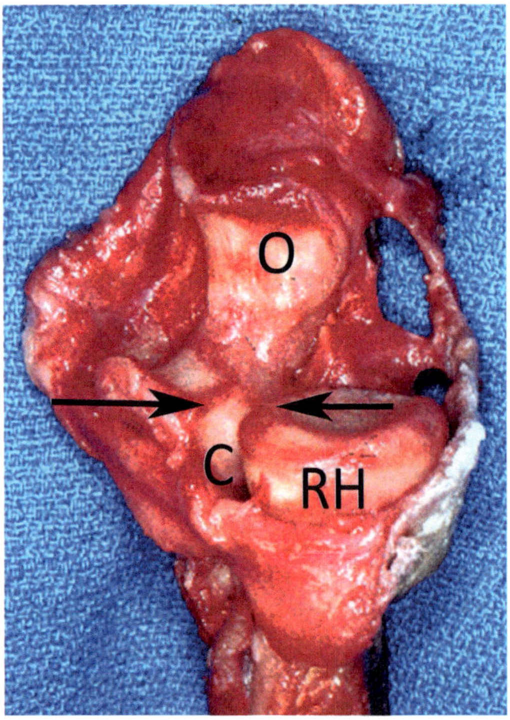


**Fig. 6.5** Cadaveric specimen showing the colinear alignment (two arrows) of the lateral coronoid facet (C) and radial head (RH). Olecranon process (O)

previously discussed, the radial head is a secondary stabilizer of the elbow, particularly to axial and posterolateral forces. Thus, in the setting of a concurrent ligamentous injury, failure to repair soft tissue structures can lead to posterolateral instability (Fig. 6.6) [50]. A study performed by Allavena analyzed bipolar prosthesis and found that in 22 patients, 6 patients demonstrated persistent posterolateral subluxation on postoperative radiographs, and 3 patients required a revision for ligamentous or capsular repair [51]. Recurrent instability is a common mode of failure following radial head arthroplasty. A literature review performed by Laumonerie found 9 cases of significant instability requiring operative revision in 80 total patients following insertion of a radial head prosthesis [18]. The surgeon must therefore critically evaluate the ligaments of the elbow and plan for concurrent reconstruction along with radial head replacement.

Finally, as discussed, both unipolar and bipolar implants have separate radial stem and head components, which allow for various combinations of head and stem sizes. A less common complication that can occur with modular implants is implant dissociation requiring implant revision (Fig. 6.7a, b). This can occur due to inappropriate sizing of the components and residual instability of the elbow allowing for significant motion of the components as well as due to mechanical failure of the linkage mechanism.

The indication and type of operative treatment for a technical failure or radial head implant failure is dependent upon the mode of failure. In cases of failure secondary to overstuffing or overlengthening of the implant without radiocapitellar arthritis or instability, options include implant revision to the appropriate size or implant removal. In elbows with radiocapitellar arthritis, the implant may be downsized or removed. In cases of elbow posterolateral instability following a radial head implant, lateral collateral ligament repair or reconstruction is warranted. Implants that have failed secondary to dissociation or breakage are generally revised or removed. In cases of implant revision, the type of implant used (standard vs. long stem) and type of fixation (cemented vs. noncemented) depend on the conditions of the proximal radius at the time of the revision (Algorithm 6.3).

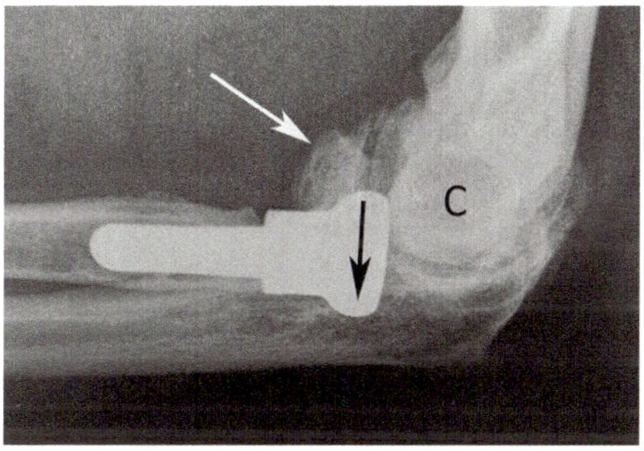


**Fig. 6.6** Lateral radiograph showing residual posterior subluxation of the radial head (black arrow). Note that there is significant periarticular elbow joint arthritis (white arrow). Capitellum (C)

## Radiocapitellar Arthritis

The radiocapitellar joint bears approximately 60% of forces transmitted through the native elbow, demonstrating its high predilection for osteoarthritis [52]. As described by Glabbeek and Cohn, radial head arthroplasty done with any change in radial length can greatly impact radiocapitellar and ulnohumeral joint pressures, which can lead to early wear and arthritic changes [46, 47]. Secondary radiocapitellar arthritis is a frequent radiographic finding after radial head arthroplasty and can lead to significant postoperative pain in some patients. Radiocapitellar arthritis has been reported in up to 70% of patients following radial head arthroplasty [15]. In a study performed by Ha et al., which evaluated 244 patients following

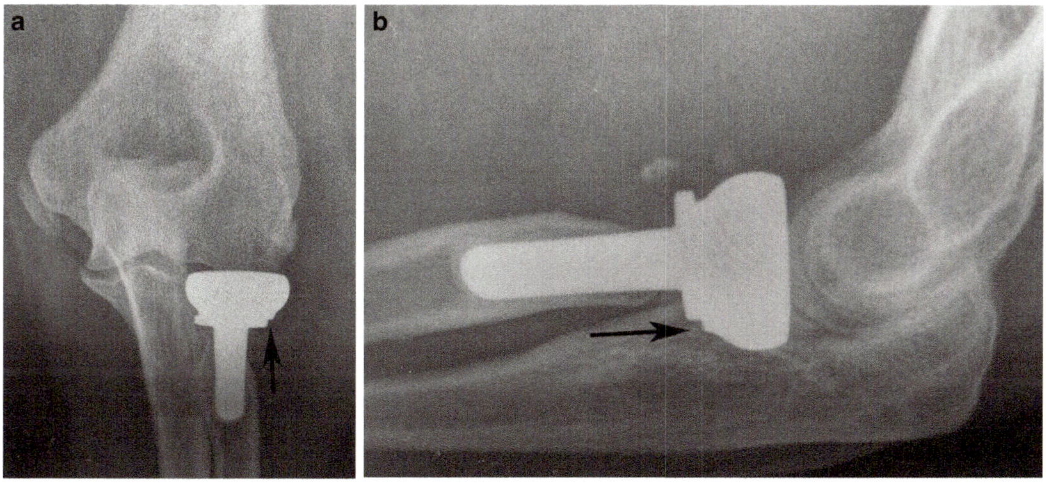


**Fig. 6.7** (**a**–**b**) Anteroposterior (**a**) and lateral (**b**) radiographs showing loosening of the radial head component relative to the stem. The radial head is slightly laterally (**a**) and posteriorly (**b**) shifted (arrows) relative to the stem

radial head arthroplasty, radiocapitellar arthritis was seen in 28% of patients and was more common in unipolar constructs when compared to bipolar constructs [25]. Bipolar constructs are designed to improve joint congruence and therefore may be less likely to impart wear on the capitellum. However, Popovic et al. reported a 58% rate of capitellar wear following the use of bipolar prosthetics indicating that the type of prosthetic may not affect wear rates [37].

Radiocapitellar arthritis is treated expectantly. If symptoms progress and begin to significantly impact quality of life, options can include downsizing of the radial head implant, a radiocapitellar joint resurfacing implant (not currently available), resection arthroplasty with anconeus interposition or tendoachilles allograft interposition, and conversion to a total elbow arthroplasty (in cases of significant ulnohumeral arthritis) (Algorithm 6.4) [53, 54].

## Infection

Deep infection is an uncommon but catastrophic complication of radial head arthroplasty. Laumonerie et al. reported 3 cases of deep infection following 80 radial head replacements; all 3 cases required explantation and revision [18]. Furthermore, Neuhaus et al. studied 14 cases requiring revision and found that 2 patients required reoperation secondary to a chronic, deep infection [55]. Lastly, Cristofaro studied 119 patients following radial head arthroplasty with only 1 patient experiencing a deep infection requiring revision [33].

Similar to other joint arthroplasty, radial head prosthetic infections can be divided into early and late infections. Early infections typically occur within the first 3 weeks of operative intervention and are directly related to surgical and sterile technique, operative time, wound closure, wound

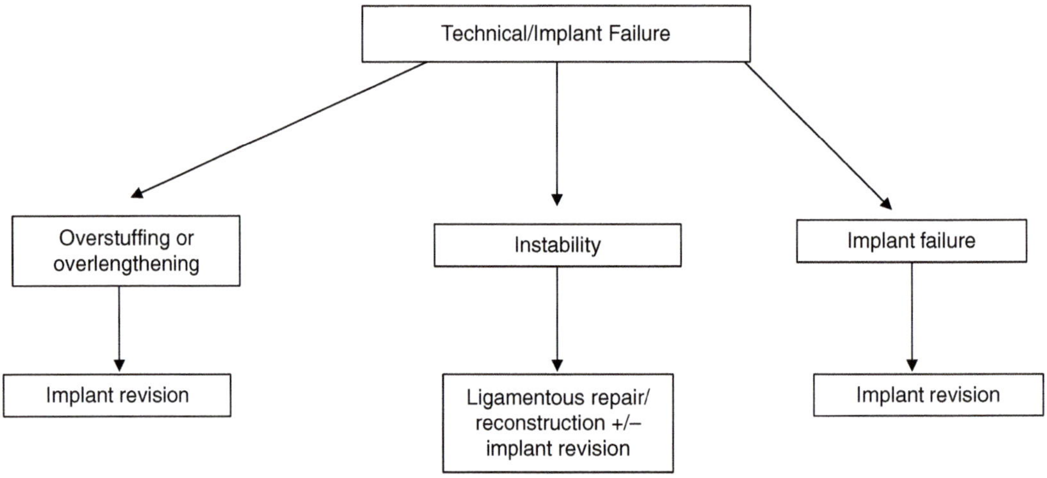


**Algorithm 6.3** Treatment algorithm for failure due to techical error or implant failure

**Algorithm 6.4** Treatment algorithm for failure due to radiocapitellar arthritis

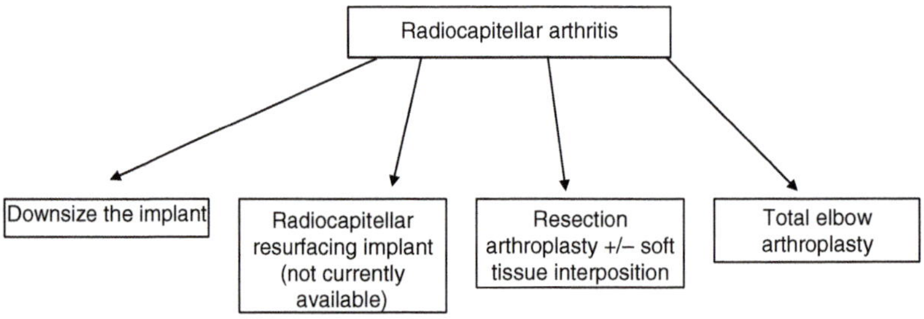

healing, open fractures and perioperative antibiotic administration [56]. If a deep postoperative infection occurs acutely, a thorough irrigation and debridement is indicated with retention of the implant. A 6-week course of microbial tailored antibiotics is typically adjunctive to the operative debridement. Superficial infections, while more common, are typically treated with a short course of oral antibiotics. Subacute infections may be best treated with implant removal with or without insertion of an antibiotic spacer and a secondary reimplantation in the setting of residual instability.

Late prosthetic infections present a far more challenging clinical scenario. No data currently exists regarding isolated radial head replacement, but the total elbow replacement literature cites *Staphylococcus aureus* as the most common microbial species in prosthetic elbow infections [57]. Late infections typically occur secondary to bacteremia or due to direct inoculation through a wound or trauma. As orthopedic implants allow for the formation of biofilms, chronic infections typically require radial head explantation, with or without an antibiotic-impregnated cement spacer, with possible revision arthroplasty following a course of IV antibiotics (Algorithm 6.5).

## Radial Head Arthroplasty Failure

Revision following a failed radial head prosthesis presents a number of challenges that require individualized consideration. Patient-specific considerations include but are not limited to age and level of activity, presence of symptoms/pain, proximal bone stock, quality of capitellar chondral surface, concomitant ulnohumeral osteoarthritis, cemented vs. press-fit implant, surgeon preference, and level of comfort performing revision procedure. Multiple options exist for revision including explantation of the prosthesis, removal of prosthesis and revision with a different radial head prosthesis, revision to total elbow arthroplasty, and revision to partial elbow arthroplasty or radiocapitellar prosthesis. Of reported revisions in current literature, 69% of revision surgeries involved isolated explantation of the prosthesis, 25% exchanged the radial head prosthesis, 3% were revised to a total elbow arthroplasty, and 3% were revised to a radiocapitellar prosthesis or partial elbow arthroplasty [35].

When determining the best option for revision, the stability of the elbow needs to be considered. A radial head prosthesis can be used to help stabi-

**Algorithm 6.5** Treatment algorithm for failure due to infection

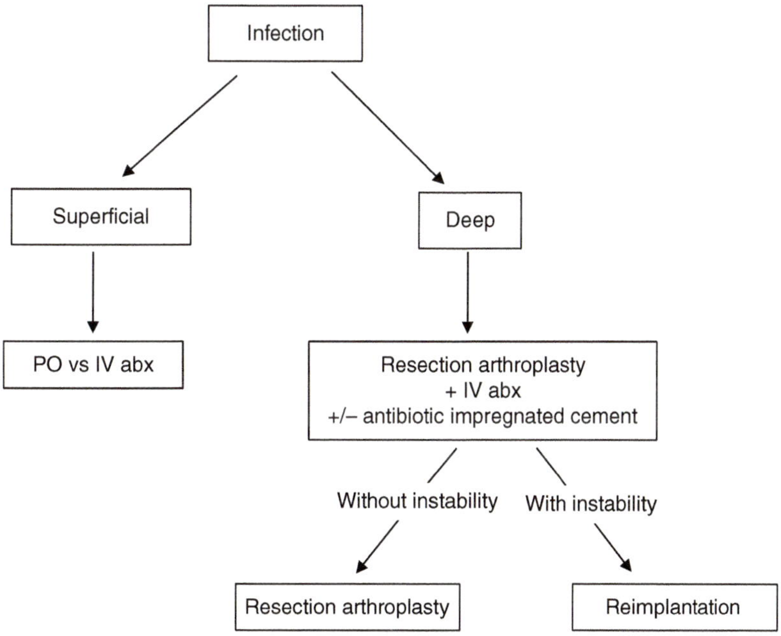

lize the elbow while the collateral ligaments heal [9, 58]. Following ligamentous healing it is safe to remove the prosthesis as subluxation or dislocation of the elbow would be very unlikely. Prior studies have demonstrated satisfactory functional outcomes in patients who undergo a radial head resection, and it is therefore reasonable to remove the prosthesis and not replace it in the setting of a stable elbow and forearm [59].

If ligamentous instability persists, exchange of the radial head prosthetic or conversion to a total elbow arthroplasty is needed. However, there is no clear consensus on the ideal management of a failed arthroplasty, and several patient-specific factors must be taken into consideration [60].

Radial head arthroplasty is an evolving technique that offers a solution to radial head and neck injuries. With numerous differing implants and multiple fixation strategies available, it is still unclear which is preferred. Although promising short- and mid-term results have been seen with radial head arthroplasty, it remains a complex procedure requiring meticulous attention to detail. An understanding of the injury pattern, patient characteristics, radiographic parameters, and implant used are required to improve outcomes and reduce complications.

## References


1. Mason M. Fractures of the head of the radius. Br J Surg. 1954;42:123–32.
2. Tejwani NC, Mehta H. Fractures of the radial head and neck: current concepts in management. J Am Acad Orthop Surg. 2007;15:380–7.
3. Swensen SJ, et al. Maximizing outcomes in the treatment of radial head fractures. J Orthop Traumatol. 2019;20:15.
4. Johnston GW. A follow-up of one hundred cases of fracture of the head of the radius with a review of the literature. Ulster Med J. 1962;31:51–6.
5. Broberg MA, Morrey B. Results of treatment of fracture-dislocations of the elbow. Clin Orthop Relat Res. 1987;216:109–19.
6. Hotchkiss R, Displaced N. Fractures of the radial head: internal fixation or excision? J Am Acad Orthop Surg. 1997;5:1–10.
7. Struijs PAA, Smit G, Steller EP. Radial head fractures: effectiveness of conservative treatment versus surgical intervention. Arch Orthop Trauma Surg. 2007;127:125–30.
8. Guzzini M, et al. Nonsurgical treatment of Mason type II radial head fractures in athletes. A retrospective study. G di Chir. 2016;37:200–5.
9. Ring D, Quintero J, Jupier J. Open reduction and internal fixation of fractures of the radial head. J Bone Jt Surg. 2002;84A:1811–5.
10. Herbertsson P, et al. Fractures of the radial head and neck treated with radial head excision. J Bone Jt Surg. 2004;86:1925–30.
11. Morrey B, Tanaka S, An K. Valgus stability of the elbow. Clin Orthop Relat Res. 1991;265:187–95.
12. Beingessner DM, Dunning CE, Gordon KD, Johnson JA, King GJW. The effect of radial head excision and arthroplasty on elbow kinematics and stability. J Bone Jt Surg. 2004;86:1730–9.
13. Ikeda M, Oka Y. Function after early radial head resection for fracture: a retrospective evaluation of 15 patients followed for 3-18 years. Acta Orthop Scand. 2000;71:191–4.
14. Harrington IJ, Sekyi-Otu A, Barrington TW, Evans DC, Tuli V. The functional outcome with metallic radial head implants in the treatment of unstable elbow fractures: a long-term review. J Trauma Inj Infect Crit Care. 2001;50:46–52.
15. Moro JK, Werier J, MacDermid JC, Patterson SD, King GJW. Arthroplasty with a metal radial head for unreconstructible fractures of the radial head. JBJS. 2001;83:1201–11.
16. Ruan HJ, Fan CY, Liu JJ, Zeng BF. A comparative study of internal fixation and prosthesis replacement for radial head fractures of Mason type III. Int Orthop. 2009;33:249–53.
17. Chen X, et al. Comparison between radial head replacement and open reduction and internal fixation in clinical treatment of unstable, multi-fragmented radial head fractures. Int Orthop. 2011;35:1071–6.
18. Laumonerie P, et al. The minimum follow-up required for radial head arthroplasty: a meta-analysis. Bone Jt J. 2017;99B:1561–70.
19. Laumonerie P, et al. Radial head arthroplasty: a historical perspective. Int Orthop. 2019;43:1643–51.
20. Speed K. Ferrule caps for the head of the radius. Surg Gynecol Obs. 1941;73:845–50.
21. Swanson AB, Jaeger SH, La Rochelle D. Comminuted fractures of the radial head. The role of silicone implant replacement arthroplasty. J Bone Jt Surg. 1981;63A:1039–49.
22. Worsing R, Engbera W, Lange T. Reactive synovitis from particular Silastic. J Bone Jt Surg. 1982;64A:581–5.
23. Mayhall WST, Tiley FT, Paluska DJ. Fracture of silastic radial-head prosthesis. Case report. J Bone Jt Surg Ser A. 1981;63:459–60.
24. Gauci MO, Winter M, Dumontier C, Bronsard N, Allieu Y. Clinical and radiologic outcomes of pyrocarbon radial head prosthesis: midterm results. J Shoulder Elb Surg. 2016;25:98–104.
25. Petscavage JM, Ha AS, Chew FS. Radiologic review of total elbow, radial head, and capitellar resurfacing arthroplasty. Radiographics. 2012;32:129–49.

26. Stuffmann E, Baratz ME. Radial head implant arthroplasty. J Hand Surg Am. 2009;34:745–54.
27. Ha AS, Petscavage JM, Chew FS. Radial head arthroplasty: a radiologic outcome study. Am J Roentgenol. 2012;199:1078–82.
28. Chanlalit C, Shukla DR, Fitzsimmons JS, An KN, O'Driscoll SW. Stress shielding around radial head prostheses. J Hand Surg Am. 2012;37:2118–25.
29. Burkhart KJ, et al. Mid- to long-term results after bipolar radial head arthroplasty. J Shoulder Elb Surg. 2010;19:965–72.
30. Bonnevialle N. Radial head replacement in adults with recent fractures. Orthop Traumatol Surg Res. 2016;102:S69–79.
31. Van Riet RP, Sanchez-Sotelo J, Morrey BF. Failure of metal radial head replacement. J Bone Jt Surg. 2010;92:661–7.
32. Duckworth AD, Wickramasinghe NR, Clement ND, Court-Brown CM, McQueen MM. Radial head replacement for acute complex fractures: what are the rate and risks factors for revision or removal? Clin Orthop Relat Res. 2014;472:2136–43.
33. Cristofaro CD, et al. High risk of further surgery after radial head replacement for unstable fractures: longer-term outcomes at a minimum follow-up of 8 years. Clin Orthop Relat Res. 2019;477:2531–40.
34. Reinhardt, D., Toby, E. B. & Brubacher, J. Reoperation rates and costs of radial head arthroplasty versus open reduction and internal fixation of radial head and neck fractures: a retrospective database study. Hand. 2019. https://doi.org/10.1177/1558944719837691.
35. Viveen J, et al. Why does radial head arthroplasty fail today? A systematic review of recent literature. EFORT Open Rev. 2019;4:659–67.
36. Flinkkilä T, Kaisto T, Sirniö K, Hyvönen P, Leppilahti J. Short- to mid-term results of metallic press-fit radial head arthroplasty in unstable injuries of the elbow. J Bone Jt Surg Ser B. 2012;94(B):805–10.
37. Popovic N, Lemaire R, Georis P, Gillet P. Midterm results with a bipolar radial head prosthesis: radiographic evidence of loosening at the bone-cement interface. J Bone Jt Surg - Ser A. 2007;89: 2469–76.
38. Dotzis A, Cochu G, Mabit C, Charissoux JL, Arnaud JP. Comminuted fractures of the radial head treated by the Judet floating radial head prosthesis. J Bone Jt Surg Ser B. 2006;88:760–4.
39. Doornberg JN, Parisien R, Van Duijn PJ, Ring D. Radial head arthroplasty with a modular metal spacer to treat acute traumatic elbow instability. J Bone Jt Surg. Ser A. 2007;89:1075–80.
40. O'Driscoll S, Herald J. Forearm pain associated with loose radial head prosthesis. J Shoulder Elb Surg. 2012;21:92–7.
41. Mellema JJ, Lindenhovius ALC, Jupiter JB. The posttraumatic stiff elbow: an update. Curr Rev Musculoskelet Med. 2016;9:190–8.
42. Veltman ES, Doornberg JN, Eygendaal D, van den Bekerom MPJ. Static progressive versus dynamic splinting for posttraumatic elbow stiffness: a systematic review of 232 patients. Arch Orthop Trauma Surg. 2015;135:613–7.
43. Salazar D, Golz A, Israel H, Marra G. Heterotopic ossification of the elbow treated with surgical resection: risk factors, bony ankylosis, and complications. Clin Orthop Relat Res. 2014;472:2269–75.
44. Yang YJ, et al. A meta-analysis of risk factors for heterotopic ossification after elbow trauma. Int J Clin Exp Med. 2016;9:5308–17.
45. Bowman SH, Barfield WR, Slone HS, Shealy GJ, Walton ZJ. The clinical implications of heterotopic ossification in patients treated with radial head replacement for trauma: a case series and review of the literature. J Orthop. 2016;13:272–7.
46. Van Glabbeek F, et al. Detrimental effects of overstuffing or understuffing with a radial head replacement in the medial collateral-ligament deficient elbow. J Bone Jt Surg. 2004;86:2629–35.
47. Cohn M, Glait SA, Sapienza A, Kwon YW. Radiocapitellar joint contact pressures following radial head arthroplasty. J Hand Surg Am. 2014;39: 1566–71.
48. Kim HM, Roush EP, Kiser C. Intraoperative fluoroscopic assessment of proper prosthetic radial head height. J Shoulder Elb Surg. 2016;25:1874–81.
49. Athwal GS, et al. Determination of correct implant size in radial head arthroplasty to avoid overlengthening: surgical technique. J Bone Jt Surg Ser A. 2010;92:250–7.
50. Marinelli A, Guerra E, Ritali A, Cavallo M, Rotini R. Radial head prosthesis: surgical tips and tricks. Musculoskelet Surg. 2017;101:187–96.
51. Allavena C, et al. Outcomes of bipolar radial head prosthesis to treat complex radial head fractures in 22 patients with a mean follow-up of 50 months. Orthop Traumatol Surg Res. 2014;100:703–9.
52. Halls AA, Travill A. Transmission of pressures across the elbow joint. Anat Rec. 1964;150:243–7.
53. Rahmi H, et al. Clinical outcomes of anconeus interposition arthroplasty after radial head resection in native and prosthetic radial heads. J Shoulder Elb Surg. 2018;27:S29–34.
54. Factor S, et al. Radial head excision and Achilles allograft interposition arthroplasty for the treatment of chronic pediatric radiocapitellar pathologies: a report of four cases. Shoulder Elb. 2020:1758573219897859. https://doi.org/10.1177/1758573219897859.
55. Neuhaus V, et al. Radial head prosthesis removal: a retrospective case series of 14 patients. Arch Bone Jt Surg. 2015;88:88–93.
56. Wang X, Fukui K, Yokoyama M, Tsuchiya M, Kaneuji A. Postoperative infection of elbow joint replacement. Transl Surg. 2013;3:57–61.
57. Kunutsor SK, Beswick AD, Whitehouse MR, Blom AW. One- and two-stage surgical revision of infected elbow prostheses following total joint replacement: a systematic review. BMC Musculoskelet Disord. 2019;20:1–9.

58. Kachooei AR, et al. Intraoperative physical examination for diagnosis of interosseous ligament rupture - cadaveric study. J Hand Surg Am. 2015;40:1785–1790.e1.
59. Antuña SA, Sánchez-Márquez JM, Barco R. Long-term results of radial head resection following isolated radial head fractures in patients younger than forty years old. J Bone Jt Surg Ser A. 2010;92:558–66.
60. Kachooei AR, Baradaran A, Ebrahimzadeh MH, van Dijk CN, Chen N. The rate of radial head prosthesis removal or revision: a systematic review and meta-analysis. J Hand Surg Am. 2018;43:39–53.e1.

# Part III

# Total Wrist Arthroplasty

# Design Considerations for Total Wrist Arthroplasty

# 7

Susanne M. Roberts, Joseph J. Crisco III, and Scott W. Wolfe

## Introduction

The history of total wrist arthroplasty (TWA) has been fraught with obstacles and continues to evolve. Despite early failures, total wrist prosthetic design has undergone a series of iterative modifications over the past 3 years that have enhanced durability and decreased complications. A firm understanding of the evolution of TWA design is central to appropriate use of the available implants and provides an important body of knowledge to advance the design of the next generation of TWA implants.

The first reported resection arthroplasty was performed in 1762 by a physician in the Prussian army, Dr. Johann Ulrich Beyer. However, the first implant arthroplasty was performed in 1890 by the German physician Dr. Themistocles Gluck. Gluck performed TWA on a 19-year-old patient with tuberculosis of the wrist using an ivory ball-and-socket design with two pegs in the metacarpals and two into the radius and ulna. Ivory was used for the design material as it was thought to incorporate into bone with minimal inflammatory response. While the patient reportedly had good pain relief and maintained a satisfactory range of motion, the wrist ultimately developed a chronic tuberculous fistula and failed [1]. Since that time, TWA has made important advancements in biocompatibility, kinematics, soft tissue management, and fixation. These innovations have gradually improved the clinical outcomes, survivorship, and decreased complication rates. Novel techniques that investigate the in vivo performance of TWA may enable the development of more durable wrist prosthetic solutions for a broad range of diagnoses.

S. M. Roberts
Division of Hand and Upper Extremity Surgery, Department of Orthopedic Surgery, Columbia University Medical Center, New York, NY, USA
e-mail: Sr3493@cumc.columbia.edu

J. J. Crisco III
Bioengineering Laboratory, Department of Orthopaedics, The Warren Alpert Medical School of Brown University and Rhode Island Hospital, Providence, RI, USA
e-mail: joseph_crisco@brown.edu

S. W. Wolfe (✉)
Hand and Upper Extremity Division, Hospital for Special Surgery, Department of Orthopedic Surgery, Weill Cornell Medicine, New York, NY, USA
e-mail: WolfeS@HSS.EDU

## First-Generation Implants

The first widely used TWA implant was designed by Swanson in 1967. Similar to current successful metacarpophalangeal implants, this design featured a one-piece implant with a distal and proximal stem and a flexible-hinged central portion composed entirely of silicone rubber [2]. The implant served primarily as an interpositional spacer to maintain radiocarpal height



G. J. W. King, M. Rizzo (eds.), *Arthroplasty of the Upper Extremity*,
https://doi.org/10.1007/978-3-030-68880-6_7

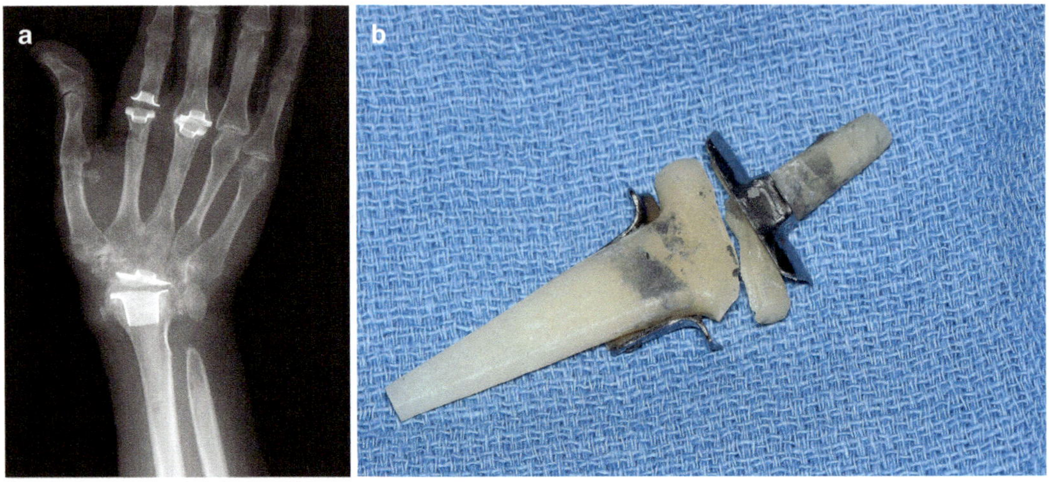


**Fig. 7.1** (**a**) A one-piece Swanson silastic wrist implant with grommets. (**b**) An excised silicone wrist implant following prosthetic fracture at the junction of the hinge and the distal stem. (With permission from Rizzo [4])

following resection of the proximal carpal row. The implant's proximal stem was inserted into the radius and the distal stem into the capitate and third metacarpal. The stems were not fixed proximally and distally, so as to "piston" within the medullary canals during flexion and extension [3]. Later iterations of the implant utilized a shorter, wider stem with metal grommets that were intended to protect the stems from wear and breakage due to bony abrasions (Fig. 7.1a).

Early results of this prosthesis were promising with regard to pain relief and range of motion. A retrospective study by Swanson of 170 silastic TWA implants in 129 patients at 4 years postoperatively showed complete pain relief in 90% of patients. The average range of motion was 34° of flexion and 26° of extension. Despite this, 25 wrists (14%) required revision surgery, 9 for implant fracture, and the remainder for tendon imbalance and synovitis [5] (Fig. 7.1b). Fatti et al. reported similar results in their short-term follow-up of 53 Swanson implants in 42 patients. In those followed less than 2.5 years, 77% had good or excellent results, while in those followed for greater than 2.5 years, only 61% had good or excellent results [6]. Longer-term results by the same authors demonstrated worsening outcomes, with silicone synovitis, implant fracture, and tendon imbalance being the prevalent complications. In a report of 39 wrists at an average of 5.8 years of follow-up, only 26% had good or excellent results. Implant fracture was seen in 14 prostheses (36%), and 9 of these required revision [7].

A study by Jolly and his colleagues similarly showed implant fracture rate of 52% in patients followed for 6 years. These fractures commonly occurred at the junction of the distal stem and the insertion point within the carpus and third metacarpal [8]. Ulnar deviation and loss of the ulnar shoulder were frequently seen with fracture of the stem, emphasizing the importance of tendon balance to the success of this implant. Silicone synovitis was reported in 30%, and was thought to be generated from particulate wear [9]. This was demonstrated radiographically as cystic changes and osteolysis about the prosthesis, and on histopathology as a foreign body reaction to refractile material that was consistent with silicone debris.

It became evident that a hinged device with a single degree of freedom (flexion-extension) is incompatible with the complex mobility of the human wrist, resulting in extreme stress on the implant with wear debris and fracture. Despite these complications, their relationship to clinical outcomes was not clear. Kistler and colleagues reviewed 27 Swanson implants at a minimum 10-year follow-up and found 19 patients reported good or excellent results despite obvious implant fractures and silicone synovitis [10]. Much like fractured MPJ and PIP hinged arthroplasties,

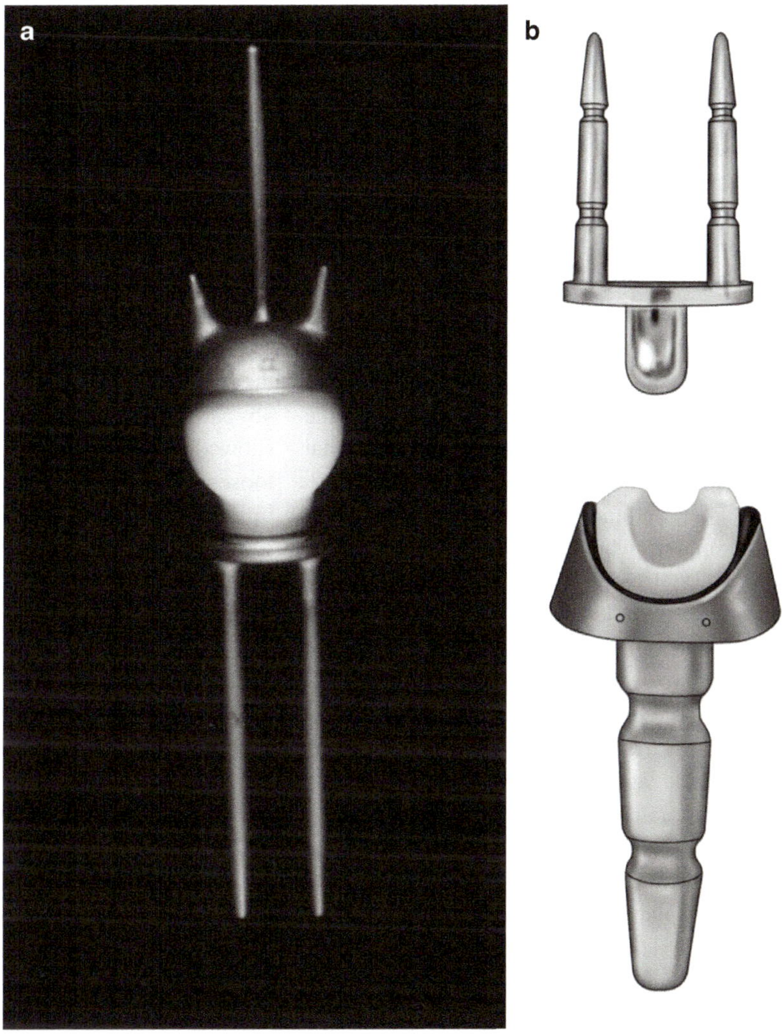


**Fig. 7.2** (**a**) Meuli III prosthesis and (**b**) Volz prosthesis (pending drawing)

those Swanson implants that survived continued to provide pain relief, and patients maintained a 43-degree arc of flexion-extension. The authors concluded that silicone implants may still be a reasonable option for very low-demand, elderly patients with rheumatoid arthritis and severe deformity or bony erosion.

## Second-Generation Implants

With the development of improved technology for metal-on-plastic total hip and knee replacements, the second generation of TWA implants attempted to reproduce this success in the wrist. Two representative examples of this generation are the Meuli prosthesis (1970) (Fig. 7.2) and the Volz (1973). The shortcomings of this generation can be attributed to their inability to reproduce normal wrist kinematics, resulting in high bone/implant interface stresses leading to component loosening, dislocation, and metacarpal cutout.

Meuli's original design consisted of a polyester ball-and-socket with malleable metal forks for distal fixation in the second and third metacarpals. The radial component was uncemented. The metal forks allowed the surgeon to flex the distal component in order to position its center of rotation (COR) more volar. His second and third iterations included ultra-high-molecular-weight polyethylene and eccentric prongs, to position the COR more ulnar [11]. Meuli's study of 41 original implants demonstrated 15 failures requiring reoperation. These were primarily attributed to technical errors in centering of the prosthesis, which was deemed critical in order to reproduce the wrist's presumed fixed center of rotation [12]. A subsequent study of the Meuli III prosthesis in 45 patients at an average of 4.5 years showed that the 11 of 49 wrists that failed due to component loosening all had malpositioning of the carpal component [13]. A study by Vogelin and Nagy of all three Meuli implant designs attributed the majority of failures to loosening of the distal component and metacarpal perforation [14]. Cooney reviewed the Mayo experience with 140 Meuli implants which demonstrated a revision rate of 33%. Complications consisted of 8.6% dislocations, 2.9% loosening, and 12.1% soft tissue contracture. The authors concluded failure of this implant to be due to three main factors: malposition of the carpal component, implant fixation, and soft tissue imbalance. They ultimately recommended against its use due to the high complication rates [15].

From a design perspective, we know now that the normal wrist has a mobile center of rotation for different planes of motion (flexion-extension, radioulnar deviation, and dart throwers) and rotation axes that shift depending on the direction of motion (coronal/sagittal or coupled motions) [16, 17]. Meuli considered the wrist to be a biaxial joint with a fixed center of rotation (COR) in the capitate head [12]. He considered his ball-and-socket design to be "unconstrained," which is technically true in rotation. But the normal wrist is not a ball-and-socket, and the considerable translational forces of normal wrist motion must be transferred to the prosthesis and to its implant-bone interface. In addition, a ball-and-socket has no restraint to axial rotation as does a normal wrist. Consequently, each of the Meuli designs had a high failure rate, which occurred predominantly with loss of fixation of the distal component.

Shortly after Meuli's initial design was released, Robert G. Volz developed a prosthesis at Arizona Medical Center that consisted of a semi-constrained, cobalt-chrome on polyethylene implant. The Volz/AMC prosthesis had a metacarpal component that fit through the capitate into the third metacarpal, featuring a cobalt-chrome hemispherical articulation with two different radii to allow for more flexion and extension than radial and ulnar deviation. This articulation was designed to constrain axial rotation. The cemented radial component had a polyethylene concave surface [18]. Volz stressed the importance of soft tissue balancing for success of the prosthesis. Volz' early study of 50 implants in 45 patients with a follow-up of 6–34 months showed good results with no reports of infection, loosening, or increased pain. There were two immediate dislocations attributed to incomplete release of the contracted volar capsule. The most prevalent complications were ulnar deviation, which was attributed to ulnar settling of the radial component, and consequent shifting of the COR. The authors recommended transfer of the extensor carpi ulnaris tendon to the base of the fourth metacarpal to lessen the ulnar moment on the prosthesis. In a later study by Volz, 25 implants in patients with rheumatoid arthritis demonstrated good results, without complications of loosening, dislocation, or imbalance in a follow-up period of 6 months to 6.7 years [19]. Gellman et al. reviewed their experience with 14 wrists which showed component migration and radiographic loosening in 7 patients with 2 dislocations. These complications were attributed to errors in soft tissue balancing and inability to match normal wrist kinematics [20].

Figgie, Ranawat, and Inglis subsequently introduced their semi-constrained "sloppy hinge" ball-and-socket Trispherical implant (Fig. 7.3). Their design consisted of a radial component featuring a spherical head articulating with a high-density polyethylene metacarpal socket and linked by a loose axle restraint, primarily oriented in the radial-ulnar direction. The axle primarily permitted flexion-extension, while the "sloppiness" of the hinge allowed radioulnar and composite motions simultaneously reducing stress on the implant. The metacarpal component was composed of large third metacarpal stem and a smaller offset stem inserted into the scaphoid

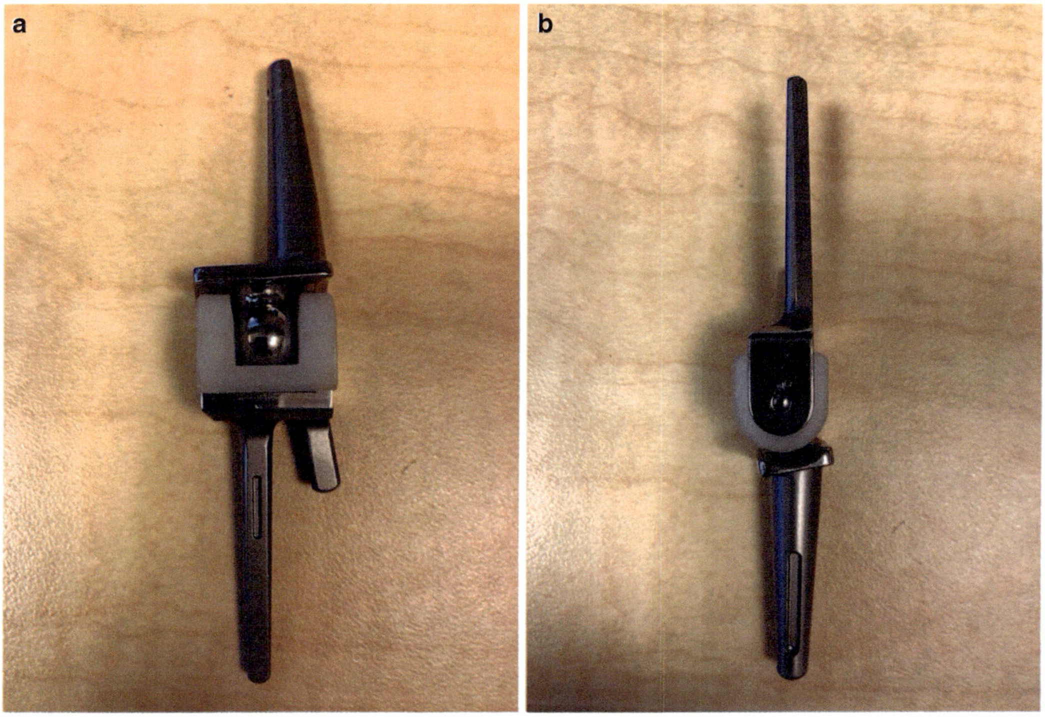


Fig. 7.3 (a) Trispherical implant with "sloppy hinge" ball-and-socket. (b) Lateral view of the Trispherical implant. Note the 12 degrees of palmar tilt of the radial implant

and second metacarpal. The radial component had a 12-degree volar tilt, and the radial stem was offset radialward, with the intent to restore the carpal COR to the proximal capitate position [21]. Both components were cemented. In their retrospective study of 35 cases with an average follow-up of 9 years, 7 patients had implant loosening and 3 with carpal component migration [22]. Their follow-up study demonstrated 8 failures out of 87 wrists, 6 of which were mechanical failures attributed to loosening and dorsal perforation of the carpal component. Ultimately, while "semi-constrained" and allowing a moving COR, these mechanisms could not replicate normal carpal kinematics, which likely was the cause of the failures.

## Third-Generation Implants

Third-generation implants improved on previous generations with the goals of minimizing bony resection and reproducing the normal wrist's normal kinematics, thus improving durability. There are three main implants that characterize this generation, the Biaxial, the Universal and related Freedom prostheses, and the ReMotion prosthesis. These implants essentially replace the radiocarpal articulation with an unlinked partially constrained articulating shape. This generation of implants shares several features: unlinked, elliptical, or toroidal articulations, screw fixation of the carpal component, and porous coating of the implant stems.

The Biaxial implant was a freely articulating cobalt-chrome on a high-density polyethylene implant (Fig. 7.4). The carpal component had one major stem in the third metacarpal and one minor stem in the trapezoid to improve rotational stability. The implant featured an ellipsoidal metallic head to articulate with a concave polyethylene bearing surface on the radial component. This ellipsoidal shape was designed in an effort to better match the predominantly biaxial radiocarpal motion. The radial component was ulnarly and palmarly offset to attempt to simulate the native

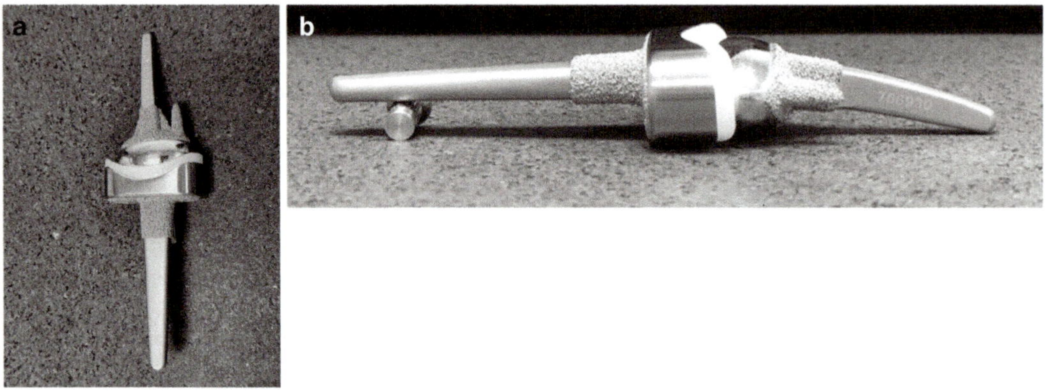


**Fig. 7.4** The Biaxial total wrist implant. Note the distal metal, proximal polyethylene configuration, and the ellipsoidal shape of the articulating surface

COR [11]. In a retrospective review of 57 cases with an average follow-up of 6.5 years, Cobb and Beckenbaugh showed improvements in pain, range of motion, and grip strength. They reported six operative complications; most of these involved stem perforation of the third metacarpal. Eleven failures were reported, including 8 cases of carpal component loosening [23]. Rizzo and Beckenbaugh also reviewed their experience in a smaller cohort of 17 patients. They were concerned that the elongated third metacarpal stem increased bone/implant stress and was technically difficult to insert [24]. A larger study by Takwale et al. in 76 implants found that the recommended alignment of the third metacarpal stem in extension leads to loosening and migration of the carpal implant [25]. Given the high percentage of distal implant loosening, the authors recommended this prosthesis only be used in very low-demand patients and with close follow-up.

The Universal 1, described by Menon in 1998, was an unlinked implant featuring a toroidal-shaped high-density polyethylene carpal component with three-screw fixation distally to help prevent loosening. The radial component stem was a tapered "T" shape in cross section, coated with titanium mesh for bony ingrowth. The distal component was anchored by a titanium plate with a central capitate screw into the third metacarpal and flanked by two screws in the second metacarpal and hamate. Like the Trispherical, the radial component had a palmar inclination to mimic the normal distal radius, and it had a deep articulating concavity to enhance stability. Menon retrospectively reviewed 37 Universal 1 implants in 31 patients with an average follow-up of 6.7 years and showed significant increases in wrist extension, radial deviation, and pain relief compared to preoperative values in 88% of patients. However, there was a 32% complication rate with 5 volar dislocations of the carpal component [26]. A prospective study by Divelbiss and colleagues of 22 implants in 19 patients with 1–2 years of follow-up showed improved range of motion, DASH scores, and pain relief but a 14% complication rate due to resorption, loosening, and dislocation [27]. A 5–10-year follow-up study by Ward et al. demonstrated a 50% revision rate in patients with rheumatoid arthritis. Equally concerning is the fact that all revised wrists showed evidence of polyethylene wear, metallosis, and component loosening [28].

The high dislocation rate, combined with loosening and particulate wear, focused attention on the shape of the articulation, prompting iterative alterations in the Universal prosthesis. The Universal 2 prosthesis, introduced in 2001, featured a distal elliptical articulating surface with increased contact surface area with the intent to distribute articular forces, decrease the stress on carpal component fixation, and produce lower polyethylene wear (Fig. 7.5a, b). In addition to these design innovations, the widespread use of

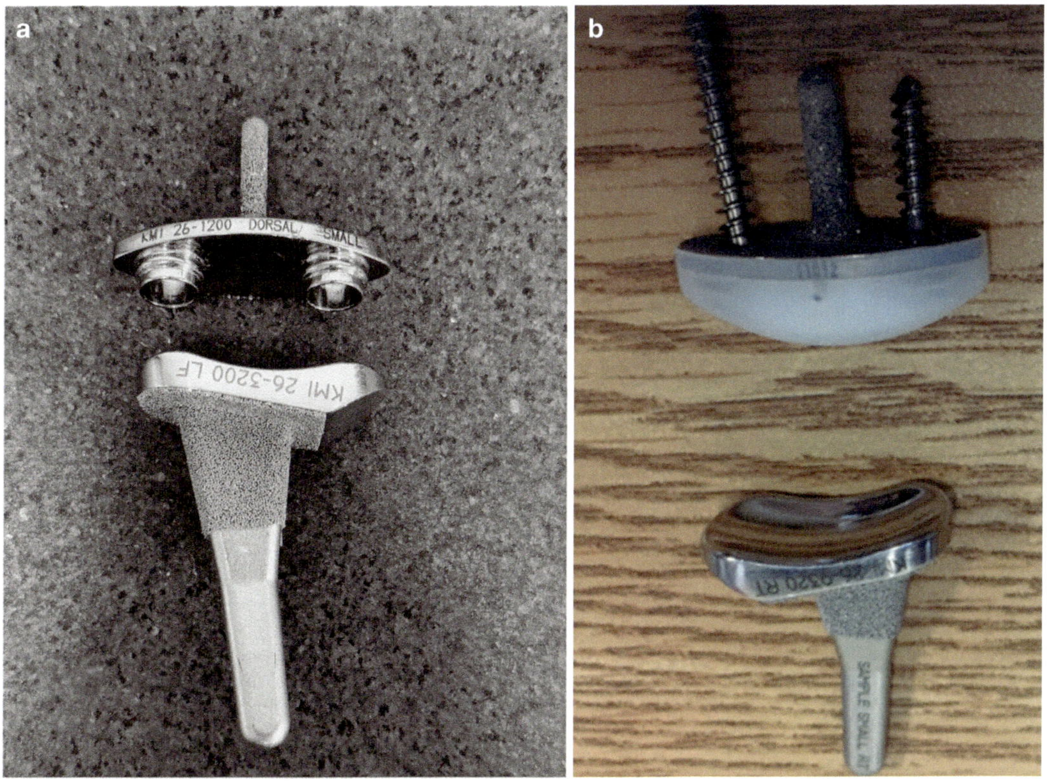


**Fig. 7.5** (**a–b**) The Universal 2 total wrist implant. (**a**) Disarticulated radial and carpal components. Note the porous coating and the central peg of the distal component. (**b**) Note the distal polyethylene ellipsoid bearing surface on the carpal component, with the two variable angle screws flanking the central peg

disease-modifying antirheumatic drugs (DMARDs) for inflammatory arthritis in the early 2000s helped to nearly eliminate implant dislocation by limiting preoperative bone erosion and soft tissue attenuation.

Comparatively, the elliptical shape of the bearing surface is the primary improvement of the Universal 2 from its predecessor. This elliptical shape improved centralization and prosthetic contact throughout the arc of motion [29]. The radial stem still featured an in-growth cobalt-chromium articular surface, while distal fixation was changed to a central, in-growth stem for the capitate instead of the central screw of the Universal 1. The central stem was bordered by two variable angle locking screws. Several small retrospective series reported improvements in outcomes with the Universal 2 system. Though mostly short- and mid-term follow-up studies (none over 5.5 years), the authors report a relatively low incidence (range 0–11%) of early loosening requiring revision, and minimal reports of instability [30–32].

The "Freedom" TWA was introduced in 2015 as third iteration of the Universal design with a narrower radial tray and modifications of the bearing surface to enable "more rotational and translational freedom" (Fig. 7.6a, b). In addition, there are locking caps for the variable angle locking screws in the carpal component to prevent loosening. We were unable to identify published data on clinical outcomes of the Freedom wrist.

The ReMotion TWA system, introduced in 2005, also relies on an elliptical articulation, intended to decrease contact stress, and incorporates a mobile bearing design on the carpal side (Fig. 7.7a, b). This "bipolar" carpal component allows for an additional 10° of axial rotation, further dispersing torsional stress in an effort to decrease distal component loosening.

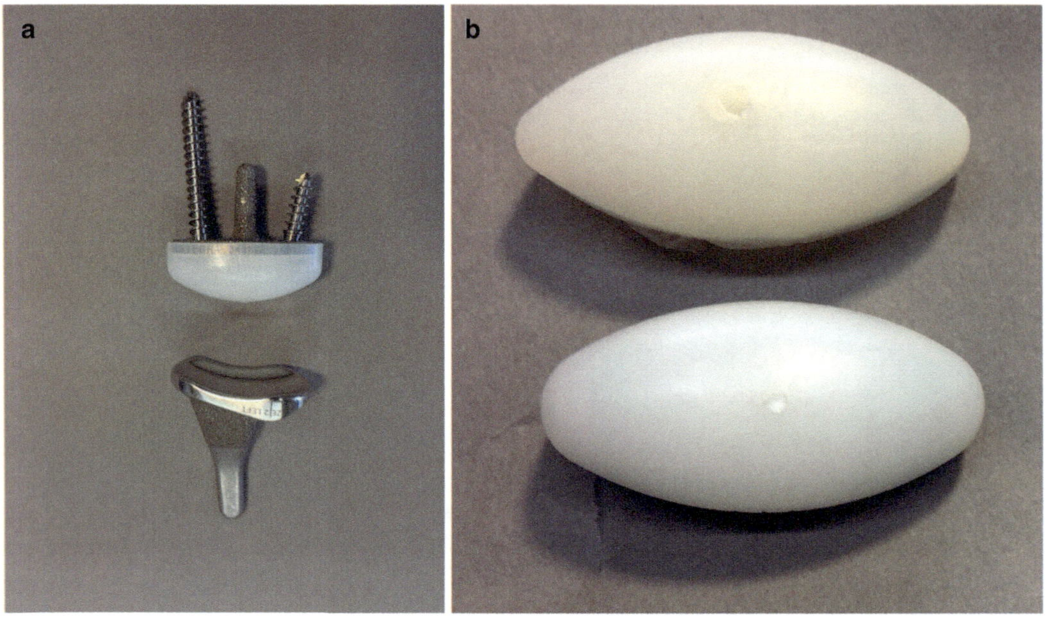


**Fig. 7.6** (**a**–**b**) The Freedom total wrist implant. (**a**) Assembled carpal and radial components. Note the more shallow radial component. (**b**) Change in shape of the bearing surface from the Universal 2 (top) to the Freedom wrist (below)

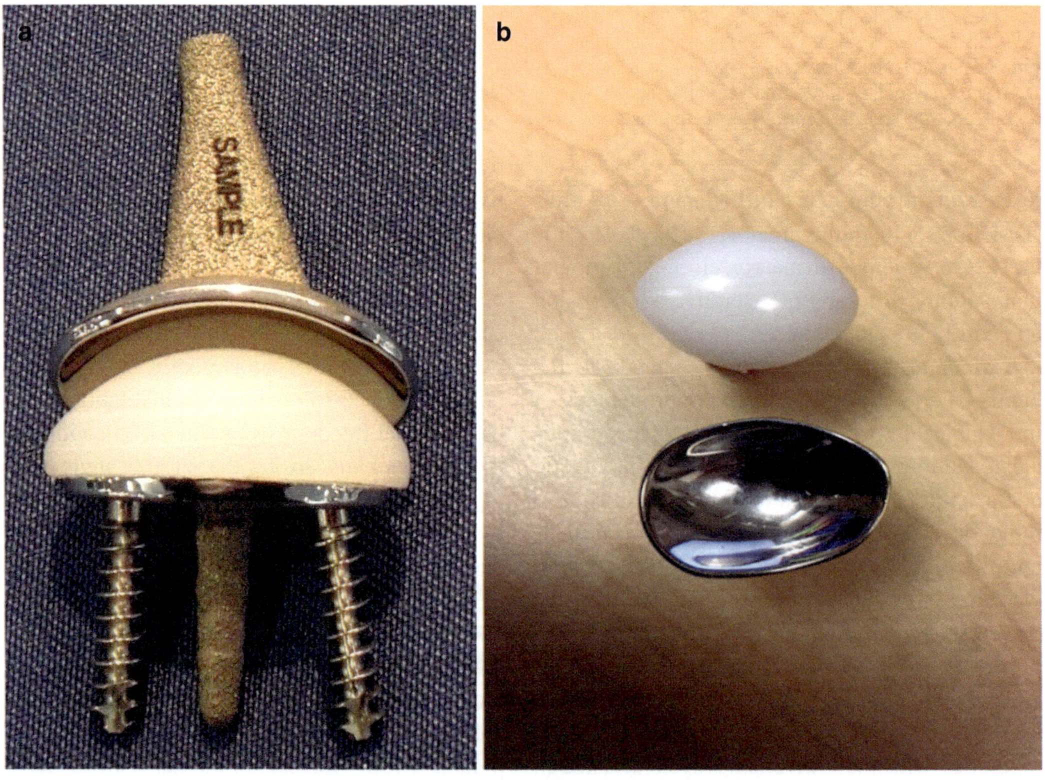


**Fig. 7.7** (**a**) The ReMotion total wrist. (With permission from Rizzo [4]) (**b**) Exploded view of the carpal bearing and the radiocarpal articulating surface

Herzberg et al. prospectively followed 129 RA and 86 non-RA patients for 2 years and reported 92% survivorship with 5 and 6% incidence of complications (defined as a return to the operating room) [33]. Boeckstyns et al. reported similar 90% survivorship at 5–9-year follow-up, a significant improvement from previous designs [34]. Both authors reported asymptomatic radiolucencies >2 mm about the radial and carpal components in 41% [35]. A subsequent histological study showed that particulate debris (polyethylene wear) was not identified in the cases with periarticular osteolysis and that most lucencies stabilized within 3 years of implantation. The authors theorized stress shielding as causation but recommended close follow-up of these cases [36].

Cooney et al. performed a comparative study between the Universal 2, ReMotion, and Biaxial TWA, and although small, the Universal 2 cohort exhibited trends of superiority via DASH. It is important to note, however, that the study was underpowered to detect differences among prostheses, so statistically backed conclusions could not be made [37]. As a group, the third-generation implants feature a biaxial articular design that replaces the radial articular surface. Consequently, normal wrist motion is replaced by motion predominantly in the orthogonal planes of flexion-extension and radioulnar deviation, with limited arcs of circumduction (20% of normal) and dart-throwing motion [38]. Replacement of the proximal carpal row with a large elliptical surface moves the center of rotation (COR) away from the anatomic center, and may increase the stresses on carpal component fixation due to a longer moment arm. Large cohorts of total wrist arthroplasty demonstrate that replacement essentially restores preoperative motion but does not increase range of motion [34]. In fact, only one design of total wrist arthroplasty, the Maestro, actually met the minimum ROM criteria for functional activities calculated by Palmer et al. [39, 40].

## Fourth-Generation Implants

Unlike modern total knee and total hip arthroplasty, which is designed by evaluation of large in vivo kinematic data sets, the evolution of total wrist arthroplasty has been largely empiric. The newest generation of TWAs departs from their predecessors focusing on restoring the complexity of native wrist kinematics. Recent computational analyses based upon detailed kinematic data captured with biplane videoradiography of patients with a representative third-generation TWA design found that the center of rotations was located at the center of curvatures of the ellipsoidal shape of the carpal component during flexion-extension and radial-ulnar deviation [17]. During coupled motions such as the "dart thrower's" motion, the COR shifts that occurred between the biaxial motions and the coupled motions were twice that of the wrists of normal volunteers. Kinematic studies of total joint prostheses in other major joints have shown that mismatches between the native and prosthetic kinematics can lead to increased loads on the implant and bone/implant interface, and are associated with component loosening and failure [41]. Attempts to more precisely recreate the native patterns of COR in total wrist design will hopefully yield better implant survivorship.

The Maestro total wrist (Biomet, Warsaw, IN) while relying on a broader contact area was designed to simulate the curvature of the distal carpal row (Fig. 7.8a, b). Like the Biaxial total wrist prosthesis and that of most major joints (hip, shoulder, knee), the Maestro has the convex cobalt-chromium articulation on the carpal side, with a broad congruent high-density polyethylene concave articulating surface on the radial side. The portion of the implants closest to the articular surfaces is porous, while the stems (both radial and capitate) are plasma-sprayed to promote bony ingrowth. While this prosthesis makes an important step toward restoring midcarpal kinematics and improving overall motion, there is no available data on its kinematic patterns during orthogonal or coupled motions. Nydick et al. reported that 75% of 23 patients experienced complete pain relief at 28-month follow-up, with a mean flexion-extension arc of 90 degrees [42]. While the Maestro showed initial early promise, it was withdrawn from the market in 2019.

The Motec total wrist (Swemac Innovation AB, Linköping, Sweden) is a cement-optional ball-and-socket arthroplasty that is available in

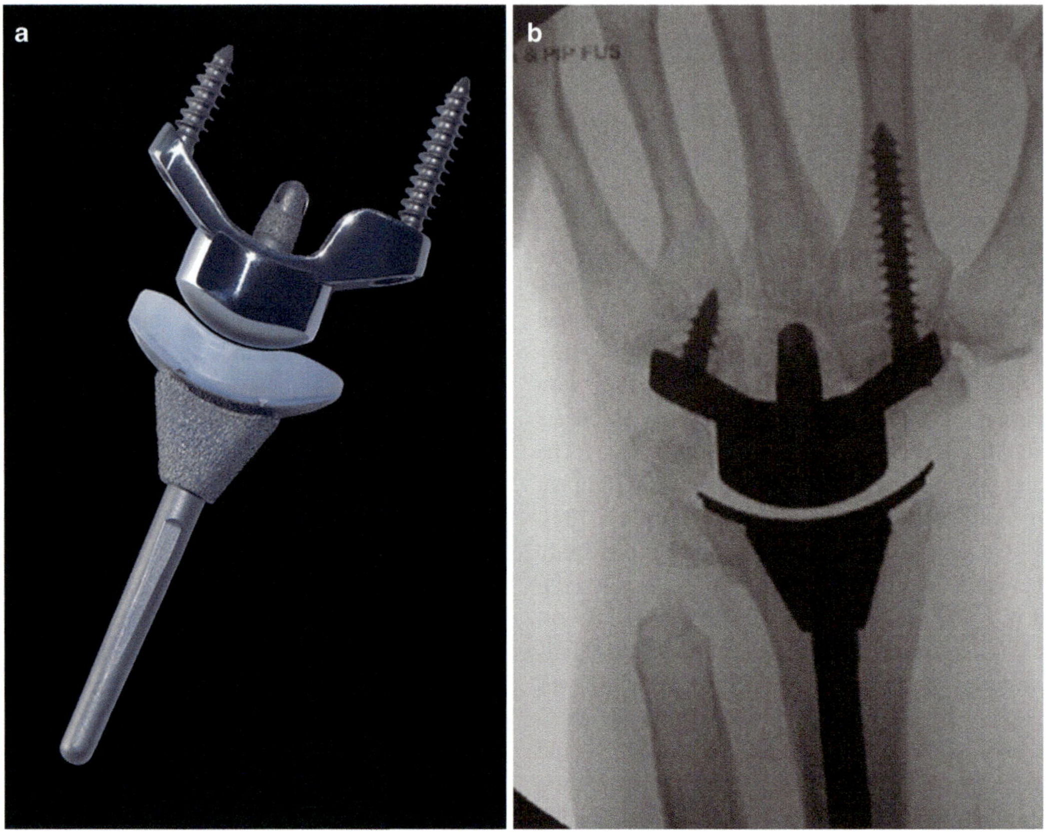

**Fig. 7.8** (**a**) The Maestro total wrist implant. Note the proximal polyethylene surface on the radial component. (Copyright Zimmer Biomet, Warsaw, IN.) (**b**) Fluoroscopic view of an implanted Maestro prosthesis, demonstrating the unique articular bearing surface, designed to better simulate the distal carpal row. (Copyright 2020, Andrew K. Palmer, MD)

both metal-on-PEEK and metal-on-metal articulations. Fixation into the radius and third metacarpal is aided by grit-blasted calcium phosphate-coated screws (Fig. 7.9a, b). Reigstad et al. performed a study in high-demand patients which demonstrated an increase range of motion and grip strength with a 10-year Kaplan-Meier survival of 86% [43]. In Yeoh and Tourret's systematic review, the Motec device had the best postoperative DASH scores of seven different modern prostheses [39]. While loosening is the most common reported complication of the Motec, metal-on-metal wear has been reported and may serve as a future weakness in this system [43, 44]. The strength of distal fixation via a long third metacarpal stem appears to be an advantage of the Motec, though the long-term fate of a ball-and-socket design remains to be seen, given the lack of rotational constraint, and the failed history of previous ball-and-socket designs.

In a starkly innovative departure from the historical implants, the Amandys Wrist Spacer (Palex Medical SA, Madrid, Spain) is a single-component interposition pyrocarbon implant (Fig. 7.10a, b). This implant has a quadri-elliptical shape, thus convex on all surfaces as opposed to distal convexity. The bony surfaces in contact with the implant are designed to slide, roll, and even rotate slightly especially at the carpal side. The implant replaces the lunate, proximal two thirds of the scaphoid and part of the capitate head only. This allows for very minimal osseous resection, especially of the distal scaphoid and triquetrum. As such, the procedure spares

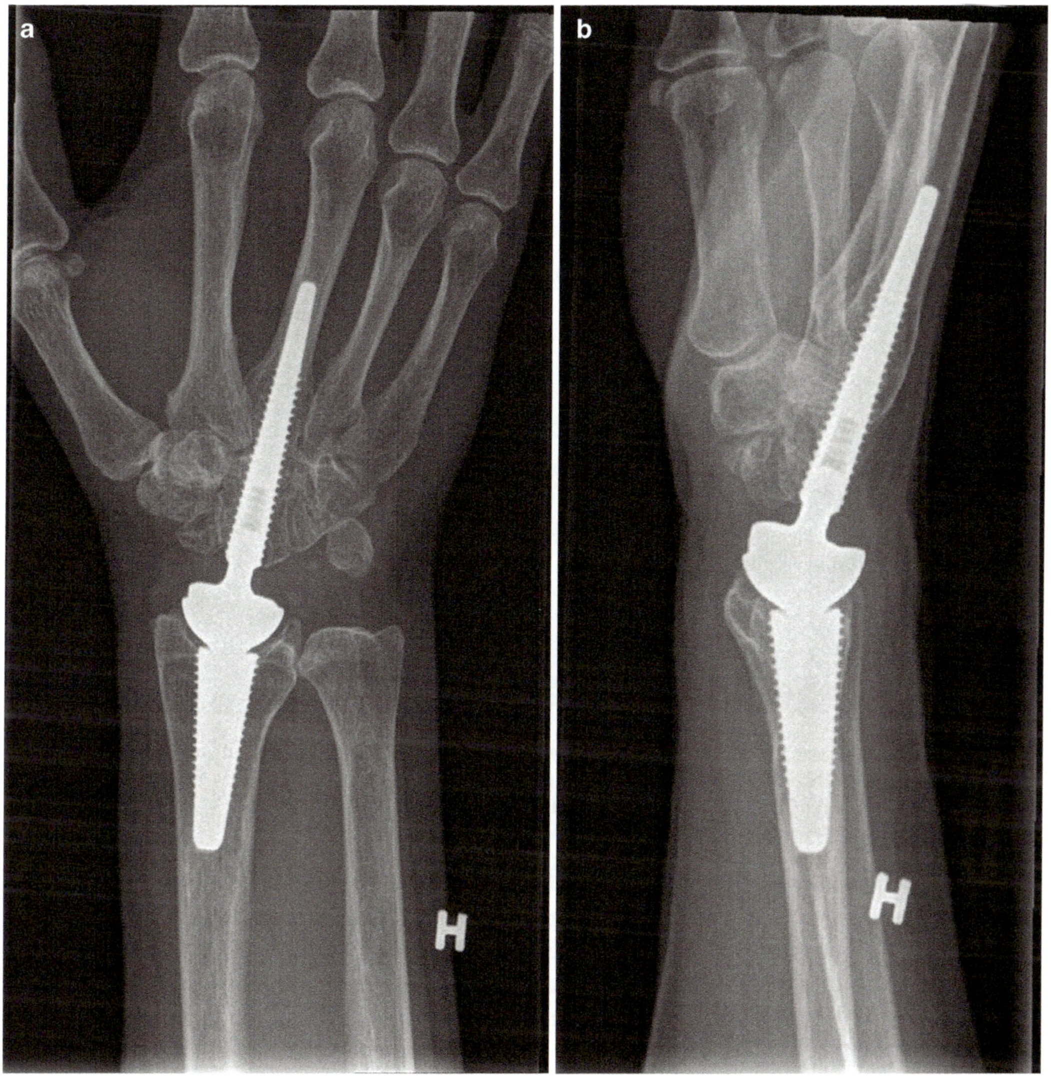


**Fig. 7.9** (**a**) Posteroanterior and (**b**) lateral radiographs of the Motec total wrist, 5 years following implantation. (Courtesy, Ole Reigstad, MD, 2020)

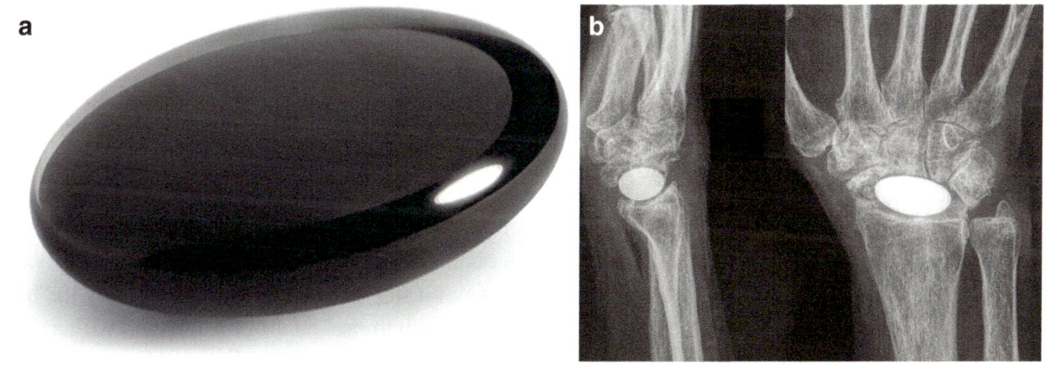


**Fig. 7.10** (**a–b**) The Amandys Wrist Spacer. (**a**) The pyrocarbon implant. (**b**) Lateral and PA of the implanted prosthesis following excision of a portion of the proximal carpal row and midcarpal joint. (Copyright, 2020, Philippe Bellemère, MD)

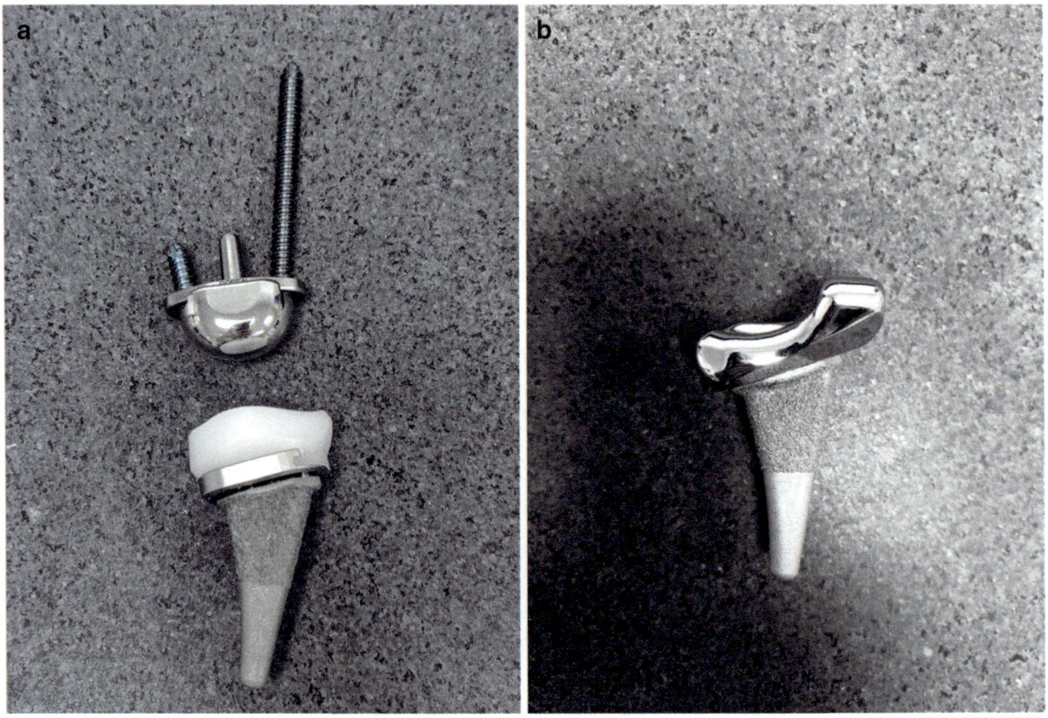

**Fig. 7.11** (**a–b**) The KinematX hemiarthroplasty shown is a monobloc design that was computer designed to mimic native midcarpal articulation. (**a**) Dorsal view. (**b**) Palmar view. Note the truncated simulation of the scaphoid tubercle. (Copyright 2020, Scott W. Wolfe, MD, Joseph J. Crisco, III., Ph.D.)

most of the extrinsic wrist ligaments with the goal of preserving the "dart thrower's" motion. Early studies did not show significant increases in range of motion or grip strength postoperatively [45, 46]. However, there were significant improvements in *Quick*DASH and PWRE pain scores [47]. Further follow-up of this design concept is needed.

Lastly, the KinematX hemiarthroplasty is a novel approach to radiocarpal arthritis that is the first solution for SLAC arthritis that increases wrist range of motion while preserving both biaxial and coupled ranges of motion [48]. It is indicated in active patients with preserved cartilage on the capitate and hamate, such as scapholunate advanced collapse (SLAC) stages I and II, and early SLAC III; Kienböck disease; and post-traumatic radiocarpal arthritis. The coated radial prosthesis is cement-optional and replaces the arthritic proximal row with a monobloc design that was computer designed to mimic the native midcarpal articulation of 25 healthy volunteers. The device mimics a radio-scapholunate fusion, and incorporates removal of the distal scaphoid (Fig. 7.11a, b) [49]. Anatomic replacement of the proximal carpal row and maintenance of the native intrinsic and extrinsic ligaments help to maintain midcarpal coupled motions of circumduction and dart-throwing motion as well as the anatomic center of wrist rotation [48]. The single-component design has the added advantage of maintaining radial length and bone stock while avoiding a distal component altogether. Its modular design allows conversion to a KinematX total wrist arthroplasty (Fig. 7.12a, b) should painful capitate arthritis develop long term, by switching out the metal concave articular surface on the proximal component for a polyethylene one, and replacing the proximal capitate with a cobalt-chromium carpal component. The advantage of a stepwise approach is the ability to "buy time" with improved motion and pain with a simple hemireplacement while avoiding the distal carpal component and its risk profile altogether.

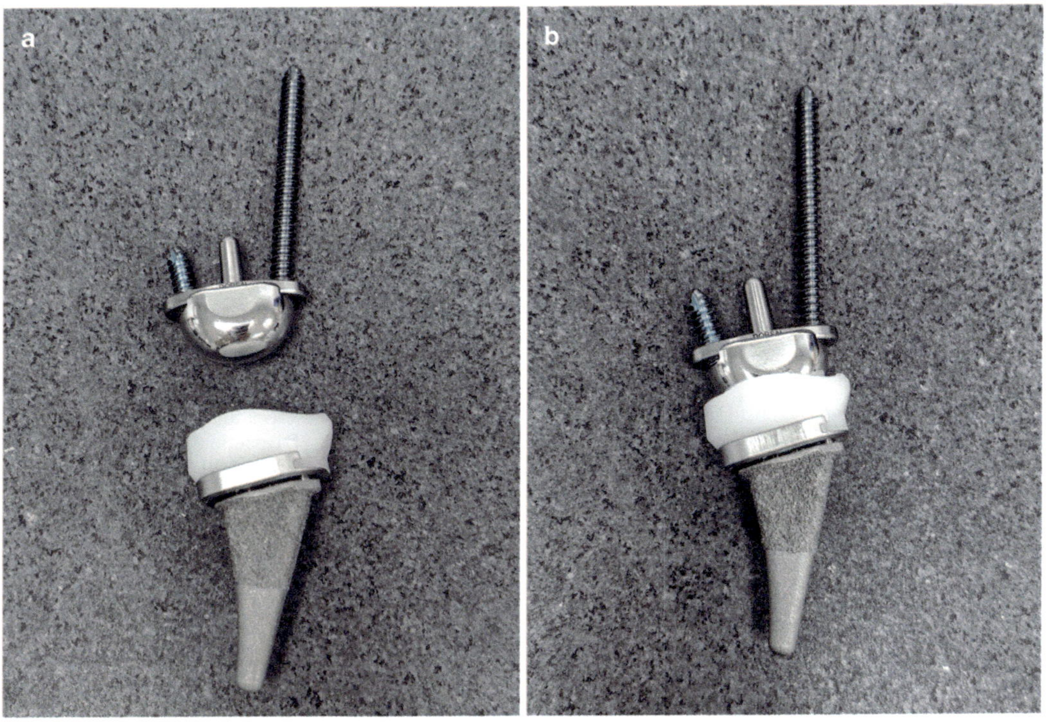

Fig. 7.12 (a–b) KinematX total wrist arthroplasty. (a) Note the distal cobalt-chrome carpal component, computer designed to emulate the midcarpal articulation. (b) The articulated modular prosthesis, with proximal polyethylene articular surface. (Copyright 2020, Scott W. Wolfe, MD, Joseph J. Crisco, III., Ph.D.)

When painful wear of the midcarpal joint becomes apparent, modular conversion to a total wrist can be performed while leaving the radial stem solidly fixed. In a prospective study of the KinematX hemiarthroplasty with 7 months of follow-up, the mean Mayo score increased from 31.9 to 58.8 postoperatively. The DASH score improved from 47.8 to 28.7 postoperatively [50]. Four-year outcomes of 20 patients demonstrated significant increases in flexion-extension and radioulnar deviation, grip strength, and Mayo and DASH scores. Two patients were converted to a total wrist arthroplasty and one to a fusion [51]. The modular procedure is promising but still relatively new and will require further long-term studies to determine its success and durability.

While the development of novel implants and the ability to measure in vivo 3D kinematics promise exciting new developments in total wrist arthroplasty, controversy remains regarding the clinical indications of TWA. Current indications include inflammatory arthritis, Kienböck disease, post-traumatic arthritis, and increasingly, SLAC arthritis. Whether durability will allow routine implantation of TWA in active and young patients remains to be seen. While TWA may not be indicated in all patients, select candidates may still benefit from achieving pain relief while maintaining wrist motion, especially in the short term. Maximizing outcomes in TWA is dependent not only on implant design, but appropriate indications and meticulous attention to bony and soft tissue reconstruction.

**Conflict of Interest** Scott W. Wolfe, MD; Joseph J. Crisco, III, Ph.D. consult for Extremity Medical, Inc. Parsippany, NJ

Note that the KinematX hemiarthroplasty, the Amandys implant, and the Motec implant are not FDA approved for implantation in the USA, while the KinematX total wrist arthroplasty is FDA approved for implantation in the USA.

## References


1. Ritt MJ, Stuart PR, Naggar L, Beckenbaugh RD. The early history of arthroplasty of the wrist. From amputation to total wrist implant. J Hand Surg Br. 1994;19(6):778–82.
2. Swanson AB. Flexible implant resection arthroplasty. Hand. 1972;4(2):119–34.
3. Swanson AB. Flexible implant arthroplasty for arthritic disabilities of the radiocarpal joint. A silicone rubber intramedullary stemmed flexible hinge implant for the wrist joint. Orthop Clin North Am. 1973;4(2):383–94.
4. Rizzo M. Wrist arthrodesis and arthroplasty. In: Wolfe SW, Hotchkiss RN, Pedersen WC, Kozin SH, Cohen MS, editors. Green's operative hand surgery. 7th ed. Philadelphia: Elsevier; 2017. p. 373–417.
5. Swanson AB, de Groot SG, Maupin BK. Flexible implant arthroplasty of the radiocarpal joint. Surgical technique and long-term study. Clin Orthop Relat Res. 1984;187:94–106.
6. Fatti JF, Palmer AK, Mosher JF. The long-term results of Swanson silicone rubber interpositional wrist arthroplasty. J Hand Surg Am. 1986;11(2):166–75.
7. Fatti JF, Palmer AK, Greenky S, Mosher JF. Long-term results of Swanson interpositional wrist arthroplasty: part II. J Hand Surg Am. 1991;16(3):432–7.
8. Jolly SL, Ferlic DC, Clayton ML, Dennis DA, Stringer EA. Swanson silicone arthroplasty of the wrist in rheumatoid arthritis: a long-term follow-up. J Hand Surg Am. 1992;17(1):142–9.
9. DeHeer DH, Owens SR, Swanson AB. The host response to silicone elastomer implants for small joint arthroplasty. J Hand Surg Am. 1995;20(3 Pt 2):S101–9.
10. Kistler U, Weiss AP, Simmen BR, Herren DB. Long-term results of silicone wrist arthroplasty in patients with rheumatoid arthritis. J Hand Surg Am. 2005;30(6):1282–7.
11. Kennedy CD, Huang JI. Prosthetic Design in Total Wrist Arthroplasty. Orthop Clin North Am. 2016;47(1):207–18.
12. Meuli HC. Arthroplasty of the wrist. Clin Orthop Relat Res. 1980;149:118–25.
13. Meuli HC, Fernandez DL. Uncemented total wrist arthroplasty. J Hand Surg Am. 1995;20(1):115–22.
14. Vogelin E, Nagy L. Fate of failed Meuli total wrist arthroplasty. J Hand Surg Br. 2003;28(1):61–8.
15. Cooney WP 3rd, Beckenbaugh RD, Linscheid RL. Total wrist arthroplasty. Problems with implant failures. Clin Orthop Relat Res. 1984;(187):121–8.
16. Crisco JJ, Heard WM, Rich RR, Paller DJ, Wolfe SW. The mechanical axes of the wrist are oriented obliquely to the anatomical axes. J Bone Joint Surg Am. 2011;93(2):169–77.
17. Akhbari B, Morton AM, Shah KN, Molino J, Moore DC, Weiss AC, et al. Proximal-distal shift of the center of rotation in a total wrist arthroplasty is more than twice of the healthy wrist. J Orthop Res. 2020;38(7):1575–86.
18. McBeath R, Osterman AL. Total wrist arthroplasty. Hand Clin. 2012;28(4):595–609.
19. Volz RG. Total wrist arthroplasty. A clinical review. Clin Orthop Relat Res. 1984;187:112–20.
20. Gellman H, Hontas R, Brumfield RH Jr, Tozzi J, Conaty JP. Total wrist arthroplasty in rheumatoid arthritis. A long-term clinical review. Clin Orthop Relat Res. 1997;342:71–6.
21. Figgie HE 3rd, Ranawat CS, Inglis AE, Straub LR, Mow C. Preliminary results of total wrist arthroplasty in rheumatoid arthritis using the Trispherical total wrist arthroplasty. J Arthroplast. 1988;3(1):9–15.
22. Figgie MP, Ranawat CS, Inglis AE, Sobel M, Figgie HE 3rd. Trispherical total wrist arthroplasty in rheumatoid arthritis. J Hand Surg Am. 1990;15(2):217–23.
23. Cobb TK, Beckenbaugh RD. Biaxial total-wrist arthroplasty. J Hand Surg Am. 1996;21(6):1011–21.
24. Rizzo M, Beckenbaugh RD. Results of biaxial total wrist arthroplasty with a modified (long) metacarpal stem. J Hand Surg Am. 2003;28(4):577–84.
25. Takwale VJ, Nuttall D, Trail IA, Stanley JK. Biaxial total wrist replacement in patients with rheumatoid arthritis. Clinical review, survivorship and radiological analysis. J Bone Joint Surg Br. 2002;84(5):692–9.
26. Menon J. Universal Total Wrist Implant: experience with a carpal component fixed with three screws. J Arthroplast. 1998;13(5):515–23.
27. Divelbiss BJ, Sollerman C, Adams BD. Early results of the Universal total wrist arthroplasty in rheumatoid arthritis. J Hand Surg Am. 2002;27(2):195–204.
28. Ward CM, Kuhl T, Adams BD. Five to ten-year outcomes of the Universal total wrist arthroplasty in patients with rheumatoid arthritis. J Bone Joint Surg Am. 2011;93(10):914–9.
29. Grosland NM, Rogge RD, Adams BD. Influence of articular geometry on prosthetic wrist stability. Clin Orthop Relat Res. 2004;421:134–42.
30. van Winterswijk PJ, Bakx PA. Promising clinical results of the universal total wrist prosthesis in rheumatoid arthritis. Open Orthop J. 2010;4:67–70.
31. Ferreres A, Lluch A, Del Valle M. Universal total wrist arthroplasty: midterm follow-up study. J Hand Surg Am. 2011;36(6):967–73.
32. Morapudi SP, Marlow WJ, Withers D, Ralte P, Gabr A, Waseem M. Total wrist arthroplasty using the Universal 2 prosthesis. J Orthop Surg (Hong Kong). 2012;20(3):365–8.
33. Herzberg G. Prospective study of a new total wrist arthroplasty: short term results. Chir Main. 2011;30(1):20–5.
34. Boeckstyns ME, Herzberg G, Merser S. Favorable results after total wrist arthroplasty: 65 wrists in 60 patients followed for 5-9 years. Acta Orthop. 2013;84(4):415–9.
35. Boeckstyns ME, Herzberg G. Periprosthetic osteolysis after total wrist arthroplasty. J Wrist Surg. 2014;3(2):101–6.

36. Boeckstyns ME, Toxvaerd A, Bansal M, Vadstrup LS. Wear particles and osteolysis in patients with total wrist arthroplasty. J Hand Surg Am. 2014;39(12):2396–404.
37. Cooney W, Manuel J, Froelich J, Rizzo M. Total wrist replacement: a retrospective comparative study. J Wrist Surg. 2012;1(2):165–72.
38. Singh HP, Bhattacharjee D, Dias JJ, Trail I. Dynamic assessment of the wrist after total wrist arthroplasty. J Hand Surg Eur Vol. 2017;42(6):573–9.
39. Yeoh D, Tourret L. Total wrist arthroplasty: a systematic review of the evidence from the last 5 years. J Hand Surg Eur Vol. 2015;40(5):458–68.
40. Palmer AK, Werner FW, Murphy D, Glisson R. Functional wrist motion: a biomechanical study. J Hand Surg Am. 1985;10(1):39–46.
41. Banks SA, Hodge WA. Implant design affects knee arthroplasty kinematics during stair-stepping. Clin Orthop Relat Res. 2004;426:187–93.
42. Nydick JA, Greenberg SM, Stone JD, Williams B, Polikandriotis JA, Hess AV. Clinical outcomes of total wrist arthroplasty. J Hand Surg Am. 2012;37(8):1580–4.
43. Reigstad O, Holm-Glad T, Bolstad B, Grimsgaard C, Thorkildsen R, Rokkum M. Five- to 10-year prospective follow-up of wrist arthroplasty in 56 nonrheumatoid patients. J Hand Surg Am. 2017;42(10):788–96.
44. Karjalainen T, Pamilo K, Reito A. Implant failure after Motec Wrist Joint Prosthesis due to failure of ball and socket-type articulation-two patients with adverse reaction to metal debris and polyether ether ketone. J Hand Surg Am. 2018;43(11):1044e1–4.
45. Pierrart J, Bourgade P, Mamane W, Rousselon T, Masmejean EH. Novel approach for posttraumatic panarthritis of the wrist using a pyrocarbon interposition arthroplasty (Amandys((R))): preliminary series of 11 patients. Chir Main. 2012;31(4):188–94.
46. Bellemere P, Maes-Clavier C, Loubersac T, Gaisne E, Kerjean Y, Collon S. Pyrocarbon interposition wrist arthroplasty in the treatment of failed wrist procedures. J Wrist Surg. 2012;1(1):31–8.
47. Bellemere P, Maes-Clavier C, Loubersac T, Gaisne E, Kerjean Y. Amandys((R)) implant: novel pyrocarbon arthroplasty for the wrist. Chir Main. 2012;31(4):176–87.
48. Wolff AHR, Hillstrom H, Lenhoff M, Zanini S, Packer G, Wolfe SW. KinematX hemiarthroplasty maintains dart-throwing coupling axis. Koloa, Hawaii: American Association for Hand Surgery; 2021.
49. Moore DC, Crisco JJ, Trafton TG, Leventhal EL. A digital database of wrist bone anatomy and carpal kinematics. J Biomech. 2007;40(11):2537–42.
50. Vance MC, Packer G, Tan D, Crisco JJ, Wolfe SW. Midcarpal hemiarthroplasty for wrist arthritis: rationale and early results. J Wrist Surg. 2012;1(1):61–8.
51. Anneberg M, Packer G, Crisco JJ, Wolfe S. Four-year outcomes of midcarpal hemiarthroplasty for wrist arthritis. J Hand Surg Am. 2017;42(11):894–903.

# Primary Total Wrist Arthroplasty

# 8

Sandra Pfanner, Giovanni Munz,
and Massimo Ceruso

## Introduction

The wrist is the joint of the upper limb most frequently involved in post-traumatic arthrosis and in immune-mediated arthritis such as rheumatoid arthritis (RA).

In the past decades, in order to obtain a stable, pain-free wrist in a patient suffering from an either degenerative or inflammatory condition where all of the bony components of the wrist joint are involved, there were no other options other than total wrist fusion. That is still now an acceptable and reliable procedure for both the patient and the surgeon. The advent of joint implant surgery in more recent years offered a new possibility in the treatment of these pathologies. The preservation of a functional range of motion and a painless wrist requires more complex technology and surgery with increased patient involvement in the aftercare.

The improvements in prosthetic design with increased strength and durability allow total wrist arthroplasty (TWA) to be considered a procedure with increasing indications due to reliable and long-lasting results [1].

S. Pfanner (✉) · G. Munz · M. Ceruso
Hand Surgery and Reconstructive Microsurgery Unit, Azienda Ospedaliero-Universitaria Careggi, Florence, Italy

The first total wrist replacement was reported to have been performed in 1891 by Themistocles Gluck [2]. The author used an ivory ball-and-socket implant in a septic arthritis in a young man with secondary tuberculosis. The range of motion was reported as good after 1 year; however, a chronic fistula persisted due to tuberculosis.

## Implants

The development of total wrist implants has been slower than other joints most likely due to the lower frequency of painful wrist osteoarthritis (OA) and the reliability of other non-substitutive treatments. Furthermore, the anatomical complexity and biomechanical peculiarities of the wrist slowed the study and progress of arthroplasty.

Modern TWA has been developed over the last few decades through a number of iterative prosthetic designs as discussed in the prior chapter. The different models were evolved by the next-generation implants. The advances of each design have not been synchronous, and it is therefore difficult to systematize the timeline in which these processes occurred [3].

In the 1980s, Menon's prosthesis, also known as Universal Wrist Implant, marks a fixed point to which to refer to the most recent prosthetic models [4, 5]. This led to the Universal 2 implant (2003) which then, in turn, evolved into the


G. J. W. King, M. Rizzo (eds.), *Arthroplasty of the Upper Extremity*,
https://doi.org/10.1007/978-3-030-68880-6_8

Freedom prosthesis (2014, Integra LifeSciences, Plainsboro, NJ, USA) to the ReMotion (2003 Avanta from 2005 Stryker, Kalamazoo, MI, USA), and Maestro implant (2004 Biomet, Warsaw, IN, USA) [6, 7].

The current generation of prostheses, defined as anatomical, was developed with the aim to more closely replicate the biomechanical features of the normal wrist.

The Universal 2 implants (Fig. 8.1) meet the characteristics of a "two-bone model" [4] because of a carpal prosthetic condyle supported by the intercarpal fusion of the residual distal carpal bones [8, 9].

The proximal component requires a minimal bone-sparing osteotomy of the distal radius in order to make a possible revision easier [4, 10]. Its stem is characterized by a volar offset to favor a correct anatomical orientation and has a titanium porous coating promoting osseous ingrowth [11]. The distal component consists of a titanium plate that is secured to the residual carpal bones with a central peg and screws, and of a polyethylene carpal condyle (UHMWPE, ultrahigh-molecular-weight polyethylene) that is fixed to it. Obtaining the intercarpal fusion of the residual distal carpal bones is mandatory in order to achieve the better support for the distal plate. Over time, the fixation system has been improved; the longer radial screw enters the second metacarpal base, while the fixation of the central peg and ulnar screw is limited to the carpal bones. In rarer cases, such as in revision surgery with soft porotic bone, the ulnar screw should be longer and penetrate the fourth metacarpal. The system permits the screws to be angled by 20°–30°. The ellipsoidal shape of the components, together with a broader concave articular surface of the proximal one, is intended to optimize stability, creating a semi-constrained system.

The U2 implants were designed to obtain an arc of motion of 40° extension, 40° flexion, and 30° radioulnar deviation. The DRUJ and TFCC may be preserved.

Loosening of the distal component is the most common reason for revision of Universal 2 [12, 13]. Kennedy studied the radiographic loosening of all the carpal components and noted 21% in central post, 21% radial screw, and 17% ulnar screw [13]. He reported on 48

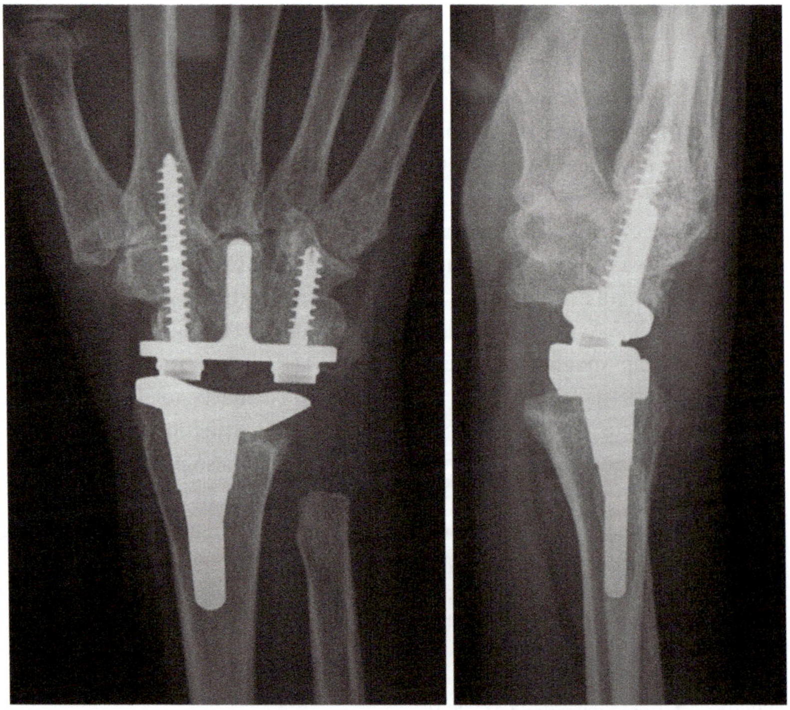

**Fig. 8.1** Universal 2 TWA in a RA 34-year-old female patient at a 3-year FU. Darrach ulnar head resection was associated

wrists with a mean follow-up of 7 years post TWA: 21% had a reoperation and 7 implants were revised [13]. Zijlker reported improved survivorship of 81% at 11 years [14]. The revision rate varies according to etiology, with a higher incidence in RA vs OA. Pfanner et al. reported a survival rate 74% in RA, in a series of 23 patients reviewed at 7 years [9].

In 2014, the U2 design was revised and renamed the Freedom Wrist Arthroplasty System (Integra LifeSciences, Plainsboro, NJ) (Fig. 8.2). This device features a cobalt-chrome-molybdenum (CoCrMo) alloy radial component with a shorter stem, and a wider ellipsoidal shaped plate, which replicates, in an increasingly anatomical way, the articular width shape of the radius. This design minimizes radial resection allowing preservation of the DRUJ and capsule. The titanium carpal plate was designed with a shorter central stem to be inserted into the capitate and two variable angle screws with a locking cap. Portions of the radial implant and carpal plate have a titanium plasma-sprayed coating for improved ingrowth. The instrument kit system has been modified to allow for a more reproducible surgical implantation.

The ReMotion TWA (Fig. 8.3) added 10° of carpal rotation in pro-supination, thereby facilitating dart throw motion, through a second articulation made between the carpal poly and the carpal plate. All components are CoCr with a titanium porous interface. The carpal part has a central porous-coated peg for the capitate, and two screws with variable angle for fixation to carpal bones only. The radial component, which sits on the lunate and scaphoid fossa, is designed to preserve the sigmoid notch and radio-carpal ligament insertions [3]. This implant has the capacity to give uniformity to the pattern of stress distribution and reduce high contact pressure [15]. With ReMotion the most common cause of failure is loosening. Radiolucency, which usually stabilizes after 3 years [16], is not directly related to loosening, but patients with signs of periprosthetic osteolysis need strict follow-up. Boeckstyns et al. found that in long-term follow-up of 6 years (5–9 years), the survivorship of implant was 90% [17]. Sagerfors at similar follow-up found 94%

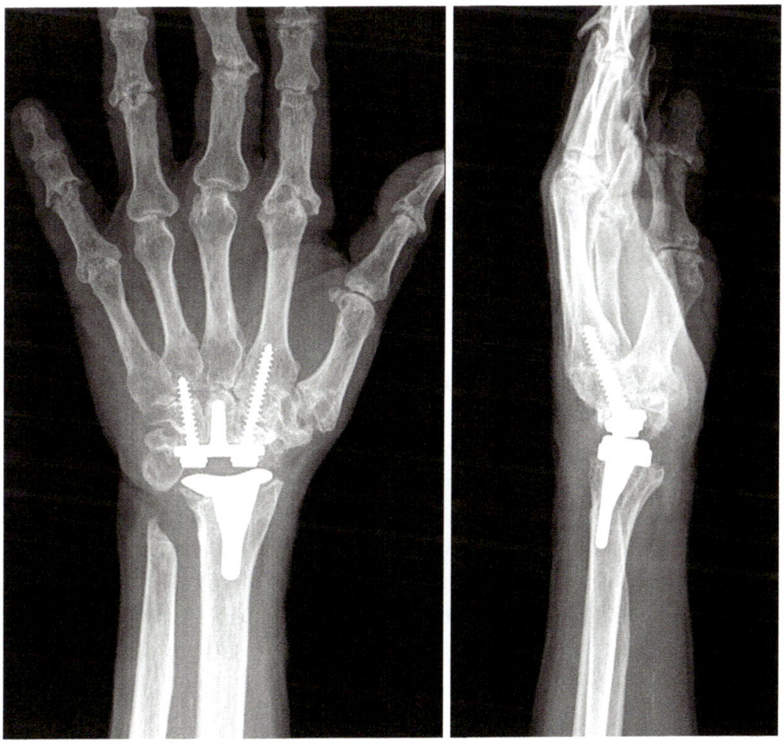

**Fig. 8.2** Freedom TWA in a RA 69-year-old male patient. X-ray control at a 2-year FU

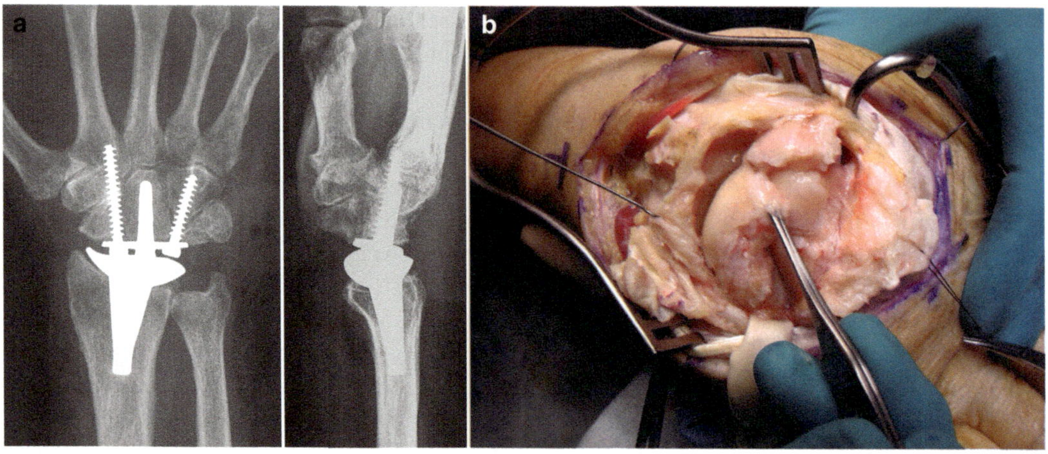


**Fig. 8.3** (**a**) SLACIII wrist treated with a ReMotion TWA in a 61-year-old male patient at a 2-year FU. (**b**) Note severe cartilage wearing of radial facets and proximal edge of scaphoid and lunate (intraoperative view)

[18]. Froschauer et al. reported a survival rate of 97% at the same follow-up in 39 OA patients [19]. Honecker et al. reported a survival rate of 82% after 10 years in a cohort composed mainly of rheumatoid patients [20].

The ball-and-socket TWA design has not been completely abandoned. Recent literature reports that the Motec prosthesis (Motec, Swemac Orthopaedics, Linköping, Sweden), a cementless modular metal-on-coated-metal ball-and-socket, has recently been revised using a new articulating material, polyether ether ketone (PEEK). This is a strong, wear-resistant polymer, but the clinical experience with it is limited [21]. Reigstad and Røkkum developed this wrist prosthesis and then modified it during a decade of trials from 1996 to 2005. The final Motec wrist prosthesis was launched in 2006. Since then, they have used it in 110 wrists from 2006 to 2018 [22]. This prosthesis gave up on the idea of anatomical design, simplifying the joint, with the aim of eliminating issues of debris and instability. The outcomes are similar to the latest anatomical implants, in terms of revision rate, pain, and AROM, with a mean follow-up of 8 years. In high-demand nonrheumatoid patients, Reigstad reported a Kaplan-Meier survival of 86% [18, 23] (Table 8.1).

## Indications

A total wrist arthroplasty should be considered in the absence of any other biologic option to restore a functional, painless, mobile wrist. In a large series of post-traumatic conditions and, to a lesser degree, even in rheumatoid patients, the extent of involvement of the carpal bones is limited either to the RC or the MC joint only. In these instances, limited carpal fusions and proximal row carpectomy are well-known reliable therapeutic procedures, which do not necessitate the use of a TWA.

A TWA is indicated for symptomatic patients with involvement of both the radio-carpal and midcarpal joints which is observed with pain and functional impairment, stiffness, or instability. This includes patients with pan-carpal OA, which is substantially a post-traumatic condition, or in nontraumatic disorders, more commonly represented by immune-mediated arthritis such as RA. Degenerative pan-carpal OA represents the late evolutionary stage of complex articular fractures or fracture dislocation of the wrist and of several ligamentous or osteo-ligamentous chronic evolutive lesions such as SLAC and SNAC wrist (Fig. 8.4) [32]. TWA may also be considered as a salvage procedure for failed treatments such as

**Table 8.1** Overview of implant outcomes

| Author | Underlying pathology | No. | Duration of follow-up (year) | ROM (F + E) | VAS 0–10 | Dash | PRWE | % Survival (*in situ) |
|---|---|---|---|---|---|---|---|---|
| *Universal 2* | | | | | | | | |
| Ferreres et al. (2011) [24] | RA, psoriatic | 19 | 5.5 | 68° (42/26) | – | – | – | 100% |
| Cooney et al. (2012) [25] | RA, OA | 8 | 6 | – | 2.3 | 20 | 25 | 87% |
| Sagerfors et al. (2015) [18] | RA, OA | 12 | 7 | Δ 0° | Δ-2.5 | 13.7 | – | – |
| Badge et al. (2016) [26] | RA | 85 | 4.5 | 50° (21/29) | – | Quick-D 46 | – | 93% |
| Gil et al. (2017) [12] | RA, OA | 39 | 9 | 66° (37/29) | 0.4 | – | – | 93% |
| Pfanner et al. 2017 [9] | RA | 23 | 6.8 | 72° | 0.8 | Quick-D 49 | – | 74% |
| Kennedy et al. (2018) [13] | RA, OA | 48 | 7 | 57° (33/24) | NA | 25.4 | – | 85% |
| Zijlker et al. (2019) [14] | RA, OA, Kienböck | 26 | 11 | NA | NA | 41 | 45 | 81% |
| Fischer et al. (2020) [27] | RA | 12 | 10 mean not reported | Δ −5° (−20/15) | Δ 0 rest | Δ −17 | Δ −43 | Kaplan-M 83% |
| *ReMotion* | | | | | | | | |
| Cooney et al. (2012) [25] | RA, OA | 22 | 6 | – | 2.3 | 37 | 32 | 100% |
| Herzberg et al. (2012) [28] | RA<br>OA | 112 | 4 | 66°<br>65° | Δ-4.8<br>−5.4 | Quick-D<br>Δ-20<br>−21 | – | 95%<br>94% |
| Boeckstyns et al. (2013) [17] | RA, OA, Kienböck | 52 | 6.5 | 60° (29/31) | 2.7 | Quick-D 42 | – | 90% |
| Sagerfors et al. (2015) [18] | RA, OA | 87 | 7 | Δ 5° | Δ-2 | 12.3 | – | 94% |
| Honecker et al. (2019) [20] | RA, OA, Kienböck | 23 | 4 | 83° (39/44) | 2.8 | Quick-D 37.9 | – | 96% |
| Chevrollier et al. (2016) [29] | RA, OA, Kienböck | 7 | 5.2 | Δ 33° | – | Δ −29% | Δ −26% | – |
| Froschauer et al. (2019) [19] | OA | 39 | 7 | 40° (20/20) | 2 | 29 | – | 97% |
| Fischer et al. (2020) [27] | RA, OA | 69 | 10 mean not reported | Δ 5° (0/5) | Δ −1.5 rest | Δ −13.5 | Δ −35.5 | Kaplan-M 94% |
| *Motec* | | | | | | | | |
| Reigstad et al. (2011) (Elos MedicalAB) [30] | OA | 8 | 7.6 | 125° (F/E+ R/U dev) | 0 median | 10.3 | – | 50% |
| Reigstad et al. (2017) [31] | OA, Kienböck | 56 | 8 | 126° (F/E+ R/U dev) | 0.8 rest 2 active | Quick-D 39 | – | 86% |
| Giwa et al. (2018) [23] | OA, RA | 25 | 5.5 | 112° | – | Quick-D 21 | – | 84% |

Underlying pathology: diagnosis ordered for frequency. *OA* including post-traumatic, *Δ* delta, difference between preoperative and postoperative, in situ, implant has not been revised at the time of follow-up

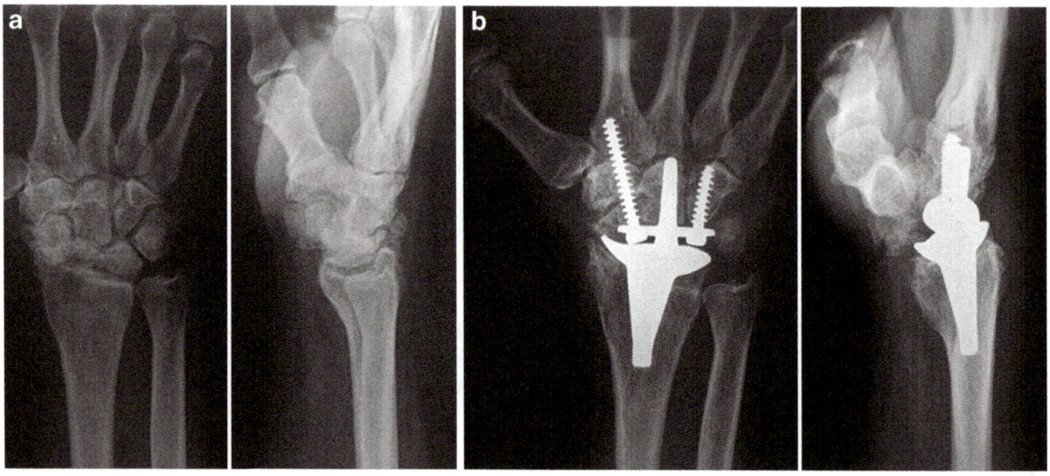

**Fig. 8.4** (**a**) SNAC wrist stage III in a 47-year-old male patient. Note pan-carpal OA (**b**) ReMotion total wrist replacement. Postoperative X-rays at a 4-year FU

proximal row carpectomy and partial wrist fusions (Fig. 8.5). Kienböck disease advanced collapse (KDAC) should likewise be included in this list (Fig. 8.6). Conversion from fusion to TWA has also been reported [33].

RA has different evolutive forms of wrist involvement that should be clearly understood before planning any surgical procedure. The Schulthess classification is a most valuable tool as it clearly outlines three different evolutive patterns based on several radiological parameters [34]. Type I has a tendency to joint ankylosis and corresponds to the juvenile or idiopathic RA (IRA) pattern. Type II is defined as reactive type and has aspects comparable to the evolution of OA conditions (Fig. 8.7). In type III, the ligamentous destructive type, the aggressive pattern of the disease on the osto-articular and ligamentous tissue, induces major instability, ulnar translocation of the carpus, and, in the most severe cases, radio-carpal dislocation. TWA should only be considered in rheumatoid wrist type I or II, as its stability is substantially dependent on a suitable quality of the capsule and periarticular soft tissue.

In RA, the effectiveness of the medical treatment is crucial also for the implant survival. Patients must be informed of the higher risk of loosening, and consequent revision, due to a possible reactivation of the autoimmune disease [9].

A very few patients have an indication for a bilateral wrist implant. They must be individually evaluated, and their personal and professional profile and expectations should be thoroughly examined.

Contraindications to TWA are irreparable tendon rupture of the radial extensors of the wrist, inadequate skin quality, and past or current infections. Moreover, major bone loss and capsule-ligamentous insufficiency are relative contraindications requiring an accurate preoperative evaluation.

## Patient's History and Objective Data

The personal profile of the patient is evaluated: age, sex, current job and possibilities for future jobs, leisure activities, and aesthetic expectations. Age is a significant factor as life expectancies increase the risk of TWA revision. Younger patients should consider arthrodesis to avoid the need for further surgery [6].

Heavy manual work is in itself a contraindication, given the limit to lift a maximum weight of 3 kg. TWA can be offered to patients who may consider switching to lighter work or who can adapt their workstation using modified tools and appropriate supports to protect the wrist during the activity.

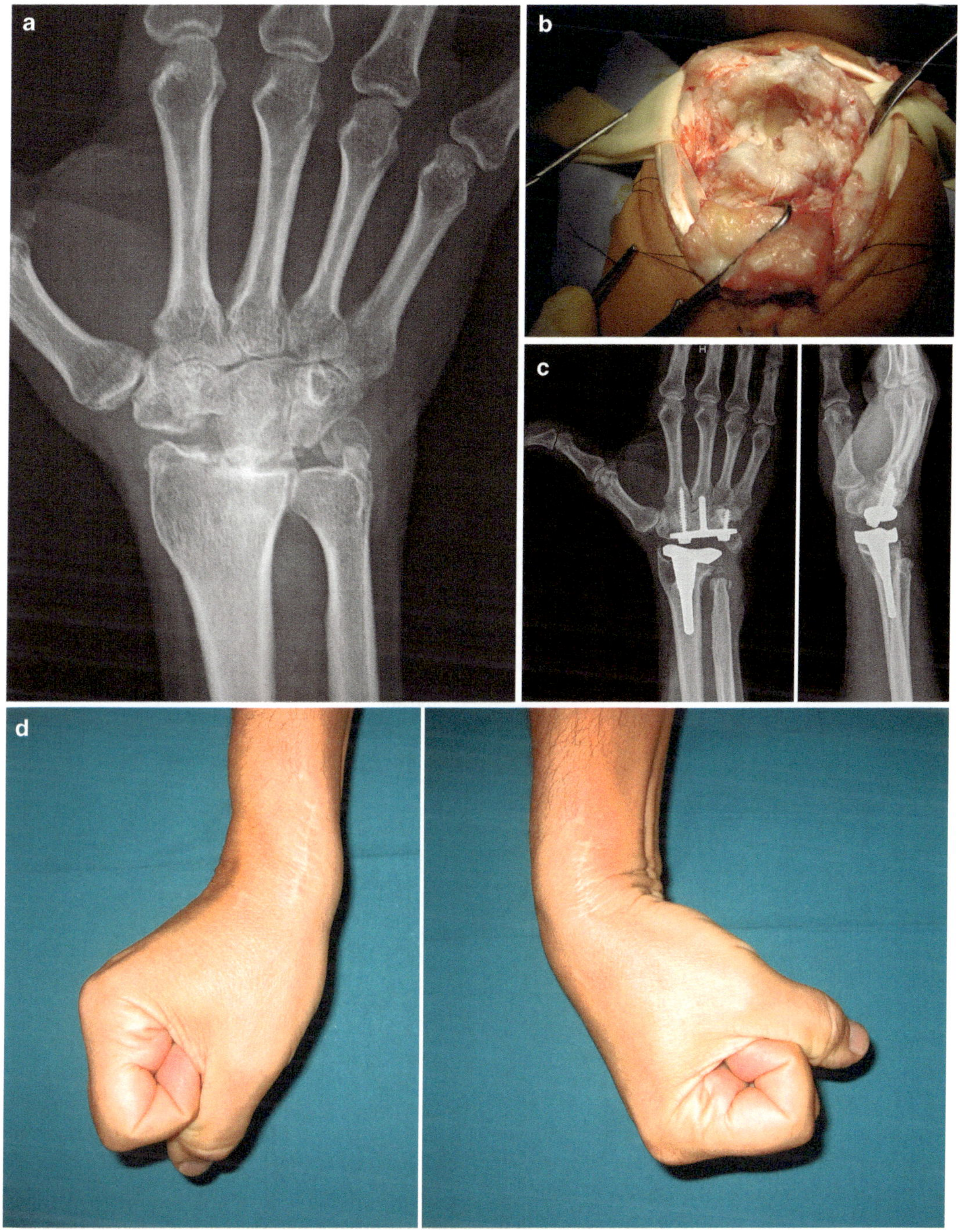


**Fig. 8.5** (**a**) Severe OA following PRC in a patient 54 y.o., formerly treated for a SNAC III wright wrist. (**a**) Preoperative X-rays (**b**) intraoperative image showing the extensive cartilage wearing of lunate fossa and capitate head. (**b**) X-rays FU at 10 years. (**c**) Clinical result

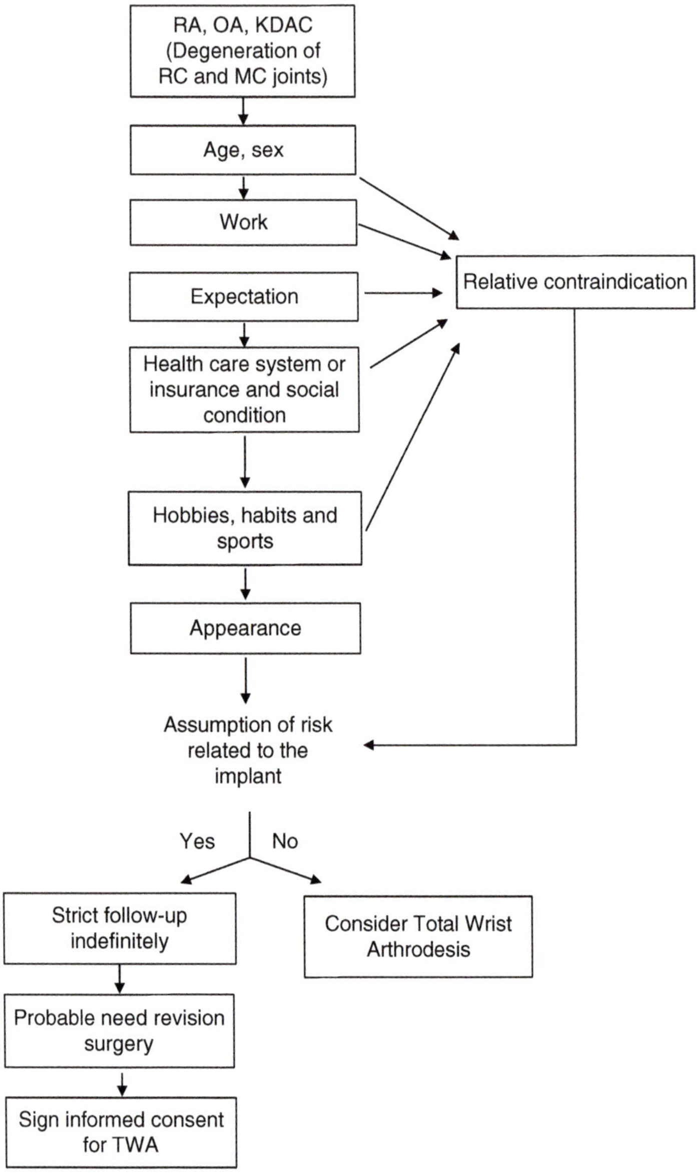


**Fig. 8.6** Flow diagram of patient evaluation information

Given the differences in the health-care system in different countries of the world, a TWA also involves economic and social considerations for each patient, and in some cases, these can be a relative contraindication [35].

Expectations for leisure activities should also be discussed, in order to cope with the wishes of the patient, who is looking for an improvement in their life. Patients should be aware of the risks associated with the procedure and the possible changes in their lifestyle including sports and hobbies required by a TWA.

Some patients are concerned about the cosmetic appearance of the wrist. Frequent questions include the surgical scar and the dorsally subluxed ulnar head which is considered non-aesthetic. The hand is the second element of interaction after face in human relationships, and it is important that patients know what they should expect. The surgical scar is long about 10–15 cm on the dorsal

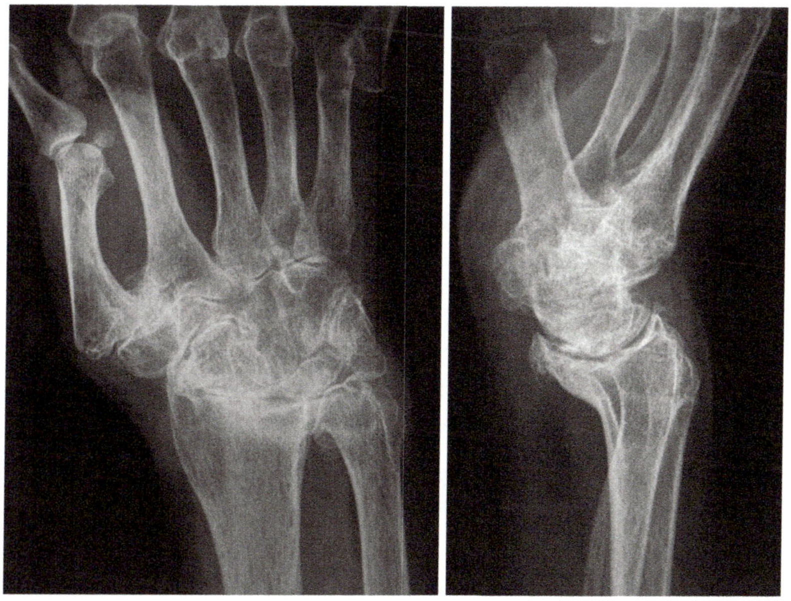

**Fig. 8.7** Schulthess Type II pan-carpal wrist RA. Note the absence of carpal translocation and a satisfactory bone stock

aspect of the wrist and will be evident. As for the prominence of the ulnar head, a Darrach procedure will result in an empty ulnar border of the wrist that may not please the patient; in these cases, an ulnar head prosthesis will maintain the anatomic wrist shape but has their own risks of potential complications.

RA patients should be informed of the possibility of a preoperative suspension of MTX, biological medications, and steroids to be discussed with their rheumatologist. TWA should also take into account if other previous surgeries, and particularly other implants, have been performed on the same or contralateral upper limb.

Pain is evaluated by the visual analogue scale (VAS) score, and standard grip strength tests are performed and compared with the contralateral side. Patients are also assessed for their function using the Quick-DASH and the Patient's Rate Wrist/Hand Evaluation (PRWHE). Active and passive flexion-extension, ulnar-radial deviation, and pro-supination are measured and recorded. In rheumatoid patients, the coexisting hand and upper limb deformities or lesions related to the disease should be noted.

A careful informed consent is obtained as the patient must be aware of risk, benefits, and alternatives, and the indications for an arthrodesis versus a TWA should be clearly discussed. The patient is informed that a specific rehabilitation protocol must be followed after surgery and that it is part of the treatment. The patient is advised they should return every year for clinical checkup and annual radiographs. The majority of patients need at least 3 months to return to previous activities, hobbies, and jobs, with limitations related to the implant characteristics, and have to accept a reduced arc of the wrist of movement is expected relative to normal.

In both scenarios, RA and OA, knowledge of the terms and informed consent is essential, as the patient must know that an implant has a certain duration and that it will likely need surgery for revision in the future.

For patients who refuse or won't fit the conditions of an arthroplasty, total wrist arthrodesis is recommended. It is explained that the procedure has a lower risk for revision, hardware does not usually have to be removed, and many heavy jobs can be performed. However, wrist motion is totally abolished, and the other joints of the upper limb and homolateral hand, as well as the contralateral wrist, will have to compensate for the loss of dexterity.

## Radiographic Assessment

### Preoperative Assessment

Besides the standard X-rays (PA and Lat views), a CT scan is helpful in better studying the extent of articular wear and bone loss and assists with planning surgery. In borderline articular conditions, CT it is particularly useful in the evaluation of RC and MC joints in order to assess whether a partial carpal fusion can still be an alternative to more extensive procedures. If in doubt, some authors advice a pre-op arthroscopy as a gold standard [23].

### Postoperative Assessment

Postoperative radiographs evaluate the implant alignment, the fusion of the residual carpal bones, and the implant-bone interface. Assess for radiolucent lines around carpal and radial components, resorption of the bone around the stem collar, migration and subsidence of the implant, and any radial stress shielding. This latter develops according to Wolff's law, and expresses the reaction of the cortical bone around the prosthesis [36]. Following the operation, X-rays are performed at 1, 6, and 12 months post-surgery and then yearly.

Among the critical X-ray findings, radiolucency is the most common. It is important to distinguish between radiolucency, which generally has a benign evolution, and loosening, whose features are angulation and subsidence of the implant, which is likely to progress to requiring surgical revision. Boeckstyns et al. reviewed a series of cases where juxta-articular radiolucency around both radial and carpal components was noted, regardless of the primary diagnosis. In most cases radiolucency stopped progressing between 1 and 3 years postoperatively and stabilized at 0.8–2.1 mm [16].

In order to predictably define the evolutionary models of TWA by correlating clinical and radiological results, we propose to classify patients into three different types [9]:

- Type A: No radiological changes in subsequent X-ray controls. Clinical outcome is stable and satisfactory.
- Type B: Progressive radiological changes in comparison with the immediate postoperative X-ray. Clinical outcome is stable. This group can be divided into two subgroups. In B1, radiological changes consist of radiolucency, sclerosis, stress shielding, osteolysis, and bony resorption. These remain unmodified on subsequent controls. Clinical outcome is stable. In B2, radiological changes consist of implant tilting, subsidence, and loosening. They progress over time. Implant migration and loosening are related to minor or no symptoms.
- Type C: Progressive radiological changes and loosening of the implant. It is a symptomatic condition with a progressive worsening of the clinical setting.
- Types A and B1 can undergo clinical and radiological follow-up once a year. In type B2 a progressive worsening of the clinical setting is predictable, and the progressive loosening observed on radiographs will require a more frequent follow-up. Type C will have to undergo a surgical revision. In these cases, a CT scan is useful for preoperative planning in order to define the extent of bone loss and implant alignment. CT scan with volume-rendered image provides good 3D definition of the implant position and bone loss (Fig. 8.8) [37].

## Surgical Technique

The patient's upper limb is positioned in 90° abduction with the palm facing downward on an arm table. A dorsal longitudinal midline skin incision, 10–15 cm long, is aligned with the third metacarpal and prolonged proximally. The skin and subcutaneous tissue are elevated together, taking care to protect the vascularization of the soft tissue and superficial radial and ulnar nerves. The extensor retinaculum is incised over the fifth compartment and is reflected to the radial side

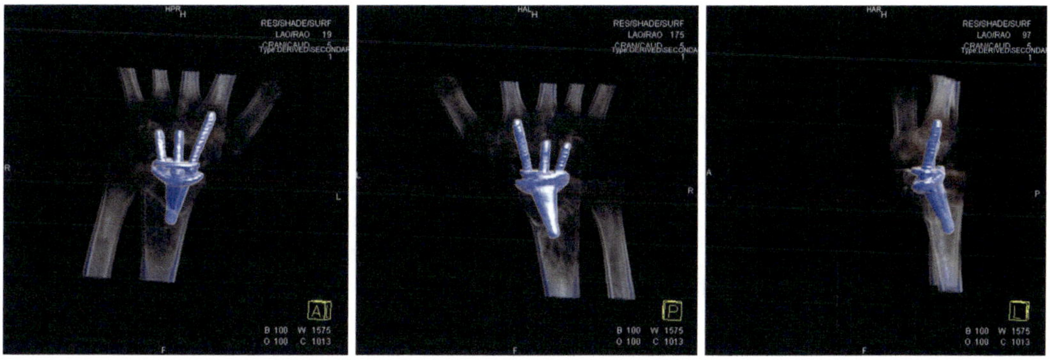

**Fig. 8.8** Preoperative volume-rendered image CT scan of a ReMotion TWA scheduled for implant revision. VRTD sequences: (**c**) anterior view (**a**) posterior view (**b**) lateral view

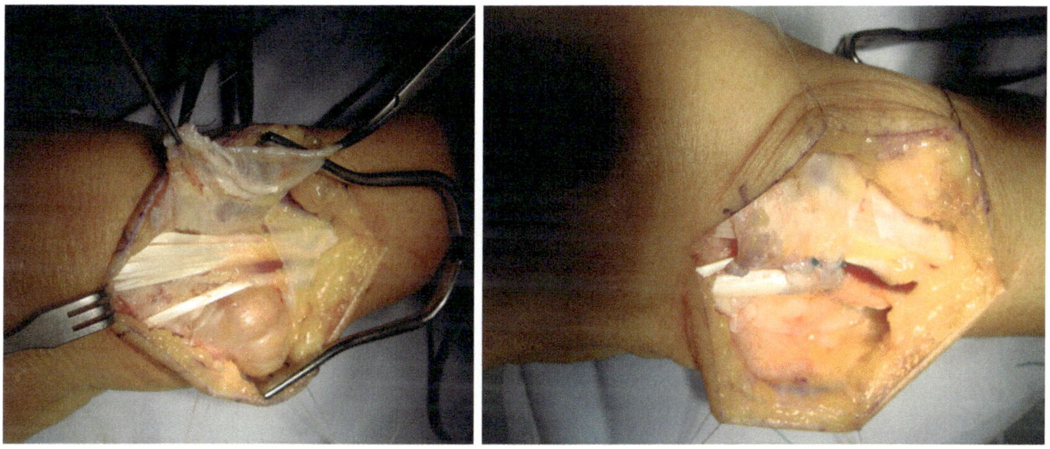

**Fig. 8.9** (**a**) Step-cut incision of the ulnar border of the extensor retinaculum in a rheumatoid wrist. (**b**) Its longest part is looped around the ECU tendon in order to restore its stabilizing effect over the ulna

exposing the extensor tendons up to the second compartment.

In rheumatoid patients, the ulnar edge of the retinacular flap is elevated from the sixth compartment with a step-cut incision so to develop two separate parts, the longest of which will be used at the end of the procedure to properly relocate the ECU tendon over the ulna; the other one will be sutured back to the remaining ulnar part of the retinaculum (Fig. 8.9) [9].

The ECR tendons are examined in order to check their continuity and condition. In case of major wearing or rupture, the ECRB must at least be intact or repairable; otherwise, a TWA is contraindicated. A segment of the posterior interosseous nerve is excised just proximal to the radio-carpal joint so to prevent the risk of a painful neuroma and to achieve a partial denervation of the wrist. The authors advise infiltrating the nerve with lidocaine before resection. The dorsal capsule is elevated as a rectangular distally based flap to obtain adequate exposure to all carpal bones.

DRUJ is left intact in the absence of instability or synovitis; the RLT capsular ligament distal to TFCC needs to be preserved [31, 38]. In the case of symptomatic instability, synovitis, impingement between the ulna and radial component, and impingement between the ulna and carpus, the procedure is extended to the DRUJ, and either an ulnar head resection is performed or one of the current ulnar prosthesis devices may be implanted depending on surgeon's preferences [11, 31, 39, 40].

Fluoroscopy is mandatory to confirm the position of the alignment guides during surgery and to check the correct rotation of the radial and carpal stem. In RA patients, the third metacarpal is often malaligned in respect to the carpus, and this can be misleading when checking the position of the guide within the capitate. The carpal stem and the radial and ulnar screws have to be centered, respectively, into the residual distal scaphoid and trapezoid, capitate and residual triquetrum, and hamate; they must also appear aligned one with the other in the lateral view (Fig. 8.10).

After the trial components have been positioned, range of motion and stability are assessed. The implant has to be stable at 35° flexion and 35° extension, and no more than 2–3 mm of laxity should be present in axial distraction. If too tight, a release of capsule and periarticular soft tissue is required, or the radius may need to be shortened. The way to establish the adequate size of the polyethylene carpal component is to test implant stability with a maneuver performed shaking the wrist in a dorso-volar direction; the prosthetic components should permit a smooth flexion-extension with no tendency to dislocate.

Press-fit cementless technique is the preferred method for primary wrist arthroplasty. To improve bone integration and stability of the carpal component, it is essential to achieve a solid intercarpal fusion of the distal row with the

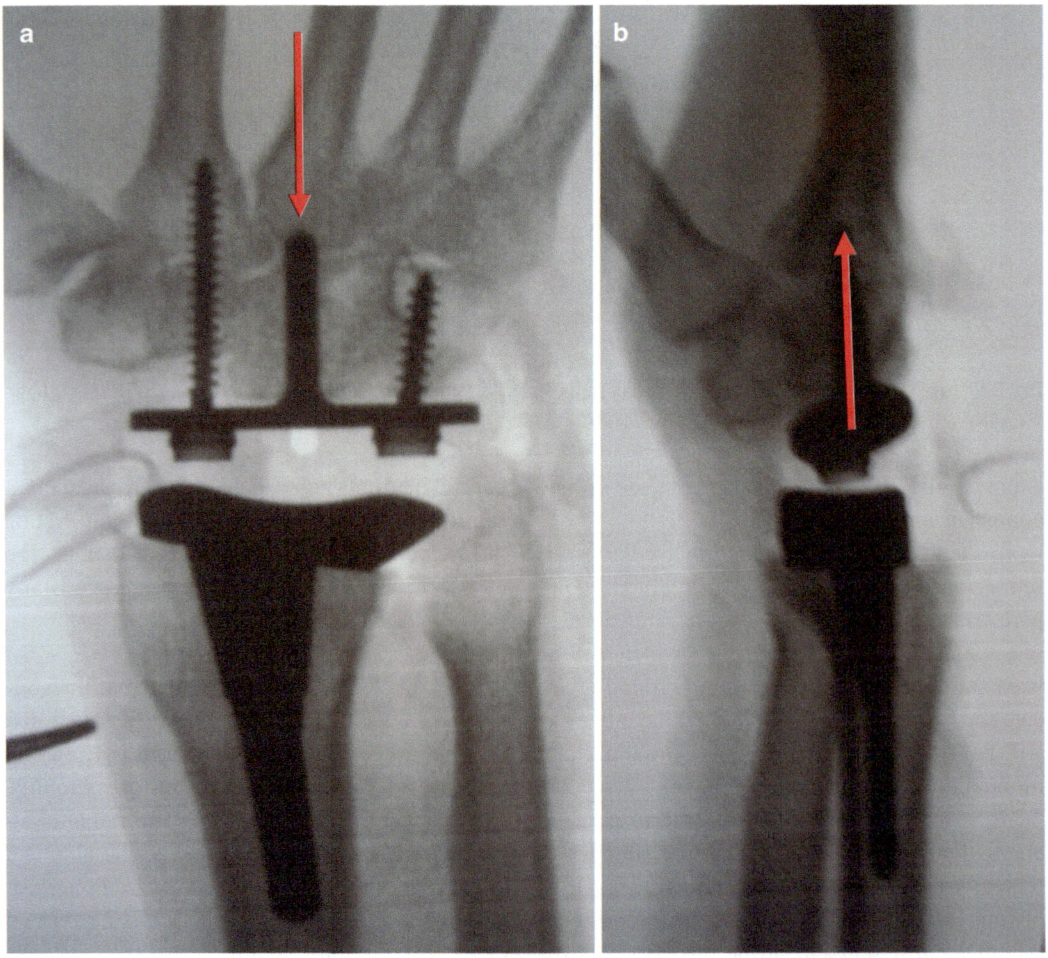


**Fig. 8.10** (**a**) Correct rotational alignment of the radial and carpal plate stems; note that fixation of the carpal stem is limited to the capitate bone; (**b**) in the lateral view, the screws are aligned parallel to each other and to the stem

impaction grafting of cancellous chips from previously resected bone. The capsular flap is sutured back to the radius using transosseous stiches. If needed, a strip of the retinaculum may be used to augment the capsular tissue length in order not to suture it too tight, which would prevent wrist flexion. In the case a Darrach procedure has been performed, DRUJ is closed by tightening of the capsular flaps with the aim of stabilizing the ulnar stump. Some authors also advise using a distally based half-slip of the ECU to improve ulnar stump stability [41–43]. Repair of the extensor retinaculum is performed over the extensor tendons. EPL is commonly left superficial to it; ECRB and ECRL can be left superficial as well, in the case the retinaculum is poor or short [44]. As described above, in rheumatoid patients one half of the ulnar margin of the retinacular flap is used to fix the ECU in its proper dorsal alignment as a DRUJ stabilizer. A surgical drain is placed and maintained for 24–48 hours. The wound is closed in layers and dressed. A short volar arm plaster splint is made in neutral position. In patients with concomitant DRUJ surgery, postoperative pro-supination is not allowed. In these cases, immobilization is obtained using an over-elbow or a sugar-tong splint.

Implant devices, instruments, and surgical procedures vary depending on the implant employed and are described in detail in the manufacturer's technical guide brochures.

## Rehabilitative Protocol

Two weeks postoperatively the plaster splint and sutures are removed, a custom-made plastic splint in a neutral position of the wrist is worn day and night; the splint allows for full flexion and extension of the fingers, and opposition of the thumb and the patient is encouraged to grip while wearing the splint. The hand therapist instructs patients to temporarily remove the splint several times a day in order to perform active flexion-extension and some radial-ulnar deviation in the absence of pain. Controlled wrist passive motion and scar treatment are also periodically done under direct control of the therapist. These treatments also aim to reduce the edema and to preserve complete finger mobility; cryotherapy may also be used to control swelling and pain. One month post-surgery, paraffin therapy, isometric contractions of the muscles of wrist and fingers, and electrotherapy in cases of limited range of motion are prescribed to increase strength. Proprioception and coordination exercises are also performed. Patients wear the splint during the night for 4 more weeks. Eight weeks after surgery, the splint is removed. Twelve weeks postoperatively patient can return to their daily activities, avoiding weights over 3 kg permanently. In case of more demanding activities such as skiing, riding scooter, and using crutches, it is recommended for the patient to wear a neoprene wrist splint or an adjustable wrist support brace.

Wrist arthroplasty nowadays seems to be more reliable; their outcomes are aligned to other major joints. Wrist prostheses make the joint stable and allow the patient to perform once again abandoned fine activities and tasks. Future direction for development of design could improve carpal component stability through knowledge of biomechanics in wrist's overload and stress shielding. A desirable progression should be the creation of revision models, with oversize components, such as longer stems and central peg.

## Wrist Hemiarthroplasty

A wrist hemiarthroplasty may be indicated when wrist OA is limited to the RC joint and the MC joint cartilage is intact. Surgical treatment options are biologic interposition arthroplasties, partial wrist fusion limited to the affected articular surfaces (such as RL and RSL fusion), and implants that include pyrocarbon spacers (such as the Amandys spacer, Tornier, Grenoble France) and prosthetic hemiarthroplasties. The advantages offered by these latter are a better ROM recovery and a shorter postoperative immobilization, when compared to the other options. Moreover, there is no risk of nonunion, and carpal bone stock and carpal height can be preserved [45, 46]. Hemi-implants are based on previous orthopedic experiences developed for the upper limb, where the possibility of keeping the cartilage articulating in direct contact with metal has already been tested in shoulder and elbow trauma salvage procedures [47].

In current wrist hemiarthroplasty, the radial articular surface is substituted. Either the proximal carpal row or the capitate head is preserved, according to pathology, and they articulate with the metallic proximal plate. A hemiarthroplasty intended for substitution only of carpal bones has been performed only with the Maestro implant, but this is reported to have a high failure rate. Huish supposes that this is due to a combination of inappropriate material and poor geometric fit with the lunate facet [48].

Indications for a wrist hemiarthroplasty are post-traumatic conditions such as displaced, impacted articular distal radius fractures with circumferential comminution, particularly in elderly people, secondary wrist OA after failed salvage treatments such as PRC, the KDAC wrist in IIIB stage Kienböck disease, and rarer oncologic conditions with involvement of the articular surface of the distal radius (Fig. 8.11) [45–47, 49–54].

Current prosthesis may be either the proximal component of a total device or hemi-prosthesis such as Cobra implant (Groupe Lépine, Lyon, France), Sophia distal radius implant (Biotech, Paris, France), KinematX midcarpal hemiarthroplasty (Extremity Medical, LLC, Parsippany, NJ), and Prosthelast (Argomedical AG, Cham, Switzerland). The latter two implants originally consisted of a radial component for hemiarthroplasty; however, a distal component was recently developed, and these devices can now be implanted as a TWA.

The proximal component of a total implant, such as Universal 2 or ReMotion, may be used off-label as a hemiarthroplasty. Only the Freedom implant has approval for both total and hemi-implants.

In 2010, Boyer and Adams published first two cases of hemi-implant associated with PRC; at 1 year, complete pain relief and a functional ROM were reported. They propose the procedure for young patients not suitable for TWA and not eligible for complete wrist arthrodesis [51].

In 2016, Gaspar et al. reviewed 52 distal radius hemiarthroplasties (13 Maestro and 39 ReMotion). At a 3-year follow-up, they report a revision rate of 29%; the most frequent complications were contracture, loosening, and infection [55]. In 2017, Anneberg et al. reported 20 cases treated with a KinematiX hemiarthroplasty prosthesis. At a mean follow-up of 4 years, ROM and grip strength were improved compared to preoperative values; two cases were converted to TWA, one due to loosening and one after CRPS; another patient underwent total wrist fusion for ulnar pain [46]. In 2012, Vance et al. published the results of 9 patients, with a mean age of 44 treated with a KinematiX implant; at a very short follow-up (8 months), they reported frequent complications, such as extensor adhesions, wrist instability, carpal impingement, and symptomatic midcarpal arthrosis [53]. Roux reports having treated comminuted distal radial fracture in elderly patients since 2005, implanting a self-designed WHA [54]. Vergnenègre treated eight patients, for distal radial fractures AO type C2 with the Sophia implant, without PRC. Their mean age was 80 years. Average time of surgery was 1 hour. Patients rapidly returned to ADL in just 3 weeks [49]. In 2019, Anger et al. implanted the Cobra device in 9 cases of AO C3 and 2 cases of AO C2, without performing PRC, and reported poor results in 4 out of 11 patients due to residual pain. The authors believe the pain is due to untreated distal ulna or the contact between proximal row and the CrCo alloy surface of prosthesis [53]. Herzberg reported his results with Cobra implant, without PRC as well, in 25 patients with a mean age of 77 years. At a follow-up of 32 months, more optimistic outcomes were observed, with AROM flexion-extension of 60° and prosupination of 150°, VAS pain 1/10. He advises hemiarthroplasty as a valid solution for irreparable fractures when osteosynthesis with a locking plate is not feasible [47].

Wrist hemiarthroplasty has promising expectations and may in the future be considered a reli-

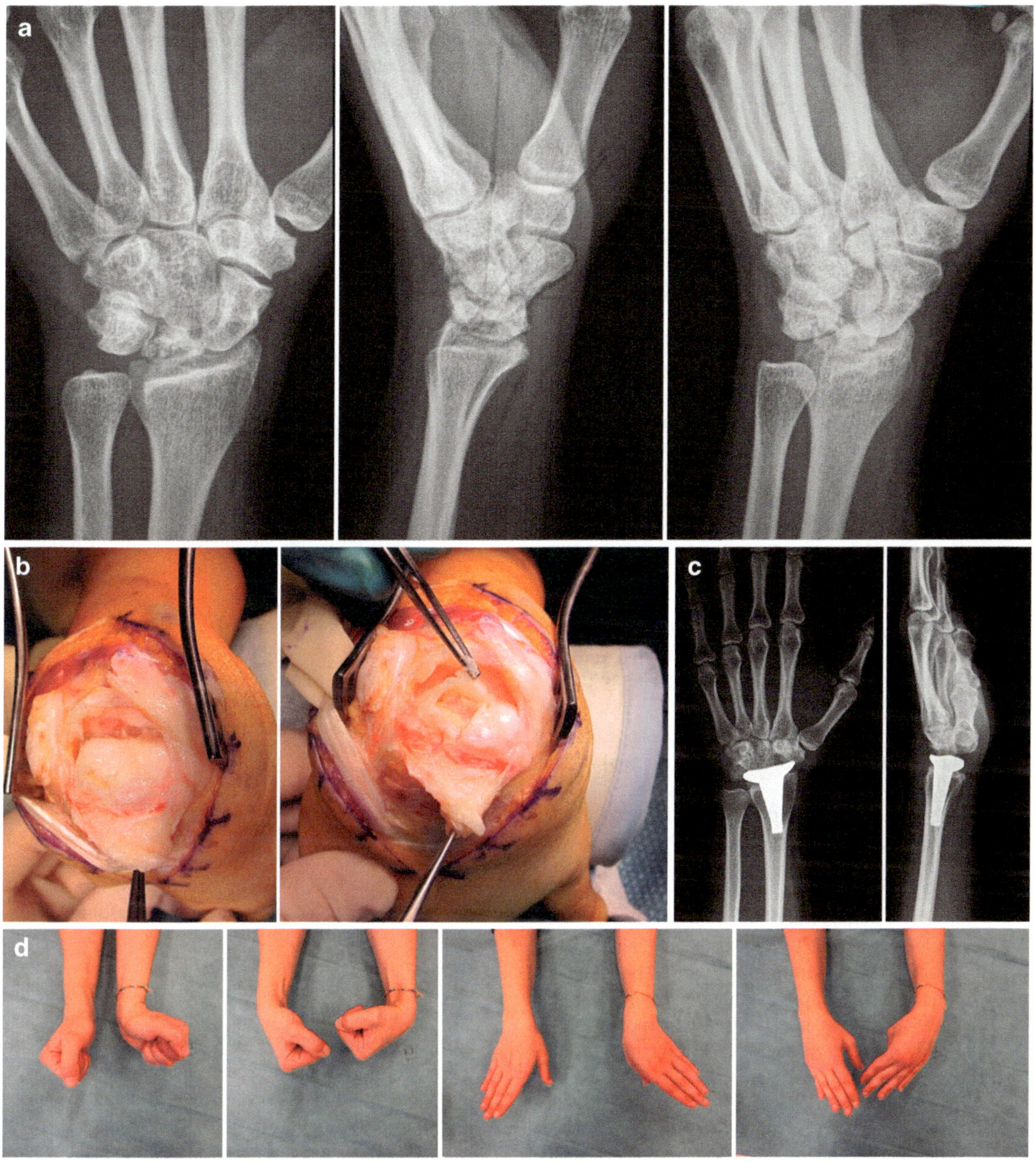


**Fig. 8.11** (**a**) Kienböck disease advanced collapse (KDAC) in a 27-year-old woman. (**b**) Intraoperative view shows cartilage wearing of radial lunate facet and lunate fragmentation. (**c**) X-ray controls (PA and Lat views) of a ReMotion hemiarthroplasty at a 7 FU. (**d**) Clinical results

able alternative to total arthrodesis and TWA in treatment of advanced stage of Kienböck disease when the lunate fossa is damaged or when lunate fossa arthrosis has developed after a PRC. WHA is also an alternative to radio-scapholunate arthrodesis in elderly patients.

Future developments may allow the surgeon to perform a reliable conversion of the WHA to a TWA. Current literature on hemiarthroplasty is limited, and the duration of follow-up remains short; further advances in these devices are likely in the years to come.

## References


1. Hindley CJ, Stanley JK. The rheumatoid wrist. Patterns of disease progression. J Hand Surg [Br]. 1991;16:275–9.
2. Ritt MJ, Stuart PR, Naggar L, Beckenbaugh RD. The early history of arthroplasty of the wrist. From amputation to total wrist implant. J Hand Surg Br. 1994;19(6):778–82.
3. Kennedy CD, Huang JI. Prosthetic Design in Total Wrist Arthroplasty. Orthop Clin North Am. 2016;47(1):207–18.
4. Menon J. Total wrist arthroplasty for rheumatoid arthritis. Hand surgery: current practice. London: Martin Dunitz; 1997.
5. Menon J. Universal total wrist implant. Experience with a carpal component fixed with three screws. J Arthroplast. 1998;13:515–23.
6. Schmidt I. Can total wrist arthroplasty be an option for treatment of highly comminuted distal radius fracture in selected patients? Preliminary experience with two cases. Case Rep Orthop. 2015;380935
7. Schmidt I. A critical appraisal to the decision by the company Zimmer Biomet to withdraw the MaestroTM Wrist Reconstructive System from the marketplace. Trauma and Emergency Care. ISSN: 2398-3345. 2018.
8. Boeckstyns ME, Herzberg G. Current European practice in wrist arthroplasty. Hand Clin. 2017;33(3):521–8.
9. Pfanner S, Munz G, Guidi G, Ceruso M. Universal 2 wrist arthroplasty in rheumatoid arthritis. J Wrist Surg. 2017;6(3):206–15.
10. Cobb TK, Beckenbaugh RD. Biaxial total wrist arthroplasty. J Hand Surg [Am]. 1996;21A:1011–21.
11. Nunez FA Jr, Wright L, Kilpatrick SE, Seitz WH Jr. Revision total wrist arthroplasty due to polyethylene wear, metallosis-induced carpal tunnel syndrome, distal ulnar impingement, and fourth carpometacarpal joint pain: case report and pitfalls to avoid. Hand (N Y). 2018;15(1):NP1–6.
12. Gil JA, Kamal RN, Cone E, Weiss AC. High survivorship and few complications with cementless total wrist arthroplasty at a mean followup of 9 years. Clin Orthop Relat Res. 2017;475(12):3082–7.
13. Kennedy JW, Ross A, Wright J, Martin DJ, Bransby-Zachary M, MacDonald DJ. Universal 2 total wrist arthroplasty: high satisfaction but high complication rates. J Hand Surg Eur Vol. 2018;43(4):375–9.
14. Zijlker HJA, Ritt MJPF, IJsselstein CB. Long-term results of universal 2 total wrist arthroplasty. J Wrist Surg. 2019;8(4):317–20.
15. Ma JX, Xu YQ. The instability of wrist joint and total wrist replacement. Chin J Traumatol. 2016;19(1):49–51.
16. Boeckstyns ME, Herzberg G. Periprosthetic osteolysis after total wrist arthroplasty. J Wrist Surg. 2014;3(2):101–6.
17. Boeckstyns ME, Herzberg G, Merser S. Favorable results after total wrist arthroplasty: 65 wrists in 60 patients followed for 5-9 years. Acta Orthop. 2013;84(4):415–9.
18. Sagerfors M, Gupta A, Brus O, Pettersson K. Total wrist arthro- plasty: a single-center study of 219 cases with 5-year follow- up. J Hand Surg Am. 2015;40:2380–7.
19. Froschauer SM, Zaussinger M, Hager D, Behawy M, Kwasny O, Duscher D. J Hand Surg Eur Vol. 2019;44(9):946–50.
20. Honecker S, Igeta Y, Al Hefzi A, Pizza C, Facca S, Liverneaux PA. Survival rate on a 10-year follow-up of total wrist replacement implants: a 23-patient case series. J Wrist Surg. 2019;8:24–9.
21. Bohler C, Kolbitsch P, Schuh R, Lass R, Kubista B, Giurea A. Midterm results of a new rotating hinge knee implant: a 5-year follow-up. Biomed Res Int. 2017;2017:7532745.
22. Reigstad O, Røkkum M. Wrist arthroplasty using prosthesis as an alternative to arthrodesis: design, outcomes and future. J Hand Surg Eur Vol. 2018;43(7):689–99.
23. Giwa L, Siddiqui A, Packer G. Motec wrist arthroplasty: 4 years of promising results. J Hand Surg Asian Pac Vol. 2018;23(3):364–8.
24. Ferreres A, Lluch A, Del Valle M. Universal total wrist arthroplasty: midterm follow-up study. J Hand Surg Am. 2011;36(6):967–73.
25. Cooney W, Manuel J, Froelich J, Rizzo M. Total wrist replacement: a retrospective comparative study. J Wrist Surg. 2012;1(2):165–72.
26. Badge R, Kailash K, Dickson DR, et al. Medium-term outcomes of the Universal-2 total wrist arthroplasty in patients with rheumatoid arthritis. Bone Joint J. 2016;98-B(12):1642–7.
27. Fischer P, Sagerfors M, Jakobsson H, Pettersson K. Total wrist arthroplasty: a 10-year follow-up [published online ahead of print, 2020 Apr 1]. J Hand Surg Am. 2020;S0363-5023(20)30084-8.
28. Herzberg G. Promising preliminary results seen with last generation wrist arthroplasty implant. Orthoped Today. 2012;32(10):18.
29. Chevrollier J, Strugarek-Lecoanet C, Dap F, Dautel G. Results of a unicentric series of 15 wrist prosthesis implantations at a 5.2 year follow-up. Acta Orthop Belg. 2016;82(01):31–42.
30. Reigstad A, Reigstad O, Grimsgaard C, Røkkum M. New concept for total wrist replacement. Motec wrist arthroplasty: 4 years of promising results. J Plast Surg Hand Surg. 2011;45(3):148–56.
31. Reigstad O, Holm-Glad T, Bolstad B, Grimsgaard C, Thorkildsen R, Røkkum M. Five- to 10-year prospective follow-up of wrist arthroplasty in 56 nonrheumatoid patients. J Hand Surg Am. 2017;42(10):788–96.
32. Trumble TE, Salas P, Barthel T, Robert KQ III. Management of scaphoid nonunions. J Am Acad Orthop Surg. 2003;11:380–91.

33. Gupta A. Total wrist arthroplasty. Am J Orthop (Belle Mead NJ). 2008;37(8 Suppl 1):12–6.
34. Flury MP, Herren DB, Simmen BR. Die Schulthess-Klassifikation der chronischen Polyarthritis am Handgelenk [The Schulthess classification of chronic polyarthritis of the wrist joint]. Orthopade. 1998;27(3):175–6.
35. Elbuluk AM, Milone MT, Capo JT, Bosco JA, Klifto CS. Trends and demographics in the utilization of total wrist arthroplasty. J Hand Surg Asian Pac Vol. 2018;23(4):501–5.
36. Wolff J. Das Gesetz von der Transformation der Knochen. Berlin: August Hirschwald; 1862.
37. Fishman EK, Ney DR, Heath DG, Corl FM, Horton KM, Johnson PT. Volume rendering versus maximum intensity projection in CT angiography: what works best, when, and why. Radiographics. 2006;26(3):905–22.
38. Halim A, Weiss AC. Total wrist arthroplasty. J Hand Surg Am. 2017;42(3):198–209.
39. Yeoh D, Tourret L. Total wrist arthroplasty: a systematic review of the evidence from the last 5 years. J Hand Surg Eur Vol. 2015;40(5):458–68.
40. Adams BD. Total wrist arthroplasty for posttraumatic arthritis with radius deformity. J Wrist Surg. 2015;4(3):164–8.
41. Matsui Y, Minami A, Kondo M, Ishikawa J, Motomiya M, Iwasaki N. A minimum 5-year longitudinal study of a new total wrist arthroplasty in patients with rheumatoid arthritis. J Hand Surg Am. 2020;45(3):255.e1–7.
42. Minami A, Kato H, Iwasaki N. Modification of the Sauvé-Kapandji procedure with extensor carpi ulnaris tenodesis. J Hand Surg Am. 2000;25(6):1080–4.
43. Minami A, Iwasaki N, Ishikawa J, Suenaga N, Kato H. Stabilization of the proximal ulnar stump in the Sauvé-Kapandji procedure by using the extensor carpi ulnaris tendon: long-term follow-up studies. J Hand Surg Am. 2006;31(3):440–4.
44. Surgical technique Integra® Freedom Wrist Arthroplasty System. 2014. https://www.smith-nephew.com/documents/nl-freedom-surgicaltechnique.pdf
45. Srnec JJ, Wagner ER, Rizzo M. Total wrist arthroplasty. JBJS Rev. 2018;6(6):e9.
46. Anneberg M, Packer G, Crisco JJ, Wolfe S. Four-year outcomes of midcarpal hemiarthroplasty for wrist arthritis. J Hand Surg Am. 2017;42(11):894–903.
47. Herzberg G, Walch A, Burnier M. Wrist hemiarthroplasty for irreparable DRF in the elderly. Eur J Orthop Surg Traumatol. 2018;28(8):1499–503.
48. Huish EG Jr, Lum Z, Bamberger HB, Trzeciak MA. Failure of wrist hemiarthroplasty. Hand (N Y). 2017;12(4):369–75.
49. Vergnenègre G, Hardy J, Mabit C, Charissoux JL, Marcheix PS. Hemiarthroplasty for complex distal radius fractures in elderly patients. J Wrist Surg. 2015;4(3):169–73.
50. Anger F, Legré R, Nguyen MK. Results of wrist hemiarthroplasty for comminuted distal radius fractures in independent elderly people: a retrospective study on eleven patients. Hand Surg Rehabil. 2019;38(3):150–6.
51. Boyer JS, Adams B. Radius hemiarthroplasty combined with proximal row carpectomy. Iowa Othop J. 2010;30:168–73.
52. Culp RW, Bachoura A, Gelman SE, Jacoby SM. Proximal row carpectomy combined with wrist hemiarthroplasty. J Wrist Surg. 2012;1(1):39–46.
53. Vance MC, Packer G, Tan D, Crisco JJ, Wolfe SW. Midcarpal hemiarthroplasty for wrist arthritis: rationale and early results. J Wrist Surg. 2012;1(1):61–8.
54. Roux JL. Replacement and resurfacing prosthesis of the distal radius: a new therapeutic concept [in French]. Chir Main. 2009;28(1):10–7.
55. Gaspar MP, Lou J, Kane PM, Jacoby SM, Osterman AL, Culp RW. Complications following partial and total wrist arthroplasty: a single-center retrospective review. J Hand Surg Am. 2016;41(1):47–53.e4.

# Revision/Failed Total Wrist Arthroplasty

9

Michel E. H. Boeckstyns

## Introduction

Fourth-generation implants for total wrist (TW) arthroplasty have been available for more than 20 years, and consequently, an increasing number need revision. The treatment options for the salvage of failed TW arthroplasty include arthrodesis, TW revision arthroplasty, resection arthroplasty, and interpositional pyrocarbon arthroplasty. TW arthrodesis is the reference treatment, but revision TW arthroplasty is an alternative option [1–5]. Interpositional and resection arthroplasties have been reported occasionally. In this chapter, published results and the author's personal experience are presented.

## Survey of the Literature

### Salvage by TW Arthrodesis

Revision of failed older-generation TW arthroplasties has been challenging due to the large bone defects resulting from the extraction of the bulky implants [4, 6–8]. Since total wrist arthrodesis was known to be a good solution for painful destroyed rheumatoid wrists, TW arthrodesis has been the most frequently used revision procedure in the days when rheumatoid arthritis was the main indication for TW arthroplasty. The technical challenges include extraction of osseointegrated components (typically the radial component), restoration of proper carpal height, and obtaining stable fixation. The radius may need to be split to facilitate removal of the implant, and cement and cerclage wires may be used to stabilize the radius in these cases. Bone grafting of the residual bony defect with an iliac crest autograft or an allograft – typically from a femoral head – is mandatory.

Intramedullary Steinmann pins, in some cases supplemented with staples, have been the most common method of fixation, but substantial complications and nonunion rates have been reported [9–12]. The series of Beer and Turner [9] included revision of eight silicone spacers and four older-generation implants. Only 7 out of 12 wrists achieved fusion, although non-fused arthrodeses could be well-tolerated. Carlson and Simmons [10] published a series of 12 wrists – 5 silicone and 7 older-generation TW arthroplasty – that were revised to a wrist arthrodesis. Complications included two patients with nonunions requiring secondary bone grafting procedures, and two patients requiring revisions of their intramedullary pins. Radmer et al. [13] revised 36 APH

M. E. H. Boeckstyns (✉)
Capio Private Hospital, Section for Hand Surgery, Hellerup, Denmark

Herlev-Gentofte University Hospital, Section for Hand Surgery, Hellerup, Denmark
e-mail: mibo@dadlnet.dk


G. J. W. King, M. Rizzo (eds.), *Arthroplasty of the Upper Extremity*,
https://doi.org/10.1007/978-3-030-68880-6_9

prostheses (APH, Implant-Service Vertriebs-GmbH, Hamburg, Germany) to arthrodesis, 25 with intramedullary nail fixation and 11 with plate and screw fixation, and obtained primary union in 34: the 2 nonunions occurred in the intramedullary nail group. Rizzo et al. [12] examined the outcomes of wrist arthrodesis for failed total wrist arthroplasty in a study of 21 wrists. The arthrodesis was stabilized with pins or plate and screws and achieved primary fusion in 11 wrists, while 10 had a nonunion.

Brase and Millender [14] reported on 16 revisions of failed silicone implants. Twelve wrists were revised to another silicone implant and four were fused. While the results after revision with another implant were discouraging and only four of the patients revised with implants reported adequate strength for most normal activities, all four patients that had an arthrodesis obtained stable, pain-free wrists [14].

Ferlic et al. [11] revised 19 wrist arthroplasties – 7 silicone implants and 12 metal-on-plastic total wrist arthroplasties. Each of the seven silicone implants was successfully revised in one operation; the four fusions and three total wrist implants were functioning 6 or more years after surgery. Nineteen operations were needed to revise the metal-on-plastic implants. All of the loose prostheses eventually required arthrodesis, but, of these two required more than one attempt [11].

More recently plate and screw fixation has been the most used fixation method (Fig. 9.1). A locking plate is preferred owing to the poor bone quality in many rheumatoid patients and the prolonged time that may be required for fusion. Adams et al. [15] published a series of 20 wrists, including 15 revisions of a fourth-generation TWA and 5 older-generation implants, one of which was a silicone spacer. All patients were treated using a dedicated wrist arthrodesis dorsal plate (Synthes, West Chester, PA) and a contoured cancellous femoral head structural allograft. Nineteen of 20 wrists fused at the first attempt at a median of 4 months. Proximal plate loosening occurred in one wrist, but the joint still fused at 6 months [15]. Reigstad et al. published a series of 11 failed Motec or Elos wrist arthroplasties (Swemac Orthopaedics AB, Linköping, Sweden) for osteoarthritis which were subsequently converted to arthrodesis using an arthrodesis plate in 8 cases or a customized peg in 3 cases. Clinical and radiological bone union was achieved in all the operated wrists.

Rizzo et al. [12] report on the functional results after TW arthrodesis for failed arthroplasty. Fourteen of 21 wrists had no pain, and there was an overall average pain score of 2.6

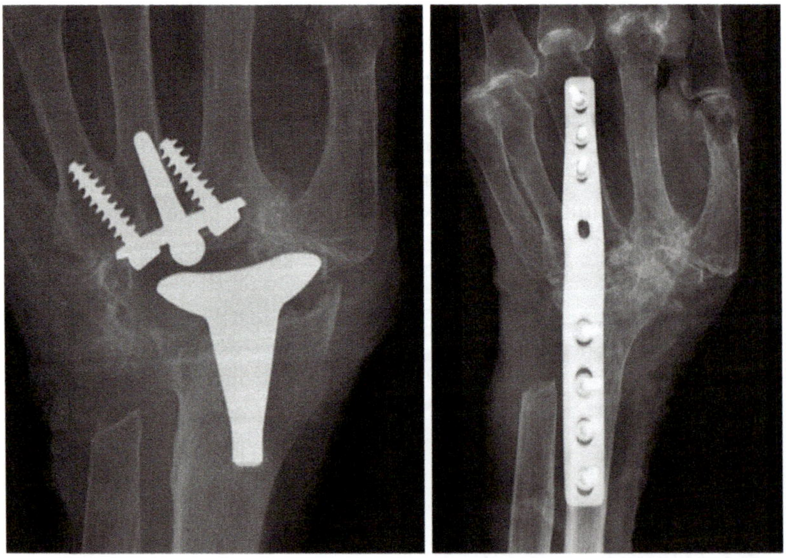

**Fig. 9.1** Revision of a failed Remotion total wrist arthroplasty to a total wrist arthrodesis

(range 0–7) on a visual analogue scale from 0 to 10. The group of patients with persistent non-union of the arthrodesis had an average pain score of 3.3 (range 0–7) versus an average pain score of 2.1 (range 0–4) in the group that fused. Overall DASH scores averaged 33 (range 11–59). The average DASH was 29 (range 11–45) in the fused group and 36 (range 13–57) in the non-union cases. Return to work data were applicable in only ten patients, of whom four were able to return to their previous level of work, four returned to work with some degree of restriction, and two either ceased work or were unable to return to work.

## Revision Arthroplasty

Rettig and Beckenbaugh used a Biaxial implant (DePuy Orthopedics, Warsaw, IN, USA) to salvage 13 failed total wrist arthroplasties of various designs, including 2 cemented Meuli (Protek AG, Bern, Switzerland), 7 Swanson Silastic (Wright Medical, Memphis, TN, USA), 2 Biaxial, and 2 Volz (Howmedica Company, Rutherford, NJ, USA) total wrist arthroplasties [2]. The distal component of the revision implant was cemented in all cases, the proximal component in 11 cases. Within a follow-up period of 31 months, two cases were converted to another prosthesis and one to a wrist arthrodesis. Two more implants showed radiographic signs of loosening. The clinical results were satisfactory in the remaining.

Cobb and Beckenbaugh published a series of ten cases of total wrist arthroplasty with a custom long-stemmed multipronged distal component, mostly a two-pronged component in the second and third metacarpal. Two had been converted to a TW arthrodesis. For the remaining eight patients, the mean follow-up period was 3.8 years (range, 3.0–4.8 years). All of the cases had functional total wrist arthroplasties at the latest follow-up evaluation [1].

Fischer et al. [16] reported on 16 revision TW arthroplasties after failure of TW arthroplasties of various designs. All patients suffered from rheumatoid arthritis. The types of revision surgery performed were exchange of the whole prosthesis in 11 cases, exchange of the proximal component in 1, and exchange of the distal component in 4. Biaxial, Remotion (Stryker, Kalamazoo, MI, USA), or Universal 2 (Integra LifeSciences, Plainsboro, NJ, USA) components were used for revision. Cement was used for fixation of the distal component of the Biaxial prosthesis in six cases. In the other cases, synthetic bone graft or allograft bone from a fresh-frozen femoral head was used to compensate for bone loss around the distal component. Four of the 16 revision arthroplasties were re-revised. Three wrists ended up with a TW arthrodesis and one with a resection arthroplasty. The 5-year cumulative implant survival was 74%, and the median DASH and PRWE scores were 60 and 37, respectively, at 5 years [16].

Pinder et al. published a series of 19 cases with various diagnoses. Five of the primary implants were silicone spacers, five were Universal 2, and eight were Biaxial. The implants used for revision were Universal 2 and Biaxial. The mean follow-up time was 10 years. The cumulative 5-year implant revision survival was 83%. Clinical outcome data were available for five patients only [17].

Talwalkar et al. report on ten failed Biaxial implants. Nine of these suffered from rheumatoid arthritis. Six underwent a revision to a second biaxial wrist replacement, three had a wrist fusion, and two were treated by excision arthroplasty. Nine of these patients were available for a clinical review. Follow-up time was 28 months. No re-revisions required further surgery or revision. Two patients with revision wrist replacements had good results, one had a fair result and one had a poor result [3].

Zijlker et al. [5] published a series of 40 wrists in 37 patients with a failed Biaxial prosthesis that were converted to a Universal 2 total wrist arthroplasty. In 24 patients the diagnosis was rheumatoid arthritis; in 11 it was osteoarthritis and in 2 Kienböck's disease. Autologous corticocancellous bone graft from the iliac crest was used in all patients. Sixteen of the 40 implants eventually failed. The cumulated 5-year survival was 87% and the 9-year survival 60%. There was no significant difference between rheumatoid and non-rheumatoid patients in terms of implant failure. Sixteen of the 24 Universal 2 implants that remained in situ after a mean follow-up of 9 years functioned satisfactorily. Patient-Rated Wrist and Hand Evaluation scores and Quick Disabilities of the Arm, Shoulder and Hand scores were 53 and 47, respectively [18].

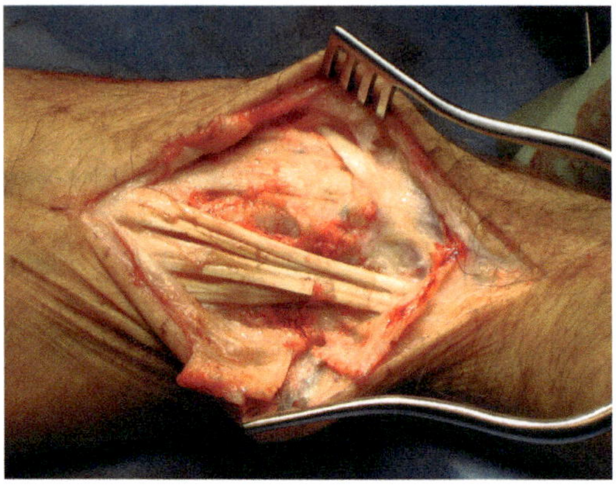

**Fig. 9.2** Intraoperative photograph showing the well-defined, reflected extensor retinaculum, divided in the fourth compartment

## Interpositional Pyrocarbon Arthroplasty

Case reports about revision of failed TW arthroplasties with the pyrocarbon radiocarpal Amandys (Tornier, Montbonnot, France) have been presented, but larger series have not been published [19].

## Resection Arthroplasty

This solution is sometimes adopted in patients who are unfit for a major procedure, or in cases where implants are excised because of infection and the result turns out to be functionally acceptable. Reports are very scarce. Both cases in the series of Talwalkar et al. had excellent results [3].

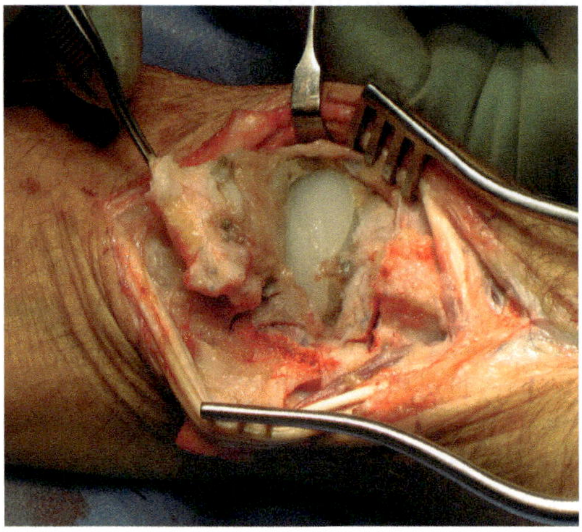

**Fig. 9.3** A distally based U-shaped capsular flap has been reflected, exposing the implant

## Author's Preferred Techniques and Personal Experience

### Technique for Revision Arthroplasty

The procedure is performed in general anesthesia or regional block and with a tourniquet applied at the upper arm. The previous skin incision over the dorsum of the hand and wrist is used. Usually the extensor retinaculum is well defined and can be divided in the fourth compartment (Fig. 9.2). The wrist capsule is opened making a U-shaped, distally based flap (Fig. 9.3). Typically, the carpal component can be removed with minimal force, especially if it is loose, which often is the case (Fig. 9.4). Removal of a well-fixed radial component can be challenging (Fig. 9.5). Burring and chiseling all around the component or an osteotomy of the radius is usually required to disrupt the osteointegration of an uncemented component or to break the cement mantle of a cemented component. Making the osteotomy at the radial side preserves the dorsal cortex. All cement, membranes, and necrotic bone are removed (Fig. 9.6). The cavities are filled with cancellous bone (Fig. 9.7). Subsequently, the radial diaphysis and the capitate are reamed (Fig. 9.8). The trial components are placed (Fig. 9.9), and their position is checked under the image intensifier. In the case of severe bone loss, a bone allograft is intercalated between the carpal plate and the reaming distal bone. The stability of the arthro-

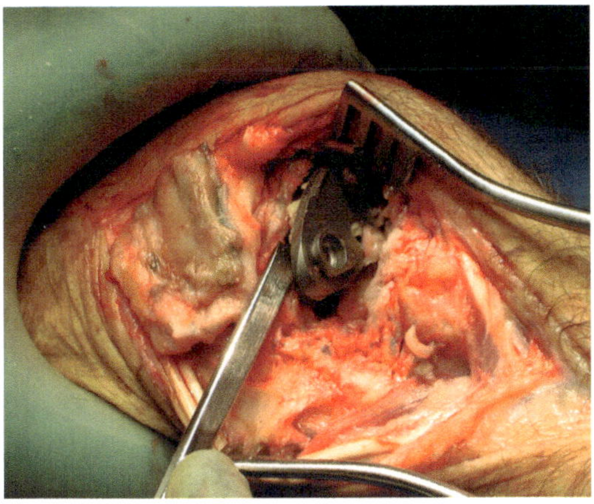

**Fig. 9.4** Removal of the distal component is usually easy

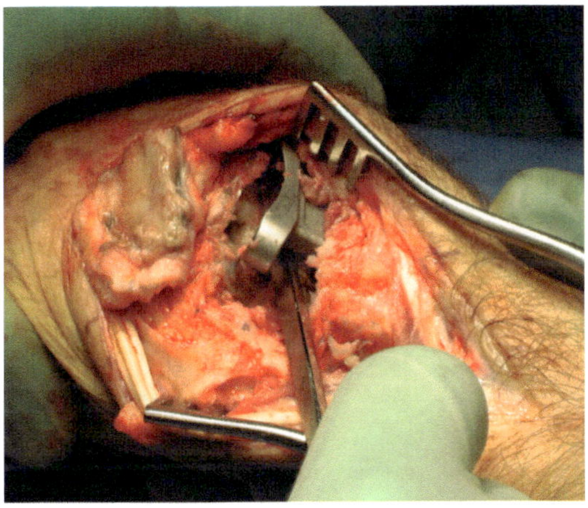

**Fig. 9.5** Removal of the loose proximal component was easy in this case, but removal of a solidly osseointegrated component can be challenging

plasty is tested during passive wrist motion as well as by longitudinal traction: this is subjective and requires experience. Finally, the implant components are impacted. I use a plastic or bony plug to obliterate the bottom of the radial cavity (Fig. 9.10) and mostly a cemented technique. Any excess cement is removed and remaining cavities are filled with cancellous bone (Fig. 9.11). A standard layered closure is performed (Fig. 9.12). The wrist is protected in a cast for 2 weeks and thereafter mobilized with gradually increasing loads. In case of a subsided

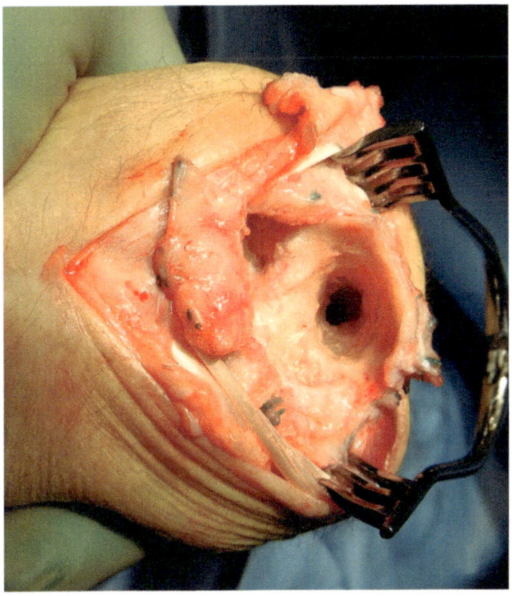

**Fig. 9.6** The radial cavity has been completely cleaned for cement, membranes, and necrotic bone

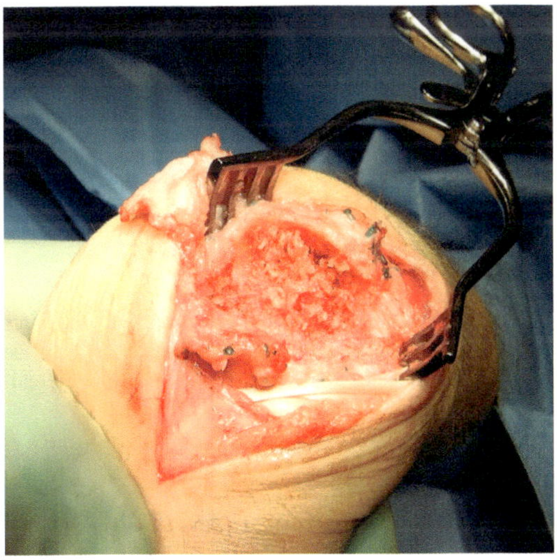

**Fig. 9.7** The radial cavity has been packed with cancellous allograft

carpal component that needs revision and a solidly implanted radial component, it suffices to exchange the carpal component alone, provided the same type of prosthesis is available.

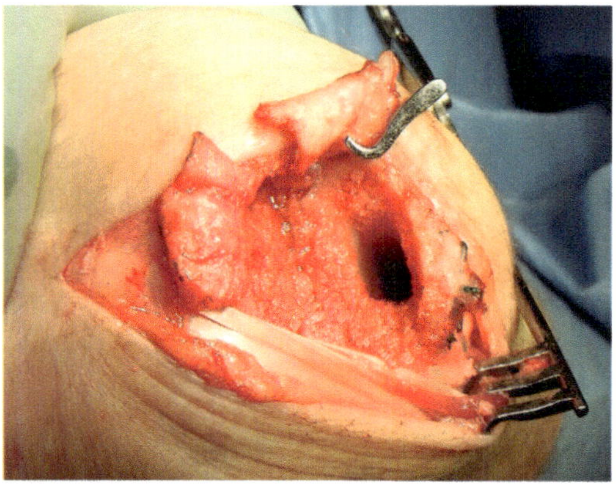

Fig. 9.8 The grafted radial cavity has been reamed

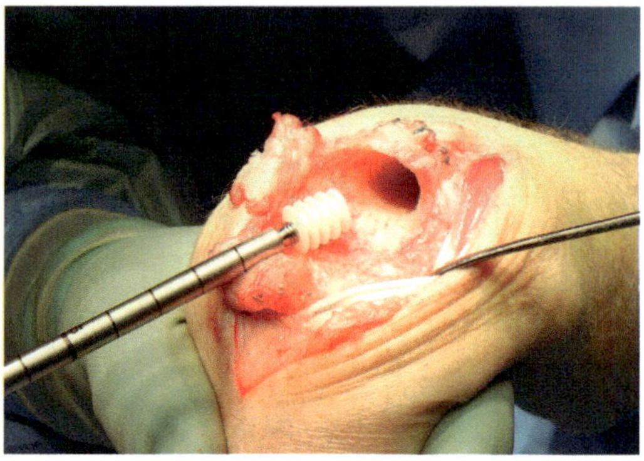

Fig. 9.10 A plastic plug is inserted to close the bottom of the radial cavity before cementation of the radial implant

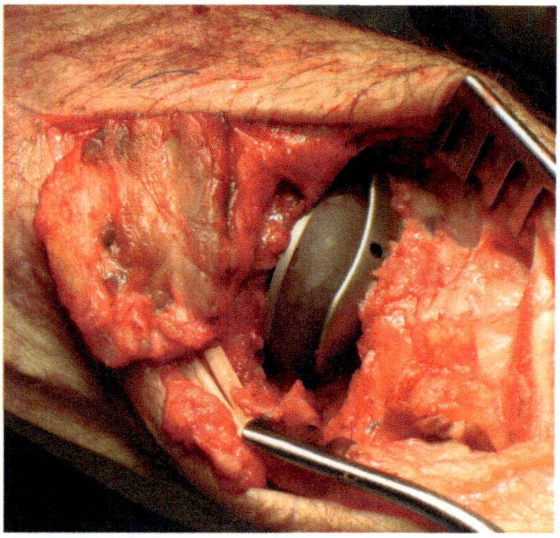

Fig. 9.9 The trial components are impacted, ready for stability testing. Carpal height and stability can be adjusted by choosing the right thickness of the intercalated carpal ball

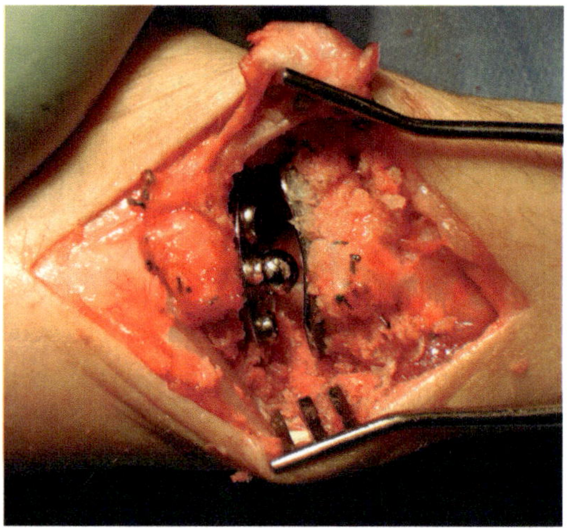

Fig. 9.11 The final components are in place, and residual bone defects have been grafted before impacting the intercalated polyethylene carpal ball

## Technique for Conversion to TW Arthrodesis

The approach and the removal of the failed components are performed as described above. A femoral head structural allograft is prepared to fit the bone defect and preserve the carpal height (Fig. 9.13). Care is taken to fuse the third carpometacarpal joint by removing its articular surfaces and packing the defect with cancellous bone. A stainless steel or titanium wrist arthrodesis plate is applied to the radial shaft and third metacarpal using a standard technique. Whenever possible, I prefer a pre-contoured plate to position the wrist in slight extension (Fig. 9.14). Screws are not inserted through the central portion of the plate in order to avoid fracture of the graft.

## Clinical Series

I reviewed a consecutive series of failed TW arthroplasties that were revised at Gentofte Hospital, Denmark, between 2008 and 2018 (Table 9.1). The primary implants were nine Remotion, two Motec, and one Universal 1.

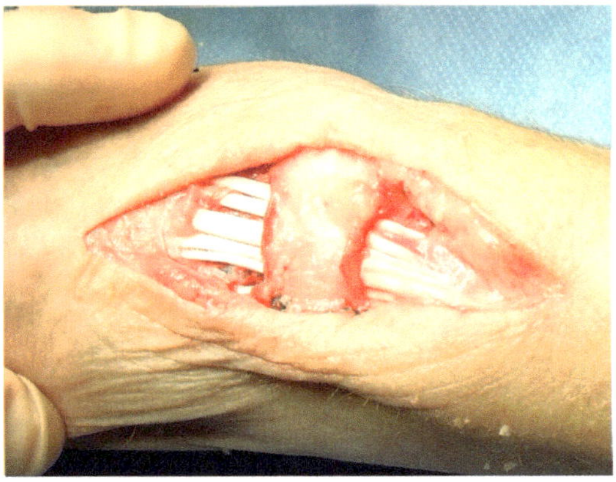

Fig. 9.12 A standard layered closure is performed

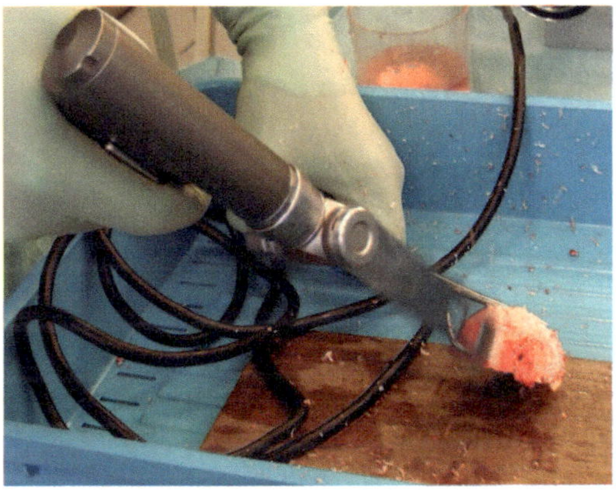

Fig. 9.13 Preparation of a fresh-frozen femoral head to fit into the defect left after extraction of the implant to be revised

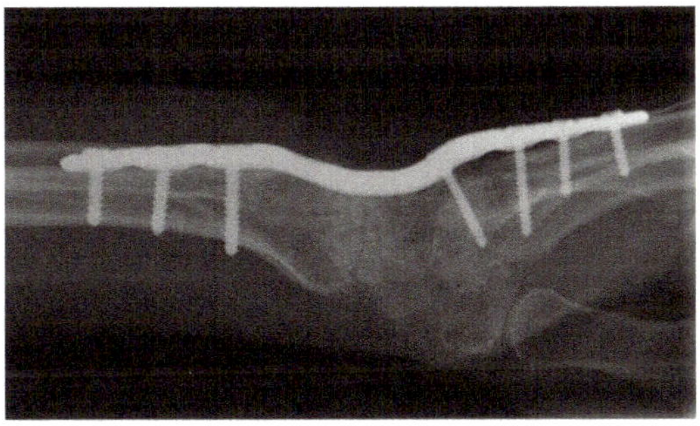

Fig. 9.14 Revision arthrodesis positioned in slight, functional extension. The degree of extension can be adjusted according to individual needs

Mean age at primary operation was 58 years (range: 28–78). The choice of revision technique was based on stability and bone stock and finally decided by shared decision-making with the informed patients. The mean follow-up time was 31 months (range 3–102). Arthrodesis was used as the first revision procedure in four cases, using plate and screw fixation. Revision arthroplasty was performed in ten cases, using a Remotion TW prosthesis (Fig. 9.15).

## Results

Five of the ten revision Remotions were re-revised and all finally ended up with a TW arthrodesis. All arthrodeses went on to fuse at the first attempt. The median QuickDASH score for patients with a functioning Remotion prosthesis was 36 at follow-up (range 18–54) and median VAS score for pain 0 (range 0–2.5). Median QuickDASH score for patients with fused wrist was 34 (range 25–63) and VAS score 2 (range 0–2). The differences of the scores between the Remotion and the fused groups were neither statistically nor clinically significant ($p = 0.23$ and 0.35, Mann-Whitney U test).

## Discussion

Total wrist arthrodesis for the salvage of failed TWA results in a complete limitation of wrist flexion/extension and radial/ulnar deviation. In order to prevent these limitations, failed implants could be salvaged by a revision implant. However, the reported implant survivals seem definitely lower compared with the survival rate in primarily implanted fourth-generation TW prostheses reported by some authors (91–100% at 8–10-year follow-up) [20–23] but not much different from the survival reported by others (50–69% at 8–10 years) [24–28]. In my personal series, half of the revised TW arthroplasties were ultimately converted to TW arthrodesis. Conversely, all

**Table 9.1** Characteristics of 14 revised wrist arthroplasties

| Patient number | Characteristic<br>Sex | Age | Diagnosis | Primary implant | Indication for revision | Revision technique | Re-revision | Final wrist status | QuickDASH score | VAS score for pain | Patient satisfaction |
|---|---|---|---|---|---|---|---|---|---|---|---|
| 1 | F | 39 | RA | Remotion | Fixed flexion deformity | Arthrodesis | No | Fused wrist | 31 | 0 | Very pleased |
| 2 | F | 56 | RA | Remotion | Loosening carpal and radial component | Cemented Remotion | No | Remotion | 36 | 2 | Very pleased |
| 3 | F | 28 | PT (SLAC) | Remotion | Malposition | Cemented Remotion | Arthrodesis | Fused wrist | 63 | 2 | Pleased |
| 4 | F | 57 | RA | Remotion | Loosening carpal component | Uncemented Remotion | Arthrodesis | Fused wrist | 54 | 2 | Pleased |
| 5 | M | 65 | RA | Remotion | Loosening radial component | Cemented Remotion | 1. Implant removal<br>2. Arthrodesis | Remotion | 16 | 2 | Pleased |
| 6 | F | 73 | OA | Remotion | Loosening carpal component | Cemented Remotion | Arthrodesis | Fused wrist | No follow-up | | |
| 7 | M | 54 | OA | Remotion | Loosening radial component | Cemented Remotion | No | Remotion | 22 | 2.5 | Pleased |
| 8 | M | 68 | SNAC | Universal 1 | Loosening radial component | Cemented Remotion | No | Remotion | 18 | 0 | Very pleased |
| 9 | F | 51 | SLAC | Motec | Loosening carpal component | Cemented Remotion | 1. Re-arthroplasty<br>2. Arthrodesis | Fused wrist | 26 | 2 | Pleased |
| 10 | F | 55 | RA | Motec | Loosening carpal component | Cemented Remotion | No | Remotion | 54 | 0 | Very pleased |
| 11 | F | 78 | RA | Remotion | Loosening carpal component | Arthrodesis | No | Fused wrist | 43 | 1 | Very pleased |
| 12 | F | 61 | Kienböck's disease | Remotion | Loosening carpal component | Cemented Remotion | No | Remotion | 36 | 0 | Pleased |
| 13 | M | 68 | OA | Remotion | Pain and osteolysis | Arthrodesis | No | Fused wrist | 36 | 2 | Pleased |
| 14 | F | 57 | PT (SLAC) | Remotion | Loosening carpal component | Arthrodesis | No | Fused wrist | 25 | 1 | Pleased |

*F* female, *M* male, *OA* osteoarthritis, *RA* rheumatoid arthritis, *PT* post-traumatic arthritis, *SLAC* scapholunate advanced collapse, *QuickDASH* short version of the Disabilities of the Arm, Shoulder and Hand questionnaire, *VAS* visual analogue scale

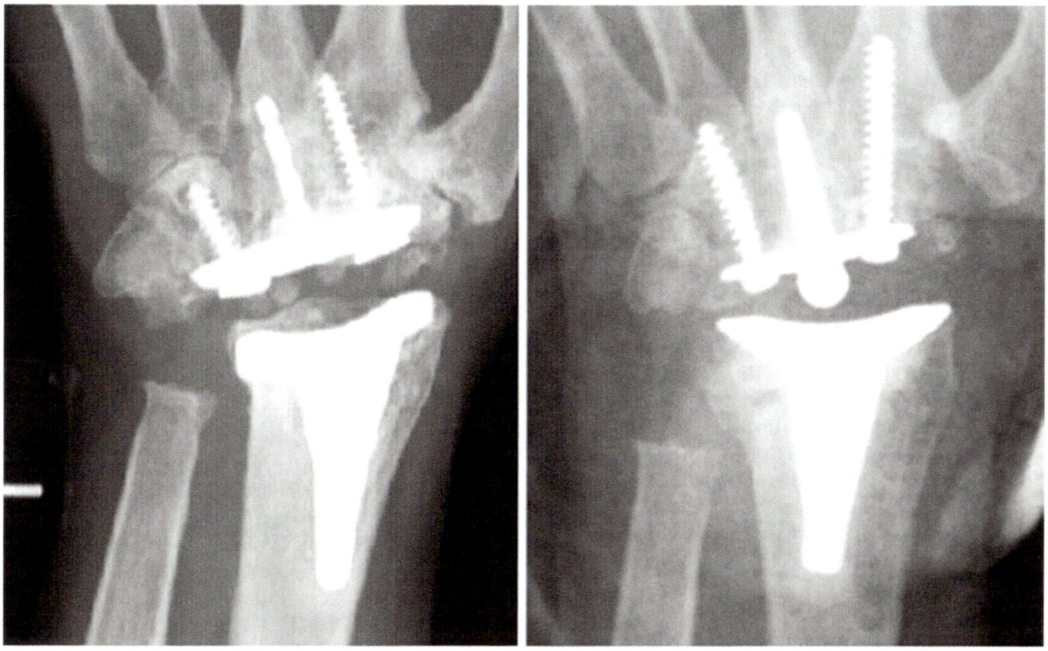

**Fig. 9.15** Pre- and postoperative radiograph of the implant exchange shown in Figure 9.2–9.14

arthrodesis healed by first intention and the patient-reported outcomes in the patient with fused wrists did not differ significantly from those in the patients with functional revision arthroplasties. The range of scores is similar to that reported by Rizzo et al. [12]. There is no doubt that the added costs, the difficulty, and the risks of each supplemental revision procedure are high. It can also be questioned whether there are patient-related factors that caused failure of the primary arthroplasty, which in turn can cause failure of a revision implant if not identified and eliminated. For these reasons, today it is my believe and current strategy that TW arthrodesis is the first choice procedure for most cases and that revision arthroplasty should be performed in very carefully selected patients only. Future studies must be carried out to identify the patients that most likely would benefit from a revision arthroplasty and which patients would be better off with an arthrodesis.

**Tips and Tricks**

- If removal of an osseointegrated radial component requires osteotomy of the radius, this can advantageously been done on the radial side, leaving the dorsal radial cortex intact for the placement of the fusion plate.
- Use plate locking screws rather than pins and staples for the fixation of an arthrodesis in osteoporotic bone.
- Weakening of finger extension and grip strength can result from reduction of carpal height and tendon bowstringing. Repair the extensor retinaculum whenever possible and restore carpal height.
- Placement of the wrist in extension and restoring carpal height favor grip strength.
- When performing re-arthroplasty, crossing the CMC joints may be necessary for the fixation of an intercalated bone graft. In these cases, the CMC joints must be fused.

## References


1. Cobb TK, Beckenbaugh RD. Biaxial long-stemmed multipronged distal components for revision/bone deficit total-wrist arthroplasty. J Hand Surg Am. 1996;21(5):764–70.
2. Rettig ME, Beckenbaugh RD. Revision total wrist arthroplasty. J Hand Surg Am. 1993;18(5):798–804.
3. Talwalkar SC, Hayton MJ, Trail IA, Stanley JK. Management of the failed biaxial wrist replacement. J Hand Surg. 2005;30(3):248–51.
4. Vogelin E, Nagy L. Fate of failed Meuli total wrist arthroplasty. J Hand Surg. 2003;28(1):61–8.
5. Zijlker HJA, Berkhout MJ, Ritt M, van Leeuwen N, CB IJ. Universal 2 total wrist arthroplasty for the salvage of failed biaxial total wrist arthroplasty. J Hand Surg Eur Vol. 2019;44(6):614–9.
6. Cooney WP 3rd, Beckenbaugh RD, Linscheid RL. Total wrist arthroplasty. Problems with implant failures. Clin Orthop Related Res. 1984;187:121–8.
7. Menon J. Total wrist replacement using the modified Volz prosthesis. J Bone Joint Surg Am. 1987;69(7):998–1006.
8. Volz RG. Total wrist arthroplasty. A clinical review. Clin Orthop Related Res. 1984;187:112–20.
9. Beer TA, Turner RH. Wrist arthrodesis for failed wrist implant arthroplasty. J Hand Surg Am. 1997;22(4):685–93.
10. Carlson JR, Simmons BP. Wrist arthrodesis after failed wrist implant arthroplasty. J Hand Surg Am. 1998;23(5):893–8.
11. Ferlic DC, Jolly SN, Clayton ML. Salvage for failed implant arthroplasty of the wrist. J Hand Surg Am. 1992;17(5):917–23.
12. Rizzo M, Ackerman DB, Rodrigues RL, Beckenbaugh RD. Wrist arthrodesis as a salvage procedure for failed implant arthroplasty. J Hand Surg Eur Vol. 2011;36(1):29–33.
13. Radmer S, Andresen R, Sparmann M. Total wrist arthroplasty in patients with rheumatoid arthritis. J Hand Surg Am. 2003;28(5):789–94.
14. Brase DW, Millender LH. Failure of silicone rubber wrist arthroplasty in rheumatoid arthritis. J Hand Surg Am. 1986;11(2):175–83.
15. Adams BD, Kleinhenz BP, Guan JJ. Wrist arthrodesis for failed Total wrist arthroplasty. J Hand Surg Am. 2016;41(6):673–9.
16. Fischer P, Sagerfors M, Brus O, Pettersson K. Revision arthroplasty of the wrist in patients with rheumatoid arthritis, mean follow-up 6.6 years. J Hand Surg. 2018;43(5):489 e481–7.
17. Pinder EM, Chee KG, Hayton M, Murali SR, Talwalkar SC, Trail IA. Survivorship of revision wrist replacement. J Wrist Surg. 2018;7(1):18–23.
18. Zijlker HJA, Ritt M, CB IJ. Long-term results of universal 2 Total wrist arthroplasty. J Wrist Surg. 2019;8(4):317–20.
19. Bellemere P. Medium- and long-term outcomes for hand and wrist pyrocarbon implants. J Hand Surg Eur Vol. 2019;44(9):887–97.
20. Badge R, Kailash K, Dickson DR, et al. Medium-term outcomes of the Universal-2 total wrist arthroplasty in patients with rheumatoid arthritis. Bone Joint J. 2016;98-b(12):1642–7.
21. Ferreres A, Lluch A, Del Valle M. Universal total wrist arthroplasty: midterm follow-up study. J Hand Surg Am. 2011;36(6):967–73.
22. Sagerfors M, Gupta A, Brus O, Pettersson K. Total wrist arthroplasty: a single-center study of 219 cases with 5-year follow-up. J Hand Surg Am. 2015;40(12):2380–7.
23. Weiss KE, Rodner CM. Osteoarthritis of the wrist. J Hand Surg Am. 2007;32(5):725–46.
24. Chevrollier J, Strugarek-Lecoanet C, Dap F, Dautel G. Results of a unicentric series of 15 wrist prosthesis implantations at a 5.2 year follow-up. Acta Orthop Belg. 2016;82(1):31–42.
25. Gaspar MP, Lou J, Kane PM, Jacoby SM, Osterman AL, Culp RW. Complications following partial and total wrist arthroplasty: a single-center retrospective review. J Hand Surg Am. 2016;41(1):47–53. e44
26. Honecker S, Igeta Y, Al Hefzi A, Pizza C, Facca S, Liverneaux PA. Survival rate on a 10-year follow-up of total wrist replacement implants: a 23-patient case series. J Wrist Surg. 2019;8(1):24–9.
27. Pfanner S, Munz G, Guidi G, Ceruso M. Universal 2 wrist arthroplasty in rheumatoid arthritis. J Wrist J. 2017;6(3):206–15.
28. Ward CM, Kuhl T, Adams BD. Five to ten-year outcomes of the universal total wrist arthroplasty in patients with rheumatoid arthritis. J Bone Joint Surg Am. 2011;93(10):914–9.

# Part IV

# Distal Radioulnar Joint Arthroplasty

# Design Considerations for Distal Radioulnar Joint Arthroplasty

# 10

Amit Gupta and Luis R. Scheker

## Introduction

The functional importance of the distal radioulnar joint has been ignored and misunderstood for a long time, resulting in the distal ulna being amputated, fused, and modified in ways that the function of the distal radioulnar joint disappeared, leaving the patient with considerable disability. Historically, it was Claude Bernard in 1851 [1] who published on the resection of the ulnar head, followed by others including Moore in 1880 [2]. Thirty years later Darrach [3] proposed that the resection be made subperiosteal. The failures of the available techniques led Kapandji, whose chief was Sauvé [4] (based on the findings of Baldwin [5] that in cases of ankylosis of the DRUJ, removing a piece of the ulnar shaft could restore pronation/supination), to perform fusion of the distal radioulnar joint with resection of a segment proximal to the head of the ulna and create a pseudoarthrosis at that point to maintain pronation and supination. However, the problem of instability of the end of the ulna persisted albeit at a more proximal level.

In the 1980s and the 1990s, interest in distal radioulnar joint (DRUJ) increased, with studies that allowed us to appreciate kinematics, biomechanics, and anatomy of DRUJ [6–13]. These studies resulted in a better understanding and a reasoned therapeutic approach to the clinical problems that affect the distal radioulnar joint.

Pathologies that affect DRUJ include arthritic problems of inflammatory, degenerative, and traumatic origin, genetic conditions such as Madelung deformity and Ehlers-Danlos syndrome, sports conditions such as epiphyseal arrest of the distal radius found in the gymnast, and arrest of the ulnar epiphysis. The innumerable techniques [14–22] that attempt to solve the problems of the distal radioulnar joint available in the literature are an indicator of the lack of a definitive solution to this problem that not only causes pain and functional disability but can also deleteriously affect the patient's quality of life and health like his/her social function (work, sports activities, relationship with friends and family), physical function, vitality, and even his state of mental function. When applicable, the patient's inability to return to work further affects his/her economic and mental well-being.

## Anatomy and Kinematics

A bicondylar joint connects the radius to the ulna through (1) the annular ligament over the head of the radius, (2) the triangular fibrocartilage complex (TFCC) (Fig. 10.1) that holds the distal radius of the ulnar head, and (3) the interosseous

A. Gupta (✉)
Department of Orthopedic Surgery, University of Louisville, Louisville, KY, USA

L. R. Scheker
Kleinert Institute, Louisville, KY, USA


G. J. W. King, M. Rizzo (eds.), *Arthroplasty of the Upper Extremity*,
https://doi.org/10.1007/978-3-030-68880-6_10

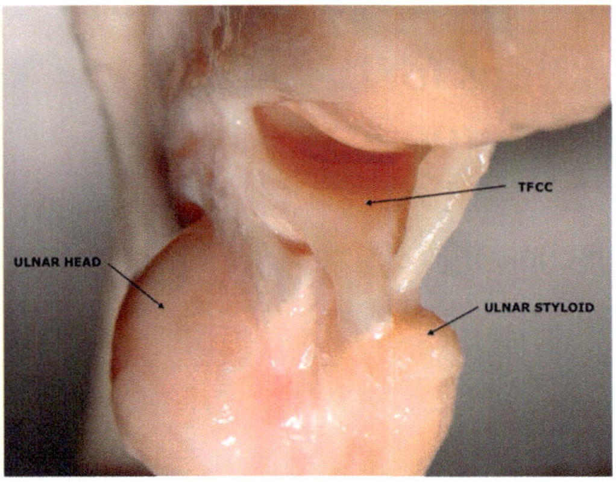


**Fig. 10.1** Anatomical specimen showing the radius, ulnar head and styloid, carpus, and TFCC

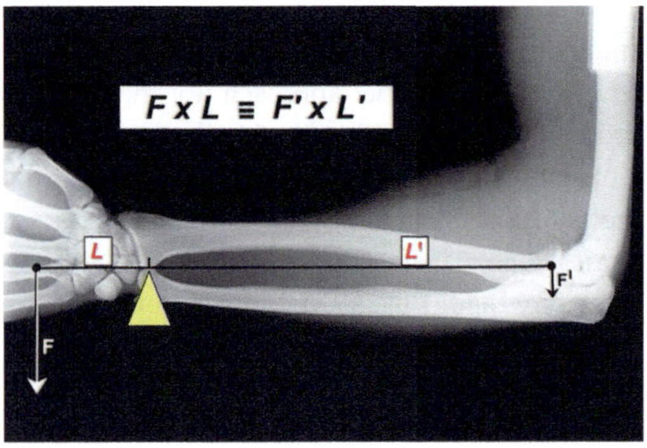


**Fig. 10.2** The axis of pronation/supination of the forearm is an imaginary line that passes through the center of the head of the radius proximally and through the fovea of the head of the ulna distally

membrane [12]. The distal radioulnar joint is in fact a "hemi-joint," with the other half being the proximal radioulnar joint (PRUJ).

Any phenomenon that alters the PRUJ or the relative length of the bones of the forearm, or that creates an abnormal angulation, can influence the functioning of the DRUJ whose axis of pronation/supination is formed by an imaginary line that passes through the center of the head of the radius proximally and through the fovea of the head of the ulna distally, such that the distal radius rotates over the ulnar head (Fig. 10.2).

The distal hemi-component of the radioulnar joint consists of bone ends and a ligament-stabilizing system. The head of the ulna and the sigmoid fossa of the radius (Fig. 10.3) constitute the articular bone elements. An important anatomical aspect is that the articular surface of the sigmoid fossa resembles an inverted hemi-cone, which prints a "corkscrew or corkscrew effect" on the head of the ulna during pronation/supination giving rise to an axial piston movement. Thus, during pronation there is a relative shortening of the radius, and as a consequence there is a relative distal axial displacement or "lengthening" of the ulnar head. In supination the opposite happens and there is a relative "shortening" of the ulnar head. In reality, the ulnar head does not move; it is the radius that shortens as it passes over the ulnar head during pronation. The radius also moves palmarly during pronation and dorsally during supination; this movement is the one that tenses the triangular fibrocartilage and limits the angle of movement.

When analyzing the articular surfaces of the DRUJ, it is observed that the sigmoid fossa is shallow with a 60-degree arc while the ulnar head arc is 105 degrees (Fig. 10.4). This makes the joint intrinsically incongruous, so that maximum joint contact exists only during the neutral or zero pronation/supination position. At maximum pronation, the radius moves, and only the deep dorsal ligament maintains it with minimal contact with the ulnar head, which makes the joint susceptible to dorsal subluxation; however, during supination, the contact between the ulna and the radius is increased because the palmar edge of the sigmoid fossa extends toward the ulnar side and the palmar ligament is stronger than the dorsal ligament, so the palmar subluxation is less frequent. It is necessary to remember that when we lift heavy objects, we supinate the forearm so that the biceps and the brachialis work in unison. In neutral or pronation position only, the brachialis flexes the elbow actively. For this reason, the anatomy of the sigmoid fossa has been created with greater contact during supination than during pronation. There are four types of sigmoid notches as described by Tolat et al. [23]: (a) flat face, (b) ski slope, (c) type C, and (d) type S.

The kinematics of the DRUJ during pronation/supination is really complex and far from a simple rotational movement of the radius over the head of the ulna. The combination of movements in the three axes of space (rotation with

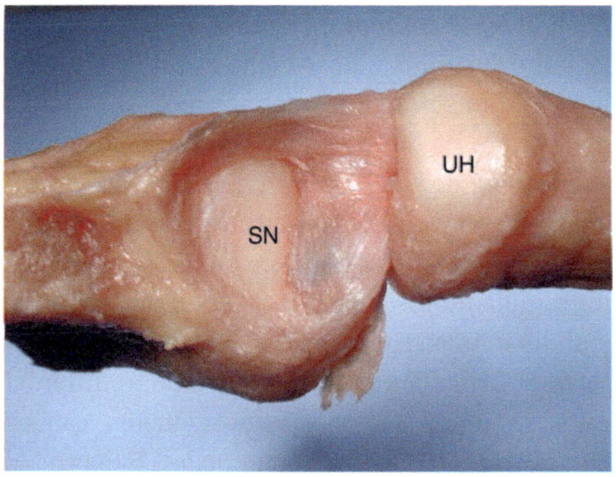


**Fig. 10.3** Anatomical specimen showing the sigmoid notch (SN) with the ulna head (UH) reflected upward

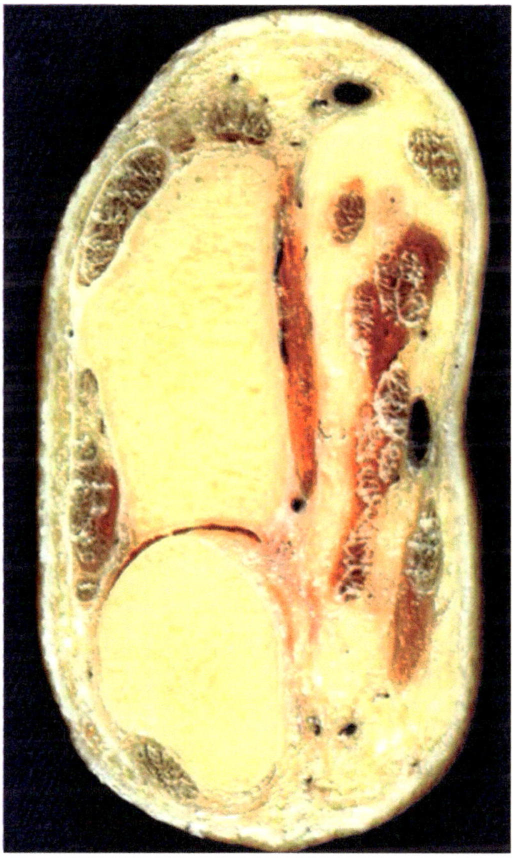

**Fig. 10.4** Anatomical specimen showing transverse section through the distal radioulnar joint showing the ulnar head and the sigmoid notch

back-palmar displacement, translation, and axial displacement or piston) is happening concurrently. There is a relative anatomical incongruity of the joint components with a tendency to subluxation in the extreme positions, more in pronation than in supination; the need for a DRUJ stabilizer is evident. This role is played by the triangular fibrocartilage complex (TFCC).

## Biomechanics

Many surgical techniques have been developed based on the concept that the main function of DRUJ is pronation and supination [3, 4, 14, 16–21]. The rotation of the radius on the head of the ulna is a function that depends on the muscular action and is not directly dependent on the joint itself. Thus, in those patients in whom this joint has been sacrificed by surgical techniques that eliminates the head of the ulna or fuses it and creates a proximal osteotomy, all have pronation and supination despite the fact that the joint has been removed. However, these patients have limited load bearing capacity, and can experience weakness if painful and even activities like lifting a glass of water can be affected. As we discussed earlier, elbow flexion and therefore weight lifting against gravity are functions of the brachialis muscle, which is inserted distal to the coronoid process. This muscle flexes the elbow in all positions of pronation and supination; however, the biceps muscle only flexes the elbow once it passes from the neutral position to the supination, and its maximum flexion force of the elbow is after complete supination. The brachioradial muscle or long supinator is only activated by trying to avoid the extension of the elbow, either with co-contraction with the triceps or by load against gravity.

Hagert in 1992 demonstrated for the first time that the main function of the DRUJ is to support weight and transmit these forces to the elbow through the ulna [12]. Thus, the hand together with the radius forms a functional unit that rests on the head of the ulna, which is "the cornerstone" that supports the weight. In the neutral position of rotation of the forearm, there is maximum articular contact between the bone ends. Hagert [11] demonstrated in cadavers that after eliminating the ulnar head, the distal end of the osteotomized ulna takes the place and function of the ulnar head. Consequently, there was a convergence and contact of the ulna toward the radius when a weight was applied.

This new concept of load articulation of the DRUJ has morphological correlation when analyzing the trabecular arrangement of the distal end of the ulna. Under normal conditions there is a close relationship of the trabecular pattern of the bone and the function it performs according to Wolff's law. Bone loading areas are characterized by a decrease in the spongy pattern with the trabeculae condensing at the cortical level. These findings agree with Hagert's theory that the ulnar head is the support point of the functional unit that forms the hand with the radius.

How is the load transmitted during prone/supination? As we saw earlier, in the extreme positions of pronation and supination, there is a tendency of subluxation of the radius in relation to the head of the ulna with little contact between the bone surfaces. If, in these situations, a load is applied (to hold a weight), dislocation would necessarily occur if the ligament components of the TFC did not come into play. The initial studies of Ekenstam and Hagert [24] on the functioning of the ligaments of the DRUJ found that the palmar radioulnar ligament tensed in pronation while the dorsal radioulnar ligament tensed in supination. Subsequently, Acosta et al. [11] showed that the ligaments that were inserted in the fovea had a totally different function. During the neutral state of rotation, in which there is maximum contact between the articular surfaces of the DRUJ, both ligament components of the TFC were in a relaxed position. As pronation was established and contact between articular surfaces with a tendency to subluxation of the distal radius was reduced following the force of gravity, the dorsal ligament component of the TFC tightened, being maximal in the extreme pronation position. During the supination, the findings were compatible; it was the palmar component that tensed.

The theory of DRUJ as a load bearing joint would be summarized as follows: in a neutral state of rotation, the large part of the load is supported by joint surfaces, in pronation where this bone contact is minimal and there is a tendency to palmar subluxation of the distal radius, the load is transmitted mainly through the dorsal component of the tightened TFC, and it undergoes stretching with deformation that is measurable, and subsequently transmits the load to the rest of the ulna. The opposite would happen during supination. Recent observations by the authors in fresh cadavers and in patients who suffered disarticulation of the wrist due to different causes showed that the previous theory can be more complex if the two components (superficial and deep fascicle) of the TFC ligaments are considered (Fig. 10.5). Probably, the tension of the dorsal ligament (deep fascicle) during pronation and the palmar (deep fascicle) during supination is the main element in the stabilization of the DRUJ. But the superficial fascicles, with less stabilizing role, may complement and help in stabilization. Thus, during pronation the deep dorsal fascicle is tensioned, which prevents palmar displacement of the radius, and the palmar superficial fascicle is wrapped around the styloid, exerting a blocking effect that supports and prevents the displacement of the radius toward the dorsum. The opposite would occur during supination, with the deep fascicle of the palmar ligament being the main actor and the dorsal superficial fascicle the secondary actor that helps in stabilization of the DRUJ.

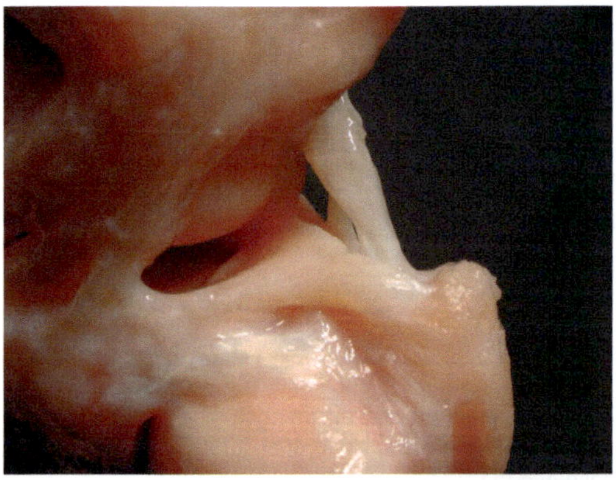

**Fig. 10.5** Anatomical dissection of the TFC showing the superficial and deep fascicles

## Design Considerations

Milch [25] recognized that amputating the head of the ulna because of length difference was not a good idea and reported removing a segment of the ulna shaft to correct this problem. In spite of his report, the procedures of Darrach [3] and Sauvé-Kapandji [4] were augmented in 1986 by Bower [16] and Watson et al. [17].

Recognition of the impingement syndrome by Bell et al. [26] and the demonstration of the dynamic impingement by Lees and Scheker [27] have shown that when the ulnar head is excised, the radius is going to fall off the stump of the ulna regardless of the procedure (Fig. 10.6 a, b, and c). To solve the impingement problems, a myriad of unipolar implants that required ligament reconstruction and the presence of the sigmoid notch were created. A large number of implants eroded into the ulnar part of the radius with loosening and dislocation of the implants.

The sigmoid notch can present with varied orientation as shown by the works of De Smet and Fabry [28] and different shapes as shown by Tolat et al. [23]. This anatomical peculiarity reduces the longevity of the hemiarthroplasties.

Confronted with patients with radioulnar impingement after salvage procedures and others with severe forearm injuries where the sigmoid notch and the radioulnar ligaments were absent where the surgical solutions were inadequate, we designed an implant that would work in conditions where there were no sigmoid notch and no radioulnar ligaments.

There was a need of an implant that would be self-stabilizing, maintaining the total range of motion and allowing weight bearing.

The original implants were made of stainless steel with an ulnar stem of 3 mm in diameter and 22 centimeters long and three-point fixation. In a subsequent modification, cobalt-chrome alloy is utilized to construct the implant, where the function of the sigmoid notch is replaced by a metal plate that contours to the ulnar border of the radius and has a distal hemi-cavity. The ulnar head function is replaced by an ulnar stem which is press fit to the ulnar medullary cavity. It has a titanium plasma spray on its distal third for bone ingrowth inside the ulnar canal and has a highly polished Morse-taper peg distally where an ultra-high molecular weight polyethylene (UHMWPE) ball is placed, which sits in the hemi-cavity, and a cover that completes the assembly.

The total Aptis arthroplasty is composed of four elements (Fig. 10.7):

1. Radial plate with 3, 4, or 5 holes depending on whether the small, medium, or large plate is used. The plates have at their distal end a small peg (radial side) that helps to position it correctly and a hemisphere (ulnar side). The plates, of three sizes, are pre-molded to be placed on the ulnar face of the radius, in 6–7 cm distal to the interosseous crest. The fixation to the radius is achieved by means of its small peg, which is introduced in the ulna-radial direction and through the holes of the plate by means of 3.5-mm screws.

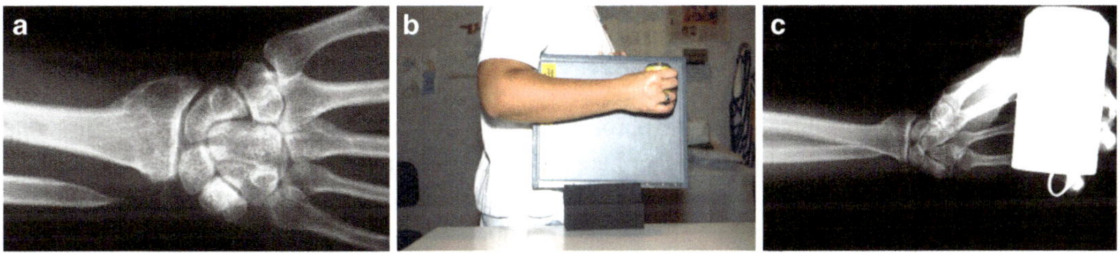


**Fig. 10.6** (**a**) PA radiograph of unloaded wrist and forearm showing the separation of the radius and the excised distal ulna. (**b**) Radiograph of the wrist and forearm of the loaded hand. (**c**) PA radiograph of the loaded wrist and forearm showing radioulnar impingement with loading

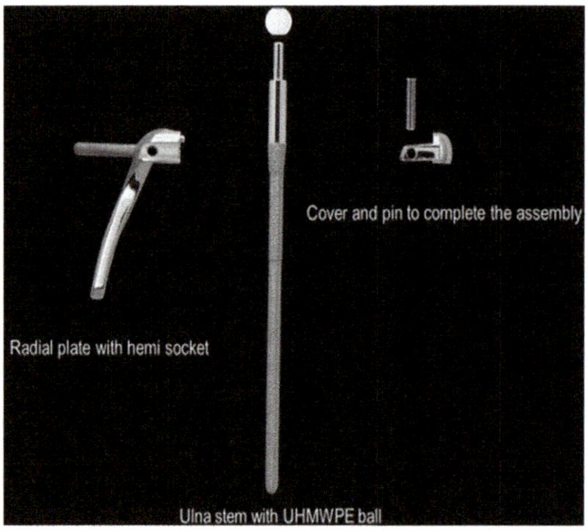


**Fig. 10.7** Components of the Aptis total distal radioulnar joint implant

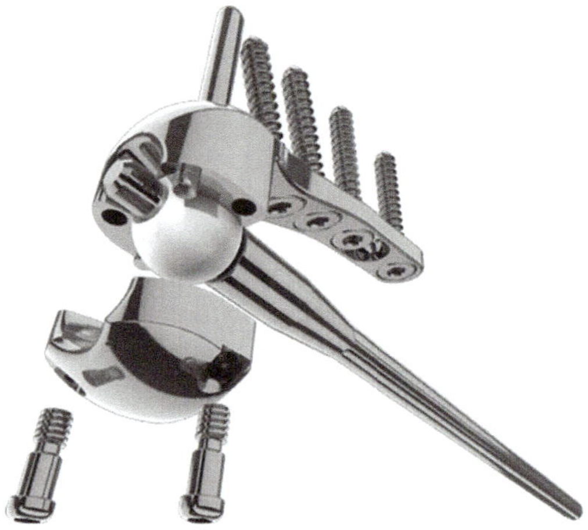

**Fig. 10.8** The components of the Aptis total distal radio-ulnar joint assembled

2. Cover with a transverse screw, which will serve as a cover to the hemisphere of the radial plate.
3. Ulnar head made of ultra-high-density polyethylene.
4. An 11-cm ulnar stem, long and with porous titanium coating on its distal third to facilitate bone incorporation. The stems have a polished extension between the base of the ball and the porous coating part to prevent the escape of bone marrow that in the past created ectopic bone (Fig. 10.8). The rod is ribbed to allow greater rotational stability and is slightly tapered to facilitate insertion. Also, at the distal end of the stem, that is, outside the ulna, a pin is incorporated, to which the prosthetic ulnar head is fitted. The ulnar stem is available in four diameters, with different neck lengths, which will be used mainly in cases where the distal ulna has been lost or it is necessary to resect a greater amount of distal ulna. Thus, the articular surface of the prosthesis is made up of the aforementioned ultra-high-density polyethylene head, inserted into the plug of the ulnar stem, and the metal surface of the plate and cover hemispheres, respectively.

The design of the implant allows full range of pronation and supination, radial migration, lifting capacity, and variable angle of rotation, and it is self-stabilizing. The implant comes in three sizes, small locking (number 10), medium locking and unlocking (number 20), and large unlocking (number 30). The stems are available in 4 diameters from 4, 4.5, 5, and 6 mm, and the length of the collar of the stems is 1–4 cm for those cases with much distal ulna excised. Originally only those cases missing the ulnar head were treated with implants, as we gained experience with its behavior; we included primary osteoarthritic patients, cases of rheumatoid arthritis, post-tumor resection, and congenital conditions like Ehlers-Danlos and Madelung deformities.

## Surgical Procedure

The procedure is generally accomplished under axillary block. An iodine plastic wrap is used to avoid contact between the implant (the stem specially) and the skin. A tourniquet is applied for visualization. A 10-cm longitudinal incision in the shape of a hockey stick is made along the ulnar border of the distal forearm, in the interval between the fifth and sixth dorsal compartments, 8 cm over the distal forearm, and 2 cm distally oblique from ulnar to radial. Care is taken to avoid damage to the sensory branch of the ulnar nerve. The skin and subcutaneous flap are elevated from the forearm fascia up to the radial wrist extensors. A rectangular ulnar-based fascia/

retinacular flap is created with enough width to cover the head of the implant; it includes the most proximal 3 mm of the extensor retinaculum. This flap will be used later to create a buffering barrier between the prosthesis and the extensor carpi ulnaris (ECU). The dissection is continued between the extensor digiti quinti minimi and the ECU until the ulna is encountered and the extensor digiti quinti minimi is elevated from the ulna together with the extensor indicis proprius (EIP); this leads us to the dorsum of the interosseous membrane which is exposed. The sensory branch of the posterior interosseous nerve is divided to avoid avulsion of the nerve from the thumb. The extensor communis is elevated by placing an elevator between the extensor mass and the radius. The ECU tendon sheet is opened completely up to its insertion at the base of the fifth metacarpal. This avoids pressure of the tendon against the distal end of the implant. The remaining head of the ulna, if present, is then excised 2 cm from the distal end of the ulnar head. At this stage, the radial attachment of the triangular fibrocartilage, if found intact, is left undisturbed. If left in situ, this structure can provide a barrier between the prosthesis and the carpal bones. The ulnar shaft is then retracted volarly, thus ensuring access to the radius. The interosseous membrane is elevated from the radius along the distal 8 cm of the interosseous crest. The radial trial plate is then placed over the interosseous crest of the radius, and its volar border is aligned with the volar surface of the radius. Care is taken to ensure that at least 3 mm of the sigmoid notch lies distal to the end of the plate. Depending on the anatomy encountered, the distal radius may require contouring. Often the volar lip of the sigmoid notch has to be removed with a saw blade or a medium-sized burr ball to create a flat surface to ensure proper seating of the radial plate. After the position of the trial plate has been deemed appropriate—meaning parallel to the volar shaft of the radius and at least 3 mm proximal to the end of the radius—a 1.4-mm (0.054-in) K-wire is inserted in one of the holes at the distal end of the trial as well as the most proximal hole. An image intensifier is used to check the position of the trial, both in anteroposterior and lateral positions. If no adjustment is needed, a 2.5-mm drill bit is used with the provided guide to drill the screw hole at the oval opening, the proper screw length is gauged, the hole is tapped, and the appropriate length 3.5-mm screw is placed. The image intensifier is used again to confirm plate positioning and proper screw length. With confirmation of the length of the screw and good plate contact with the bone, the distal K-wire is removed, and the hole for the radial peg is drilled with appropriate drill bit. When the surgeon is satisfied, the trial component is removed, the area profusely is irrigated, and the prosthesis radial component is installed. If necessary, a soft mallet is used to achieve good contact between the radial plate and the ulnar border of the radius. After the last screw is placed in position, a final check of the radial plate to confirm screw length and position is performed with the image intensifier. Attention is now turned to the ulna. With the forerarm fully pronated, a measuring device with an appropriate colored ball (blue for large implant; black for medium sized and small implants) is positioned such that the ball is fitting into the hemi socket of the radial component and the measuring device is juxtaposed aginst the ulnar shaft. This enables the surgeon to assess the exact amount of ulna to be resected. After final resection of the distal ulna, a 2.3-mm (0.090-in) guide wire is inserted into the ulnar medullary canal to act as a centralizer for a cannulated drill bit of the predetermined size. It is important that the guide wire surpass the length of the drill bit to avoid penetrating the ulnar cortex. The cannulated drill bit is introduced for a length of 11 cm. Next, a medullary broach of appropriate size is inserted into the canal to bevel the distal ulna and plane its distal end. The medullary canal is now thoroughly irrigated, and the stem of the ulnar component is introduced leaving the polished peg showing distal to the rim of the socket. The UHMW polyethylene ball is placed over the distal peg or pivot, and the ulnar component is positioned within the hemi-socket of the radial component. Finally, the other half of the radial socket or cover is positioned and secured with a transverse screw. The image intensifier is once again used to confirm adequacy of the overall position. Full range of motion is confirmed. The fascia/retinacular flap is placed between the prosthesis and the ECU tendon and sutured to the radius. This prevents tenosynovitis of the ECU and provides a cushion over the implant, especially for a patient with little subcutaneous adipose tissue. The tourniquet is released, and complete hemostasis is secured. The skin is then closed with interrupted sutures and a bulky soft dressing is applied.

## Postoperative Protocol

The wound is kept dry and clean in a bulky soft dressing for 2 weeks, at which time the skin sutures are removed. Immediate full range of motion is encouraged. Lifting is allowed as soon as the patient has recovered from the anesthetic, and after full recovery is limited to 20 lb (9 kg). In vitro testing showed that ultimate load to failure was between 148 and 186 lb with an average of 169 lb (76 kg), at which point the highly polished peg and the end of the ulna stem bent. By limiting lifting to no more than 20 lb, the patient has a margin of safety of seven times.

## **Results** (Figs. 10.9 and 10.10)

Our combined cases surpass 400 patients; of those 263 have more than 5 years of follow up, and 128 had more than 2 procedures before the total DRUJ was implanted. The average preoperative grip strength measured with a dynamometer (Jamar II, Jamar Dynamometer, Bolingbrook, IL) was 38.3 lb (17.4 kg) on the affected side and 70 lb (32 kg) on the opposite side. The postoperative grip strength increased to a mean of 44.5 lb (20.2 kg) on the operated side. Mean postoperative grip strength, evaluated with a dynamometer (Jamar II, Jamar Dynamometer), was 63.4% of the contralateral unaffected side. Before surgery, patients could lift an average of 2.6 lb (1.2 kg) with the affected side, limited by pain; after surgery, they were able to lift an average of 11.6 lb (5.3 kg). Patients subjectively scored preoperative pain on a scale from 0 to 5 at an average of 3.8, and postoperative pain at a mean of 1.3. Mean pronation was 79° (range 15–90°) and mean supination was 72° (range 30–90°) at final follow-up. Seventy percent of our patients have had at least one previous procedure; some had failed "ulna stabilization" with tendon sling procedures, allograft tendon interposition, and failed ulnar head replacement. Of this group of patients, 1 had 14 previous procedures. Most of these patients have been incapacitated for a prolonged period of time because of pain. This has led to a lack of use, causing muscle atrophy in both the arm and the forearm. For this reason, these previously operated patients were often weaker than those who received the device as their first procedure or those on whom the replacement was performed shortly after the failed previous procedure. Rampazzo et al. [29] noticed while evaluating those patients with implants under the age of 40 years that when the implant was performed, primarily the results were much better in regard to postoperative pain, strength, and speed of recovery. Postoperative complications were seen in 26 cases. Two patients had low-degree soft tissue infection that resolved with antibiotic treatment. Both patients had multiple previous operations. Two patients had ECU tenosynovitis due to too large implant; now we have a smaller implant for those cases. This was successfully treated by creating a fascial flap that was interposed between the implant and the ECU tendon. A fascial flap is now performed routinely at the initial implantation surgery. Eight patients had ectopic bone formation around the distal ulna and were treated successfully with surgical excision. This ectopic calcification was caused by the bone marrow escaping around the original stem that had no extended collar. After the stem had 1-cm extended collar, the ulnar canal is sealed, and no other cases of ectopic bone have been seen. Of the patients with ectopic bone formation, six patients had ECU tendinitis that settled after excision of the ectopic bone. One patient, at the 1-year follow-up X-ray, was noticed to have some ulna resorption in the distal segment of the ulna where she had an ulna shortening 6 months before the replacement arthroplasty. At present, the ulna stem remains well secured and she is symptom-free.

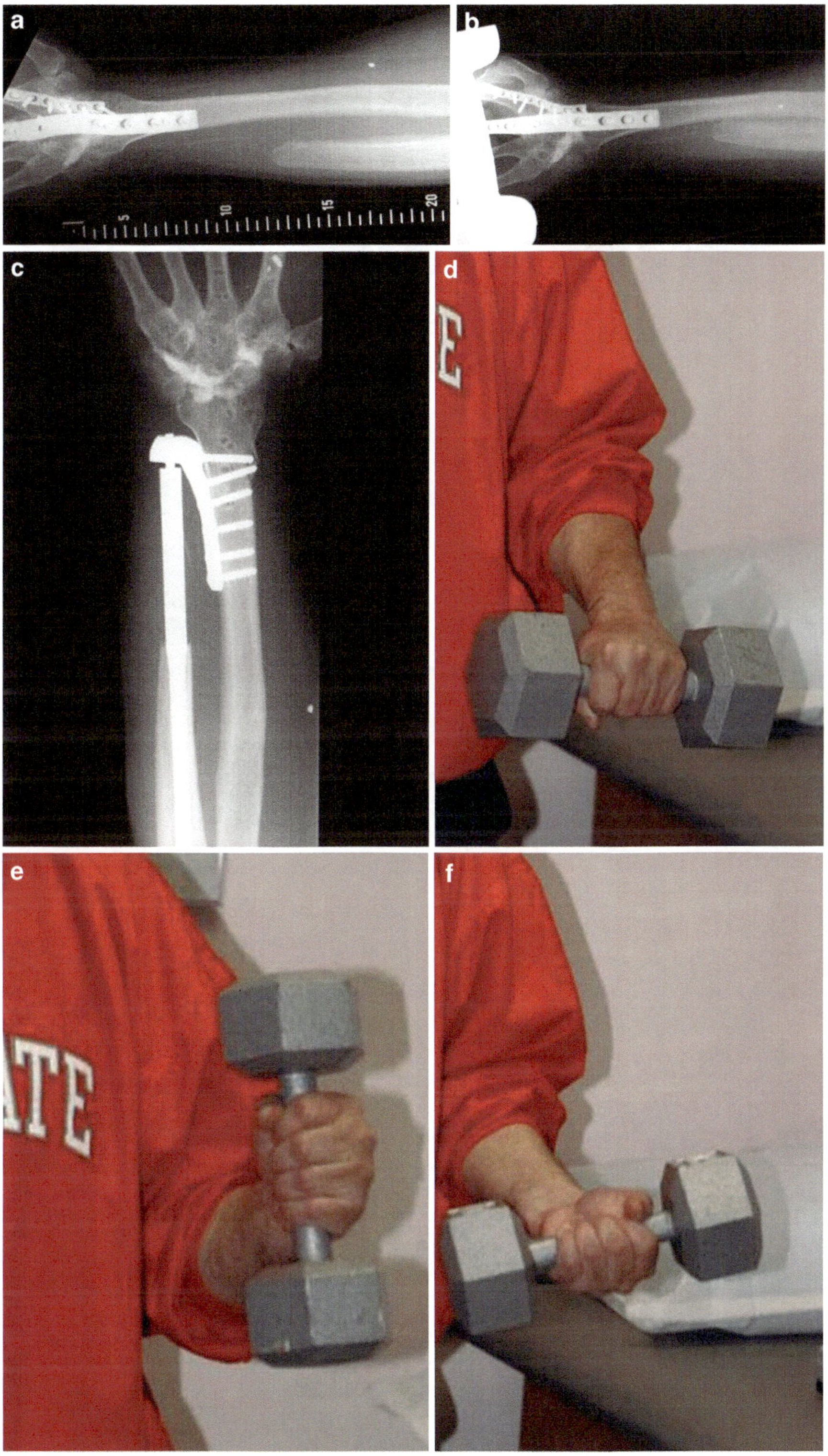

**Fig. 10.9** (**a**) This patient had wrist arthrodesis with wide excision of the distal ulna. There is no radioulnar impingement in the unloaded position. (**b**) However, with load bearing, there is radioulnar impingement that causes pain and weakness of grip. (**c**) Radiograph of DRUJ replacement arthroplasty with Aptis implant showing the implants in good alignment. (**d**, **e**, and **f**) The patient is now able to lift weights that he was unable to do

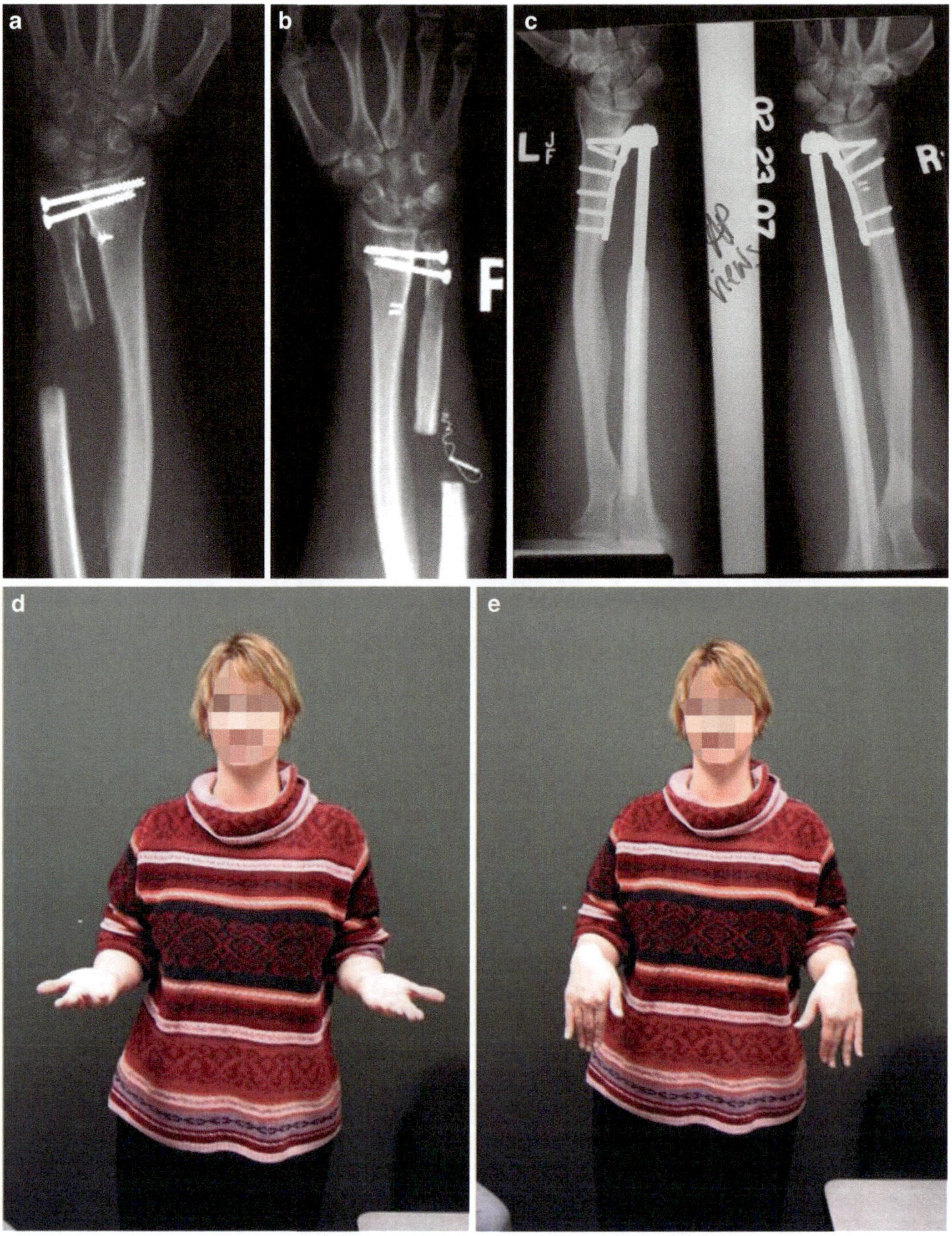


**Fig. 10.10** (**a** and **b**) This young patient underwent attempted bilateral Sauvé-Kapandji procedures with severe disability. (**c**) Radiographs showing bilateral Aptis total distal radioulnar joint implants. (**d** and **e**) Full restoration of function with load bearing capacity was possible after Aptis total distal radioulnar joint replacement arthroplasties

At the time of this writing, the longest follow-up with the Aptis DRUJ prosthesis is 15 years. No prosthesis had to be removed because of excessive wear, loosening, or material failure. There have been four implants removed because of unknown preoperatively allergy three to nickel and one to cobalt-chrome and three due to late infections, requiring those of allergies to be replaced by implants made of titanium. Those with infections were treated by removing the implants, extensive curettage, and bone substitute with antibiotic inserted in the defects, replacing the implants 3–6 months later. Galvis et al. [30] reported excellent recovery in cases of rheumatoid arthritis with dislocated distal radius and ruptured tendons. The Aptis DRUJ prosthesis is an alternative to the other salvage procedures that allows full range of motions as well as the ability to grip and lift weights encountered in daily living.

## Conclusions

The distal radioulnar joint is a weight bearing joint and together with the proximal radioulnar joint forms a complete unit that helps in load transmission from the hand and wrist to the elbow. Although the ability to pronate and supinate is important, it has the ability to lift loads that helps better define function. When this joint is affected by injury or disease, it is important to reconstruct the DRUJ and restore the loading capacity of the joint. The Aptis total distal radioulnar joint replacement system was designed to help in restoring the load bearing capacity of the forearm, and our clinical experience shows that it has been successful in this endeavor.

## References

1. Bernard CH, Huette CH. In: Buren WHV, Isaacs CE, editors. Illustrated manual of operated surgery and surgical anatomy. New York: HBailliere; 1857.
2. Moore EM. Three cases illustrating luxation of the ulna in connection with Colles' fracture. Med Record. 1880;17:305.
3. Darrach W. Forward dislocation at the inferior radioulnar joint with fractures of the lower third of radius. Ann Surg. 1912;56:801.
4. Sauvé L, Kapandji M. Nouvelle technique de traitement chirurgical des luxations récidivantes isolées de l'extrémité inférieure du cubitus. J Chir. 1936;7:589.
5. Baldwin W. Orthopaedic surgery of the hand and wrist. London: Henry Frowde, Hodder & Stoughton; 1921. p. 241–82.
6. Palmer AK, Werner FW. The triangular fibrocartilage complex of the wrist- anatomy and function. J Hand Surg. 1981;6A:153–72.
7. Palmer AK, Werner FW. Biomechanics of the distal radioulnar joint. Clin Orthop. 1984;187:26–35.
8. Thiru RG, Ferlic DC, Clayton ML, McClure DCT. Arterial anatomy of the triangular fibrocartilage of the wrist and its surgical significance. J Hand Surg (Am). 1986;11(2):258–63.
9. Mikic ZD. Detailed anatomy of the articular disc of the distal radioulnar joint. Clin Orthop. 1989;245:123–32.
10. Chidgey LK. Histologic anatomy of the triangular fibrocartilage. Hand Clinic. 1991;7:249–62.
11. Acosta R, Hnat B, Scheker LR. Distal radio-ulnar ligament motion during supination and pronation. J Hand Surg. 1993;18B:502–5.
12. Hagert CG. The distal radioulnar joint in relation to the whole forearm. Clin Orthop. 1992;275:56–64.
13. Linscheid RL: Biomechanics of. the distal radioulnar joint. Clin Orthop. 1992;275:46–55.
14. Kessler I, Hecht O. Present application of the Darrach procedure. Clin Orthop. 1970;72:254–60.
15. Tsai TM, Stillwell JH. Repair of chronic subluxation of the distal radioulnar joint (ulnar dorsal) using flexor carpi ulnaris tendon. J Hand Surg. 1984;9B:289–94.
16. Bowers WH. Distal radio-ulnar joint arthroplasty: the hemi-resection interposition. J Hand Surg. 1985;10A:169–72.
17. Watson HF, Ryu J, Burgess RC. Matched distal ulnar resection. J Hand Surg. 1986;11A:812–7.
18. Breen TF, Jupiter JB. Extensor carpi ulnaris and flexor carpi ulnaris tenodesis of the unstable distal ulna. J Hand Surg. 1989;14A:612–7.
19. Leslie BM, Carlson G, Ruby LK. Results of ECU tenodesis in rheumatoid wrist undergoing a distal ulnar resection. J Hand Surg. 1990;15A:547–51.
20. Sanders RA, Frederick HA, Hontas R. The Sauvé-Kapandji procedure: a salvage operation for the distal radio-ulnar joint. J Hand Surg. 1991;19A:1125–9.
21. Tsai TM, Shimizu H, Adkins P. A modified extensor carpi ulnaris tenodesis with Darrach procedure. J Hand Surg. 1993;18A:697–702.
22. Scheker LR, Severo A. Ulnar shortening for the treatment of early Post-traumatic osteoarthritis at the distal Radioulnar joint. J Hand Surg. 2001;26B(1):41–4.
23. Tolat AR, Stanley JK, Trail IA. A cadaveric study of the anatomy and stability of the distal radioulnar joint in the coronal and transverse planes. J Hand Surg Br. 1996;21(5):587–94.

24. af Ekenstam FW, Hagert CG. The distal radioulnar joint. The influence of geometry and stability of the distal radioulnar joint. Scand J Plast Reconstr Surg. 1985;19:27.
25. Milch H. So called dislocation of the lower end ulna. Ann Surg. 1942;116:282–92.
26. Bell MJ, Hill RJ, McMurtry RY. Ulnar impingement syndrome. J Bone Joint Surg. 1985;67B:126–9.
27. Lees VC, Scheker LR. The radiological demonstration of dynamic ulnar impingement. J Hand Surg. 1997;22B:448–50.
28. De Smet L, Fabry G. Orientation of the sigmoid notch of the distal radius: determination of different types of the distal radioulnar joint. Acta Orthopaedica Belgica. 1992;59(3):269–72.
29. Rampazzo A, Gharb BB, Brock G, Scheker LR. Functional outcomes of the Aptis-Scheker distal radioulnar joint replacement in patients under 40 years old. J Hand Surg Am. 2015;40(7):1397–403.
30. Galvis EJ, Pessa J, Scheker LR. Total joint arthroplasty of the distal radioulnar joint for rheumatoid arthritis. J Hand Surg Am. 2014;39(9):1699–704.

# 11 Primary Distal Radioulnar Joint Arthroplasty

Logan W. Carr and Brian Adams

## Introduction

The distal radioulnar joint (DRUJ) plays a key role for upper extremity function, including forearm rotation, forearm and wrist stability, and transmission of load across the wrist. The minimal osseous constraint provided by the sigmoid notch increases the risk for DRUJ instability and likely contributes to developing osteoarthrosis and post-traumatic arthrosis. Distal radius fractures often involve the sigmoid notch, which can disrupt joint conguity leading to instability and abnormal articular contact stresses. Madelung's deformity and other congenital conditions can severely affect the congruity and alignment of the joint leading to degenerative changes. Because the joint has robust synovium, it is also susceptible to inflammatory arthritis. A variety of surgical techniques are described for the treatment of arthritis, ranging from ablation using the Darrach procedure for low-demand patients to anatomic reconstruction with joint replacement to maintain a more natural function. The aim of this chapter is to review the role of primary arthroplasty in the management of DRUJ arthritis.

**Supplementary Information** The online version of this chapter (https://doi.org/10.1007/978-3-030-68880-6_11) contains supplementary material, which is available to authorized users.

L. W. Carr · B. Adams (✉)
Department of Orthopedic Surgery, Baylor College of Medicine, Houston, TX, USA
e-mail: Brian.Adams@bcm.edu

## Anatomy

The sigmoid notch of the radius is shallow and has a much greater radius of curvature than the ulnar head, resulting in little inherent stability [1]. Joint geometry provides approximately 20% of the DRUJ stability, leaving the surrounding soft tissues responsible for the vast majority [2]. The triangular fibrocartilage complex (TFCC) is located between the carpus and distal ulna, being comprised of the radioulnar ligaments, articular disc, meniscus homolog, ulnocarpal ligaments, and the extensor carpi ulnaris (ECU) subsheath (Fig. 11.1). The TFCC provides both ligamentous functions for wrist and forearm stability and transmits substantial axial load between the carpus and forearm as well as sagittal loading during lifting [3].

DRUJ stabilizers can be described as extrinsic or intrinsic in relation to its capsule. Extrinsic stability is provided dynamically by the ECU tendon and pronator quadratus, while the distal interosseous membrane (IOM) and ECU subsheath provide static constraint [4]. The stout radioulnar ligaments, which comprise the volar and dorsal margins of the TFCC, are the most important intrinsic soft tissue stabilizers [5]. Each radioulnar ligament includes a superficial


G. J. W. King, M. Rizzo (eds.), *Arthroplasty of the Upper Extremity*,
https://doi.org/10.1007/978-3-030-68880-6_11

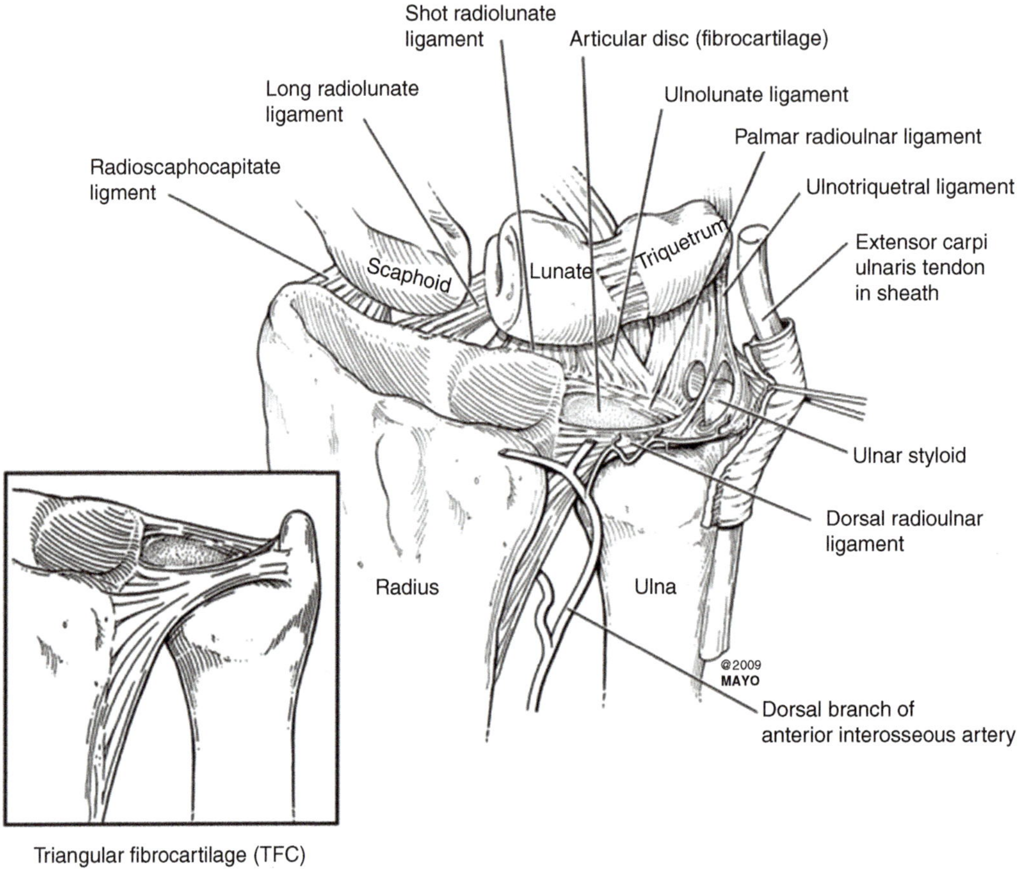


**Fig. 11.1** Anatomy of the TFCC and soft tissue stabilizing structure: many operations involving the ulnar head sacrifice, stabilize, or preserve the structures of the TFCC. (Reproduced with permission from Carlsen et al. [31])

and deep component. The deep fibers (ligamentum subcruentum) attach to the fovea, through which the axis of forearm motion passes.

## Causes of Arthritis

The DRUJ is susceptible to both osteoarthrosis and post-traumatic arthrosis. Distal radius fractures extending into the sigmoid notch can cause chondral damage or create an articular step-off resulting in degeneration. Malunion of either the distal radius or the ulna can substantially alter joint contact resulting in degeneration (Fig. 11.2). Similarly, forearm fractures in children can lead to growth disturbances and subsequent arthrosis. Congenital conditions, such as Madelung's deformity, may present with delayed arthrosis due to altered joint loading. The DRUJ is particularly susceptible to cartilage and ligamentous damage caused by chronic synovitis from rheumatoid arthritis and other inflammatory conditions.

## Diagnosis (Physical Examination and X-ray)

The onset of symptoms caused by DRUJ arthrosis is often gradual over a course of years and may not be apparent until an aggravating injury or over-use event occurs. The physical examination starts with inspection of both wrists to detect asymmetry at resting posture. An asymmetrical, prominent ulna indicates possible instability, malunion, or inflammatory arthritis. Precise

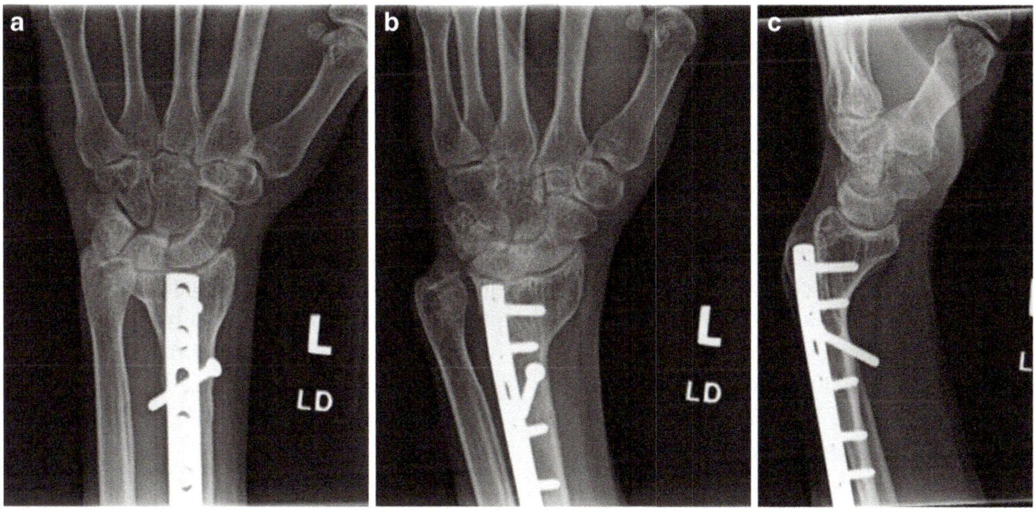


**Fig. 11.2** Distal radius malunion following fixation showing DRUJ instability and arthritis. Lateral, oblique, and posteroanterior X-rays of the patient illustrated in Video 11.1

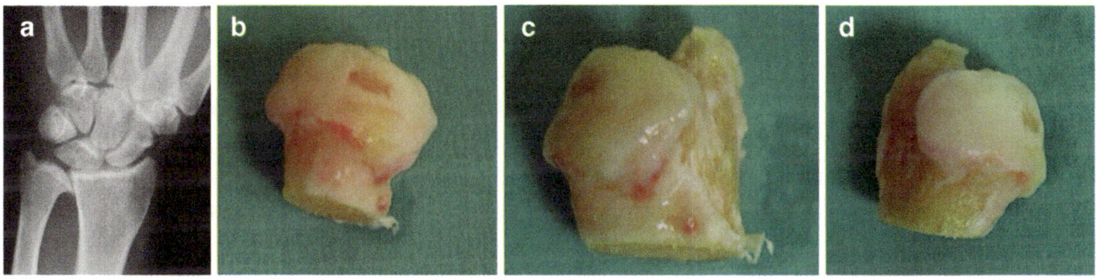


**Fig. 11.3** Radiograph shows joint space narrowing, osteophytes, and sclerosis consistent with DRUJ arthritis. Clinical photographs show eburnation of cartilage and osteophytes of the ulnar head

palpation can isolate tenderness involving the ECU tendon sheath, the ulnar styloid, or the fovea. TFCC injury, ECU tendonitis or subluxation, and ulnar impaction are not mutually exclusive. Pain and crepitus are commonly elicited during rotation, especially when combined with manual joint compression. DRUJ instability is typically confirmed by finding increased translation of the ulna relative to the radius during manipulation of the joint in multiple positions; however, this must be compared to the contralateral side to confirm the laxity is pathologic. In performing this maneuver, the ulnar should be grasped proximal to the DRUJ to avoid misinterpreting joint pain for pain caused by joint translation. The modified press test described by Adams can demonstrate dynamic volar instability [6] (Video 11.1).

Imaging studies are an adjunct to a careful history and physical examination. Plain X-rays will show sequelae of arthrosis, such as joint space narrowing, sclerosis, subchondral cysts, and osteophytes (Fig. 11.3). Malunion, DRUJ subluxation, and other pathology may also be seen. CT will further delineate articular congruity, joint deformity, and arthrosis, which is most useful when including the contralateral wrist in mirrored and multiple positions. MRI is most useful for soft tissue pathology including TFCC integrity, but can also show signs of arthrosis and subluxation.

## Treatment

Initial management can be nonsurgical, especially when instability, pain, and/or arthritis is mild, and includes activity modification, strengthening exercises, anti-inflammatory drugs, brace support, and possible limited or intermittent immobilization. While it is appropriate to begin with nonsurgical treatment, these methods typically have variable and often limited long-term success. There are three broad categories of surgical treatment, with technical variations in each category: partial or complete resection of the distal ulna (hemiresection with soft tissue interposition or the Darrach procedure), arthrodesis of the DRUJ with ulnar neck resection (Sauve-Kapandji procedure), and partial or complete arthroplasty (ulnar head replacement or total DRUJ replacement).

## Surgical Exposure

Perhaps the most utilitarian approach to the DRUJ is dorsally through the fifth extensor compartment or between the fifth and sixth extensor compartments, with preservation of the radioulnar ligaments and other TFCC components. Alternatively, particularly for revision surgery or severe trauma, a lateral approach can be made in the interval between the ECU and flexor carpi ulnaris (FCU). In either approach, the dorsal sensory branch of the ulnar nerve is protected. For the dorsal approach, a 4–6 cm skin incision is made between the fifth and sixth extensor compartments, extending proximally from the level of the ulnar styloid (Fig. 11.4a). The fifth compartment is opened, except for its distal portion, and the extensor digiti minimi (EDM) tendon is retracted.

An ulnar-based rectangular-shaped flap is created in the DRUJ capsule, beginning just proximal and parallel to the dorsal radioulnar ligament, continuing along the dorsal rim of the sigmoid notch leaving a small cuff, and then extending over the ulnar neck (Fig. 11.4b). Care is taken not to cut the dorsal radioulnar ligament (Fig. 11.4c). Retraction of this flap exposes the articular surfaces of the distal radioulnar joint and the proximal surface of the TFCC (Fig. 11.4d). The integrity of the TFCC is assessed. Unless greater

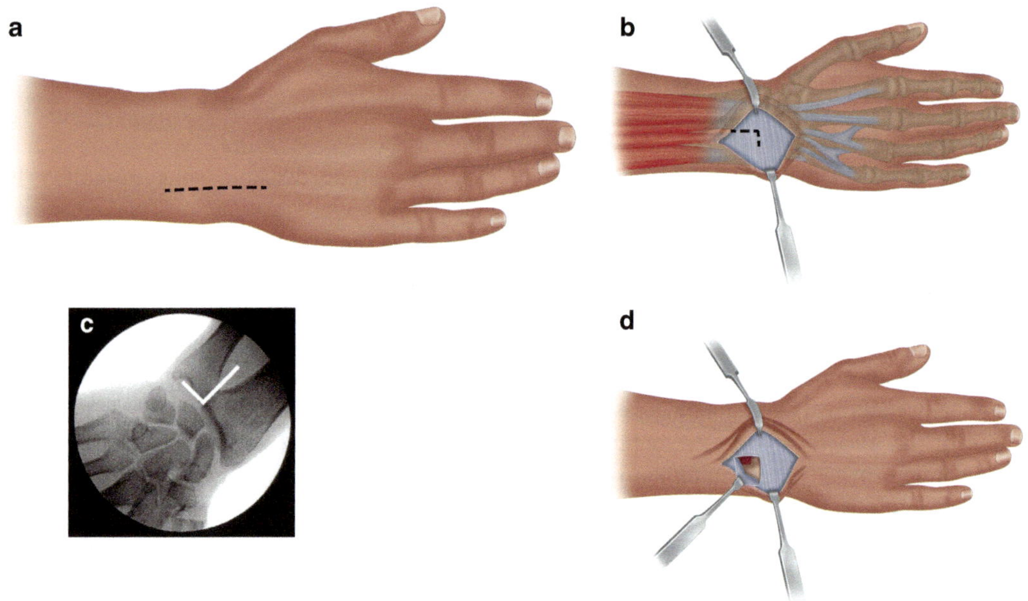


**Fig. 11.4** Surgical exposure: (**a**) incision overlying the septum dividing the fourth and fifth extensor compartment. (**b**) An L-shaped or rectangular flap is designed in the DRUJ capsule. (**c**) The transverse limb of the capsular flap is proximal to the TFCC to preserve the radioulnar ligaments. (**d**) Retraction of the flap allows visualization of the DRUJ and ulnar head. (Reproduced with permission from Integra LifeSciences, Princeton, NJ)

exposure is needed, the ECU sheath should not be opened or elevated from the ulnar groove, as preserving the sheath will maintain its important stabilizing function for the ulnocarpal joint. At completion of the bony procedure, the dorsal DRUJ capsule and retinaculum are closed together with only slight imbrication to avoid loss of motion. The EDM is left subcutaneous. The technique for constrained total DRUJ replacement requires a more extensive exposure and dissection.

## Surgical Treatment: Resection Arthroplasty

### Distal Ulna Resection Arthroplasty (Darrach)

Distal ulna resection was described by Darrach in 1912 [7]. The procedure was widely used for chronic instability and arthrosis before the indications were refined. The entire ulnar head is removed while preserving the surrounding soft tissue envelope (Fig. 11.5). The ulnar head is resected just proximal to the sigmoid notch with a slightly angled osteotomy to help preserve more soft tissue. Sharp edges are removed with a file or rongeur to reduce potential adjacent tendon wear, particularly the ECU and EDM tendons. Prono-supination is performed to assess stump stability. The volar DRUJ capsule can be sutured to the ulnar stump using transosseous sutures and the dorsal capsule imbricated during closure to improve stability.

If the ulnar stump is prominent or demonstrates substantial instability during forearm rotation, then additional stabilizing techniques can be used. Common methods use strips of the ECU and FCU tendons secured to the ulna by means of bone tunnels or suture anchors [8]. Another technique uses the pronator quadratus (PQ) as an interposition and stabilizer by suturing it to the ulnar stump or dorsal capsule.

Tendon allograft interposition provides more bulk to reduce the problem of radioulnar impingement. One technique uses an Achilles tendon allograft that is folded to create a large buffer between the radius and ulna and sutured to each bone to add stability [9]. Long-term follow-up has shown satisfactory results, particularly as a salvage technique for failed distal ulna resections [10]. Tendon transfers and allografts have also been used to augment DRUJ stability during revision surgery for complications following ulnar resections and implant arthroplasty [11, 12].

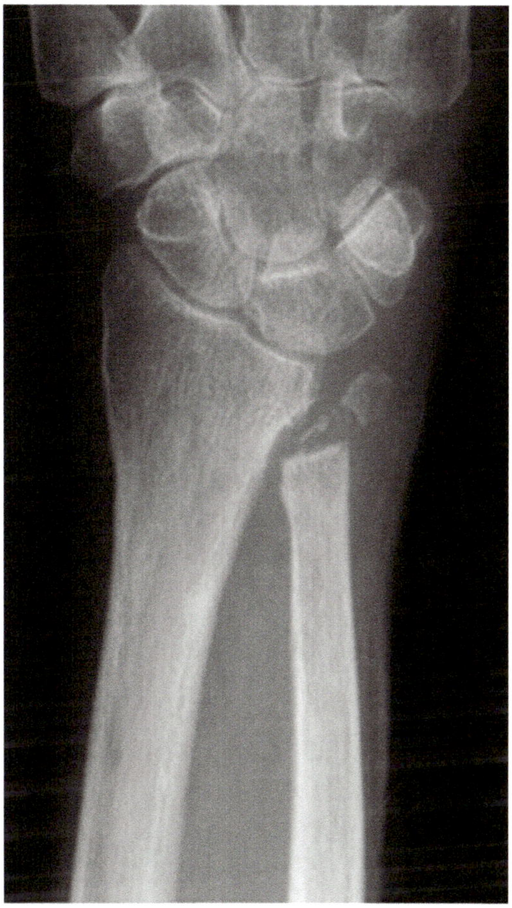

**Fig. 11.5** Ulnar head resection arthroplasty (Darrach): radioulnar convergence has resulted in impingement by the ulnar stump and scalloping of the adjacent radius

The Darrach procedure yields satisfactory results in the low-demand patients [13, 14]. Younger or more active patients may continue to have painful clicking, instability, and weakness that are associated with radioulnar convergence as evidenced by scalloping on X-rays (Fig. 11.5) [15].

## Partial Distal Ulnar Head Resection (Hemiresection Arthroplasty)

The classic hemiresection arthroplasty procedure involves resection of the articular portion of the distal ulna with preservation of the surrounding soft tissues, including the TFCC, for stabilization. Bowers described resection of a portion of the head including the articular surface combined with tendon interposition and capsule reconstruction [16]. The technique is commonly referred to as the hemiresection interposition arthroplasty or HIT procedure. Although initially described for treatment of rheumatoid arthritis, the procedure has been used for all types of arthritis.

A rounded contouring of the distal ulna is done to match the obliquity of the sigmoid notch while preserving the TFCC attachment to the ulnar styloid (Fig. 11.6). Ulnocarpal impingement between the remaining ulnar styloid and the triquetrum can be a problem, particularly with positive ulnar variance; a shortening osteotomy through the remaining ulnar head may be necessary [17].

## Sauve-Kapandji Procedure

When there is loss of the distal radioulnar articulation, the dynamic stabilizers are unopposed. This results in convergence of the radius and the ulna, slack in the static stabilizing structures, and progressive instability. The Suave-Kapandji procedure involves arthrodesis of the DRUJ and a proximal osteotomy to allow forearm rotation (Fig. 11.7). It is an attempt to correct the aforementioned complications related to resection arthroplasty.

Early complications were attributable to nonunion and radioulnar impingement. Tenuous

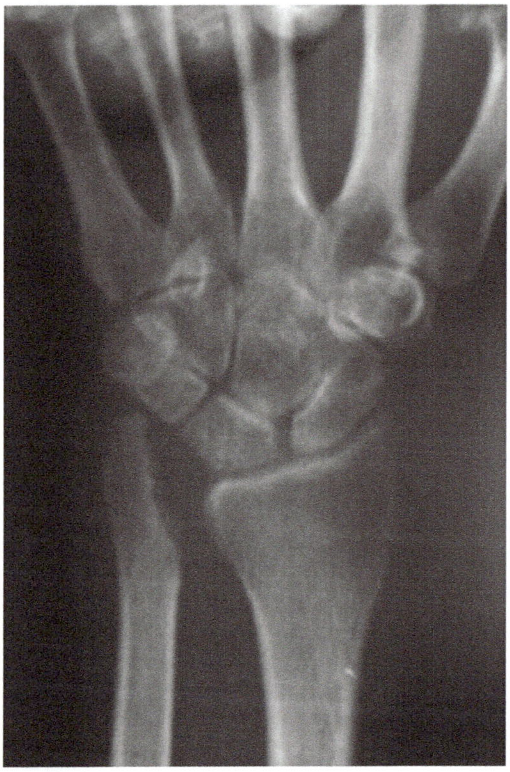

**Fig. 11.6** Hemiresection interposition arthroplasty (HIT) with residual stylocarpal impingement due to preoperative positive ulnar variance

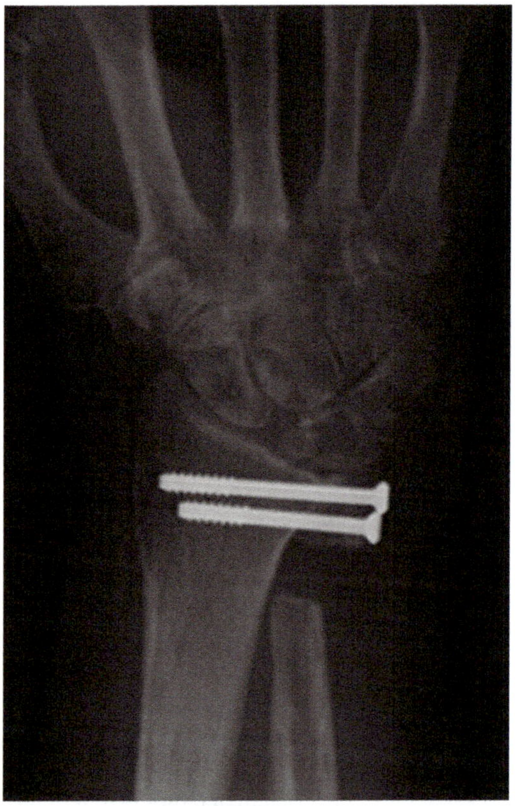

**Fig. 11.7** Suave-Kapandji procedure with radioulnar convergence but no radiographic signs of impingement

single-point fixation and a large segment of bone resected led to these respective complications. Current techniques use two points of fixation, most commonly with cancellous screws in compression. Ten to fifteen millimeters is resected with interposition of the pronator to prevent ossification across the gap. Fujita et al. described a modified technique to improve stability and union rate [18]. A 30 mm distal ulna segment is rotated 90 degrees and inserted into a hole created in the sigmoid notch. The objectives are to improve union and prevent ulnar translation of the wrist. Many soft tissue stabilizing procedures have been described to prevent radioulnar impingement; however, the appropriate vector to maintain separation has not been achieved [19, 20].

## Surgical Treatment: Implant Arthroplasty

### Total Ulnar Head Arthroplasty

Total ulnar head arthroplasty replaces the entire ulnar head including the ulnar styloid with a stemmed implant (Fig. 11.8). The technique is most commonly used for a failed Darrach procedure, but has also been used for a failed HIT procedure, ulnar head fracture, and primary treatment for rheumatoid arthritis and osteoarthritis or even in extensive trauma. Like the Darrach procedure, all soft attachments to the distal ulnar must be released. The implant relies on the surrounding soft tissue envelope for joint stability. Although preoperative DRUJ instability is usually a contraindication for primary total ulnar head arthroplasty, if used after a failed resection arthroplasty due to radioulnar impingement, there will often be sufficient scar tissue that stabilizes the ulna after implantation [21]. Moreover, radiographic and clinical instability cannot consistently be correlated to clinical outcomes [22].

In the initial technique for a total ulnar head replacement, the sigmoid notch was deepened and contoured to match the radius of curvature of the implant head to improve joint stability; however, this technique is no longer commonly performed due to the increased risk of greater sigmoid notch erosion. In fact, sigmoid notch erosion is common even if the notch is not altered, but typically stabilizes by the second year and is not consistently symptomatic [22]. Resurfacing the sigmoid notch with an implant in an unconstrained fashion did not consistently improve outcomes and was associated with joint instability. Recently, Kakar et al. used lateral meniscal allograft to create a labrum to receive the ulnar

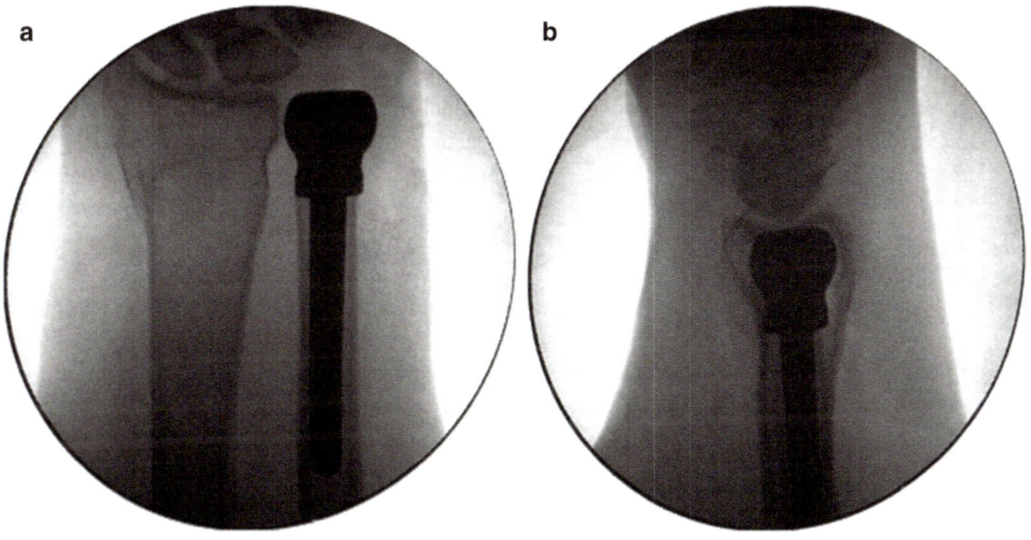

Fig. 11.8 Total ulnar head replacement

head implant [23]. While none of the four patients in this study were unstable postoperatively, only two had preoperative instability. Furthermore, the study lacked standardized outcomes, independent reviewers, objective measures of stability, patient numbers and was retrospective.

Ulnar neck resorption beneath the implant head is also common, which is likely caused by stress shielding, but this rarely causes implant loosening. Early implants with an extended collar showed higher rates of radiolucency, loosening, and subsequent failure [24]. This study also revealed that a pedestal at the proximal aspect of the implant stem results in a poor functional outcome.

Survivorship varies widely in definition, but is commonly defined as complications resulting in surgical removal. Sabo reported 90% survival in 74 patients at 5 and 15 years with an average follow-up of 7 years [25]. Patients in this study had improved patient-reported outcomes. In addition, the vast majority of patients would have the procedure again and recommend it to others. Interestingly, patients who had ulnar implant arthroplasty for post-traumatic conditions were less satisfied and had higher disability than patients who received the implant for arthritic conditions.

A systematic analysis that compiled over 150 wrists demonstrated high longevity and patient satisfaction [26]. Another systemic review found a low complication rate, and improved grip strength, pain, motion, and DASH scores [27]. While the data includes different implants from different manufacturers, implant designs are similar.

## Partial Ulnar Head Arthroplasty

Isolated DRUJ arthritis without instability can be treated with a partial ulnar head replacement arthroplasty (Fig. 11.9a). The technique can be used as a primary treatment for osteoarthritis, a failed wafer resection, a failed HIT procedure, or a comminuted ulnar head fracture. Because only the articular portion of the head is resected, the kinematics of the joint are minimally altered [28]. Furthermore, modular partial head implant designs closely mimic the radiograph of an actual closely mimic the radiograph of an actual ulnar head in all dimensions. [29].

First Choice (Integra, Princeton, NJ) is the only partial ulnar head implant currently available in the USA (Fig. 11.9b–d). With this technique, the ECU tendon and its subsheath, TFCC attachment to the ulnar styloid, and ulnocarpal ligaments are preserved, which provide continued stability to the DRUJ. To insert the implant, the medullary canal is entered through the fovea and reamed to cortical contact for eventual press-fit implant fixation. A cutting jig is applied to the reamer to create a precise implant fit against the remaining head. This product is modular with three stem sizes and four head sizes.

Sigmoid notch erosion does occur, but is less than total ulnar head arthroplasty [21, 27]. Ulnar neck resorption also occurs, but did not result in implant loosening in a series of 18 patients with an average of 4.6 years of follow-up [21]. Partial ulnar head replacement lacks long-term data, but preliminary results are promising.

## Semi-constrained Total DRUJ Arthroplasty

A semi-constrained, bipolar, modular DRUJ implant (Aptis Medical, Louisville, KY) was designed for the treatment of a failed Darrach procedure but later used for a variety of DRUJ conditions that include an unstable arthritic joint, particularly after failed surgery, and has also been used for primary treatment [3].

The Aptis arthroplasty replaces the DRUJ with a small ball-in-socket mechanism that provides intrinsic stability, which is supported by a radial plate and ulnar stem (Fig. 11.10). Preoperative planning estimates the size and location of the implant. A press-fit ulnar stem is selected based on the width of the medullary canal. The position of the articulation depends on

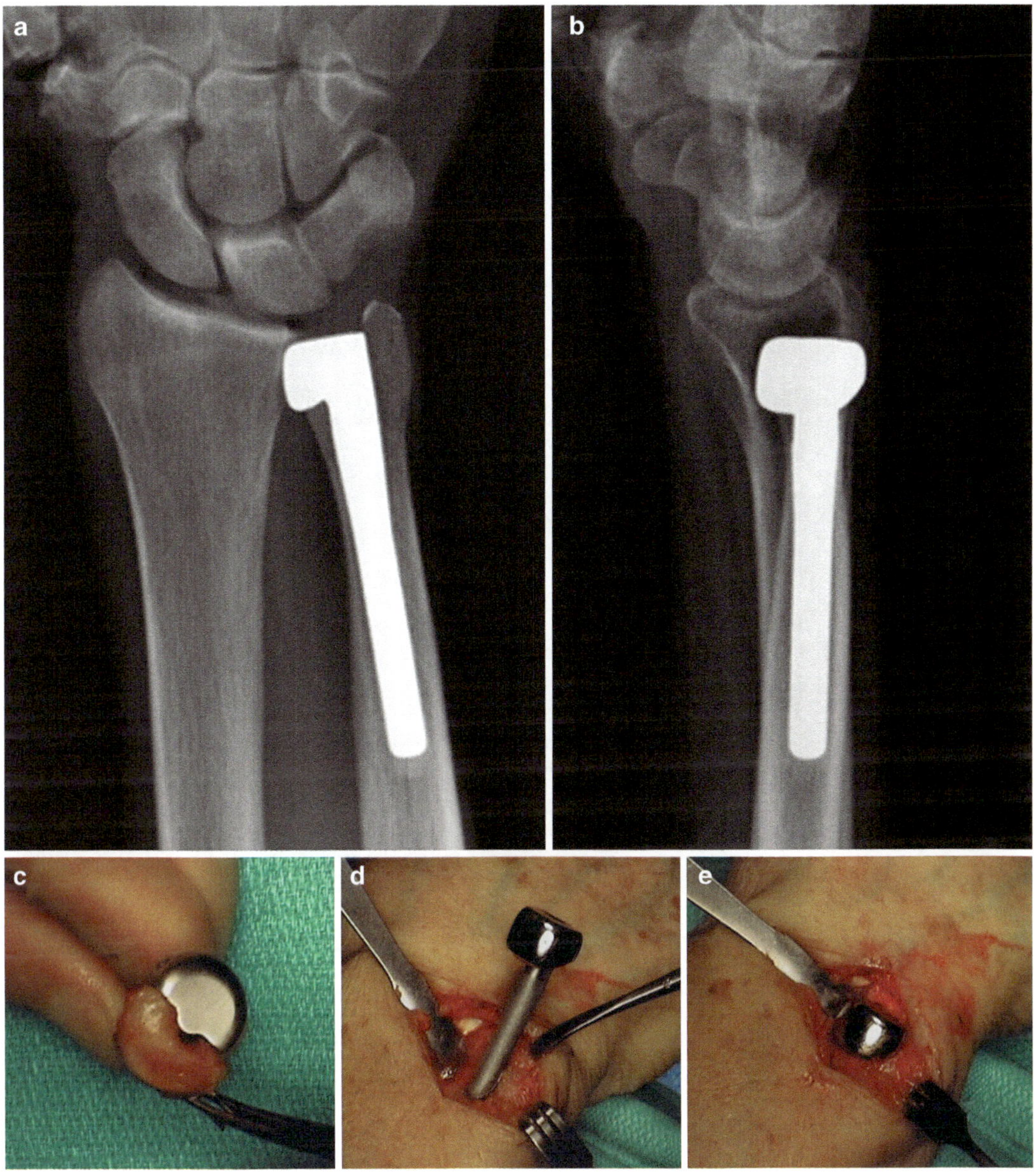


**Fig. 11.9** (**a**–**e**) Partial ulnar head replacement

the condition being treated. Precise implantation is necessary to avoid potential mechanical problems and soft tissue irritation. In particular, the extensor tendons should be protected using a retinacular flap.

The majority of studies show improved motion with favorable patient-reported outcomes including pain scores [12, 27]. Because this implant is used mainly as a salvage procedure, wound healing and soft tissue complications are common [12], which are worse in patients with rheumatoid arthritis or immunosuppression. While successful in properly selected younger patients, with an implant survival rate of 96% at 5 years in one series, ECU tendonitis was a common complication [30].

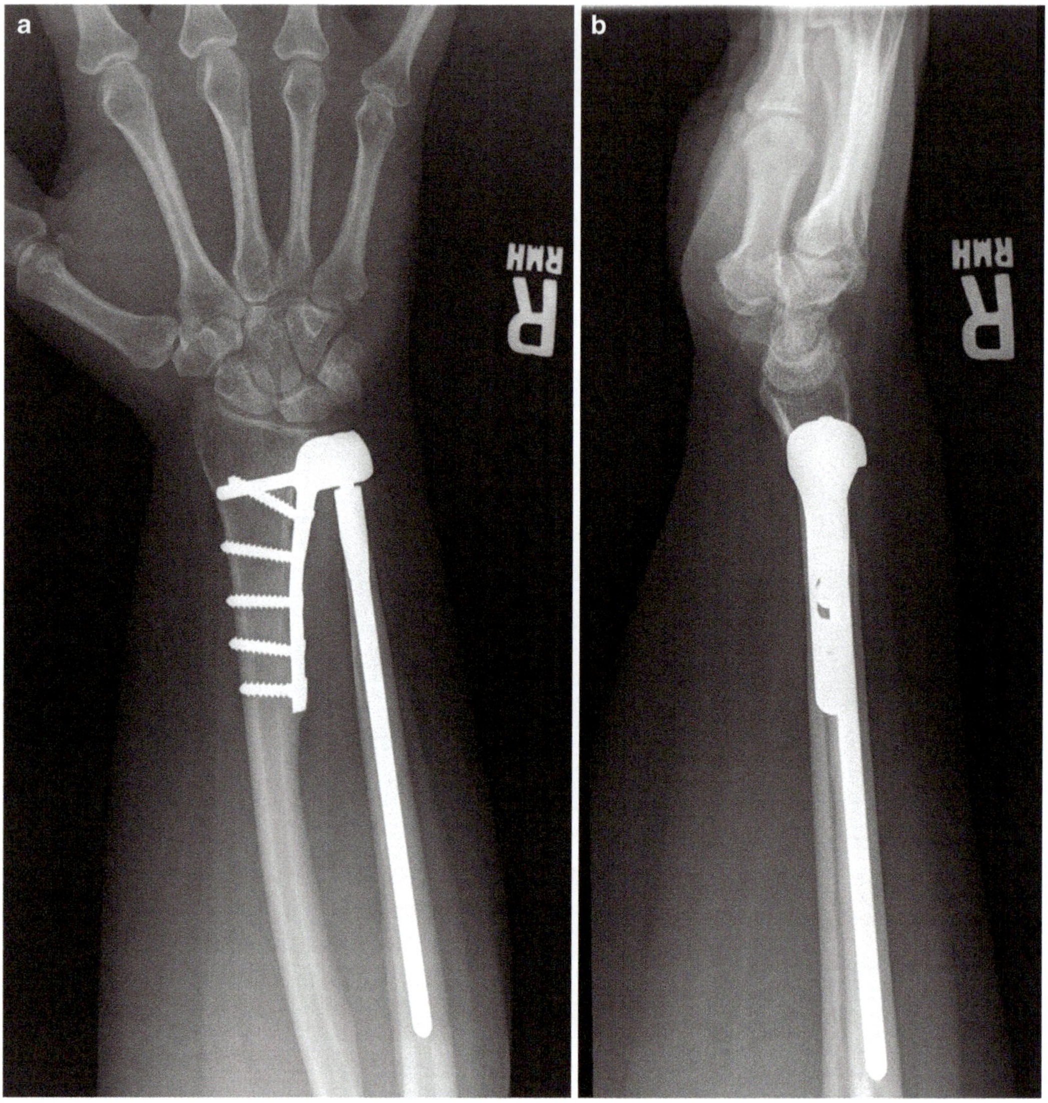


Fig. 11.10 Constrained arthroplasty

## Conclusion

DRUJ arthritis can cause substantial pain and functional limitation. There are many surgical options available, ranging from resection arthroplasties to implant arthroplasties. Resection arthroplasties are complicated by instability that is most pronounced in active patients. Implant arthroplasties vary from partial ulnar head replacement to total joint replacement. Total ulnar head replacement has potentially broad indications, albeit achieving joint stability can be challenging. Partial ulnar head replacement maintains more natural joint kinetics, but has narrower indications. Total joint replacement obviates instability, but requires extensive dissection and results in more soft tissue complications. All techniques and implants have been used successfully for primary treatment and as a salvage operation.

## References


1. af Ekenstam F, Hagert CG. Anatomical studies on the geometry and stability of the distal radio ulnar joint. Scand J Plast Reconstr Surg. 1985;19(1):17–25.
2. Stuart PR, Berger RA, Linscheid RL, An KN. The dorsopalmar stability of the distal radioulnar joint. J Hand Surg Am. 2000;25(4):689–99.
3. Scheker LR, Babb BA, Killion PE. Distal ulnar prosthetic replacement. Orthop Clin North Am. 2001;32(2):365–76, x.
4. Hotchkiss RN, An KN, Sowa DT, Basta S, Weiland AJ. An anatomic and mechanical study of the interosseous membrane of the forearm: pathomechanics of proximal migration of the radius. J Hand Surg Am. 1989;14(2 Pt 1):256–61.
5. Kleinman WB. Stability of the distal radioulnar joint: biomechanics, pathophysiology, physical diagnosis, and restoration of function what we have learned in 25 years. J Hand Surg Am. 2007;32(7):1086–106.
6. Adams BD. Anatomic reconstruction of the distal radioulnar ligaments for DRUJ instability. Tech Hand Up Extrem Surg. 2000;4(3):154–60.
7. Jupiter JB, Ring D. A comparison of early and late reconstruction of malunited fractures of the distal end of the radius. J Bone Joint Surg Am. 1996;78(5):739–48.
8. Breen TF, Jupiter JB. Extensor carpi ulnaris and flexor carpi ulnaris tenodesis of the unstable distal ulna. J Hand Surg Am. 1989;14(4):612–7.
9. Sotereanos DG, Göbel F, Vardakas DG, Sarris I. An allograft salvage technique for failure of the Darrach procedure: a report of four cases. J Hand Surg Br. 2002;27(4):317–21.
10. Sotereanos DG, Papatheodorou LK, Williams BG. Tendon allograft interposition for failed distal ulnar resection: 2- to 14-year follow-up. J Hand Surg Am. 2014;39(3):443–8.e1.
11. Allende C. Allograft tendon interposition and brachioradialis tendon stability augmentation in revision surgery for failed Darrach distal ulna resections. Tech Hand Up Extrem Surg. 2010;14(4):237–40.
12. DeGeorge BR, Berger RA, Shin AY. Constrained implant arthroplasty for distal radioulnar joint arthrosis: evaluation and management of soft tissue complications. J Hand Surg Am. 2019;44(7):614.e1–9.
13. Grawe B, Heincelman C, Stern P. Functional results of the Darrach procedure: a long-term outcome study. J Hand Surg Am. 2012;37(12) 2475–:80.e1–2.
14. Faucher GK, Zimmerman RM, Zimmerman NB. Instability and arthritis of the distal radioulnar joint: a critical analysis review. JBJS Rev. 2016;4(12):1–9
15. Field J, Majkowski RJ, Leslie IJ. Poor results of Darrach's procedure after wrist injuries. J Bone Joint Surg Br. 1993;75(1):53–7.
16. Bowers WH. Distal radioulnar joint arthroplasty: the hemiresection-interposition technique. J Hand Surg Am. 1985;10(2):169–78.
17. Glowacki KA. Hemiresection arthroplasty of the distal radioulnar joint. Hand Clin. 2005;21(4):591–601.
18. Fujita S, Masada K, Takeuchi E, Yasuda M, Komatsubara Y, Hashimoto H. Modified Sauvé-Kapandji procedure for disorders of the distal radioulnar joint in patients with rheumatoid arthritis. J Bone Joint Surg Am. 2005;87(1):134–9.
19. Sauerbier M, Berger RA, Fujita M, Hahn ME. Radioulnar convergence after distal ulnar resection: mechanical performance of two commonly used soft tissue stabilizing procedures. Acta Orthop Scand. 2003;74(4):420–8.
20. Bieber EJ, Linscheid RL, Dobyns JH, Beckenbaugh RD. Failed distal ulna resections. J Hand Surg Am. 1988;13(2):193–200.
21. Adams BD, Gaffey JL. Non-constrained implant arthroplasty for the distal radioulnar joint. J Hand Surg Eur Vol. 2017;42(4):415–21.
22. Axelsson P, Sollerman C, Kärrholm J. Ulnar head replacement: 21 cases; mean follow-up, 7.5 years. J Hand Surg Am. 2015;40(9):1731–8.
23. Kakar S, Noureldin M, Elhassan B. Ulnar head replacement and sigmoid notch resurfacing arthroplasty with a lateral meniscal allograft: 'calamari procedure'. J Hand Surg Eur Vol. 2017;42(6):567–72.
24. Kakar S, Swann RP, Perry KI, Wood-Wentz CM, Shin AY, Moran SL. Functional and radiographic outcomes following distal ulna implant arthroplasty. J Hand Surg Am. 2012;37(7):1364–71.
25. Sabo MT, Talwalkar S, Hayton M, Watts A, Trail IA, Stanley JK. Intermediate outcomes of ulnar head arthroplasty. J Hand Surg Am. 2014;39(12):2405–11.e1.
26. Calcagni M, Giesen T. Distal radioulnar joint arthroplasty with implants: a systematic review. EFORT Open Rev. 2016;1(5):191–6.
27. Moulton LS, Giddins GEB. Distal radio-ulnar implant arthroplasty: a systematic review. J Hand Surg Eur Vol. 2017;42(8):827–38.
28. Garcia-Elias M. Eclypse: partial ulnar head replacement for the isolated distal radio-ulnar joint arthrosis. Tech Hand Up Extrem Surg. 2007;11(1):121–8.
29. Conaway DA, Kuhl TL, Adams BD. Comparison of the native ulnar head and a partial ulnar head resurfacing implant. J Hand Surg Am. 2009;34(6):1056–62.
30. Rampazzo A, Gharb BB, Brock G, Scheker LR. Functional outcomes of the Aptis-Scheker distal radioulnar joint replacement in patients under 40 years old. J Hand Surg Am. 2015;40(7):1397–403.e3.
31. Carlsen BT, Rizzo M, Moran SL. Soft-tissue injuries associated with distal radius fractures. Oper Tech Orthop. 2009;19(2):107–18. https://doi.org/10.1053/j.oto.2009.05.003.

# Revision/Failed Distal Radioulnar Joint Arthroplasty

# 12

Chelsea Boe, Abhiram R. Bhashyam, and Doug Hanel

## Introduction

A painful, dysfunctional, or severely arthritic distal radioulnar joint (DRUJ) can be reconstructed by fusion, resection arthroplasty with or without soft tissue interposition, or prosthetic joint arthroplasty [1–4]. Unfortunately, patients may still develop persistent dysfunction following these procedures due to the inherent stresses on across the DRUJ during functional motion of the forearm and wrist [1, 3]. The loss of the bony buttress on the ulnar side of the wrist and/or failure to recreate that support with an appropriately positioned and tensioned arthroplasty alters loading across the DRUJ and allows for convergence of the radius and ulna with contraction of the pronator quadratus, abductor pollicis longus, and extensor pollicis brevis [5, 6].

Failures of previous arthroplasty procedures represent a difficult problem in a particularly complex patient population. Typically, these patients are encountered after several prior surgeries with complaints such as persistent pain, instability, and general wrist dysfunction. Treatment and patient education about expected outcomes are a further challenge given the limited body of evidence on managing complications or failure of DRUJ arthroplasty. The larger published series assessing outcomes following DRUJ arthroplasty include 30–50 patients, the largest published to date including just 52 total patients. Complication rates in these cohorts ranged from 30% to 40%, with limited description of patient evaluation and treatment of these complications [7–12]. Further contributing to the paucity of data is the limited number of providers who have the experience and willingness to tackle these complex problems. Given the inherent heterogeneity of this population in addition to the previously described factors, application of the evidence is prone to subjectivity. As such, this review stems from a compilation of available evidence and nearly four decades of experience in treating these patients at tertiary referral centers.

In presenting their approach to the challenging problem of ulnar-sided wrist pain, Kakar and Garcia-Elias define pathology from four interrelated zones, each associated with treatments specific to that zone [3]. Identifying the involved zone(s) and applying appropriate treatment while remaining respectful of the potential for interrelated problems is essential to successful resolution of primary DRUJ pathology. We propose that the concept of using a mental algorithm for processing interrelated pathology on the ulnar side of the wrist can also be adapted to failed DRUJ arthroplasty. In this setting, the zones are unique as while there is no longer a TFCC, articular

C. Boe · A. R. Bhashyam · D. Hanel (✉)
Department of Orthopaedics and Sports Medicine, University of Washington, Seattle, WA, USA
e-mail: abhiramb@uw.edu; dhanel@uw.edu


G. J. W. King, M. Rizzo (eds.), *Arthroplasty of the Upper Extremity*,
https://doi.org/10.1007/978-3-030-68880-6_12

surface, or cartilage interface, there exists the potential for new pathology related to the prior operation(s).

Previous authors have identified multiple potential sources of pain and dysfunction following procedures for resection of the distal ulna, including neurogenic pain, tendinitis, tenosynovitis, and radiocarpal arthritis [13]. By expanding and regrouping those potential pain generators, we propose six interrelated zones to frame evaluation of the failed DRUJ arthroplasty. The zones are nerve, tendon, adjacent arthritis, impingement, implant complication/instability, and infection. Applying the useful framework proposed by Kakar and Garcia-Elias [3], the four-leaf clover becomes a multi-petal flower, distilling complex problems into discrete arenas with succinct and specific solutions (Fig. 12.1). Each of these zones should be individually considered when evaluating a new patient with a failed DRUJ arthroplasty and each zone specifically interrogated to gain a comprehensive understanding of pathology, such that targeted and comprehensive treatment can be determined and performed.

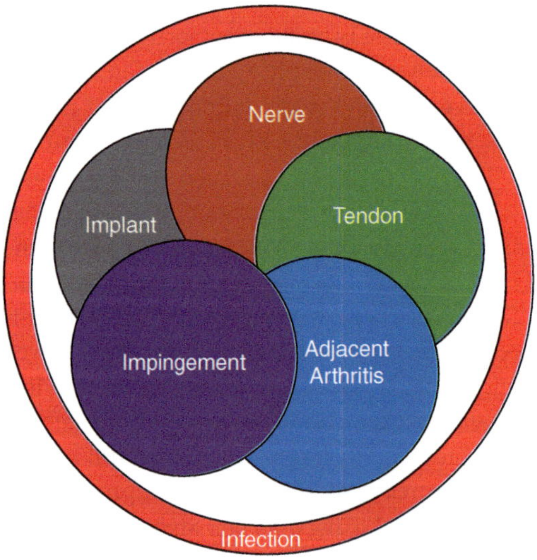


**Fig. 12.1** Six zone algorithm for evaluating potential sources of pain and dysfunction following DRUJ arthroplasty

## Clinical Presentation

### Patient History

Each patient requires holistic review, avoiding the temptation to focus on the most recent procedure. This entails a thorough history and physical with special emphasis on the unique functional demands specific to each patient, including a review of previous pathology and procedures on the extremity. The critical information to glean is the connection between the patient's symptoms prior to an intervention and how the intervention changed those symptoms. The time course is important as problems that developed insidiously following intervention suggest a different etiology than problems which preceded or developed abruptly following intervention. Another critical point is confirming that physical and radiological exam findings are in fact representative of the specific complaints that affect the patient in their day-to-day life. For example, all distal ulnar resections will have convergence, but this finding may not correlate with the pain which limits function and prompted presentation to clinic [13, 14].

### Physical Examination

The physical examination begins with a general inspection of traumatic and surgical scars, obvious deformity such as subluxated tendons, and the defect created by the absence of the ulnar head.

Range of motion of the shoulder, elbow, and hand is assessed. A cursory way to confirm a functional range of motion of the shoulder and elbow is to ask the patient to place their hands to their mouth, to their ear, to the back of their head, and behind their back in the region of the lumbar spine. This simulates self-cares and basic functional needs, including performing personal hygiene, feeding independently, and using a cell phone. Wrist flexion and extension are measured with the elbow flexed to 90° and resting on the exam table. The contralateral side is similarly measured and recorded for comparison. Digit range of motion is assessed by asking the patient to transition from holding their digits in full extension to full composite flexion ("make a fist"). This confirms the presence or absence of hand pathology that may need to be addressed in conjunction with the DRUJ. Pain and crepitus with range of motion of the radiocarpal joint, the hand, elbow, or shoulder may direct more thorough evaluations of these joints to identify adjacent joint arthritis that may contribute to DRUJ dysfunction or be exacerbated by any intervention to the DRUJ.

Palpation of adjacent joints is critical, as active range of motion may be insufficient to reveal pathology. The radiocarpal joint is palpated, first by identifying Lister's tubercle and rolling the examiner's thumb distal to the radiocarpal articulation. Pain more radially over the radial styloid may suggest underlying arthritic changes, while pain more proximally may suggest either tenosynovitis or prominent radial hardware in the setting of a previous constrained arthroplasty. A shearing compressive force at the pisotriquetral joint also suggests an arthritic joint (Fig. 12.2).

A complete peripheral nerve examination is performed with objective measures of motor strength and sensibility recorded. Special attention is paid to the dorsal cutaneous branch of the ulnar (DCBrUN) which can be injured by traction or transected in a dorsally based approach to the DRUJ. Each nerve distribution, especially the DCBrUN, should be palpated to assess hypersensitivity. Tinel's sign can be assessed to elucidate and pinpoint an area of maximal tenderness that may correlate with neuroma formation from a prior procedure. Compressive provocative testing can also quickly and easily be performed to confirm the baseline function of the median nerve at the wrist and the ulnar nerve at the elbow and Guyon's canal. Sensibility is objectively recorded by measuring static two-point discrimination on the radial and ulnar aspect of each digit as well as monofilament testing in the same distribution. Strength is evaluated by testing of grip, appositional ("key") pinch and oppositional pinch.

Having completed the above, the DRUJ is assessed. The patient's arm is placed by their side with the elbow flexed 90° to limit shoulder motion. The patient is asked to move the forearm from maximum supination to maximum pronation and describe the amount and quality of pain that is occurring at the distal end of the ulna. If the motion is pain-free, then the patient is asked to hold a 5 kg weight, repeat the pronation supina-

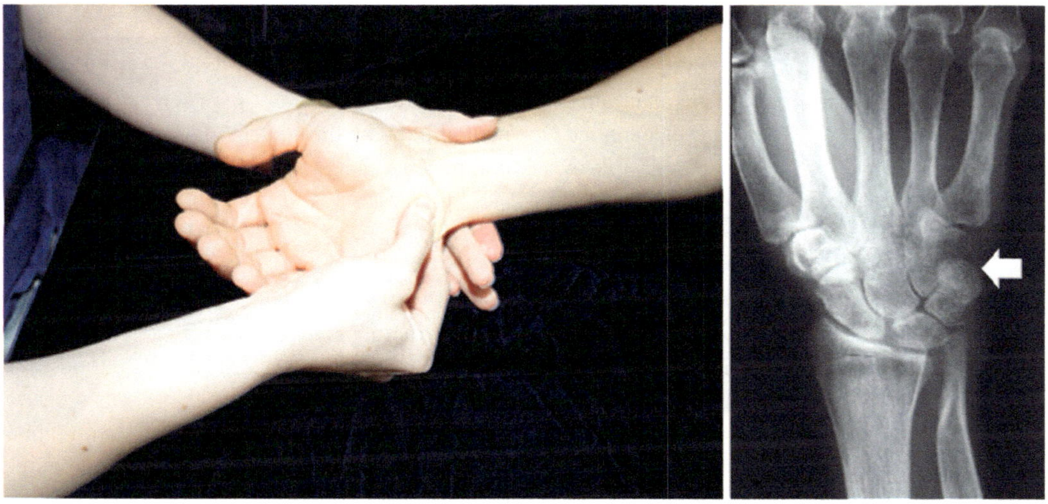

**Fig. 12.2** Clinical and radiographical evaluation of the pisotriquetral joint with arthritic changes suggestive of pisotriquetral arthrosis

tion action, and describe any accompanied pain. Translation is assessed with the patient's elbow resting on the exam table. The examiner translates the ulna in a volar-dorsal direction while stabilizing the radius. This is performed in neutral, full pronation and full supination. Finally, a compression test is performed with a grasping maneuver that pushes the end of the ulna against the radius while pronating and supinating the forearm. This latter examination can be quite uncomfortable and should be performed gently and discontinued if particularly painful (Fig. 12.3).

Maneuvers designed to identify irritation of the flexor carpi ulnaris (FCU) and irritation or subluxation of the extensor carpi ulnaris (ECU) are performed. With the patient's elbow flexed and resting on the exam table, the patient is asked to maintain a neutral position while the examiner applies a gentle extension force. This causes tension and prominence of the FCU, which can then be palpated from the mid forearm into the base of the palm, where it envelops the pisiform, before inserting into the base of the fifth metacarpal. Swelling and tenderness along the FCU tendon may be noted.

Examining the ECU has been described with various maneuvers that reveal the tendon perching or subluxating from the sixth dorsal extensor compartment. In the setting of failed DRUJ surgery, tendon subluxation is not subtle. The subluxation can be presented by placing the wrist in extension and rotating the forearm through a complete range of pronation and supination while palpating the sixth dorsal extensor compartment at the ulnar head. The maneuver is then repeated with the wrist in flexion and again in extension. The subluxation can be exaggerated by having the patient resist counter pressure placed on the wrist by the examiner, relying on the principle of co-contraction of the ECU and FCU to maintain neutral wrist position in the face of directional force. It has been argued that this maneuver also stresses the TFCC, LT ligament, and ulnocarpal articulation and may be less specific for ECU pathology. Thus, we also routinely perform the "synergy test" to specifically assess ECU tendonitis, as elegantly described by Ruland and Hogan (Fig. 12.4) [15]. This is performed with the patient's elbow flexed and resting on the exam table, the wrist positioned in neutral and maximal supination, and the digits fully extended. The examiner attempts to compress the patient's thumb and long finger while the patient resists this effort. A positive test elicits characteristic pain at the sixth dorsal extensor compartment radiating along the ECU tendon proximally and/or palpable subluxation of the ECU tendon. This can be especially helpful in elucidating a potential cause of mild pain over the

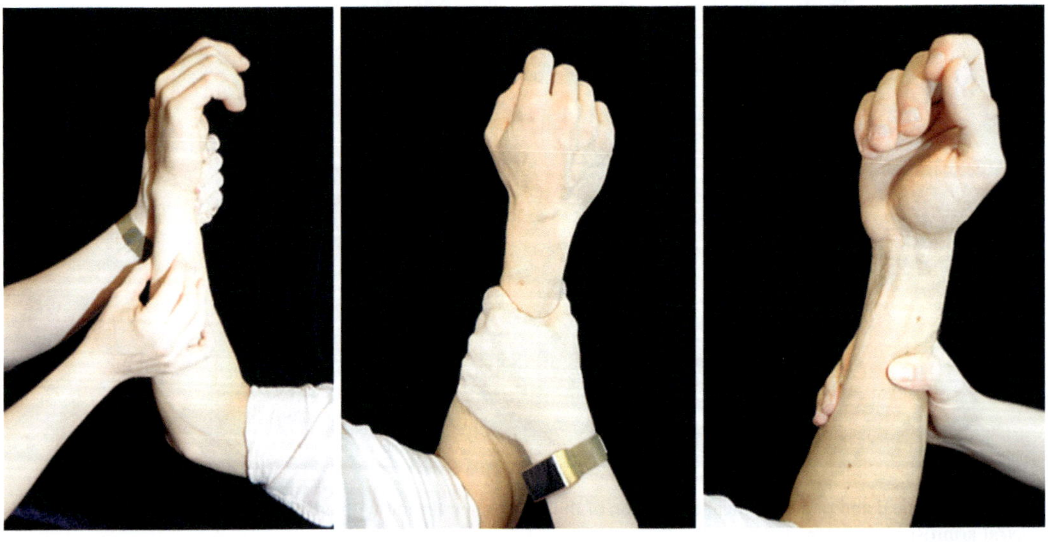

**Fig. 12.3** Provocative testing of DRUJ pain: translation, compression in pronation, compression in supination

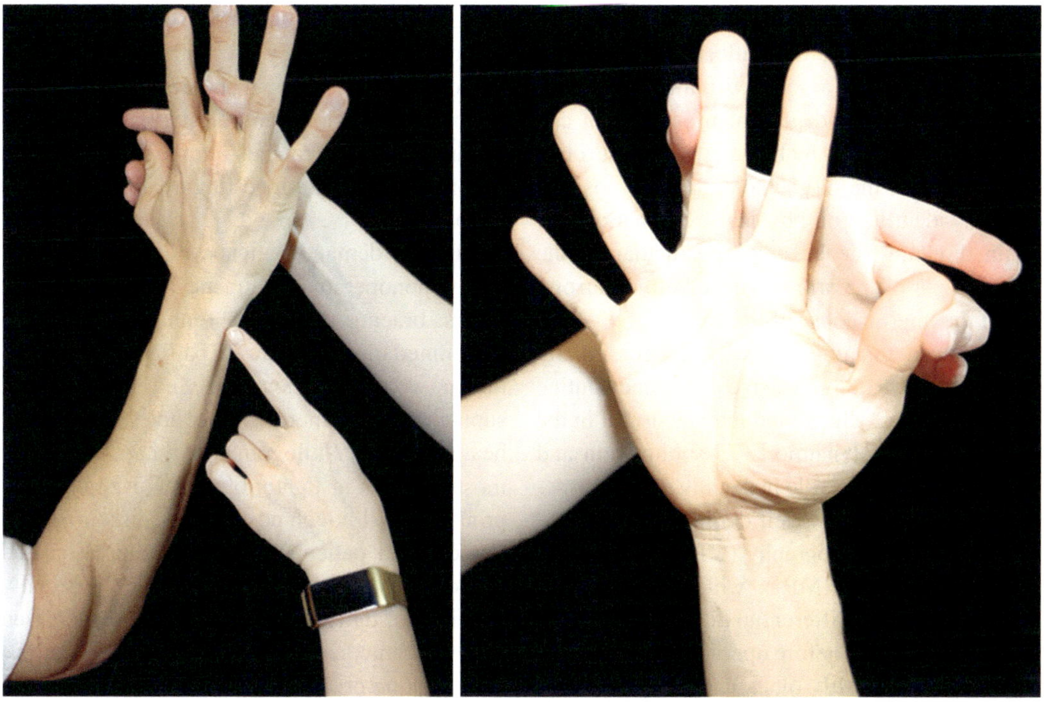

**Fig. 12.4** Provocative testing for ECU subluxation using the "synergy" test

prominence of a metallic implant in an otherwise stable DRUJ after reconstruction.

## Diagnostic Studies

Radiographs of the elbow, forearm, and wrist should be taken in posteroanterior (PA), lateral, and oblique projections, including an oblique view of the proximal radioulnar joint (PRUJ). As the majority of these patients have undergone some sort of ulnar head resection, the ECU sulcus cannot be used to determine a true PA projection of the DRUJ as previously described [16]. Thus, a PA will need to be approximated by abducting the shoulder to 90°, flexing the elbow to 90° and positioning the forearm in neutral with the forearm and hand flat on the cassette. A true lateral of the wrist can be obtained without the ulnar head, and the accuracy of the projection is confirmed by using the scaphopisocapitate (SPC) alignment criteria described by Yang et al. [17]. This image is essential for assessing the correct placement of constrained metallic arthroplasties.

The radiographs are scrutinized for adjacent joint osteoarthritis, fractures, and carpal malalignment. Radiographs of the elbow are used to predict the potential exacerbation of arthritic conditions upon correction and increased used of the limb after DRUJ reconstruction. In some cases, DRUJ and PRUJ pathology will need to be addressed simultaneously. In the setting of ulnar head arthroplasty, the ulnar cortex of the radius is assessed for signs of scalloping suggesting erosion from contact with the distal end of the ulna. Implant arthroplasties are assessed for alignment and cortical erosion, lucent lines around the implant, and stress reaction, which may suggest underlying or impending stress fracture or indolent infection.In the setting of previous ulnar head resection arthroplasty, special radiographs to assess for radioulnar instability are indicated. As described by Lees and Scheker, the image is obtained with the patient's arm at their side, elbow flexed to 90°, and forearm in neutral. A cassette is placed between the forearm and the body, while the patient holds a 2.2 Kg (5 lb) weight. The beam of the radiograph is directed perpendicular to the forearm in the coronal plane [13]. The radiograph will reflect the amount of convergence that is associated with resection of the ulnar head. The degree of impingement can be further augmented by having the patient rotate the forearm in the most uncomfortable position that was identified on physical examination and again directing the beam perpendicular to the coronal axis of the arm to visualize the narrowing of the interosseous space.

Advanced imaging studies are occasionally indicated after comprehensive exam and routine imaging studies. Ultrasound may be useful in the identification of dynamic ECU subluxation and tenosynovitis, but its role in dealing with this specific population is not well defined in the literature. Computed tomography (CT) and magnetic resonance imaging (MRI), which are essential contributors to the differential diagnosis of DRUJ pain and instability before operative intervention, play a more limited role after an arthroplasty procedure. CT and MRI after arthroplasty can be used to define the integrity of the medullary canals of the forearm bones, document the extent of static displacement of the remaining ulna, and help delineate the role of tenosynovitis, carpal necrosis, intercarpal arthrosis, implant loosening, and infection, although artifact can limit interpretation of these studies. If physical examination reveals decreased sensibility and grip strength weakness that is suggestive of pathology more substantial than pain limitation, electrodiagnostic testing will help identify the extent and location of any nerve injury, as well as help differentiate weakness secondary to nerve injury.

## Principles of Management

The overall treatment of a failed DRUJ arthroplasty must be inclusive of all pathology and comprehensive in addressing each specific pathology. The six zones (nerve, tendon, adjacent arthritis, impingement, implant complication/instability, and infection) allow a formulaic pattern of examination and framework for thoughtful treatment of this patient population. The final intervention should incorporate treatment targeted at each contributing pathology. Except for isolated tendon or nerve problems, there are limited surgical options for revision arthroplasty. Functional status and physical demands are the critical factors in formulating and suggesting treatment plans to the patient.

For low-demand patients, our first option is always nonoperative treatment. We use mild analgesics, bracing that limits forearm motion and accommodative strategies to palliate pain. In particular, we teach patients to avoid pronation and supination movements while holding anything heavier than a 2-kilogram weight, as this is the most common instigator of pain. Revision DRUJ procedures, although possible, are discouraged in low-demand patients because of the associated loss of independence during recovery, especially activities of daily living, as well as the increased risk of immediate postoperative complications necessitating prolonged immobilization.

In general, higher-demand patients are more clinically challenging secondary to the higher expectations and anticipated ongoing use of the extremity. In higher-demand patients with a failed ulnar head resection, options include further ulnar shortening or soft tissue interposition arthroplasty. Wolfe et al. advocated further shortening of the ulna to minimize distal impingement. In their study, they reported substantial pain relief, though admittedly with persistent proximal impingement and volar-dorsal translation [18]. Garcia-Elias et al. have suggested that extensive ulnar resection risks further destabilization of the ulna by further resecting the interosseous ligament and increasing reliance on dynamic secondary stabilizers [19]. Perhaps for this reason, further reports of wide resection of the ulna have not been repeated in the literature. Soft tissue interposition arthroplasty as advocated by and eponymously named for Sotereanos, which entails complete ulnar head resection and placement of allograft between the radius and ulna, has been advocated as a method to provide a physical barrier between the radius and ulna which simultaneously tensions the interosseous ligaments conferring increased stability to the ulna [20]. As a primary intervention, this procedure is effective in alleviating pain, with greater than 80% of patients reporting significant reduction in pain related to impingement in the early postoperative period [21–24]. However, results in the setting of previous resection arthroplasty demonstrate less reliable pain relief and improvement of overall function [23, 24].

In the setting of high-demand patients with failed previous arthroplasty, one would anticipate simple resection arthroplasty and procedures which do not recreate the stability of the distal radioulnar joint DRUJ to be prone to failure. Regardless, we always discuss nonoperative management. Depending on the degree of dysfunction and the patient's specific goals for functional improvement, satisfying expectations may not be possible. This can be a difficult discussion of realistic goals, and the treating provider has a responsibility to clarify and temper appropriate expectations. We often encourage patients in this population to think critically about their willingness to curtail activities that place high demands on the extremity and prolong nonoperative management for as long possible. We often do our best to remember and convey that there is no situation which cannot be made worse with operative intervention.

Admittedly, this high-demand group is often resistant to living with dysfunction and unwilling to make dramatic, lifelong changes in activities or occupation. There are two procedures that we consider in this setting. The first is the previously described Sotereanos procedure, which uses a large interposition allograft as a spacer and interosseous membrane (IOM) tensioning device [20]. In this procedure, a large bulk allograft is secured with suture anchors placed between the radius and the ulna. With a 14-year follow-up, the initial reports presented by Sotereanos et al. are promising [24]. We use this technique in young patients with the anticipation that when it fails, the procedure can be repeated or revised with a semi-constrained arthroplasty. It is tempting to envision interposition arthroplasty as "no bridges burned," but additional surgeries always carry potential for complications. The durability of interposition arthroplasty in the setting of previously performed and now failed arthroplasty is not well-known, yet this remains a consideration for appropriately selected patients who may be very young or unwilling to accept an arthroplasty procedure.

The second procedure considered for high-demand patients with failed previous arthroplasty is revision to semi-constrained arthroplasty as advocated by Scheker [11]. Revision to a semi-constrained arthroplasty is the preferred definitive intervention as it most closely recreates the normal dynamic motion of the forearm. Patients report a forearm that feels essentially normal to them [10, 11]. While the manufacturer recommends restrictive life-long weight limits and activity restrictions, patients routinely exceed these and use the extremity normally [7, 8, 11]. This surgical option is highly attractive to patients who have been severely limited and for whom expectations include returning to vocations and hobbies that require dynamic pronation and supination of both hands. Technically this is accomplished with revision utilizing longer ulnar stems or impaction grafting for bone loss in the ulnar diaphysis (Fig. 12.5).

For cases in which there is extensive bone loss, deformity that cannot be corrected, an infection that cannot be cleared, or an occupation that places heavy load on the extremity, we recommend creation of a single bone forearm (Fig. 12.6). This is particularly suited for the patient who presents with pain throughout the range of motion of the DRUJ and has gross multiplanar instability and an occupation or geographic location that precludes the necessary therapy, follow-up, or restrictions associated with interposition or semi-constrained arthroplasty. As such, the only option for pain relief is a one bone forearm. This is a hyper-select group of patients which is definitively not well captured in the literature. In general, patient function after creation of a one-bone forearm is adequate and satisfaction only moderate [7, 25]. However, our experience suggests that for the appropriately selected patient, this is a very reliable option that is well tolerated with acceptable outcome from the perspective of both patient and physician.

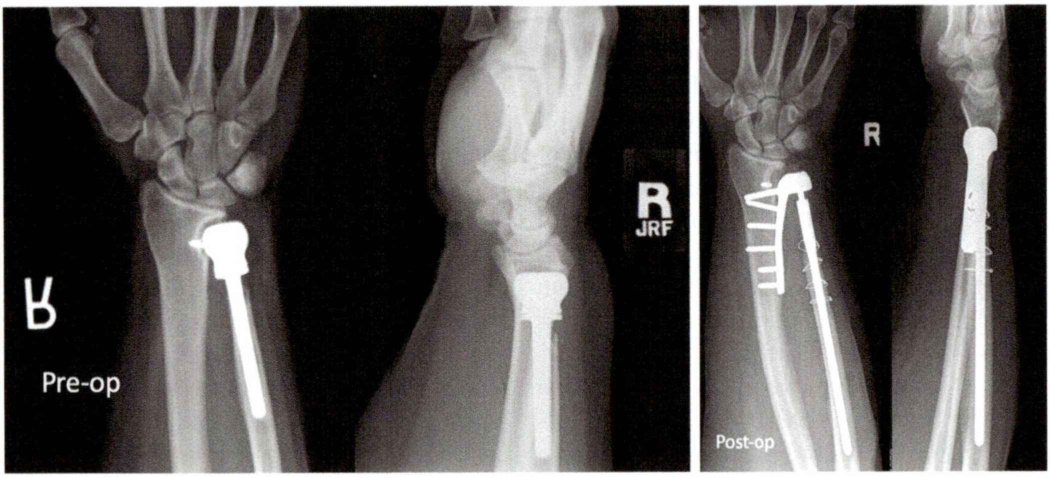


**Fig. 12.5** Revision of a prior failed ulnar head hemiarthroplasty to a semi-constrained Aptis-Scheker arthroplasty with 8 years of follow-up

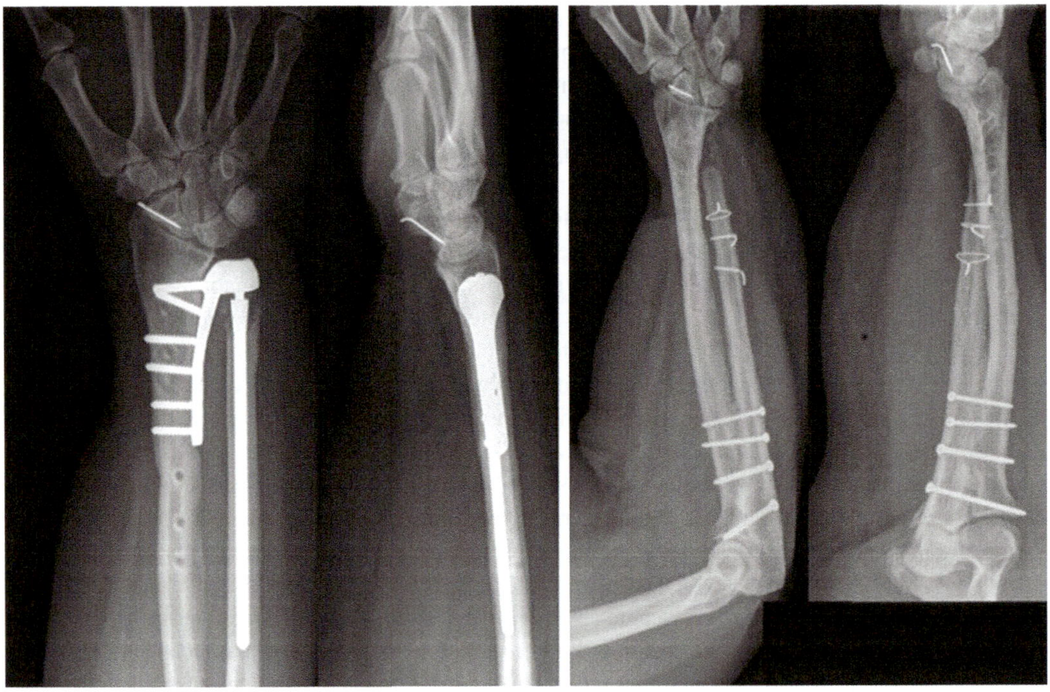

**Fig. 12.6** Creation of a single bone forearm in the setting of bone loss and infection

## Treatment Algorithm by Zone of DRUJ Pathology

### Zone 1: Nerve

Nerve injury and the resultant neurogenic pain can negate an otherwise acceptable DRUJ arthroplasty and result in profound dysfunction. The DCBrUN travels in the subcutaneous tissue as it traverses the ulnar neck and head from proximal volar to distal dorsal. This passage makes it prone to transection when the DRUJ is approached through a skin incision along the subcutaneous border of distal ulna, as well as by traction injury when the dorsal skin flaps are elevated to expose the DRUJ. The incidence of nerve injury with this approach is not well defined. While the original descriptions of DRUJ approaches for reconstruction do not mention neurologic injury, recent articles have reported a frequency of nerve complications that is not insignificant [7, 26–28].

Palliating neurogenic pain may be all that is needed to salvage a "failed reconstruction." If present, it is critical to address neurogenic pain to optimize outcome even in the setting of other contributing pain generators. The relative contribution of an injured nerve to the patient's pain can be estimated using a diagnostic injection of local anesthetic. The response to injection should be assessed with regard to pain as well as functional improvement. If the diagnostic injection is accompanied by return to normal function, however transient, then addressing the nerve injury alone may be sufficient. If not, then the additional causes of pain must be addressed. If the pain is significantly improved with the injection, then directed treatment is first predicated upon the length of time from injury. Observation should be recommended if the patient presents within 3 months of their last procedure or time of nerve injury, as many nerve-related symptoms in this time period are neuropraxic in nature and will resolve spontaneously [8]. Additionally, nonoperative management in the form of structured and supervised desensitization should be undertaken. If the injury is greater than 3 months old and nonoperative desensitization has failed to improve symptoms, then operative intervention is warranted.

Operative intervention for DCBrUN dysfunction entails thorough neurolysis and consideration of nerve wrapping with vein grafts, collagen conduits, or silicone sleeves. These wraps are well described in treatment of peripheral neuritis and treatment of neuromas in continuity. However, benefits specific to traumatic neuritis of the DCBrUN have not been reported, and our personal experience has not demonstrated appreciable benefit [7]. Our preferred treatment is neurolysis and neurectomy, with implantation of the transected free nerve end into an adjacent muscle belly, namely, the ECU or FCU, as has been described for painful neuromas of the sensory branch of the radial nerve (Fig. 12.7) [29].

## Zone 2: Tendon

Tendon-related problems can include tenosynovitis, tendonitis, adhesions, and tendon subluxation. Resection of the ulnar head can be associated with irritation of the ECU, though it has been noted infrequently after placement of a bipolar, semi-constrained, modular implant such as the Aptis DRUJ prosthesis (Aptis Medical, Glenview, KY) [7, 10, 26, 27]. The discomfort can be substantial and sufficient to compromise an otherwise good result. The common clinical finding is a painful ECU tendon as it translates over ulnar head component of the prosthesis. Swelling of the ECU tendon may be noted but a fulminant tenosynovitis rarely occurs. The diagnosis is readily confirmed with relief after injection of local anesthetic adjacent to the tendon

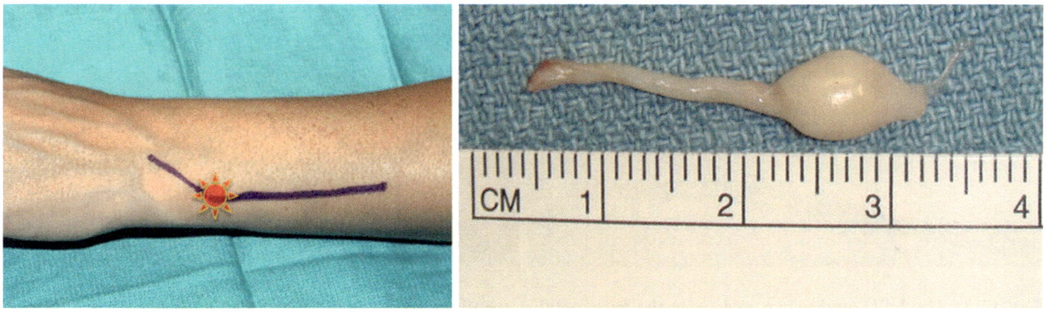


Fig. 12.7 Painful neuroma of the dorsal cutaneous branch of the ulnar nerve that was treated with neurolysis, neurectomy, and implantation of the free nerve ending into the adjacent muscle belly

and ulnar head component. Ultrasound may also be helpful in demonstrating inflammation about the tendon and/or subtle subluxation. Treatment is surgical with stabilization of the ECU with capsular interposition to prevent the ECU tendon from gliding over the bare metal of the ulnar head component (Fig. 12.8). Despite this direct irritation of the ECU, tendon rupture has not been reported.

The developers of this implant recognized this potential problem and recommend that an ulnar based flap of extensor retinaculum be elevated in the exposure of the joint and then placed between the ulnar head component and the ECU tendon at the time of initial arthroplasty. When this device is being used to salvage a previous DRUJ resection, the scar formed by prior surgery may prevent the retinacular flap from being raised [27]. In this case, the DRUJ is reconstructed with the Aptis prosthesis, tenolysis of the ECU is performed, and a dermoadipose graft is harvested from the groin and interposed between the prosthesis and the tendon (Fig. 12.8).

Tenosynovitis of the extensor digiti communis (EDC) tendons has been reported after successful DRUJ reconstruction with the Aptis prosthetic. The frequency of this complication is unknown. In one such case, fascia lata allograft was interposed with resolution of symptoms [26].

## Zone 3: Adjacent Joint Arthritis

The wrist includes numerous local articulations with propensity for degenerative change which can complicate the evaluation of a painful DRUJ. The radiocarpal, midcarpal, and pisotriquetral joints are not uncommonly degenerative, especially in situations where the degree of degeneration and dysfunction of the DRUJ has

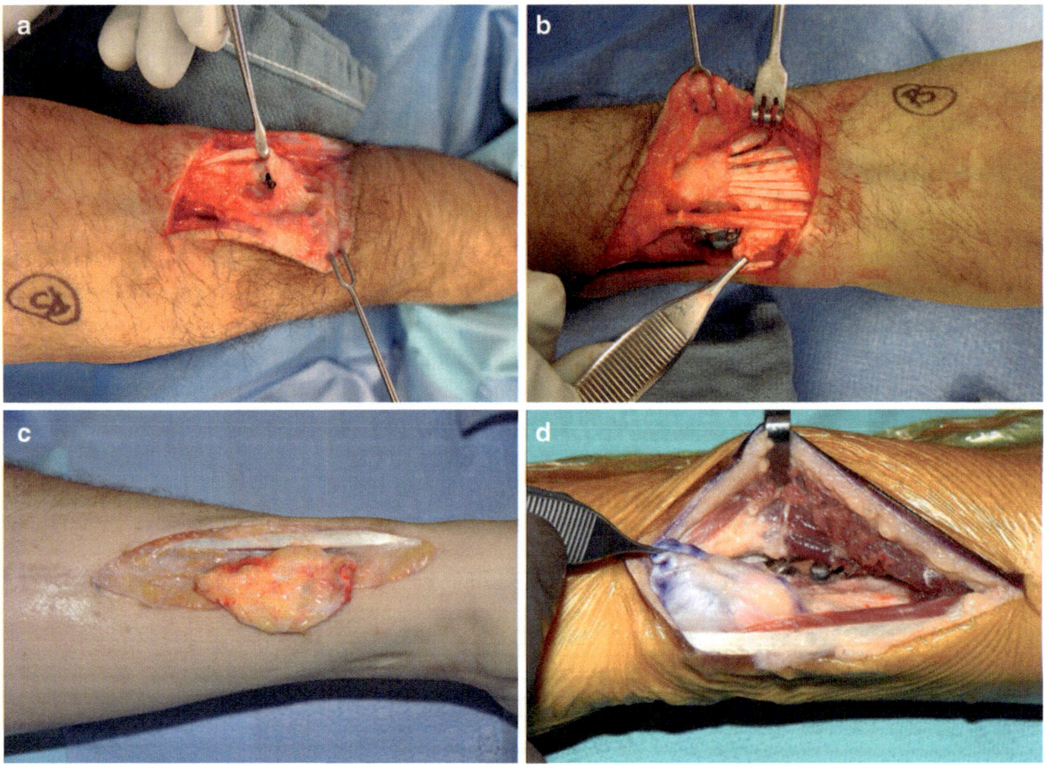


**Fig. 12.8** The ECU tendon can glide over the bare metal of the ulnar head component (**a**). In these cases, this can be treated with an ulnar-based flap of the extensor retinaculum (**b**) or a dermoadipose graft (**c**). It is currently recommended to use an ulnar-based extensor retinaculum flap at the primary operation (**d**)

become so severe as to necessitate at least one if not multiple arthroplasty attempts. It underscores the critical need to assess the specific pain complaints of the patient and correlate that pain to both in the history and physical exam.

Radiocarpal arthritis is often diagnosed with localization of pain to the radial side of the wrist and reproduction of pain with wrist flexion and extension. This can be managed in similar fashion to radiocarpal arthritis in the absence of a DRUJ arthroplasty. A similar approach can be undertaken with midcarpal arthritis. With regard to pisotriquetral arthritis, compression of this joint is painful on exam, and tangential shearing force reproduces discomfort that is limiting for the patient. This can be addressed with pisiform excision with reliable relief of pain [27].

Elbow arthritis, specifically with involvement of the PRUJ, can play a role in upper extremity limitation and pain. Physical exam of the elbow and proximal localization of pain with attempted pronation and supination can identify potential contributing pathology from these proximal articulations. Treatment is indicated in similar fashion to patients without DRUJ arthritis, but it remains critical to appreciate the role that these limitations can play on overall dysfunction of the extremity, especially in consideration of radial head resection.

## Zone 4: Impingement

Impingement can occur in the dorsal-volar direction, often described as translational, as well as in the radial-ulnar direction, described as impingement. Impingement of the radius and ulna after resection is inevitable with the loss of the distal radioulnar articulation, as in the setting of resection arthroplasty [18, 22, 30]. However, this impingement does not always translate to pain and dysfunction, emphasizing the importance of correlating physical exam and imaging findings with clinical complaints. Common complaints include the inability to perform gripping activities or lift anything with the hand of the affected extremity. Often these patients report using their forearm as a hook to carry objects such as grocery bags to avoid compressive forces across the DRUJ. They may also report performing activities with the wrist locked in full pronation or full supination. The degree of pathology can easily be identified with weighted radiographic evaluation, but this must be correlated with replication of pain and dysfunction with compression on physical exam [13, 14, 22].

Treatment of impingement is targeted at supporting the resected ulnar stump. Numerous procedures have been described to support the distal ulna and resist translational instability, often involving use of slips of the ECU or FCU for dynamic support and recreation of forces resisting excessive motion in the sagittal plane. Unfortunately, these procedures have not demonstrated durable long-term correction of ulnar stump instability, and recurrent translation or impingement occurs in the majority of cases when followed for greater than 5 years [31, 32].

Direct support of the ulnar stump can be accomplished with a physical barrier between the two bones which resists direct compression of the ulnar head against the radius and additionally tensions the interosseous ligaments supporting the translation of the ulnar stump in all planes in the form of a Sotereanos procedure [21, 22, 24]. However, the definitive treatment for instability in both the volar-dorsal and radioulnar planes is recreation of the distal radioulnar joint articulation by insertion of a semi-constrained implant [11]. This stabilizes the ulnar stump and prevents painful impingement by buttressing the ulnar diaphysis against the ulnar cortex of the radius.

## Zone 5: Implant Complications

A well-functioning DRUJ prosthesis is dependent on numerous aspects of implantation technique as well as design of the implant itself. Older generation implants suffered from significant flaws that led to progressive loosening or disengagement of the radial plate from the ulnar head [11]. Modern implants appear to have solved these early design flaws, and results demonstrate revision-free survival of greater than 95% at 5 years [7, 10, 28].

The technique of implantation is dependent on appropriate imaging as the primary determinant of alignment and center of rotation. Inappropriately aligned implants (with center of rotation deviated from the true center of the previous ulnar head) lead to continuous translational force and painful stress along the ulnar implant and the radioulnar articulation. This can lead to progressive loosening, cortical erosion, or stress reaction along either the ulnar cortex or radial plate [7]. In addition to stress reaction related to inappropriate alignment, the rigidity of the implant itself can lead to stress risers and potential stress fracture. The rigid medullary canal filling implant which abruptly ends in the middle of the ulnar diaphysis and rigid radial plate ending in the diaphysis of the radius represent stress risers. With significant impact loading, radial stress fractures may occur as early as within the first 6 weeks of the primary procedure, even when the proximal most screw is deliberately unicortical to minimize the stress riser [7].These can be treated with compression plating (Fig. 12.9).

## Zone 6: Infection

In the setting of multiple surgeries and certainly with implant arthroplasty, infection must always be a consideration. The highly vascular nature of the upper extremity relative to other privileged joint sites potentially makes upper extremity arthroplasty more vulnerable to hematogenous spread [7]. For this reason, we routinely recommend prophylaxis to patients with DRUJ arthroplasty undergoing invasive or dental procedures for their lifetime, similar to multiply revised lower extremity arthroplasties [33].

When examining a previous arthroplasty, the soft tissues and images are thoroughly scrutinized for reactive changes suggestive of infection. The interview is aimed at a thorough understanding of any delayed healing or postoperative wound complications that could suggest indolent infection. If any lucency, erosion, or widening around the implant is noted on the images, especially if there is a history of wound complications or concerns with the soft tissue exam such as erythema or chronic swelling or there is unexplained pain in the setting of an implant which is localized to the DRUJ, then screening labs are obtained. We routinely obtain a complete blood count with differential, erythrocyte sedimentation rate, and C-reactive protein. If the serologic exam is abnormal, clinical exam or history is highly suggestive, or no other explanation for ongoing pain can be found, we perform open tissue biopsy. This is performed as an independent procedure such that chance for propagating low-grade infection to revision implants is minimized.

Treatment is dependent on function, level of pain, and patient-specific factors. Resection of implants with antibiotic spacer placement and a 6-week course of intravenous antibiotics is the

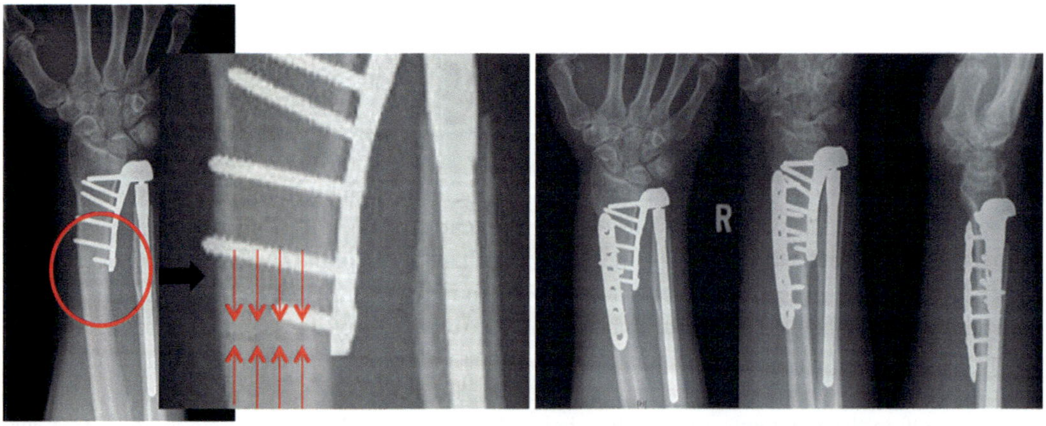


**Fig. 12.9** Radius stress fractures can occur with impact loading and can be treated with compression plating

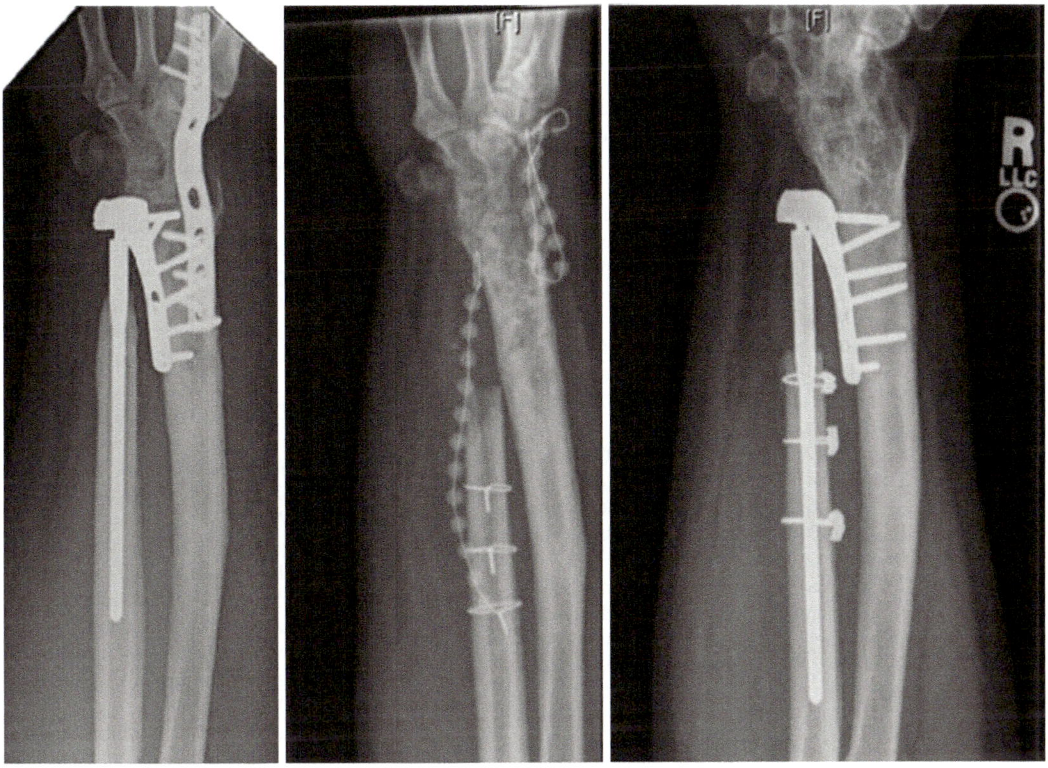

**Fig. 12.10** Case example of a DRUJ arthroplasty that became infected after a routine dental procedure. The patient was treated with implant resection and antibiotic spacer placement with a six-week course of intravenous antibiotics, followed by revision implantation

standard of care for an acute infection. Revision to new constrained implant can be considered once infection has been thoroughly treated (Fig. 12.10). Lifelong suppression with antibiotics can also be considered for those patients who cannot undergo a two-stage procedure related to underlying medical status, soft tissue, and/or bone stock concerns.

## Conclusion

DRUJ dysfunction alone is a challenging problem to address. Patients with previous DRUJ arthroplasty and persistent pain and dysfunction are a complex patient population with limited options for management. A thorough and holistic evaluation of all aspects of the patient and extremity are critical for successful treatment. We propose framing this evaluation in six interrelated zones to identify less obvious potentially contributing pathology. Treatment is then designed based on patient-specific factors such as level of demand and the quality of the tissues, with mindfulness to include all relevant pathology identified in careful consideration of each of the six zones. The outcomes for this group are difficult to articulate due to the extreme heterogeneity and rarity of these patient encounters, even at tertiary referral centers. However, careful evaluation and cognizance of patient goals with grounded and realistic management of expectations can yield high patient satisfaction despite the enormous challenge of tackling these complex clinical scenarios.

## References


1. Adams B, Berger R. An anatomic reconstruction of the distal radioulnar ligaments for posttraumatic distal radioulnar joint instability. J Hand Surg Am. 2002;27:243–51.
2. George MS, Kiefhaber TR, Stern PJ. The Sauve-Kapandji procedure and the Darrach procedure for distal radio-ulnar joint dysfunction after Colles' fracture. J Hand Surg Br. 2004;29(6):608–13. https://doi.org/10.1016/j.jhsb.2004.08.001.
3. Kakar S, Garcia-Elias M. The "four-leaf clover" treatment algorithm: a practical approach to manage disorders of the distal radioulnar joint. J Hand Surg [Am]. 2016;41(4):551–64. https://doi.org/10.1016/j.jhsa.2016.01.005.
4. Willis AA, Berger RA, Cooney WP 3rd. Arthroplasty of the distal radioulnar joint using a new ulnar head endoprosthesis: preliminary report. J Hand Surg [Am]. 2007;32(2):177–89. https://doi.org/10.1016/j.jhsa.2006.12.004.
5. Kaiser GL, Bodell LS, Berger RA. Functional outcomes after arthroplasty of the distal radioulnar joint and hand therapy: a case series. J Hand Ther. 2008;21(4):398–409. https://doi.org/10.1197/j.jht.2008.06.002.
6. Kakar S, Fox T, Wagner E, Berger R. Linked distal radioulnar joint arthroplasty: an analysis of the APTIS prosthesis. J Hand Surg Eur Vol. 2014;39(7):739–44. https://doi.org/10.1177/1753193414523189.
7. Bellevue KD, Thayer MK, Pouliot M, Huang JI, Hanel DP. Complications of semiconstrained distal radioulnar joint arthroplasty. J Hand Surg [Am]. 2018;43(6):566 e1–9. https://doi.org/10.1016/j.jhsa.2017.11.004.
8. Galvis EJ, Pessa J, Scheker LR. Total joint arthroplasty of the distal radioulnar joint for rheumatoid arthritis. J Hand Surg [Am]. 2014;39(9):1699–704. https://doi.org/10.1016/j.jhsa.2014.03.043.
9. Laurentin-Perez LA, Goodwin AN, Babb BA, Scheker LR. A study of functional outcomes following implantation of a total distal radioulnar joint prosthesis. J Hand Surg Eur Vol. 2008;33(1):18–28. https://doi.org/10.1177/1753193408087118.
10. Rampazzo A, Gharb BB, Brock G, Scheker LR. Functional outcomes of the Aptis-Scheker distal radioulnar joint replacement in patients under 40 years old. J Hand Surg [Am]. 2015;40(7):1397–403 e3. https://doi.org/10.1016/j.jhsa.2015.04.028.
11. Scheker LR. Implant arthroplasty for the distal radioulnar joint. J Hand Surg [Am]. 2008;33(9):1639–44. https://doi.org/10.1016/j.jhsa.2008.08.014.
12. Scheker LR, Martineau DW. Distal radioulnar joint constrained arthroplasty. Hand Clin. 2013;29(1):113–21. https://doi.org/10.1016/j.hcl.2012.08.023.
13. Lees VC, Scheker LR. The radiological demonstration of dynamic ulnar impingement. J Hand Surg Br. 1997;22B(4):448–50.
14. Bell MJ, Hill RJ, McMurtry RY. Ulnar impingement syndrome. J Bone Joint Surg Br. 1985;67(1):126–9.
15. Ruland RT, Hogan CJ. The ECU synergy test: an aid to diagnose ECU tendonitis. J Hand Surg [Am]. 2008;33(10):1777–82. https://doi.org/10.1016/j.jhsa.2008.08.018.
16. Levis CM, Yang Z, Gilula LA. Validation of the extensor carpi ulnaris groove as a predictor for the recognition of standard posteroanterior radiographs of the wrist. J Hand Surg [Am]. 2002;27(2):252–7. https://doi.org/10.1053/jhsu.2002.31150.
17. Yang Z, Mann FA, Gilula LA, Haerr C, Larsen CF. Scaphopisocapitate alignment: criterion to establish a neutral lateral view of the wrist. Radiology. 1997;205(3):865–9.
18. Wolfe SW, Mih AD, Hotchkiss RN, Culp RW, Keifhaber TR, Nagle DJ. Wide excision of the distal ulna: a multicenter case study. J Hand Surg [Am]. 1998;23(2):222–8. https://doi.org/10.1016/s0363-5023(98)80117-2.
19. Garcia-Elias M. Failed ulnar head resection: prevention and treatment. J Hand Surg Br. 2002;27(5):470–80. https://doi.org/10.1054/jhsb.2002.0815.
20. Greenberg JA, Sotereanos D. Achilles allograft interposition for failed Darrach distal ulna resections. Tech Hand Up Extrem Surg. 2008;12(2):121–5. https://doi.org/10.1097/BTH.0b013e3181640346.
21. Bain GI, Pugh DM, MacDermid JC, Roth JH. Matched hemiresection interposition arthroplasty of the distal radioulnar joint. J Hand Surg Am. 1995;20:944–50.
22. Nawijn F, Verhiel S, Jupiter JB, Chen NC. Hemiresection interposition arthroplasty of the distal radioulnar joint: a long-term outcome study. Hand (N Y). 2019:1558944719873430. https://doi.org/10.1177/1558944719873430.
23. Papatheodorou LK, Rubright JH, Kokkalis ZT, Sotereanos DG. Resection interposition arthroplasty for failed distal ulna resections. J Wrist Surg. 2013;2(1):13–8. https://doi.org/10.1055/s-0032-1333062.
24. Sotereanos DG, Papatheodorou LK, Williams BG. Tendon allograft interposition for failed distal ulnar resection: 2- to 14-year follow-up. J Hand Surg [Am]. 2014;39(3):443–8 e1. https://doi.org/10.1016/j.jhsa.2013.11.004.
25. Devendra A, Velmurugesan PS, Dheenadhayalan J, Venkatramani H, Sabapathy SR, Rajasekaran S. One-bone forearm reconstruction: a salvage solution for the forearm with massive bone loss. J Bone Joint Surg Am. 2019;101(15):e74. https://doi.org/10.2106/JBJS.18.01235.
26. DeGeorge BR Jr, Berger RA, Shin AY. Constrained implant arthroplasty for distal radioulnar joint arthrosis: evaluation and management of soft tissue complications. J Hand Surg [Am]. 2019;44(7):614 e1–9. https://doi.org/10.1016/j.jhsa.2018.09.003.
27. Lans J, Chen SH, Jupiter JB, Scheker LR. Distal radioulnar joint replacement in the scarred wrist.

J Wrist Surg. 2019;8(1):55–60. https://doi.org/10.1055/s-0038-1670681.
28. Reissner L, Bottger K, Klein HJ, Calcagni M, Giesen T. Midterm results of semiconstrained distal radioulnar joint arthroplasty and analysis of complications. J Wrist Surg. 2016;5(4):290–6. https://doi.org/10.1055/s-0036-1583303.
29. Dellon AL, Mackinnon SE. Treatment of the painful neuroma by neuroma resection and muscle implantation. Plast Reconstr Surg. 1986;77(3):427–38. https://doi.org/10.1097/00006534-198603000-00016.
30. Grawe B, Heincelman C, Stern P. Functional results of the Darrach procedure: a long-term outcome study. J Hand Surg [Am]. 2012;37(12):2475–80. e1–2. https://doi.org/10.1016/j.jhsa.2012.08.044.
31. Kleinman WB, Greenberg JA. Salvage of the failed Darrach procedure. J Hand Surg Am. 1995;20:951–8.
32. Leslie BM, Carlson G, Ruby LK. Results of extensor carpi ulnaris tenodesis in the rheumatoid wrist undergoing a distal ulnar excision. J Hand Surg [Am]. 1990;15(4):547–51. https://doi.org/10.1016/s0363-5023(09)90013-2.
33. Matar WY, Jafari SM, Restrepo C, Austin M, Purtill JJ, Parvizi J. Preventing infection in total joint arthroplasty. J Bone Joint Surg Am. 2010;92 Suppl 2:36–46. https://doi.org/10.2106/JBJS.J.01046.

# Part V

# Carpometacarpophalangeal Joint Arthroplasty

# Design Considerations for Carpometacarpophalangeal Joint Arthroplasty

13

Amy L. Ladd, Avi D. Goodman, and Arnold-Peter C. Weiss

## Introduction

The thumb is crucial for a patient's well-being, providing approximately 40% of hand function, and over 20% of body function [1]. In turn, this function depends on a thumb carpometacarpal (CMC) joint that is both stable and mobile, allowing for an impressive array of motion. The CMC is also tied intimately to the surrounding joints, including the trapeziotrapezioid, scaphotrapezial (ST), scaphotrapezial-trapezoid (STT), and trapezium-index metacarpal joints.

## Epidemiology

The thumb CMC joint is the second most common site of arthritis in the hand (following the distal interphalangeal joints), and more commonly affects women than men, up to seven times as frequently [2]. Like other forms of arthritis, it is strongly associated with aging; advancing age is the strongest risk factor [3]. At age 75, the prevalence of the radiographic thumb CMC arthritis in women is at least 40%, compared with approximately 25% in men [4]. The severity also increases with age, and the prevalence of severe arthritis approaches 70% in women older than 80 years of age [2]. The gender differences may be due, in part, to the influence of ligamentous laxity and hormones, and less so anatomy [5, 6].

When affected by osteoarthritis, a number of treatment options exist, including CMC arthroplasty. While this term encompasses a large variety of procedures, from simple trapeziectomy, ligament reconstruction and tendon interposition, to prosthetic replacement, the goals remain the same: pain relief, motion to perform everyday tasks, preventing deformity at adjacent joints, and immediate and long-term stability [7].

## Clinical Presentation

Symptoms typically include the insidious onset of progressive basilar thumb pain, worse with forceful pinch grasp. Physical exam demonstrates a positive CMC grind test, reproducing pain with passive joint motion under axial load; this test is quite specific (97%) but not very sensitive (30%). The traction-shift test, in which subluxation and relocation reproduces and then

A. L. Ladd (✉)
Chase Hand and Upper Limb Center, Department of Orthopaedic Surgery, Palo Alto, CA, USA
e-mail: alad@stanford.edu

A. D. Goodman · A.-P. C. Weiss
Department of Orthopaedics, Rhode Island Hospital/Brown University, Providence, RI, USA

Alpert Medical School of Brown University, Providence, RI, USA
e-mail: avi_goodman@brown.edu; apcweiss@brown.edu


G. J. W. King, M. Rizzo (eds.), *Arthroplasty of the Upper Extremity*,
https://doi.org/10.1007/978-3-030-68880-6_13

lessens pain, is more sensitive (67%) and specific (100%) [8]. Tenderness at the CMC joint is common. A compensatory hyperextension deformity of the metacarpal (Z-deformity) may be present, especially in longer-standing CMC arthritis with limited abduction [9].

## Eaton-Glickel Staging

In addition to the clinical symptoms, thumb CMC arthritis may be evaluated radiographically with the Eaton-Glickel classification system [10]. Stage I involves slight joint widening, while Stage II progresses to joint space narrowing and adds minimal subchondral sclerosis and joint debris <2 mm. Stage III demonstrates significant narrowing or obliteration of the joint space, along with joint debris >2 mm, sclerotic bone, cystic changes, and varying degrees of dorsal subluxation. Stage IV includes major subluxation, scaphotrapezial joint involvement, and significant sclerotic, cystic, and osteophytic formation. Although useful for discussion, the Eaton-Glickel classification has a poor correlation with symptoms and only poor-to-fair interrater reliability (Table 13.1) [11–13].

**Table 13.1** The Eaton and Littler radiographic staging system for basal thumb osteoarthritis

| Stage | Radiographic findings |
|---|---|
| I | Normal articular contours; slight widening of joint space (joint capsule distension)[a] |
| II | Slight narrowing of joint space; calcific/bony debris <2 mm in diameter; minimal sclerotic changes[a] |
| III | Marked joint space narrowing; sclerotic bone and cystic changes; varying degrees of subluxation; debris >2 mm in diameter; STT joint spared[a] |
| IV | Obliteration of TMCJ as in stage III with STT joint narrowing associated with sclerosis and cystic changes[a] |
| V | Pantrapezial arthritis[b] |

From: Berger et al. [12] (with permission)
*STT* scaphotrapezial trapezoid, *TMCJ* trapeziometacarpal joint
[a]From Wajon et al. [16]
[b]From Tomaino [83]

## Indications for Surgery

Initial treatment for basilar thumb arthritis is conservative, with activity modification, brace use, therapy, and oral (or topical) nonsteroidal anti-inflammatories [14–17]. If pain continues, injections of corticosteroids (or hyaluronic acid, although only preliminary data exist) may be considered [14, 18–22]. Pain and loss of function that is refractory to these conservative measures is the relative indication for surgery. Other considerations for the choice of surgical management include MCP joint instability and STT joint involvement.

## History of CMC Arthroplasty

In 1949, Gervis et al. recommended simply removing the trapezium as treatment for painful basilar thumb arthritis [23]. One particular concern with simple trapeziectomy is the risk of metacarpal subsidence, with a potential loss of strength and first ray length. Although many techniques have subsequently been described and have increased in popularity, no one specific method had shown to have a convincing clinical benefit to justify extra surgical time, morbidity, and expense. The simple trapeziectomy is certainly not perfect, with a loss of strength, but does reliably restore motion and decrease pain [24]. A number of recent systematic reviews and meta-analyses, including a Cochrane Database review, showed no superior procedure with regard to pain, physical function, motion, or global assessment [16, 17, 25–27]. When considering new designs for CMC arthroplasty, simple trapeziectomy may be regarded as the standard.

To prevent subsidence, the metacarpal should be suspended or supported in some manner. Froimson suggested placing a ball of tendon (harvested from the forearm) into the space formerly occupied by the trapezium [28]. In 1973, Eaton described a ligamentous reconstruction, using a tendon (again harvested from the forearm) to reconstruct the ligaments between the first and second metacarpal bases to suspend the thumb metacarpal in two planes and reinforce the lax volar ligaments [29].

These two ideas were combined in 1986 by Burton and Pelligrini, with the ligamentous reconstruction and tendon interposition (LRTI) procedure, first performing a trapeziectomy, and then using a forearm tendon to reconstruct the ligament, and finally forming it into a space-occupying ball (Fig. 13.1) [30]. This has become the most commonly performed method of surgical management in the United States and has generally enjoyed a high rate of satisfaction, good pain relief, and minimal subsidence [14]. However, there remain concerns about the morbidity of tendon harvest, as well as operative time. This may also be achieved by a hematoma distraction arthroplasty, in which the thumb metacarpal is temporarily pinned to the second metacarpal for 4–6 weeks, and a hematoma is allowed to form and consolidate.

The thumb metacarpal may also be suspended through synthetic means. Suture suspensionplasty, in which the flexor carpi radialis (FCR) and abductor pollicis longus (APL) tendons are sutured together with nonabsorbable suture, has been recently described and popularized and may represent a cost-effective strategy to maintain ray length with minimal morbidity [31–33]. Suture-button suspensionplasty, using a suture-button implant (i.e., EndoButton, Arthrex, Naples, FL), has been another recent innovation. By providing a robust mechanism for suspending the thumb metacarpal to the second metacarpal, this may allow for earlier rehabilitation and loading of the joint with less subsidence (Fig. 13.2); however, there have also been early reports of metacarpal fractures through drill holes [34–37].

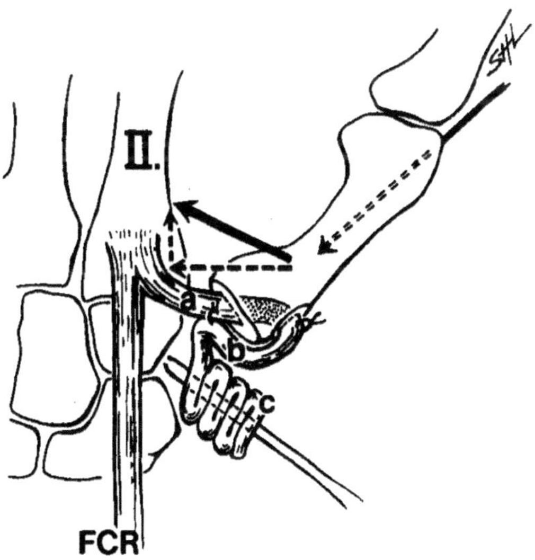


Fig. 13.1 Schematic representation of ligament reconstruction with tendon interposition arthroplasty. The forces in function producing proximal migration and radial subluxation of the metacarpal are neutralized by ligament reconstruction as indicated in the vector diagram. *Key: a,* ligament reconstruction, *b,* metacarpal resurfacing; *c,* tendon arthroplasty spacer. (From: Burton et al. [30] (with permission))

Management of basilar thumb arthritis does not necessarily demand a full trapeziectomy. For early-stage disease with normal articular surfaces and symptomatic volar ligament laxity, an isolated volar ligament reconstruction (using FCR or APL) may be appropriate. Arthroscopic debridement has shown to improve pain and satisfaction, albeit with no differences in objective measures; this technique is relatively new, and longer-term follow-up is needed for a full evaluation [38–40]. Metacarpal extension osteotomy, which may involve load transfer and diminished laxity by placing the thumb base in 30° of extension, may be useful for patients with mild to moderate disease [41, 42]. Arthrodesis of the CMC joint may be indicated for young patients with significant demands of their hands, such as laborers, and should not be used for patients with scaphotrapezial arthritis (as this transfers axial loading to the scaphotrapezial joint) [25, 38, 43, 44].

Lastly, a number of prosthetic implants have been designed, with varying degrees of success. These include interposition-type designs, hemiarthroplasty, and total joint arthroplasty. Please see section "Prosthetic Designs" for further detail. A recent systematic review and meta-analysis demonstrated a significantly higher incidence of failure for implant-based arthroplasties, when compared to non-implant procedures (simple trapeziectomy, LRTI, fusion) [45].

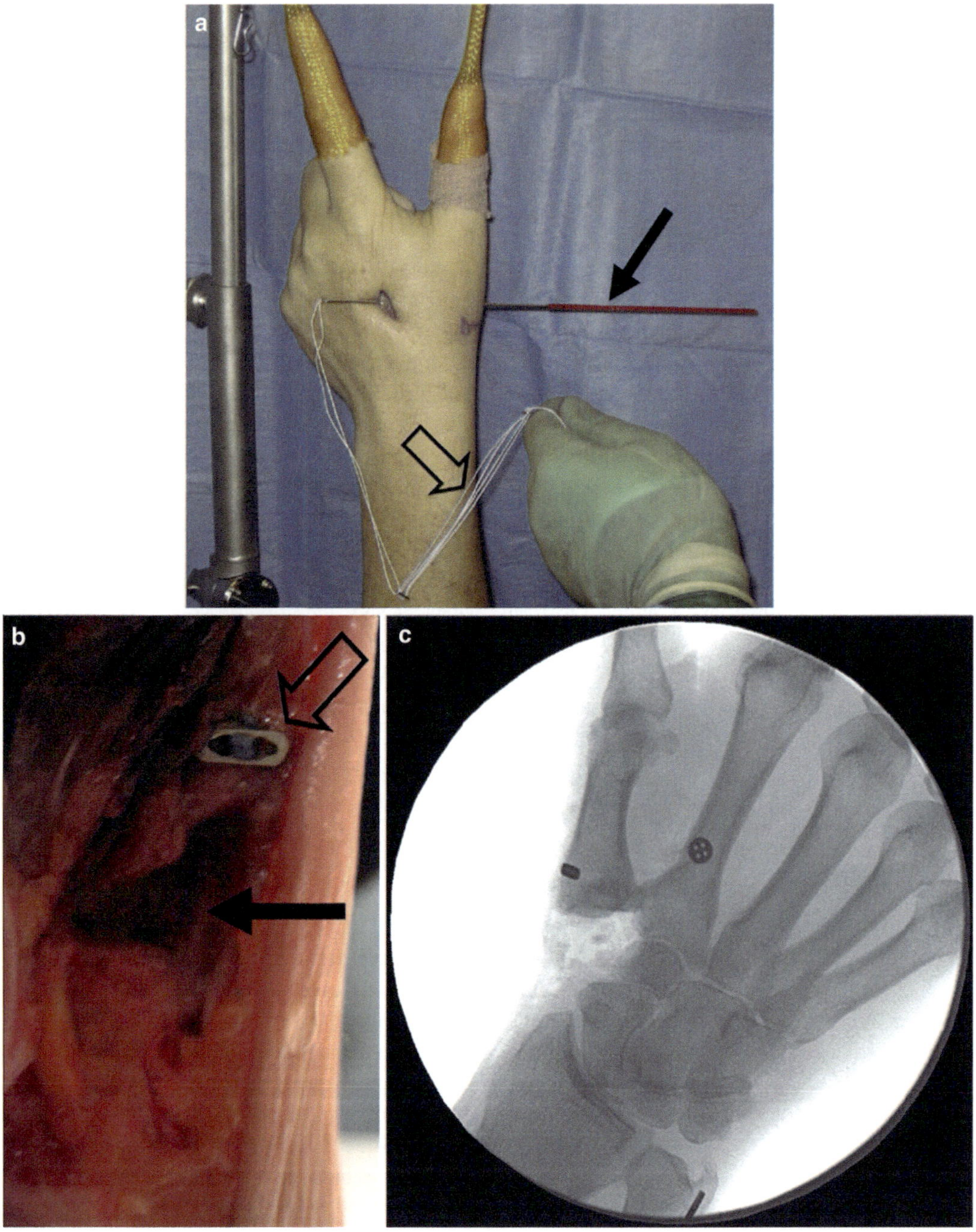


**Fig. 13.2** (**a**) Clinical photograph. Solid arrow indicates suture passer passing through the base of the first metacarpal and exiting through the dorsal accessory incision. Open arrow indicates the suture button device. (**b**) Cadaveric photograph. Solid arrow indicates the trapeziectomy site. Open arrow indicates the suture button device implanted at base of the thumb metacarpal. (**c**) Fluoroscopic image of the suture button device in situ. The two stainless steel buttons are secured on the ulnar aspect of the second metacarpal diaphysis and the radial base of the thumb metacarpal. The radiolucent sutures are not visible. (From: Yao et al. [35] (with permission))

## Anatomy

### Bony Anatomy

The bony anatomy of the thumb CMC joint is complex, and although it has been studied and admired for thousands of years, novel aspects continue to be discovered. Noted by scholars dating back to Aristotle, the thumb drives prehension, primarily through opposition [46]. This mechanism, which positions the thumb tip opposite the tips of other digits, comprises rotation and translation along multiple axes.

The CMC joint has a biconcave-convex (reciprocal interlocking saddle) shape, which provides little inherent static stability. The articular surfaces are also not size-matched; the diameter of the trapezial surface is approximately 34% smaller than the metacarpal base diameter [47, 48].

The architecture of the trapezium dictates that the axis of the thumb at the CMC joint rests in pronation and approximately 80 degrees of flexion (relative to the plan of the finger metacarpals) [49]. This position in space optimizes the ability of the thumb to perform opposition. The unique bony morphology of the thumb allows motion including flexion, extension, abduction, adduction, hitchhiker, circumduction, and opposition. Opposition includes a screw-home torque rotation in its final phase, which greatly enhances the stability [50]. These motions combine to create functional movements, such as power grip, power pinch, and precision pinch.

When considering the design of a CMC arthroplasty, this balance between a lack of inherent instability and wide range of motion much be carefully considered, balancing stability and mobility [9]. This may be particularly important with prosthetic implants, but also remain important concerns when designing a ligamentous reconstruction.

### Ligamentous Anatomy

The ligamentous anatomy is critical to the stability of the CMC joint. As few as 3 and as many as 16 ligaments have been described as primary stabilizers of the joint and are generally thicker dorsally and thinner volarly (Fig. 13.3) [46, 50, 51]. Although the volar anterior oblique ("volar beak") ligament was previously thought to be a primary stabilizer, more recent studies have demonstrated that this is primarily a capsular structure, with a mean thickness of 0.71 mm [52].

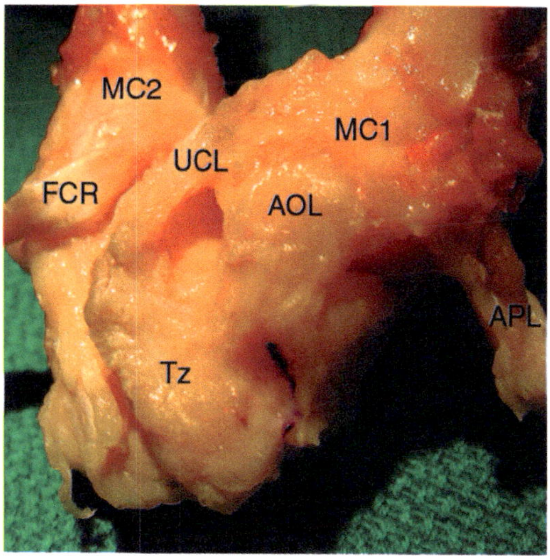


**Fig. 13.3** The volar thumb CMC ligaments from a right hand, showing the attenuated volar anterior oblique ligament (AOL) and ulnar collateral ligament (UCL), which course from the trapezial ridge (Tz) onto the volar base of metacarpal 1 (MC1). Also seen are the abductor pollicis longus (APL) and the flexor carpi radialis (FCR) tendons, as well as the base of metacarpal 2 (MC2). (Courtesy of Amy Ladd, MD, and Stanford University, Palo Alto, CA)

In contrast, the dorsal deltoid (dorsoradial) ligament is comprised of three thicker (mean 1.85 mm) ligaments, with an ultrastructure of grouped collagen bundles, consistent with a role of primary stabilizer of the CMC joint [52, 53]. Arising from the dorsoradial tubercle of the trapezium and inserting broadly onto the dorsal base of the metacarpal, this ligament primarily resists dorsal and dorsoradial forces and plays an important role in any reconstructive procedure (Fig. 13.4). The thumb ulnar collateral ligament is extracapsular and acts to prevent volar subluxation of the metacarpal base [47, 52].

The intermetacarpal ligament, running between the thumb and index metacarpal, helps to stabilize the CMC joint if both the dorsal and volar ligament complexes are incompetent. This

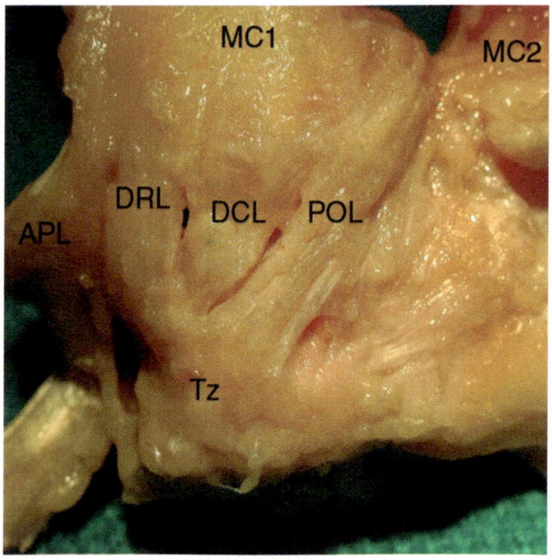


**Fig. 13.4** The dorsal thumb CMC ligaments from a right hand showing the dorsal deltoid ligament complex consisting of the dorsal radial ligament (DRL), dorsal central ligament (DCL), and posterior oblique ligament (POL), all emanating from the dorsal tubercle of the trapezium (Tz). Also seen are the dorsal bases of metacarpal 1 and 2 (MC1, MC2) and the abductor pollicis longus (APL). (Courtesy of Amy Ladd, MD, and Stanford University, Palo Alto, CA)

ligament is recapitulated in a ligament reconstruction or suspensionplasty procedure after a trapezium excision, usually a tenodesis between the FCR and APL tendons.

Ligament physiology may differ between the sexes (unlike the bony morphology) and can be affected by systemic pathology. Various studies have shown a correlation between joint hypermobility, as with Ehlers-Danlos syndrome, and CMC arthritis [54, 55]. Reproductive hormones such as relaxin may influence ligamentous laxity (and therefore predispose to ligament attenuation and then arthritis), although this has not been fully demonstrated in the CMC joint [56, 57].

## Biomechanics

With the length of the thumb as a lever arm, thumb CMC joint experiences a considerable amount of force. Compared with the pinch force at the thumb tip, the CMC joint undergoes a force that is up to 13.4× greater, while the shear stresses are 2.5× the applied force [50]. Normal grasping activities can have an applied force of 20 kg, while power grasp may generate a deforming force of 120 kg.

The unique morphology of the CMC joint dictates that the mechanical load transmission are complex, are dynamic through the range of motion, and may change with abnormalities of structure (i.e., arthritis) or physiology (i.e., hyperlaxity). Cantilever bending produces forces that are directed dorsally and radially at the base of the metacarpal, which results in shear forces. An increased load is borne by the volar surface, which correlate to the radiographic, surgical, and cadaveric findings of the "cirque" pattern of preferential volar wear [9, 46, 58–64].

## Kinematics

The thumb CMC joint facilitates a variety of motions important for day-to-day function. The arcs of motion include flexion-extension, abduction-adduction, and pronation-supination (Fig. 13.5). In healthy adults, key pinch involves volar translation of the metacarpal, as well as internal rotation, and flexion relative to the distal trapezial surface. For object grasp, the thumb metacarpal progresses through ulnar translation of the metacarpal, flexion, and abduction on the distal trapezial surface. For each of these tasks, it is important to appreciate a coupling of the flexion-extension and abduction-adduction arcs; extension of the thumb metacarpal is associated with adduction, while flexion is associated with abduction [9, 63, 65, 66].

During the "screw-home" mechanism in terminal opposition, the dorsal ligament complex tightens and the volar ligament complex becomes lax, compressing the volar beak of the thumb metacarpal into the recess area of the trapezium (the pivot point, Fig. 13.6) [50]. Anatomically, this compression changes the CMC joint from incongruous to congruous and, functionally, from unstable to stable. This screw-home mechanism is therefore the key to opposition and in turn permits such other motions as power pinch, lateral pinch, thumb-to-tip pinch, three-jaw chuck

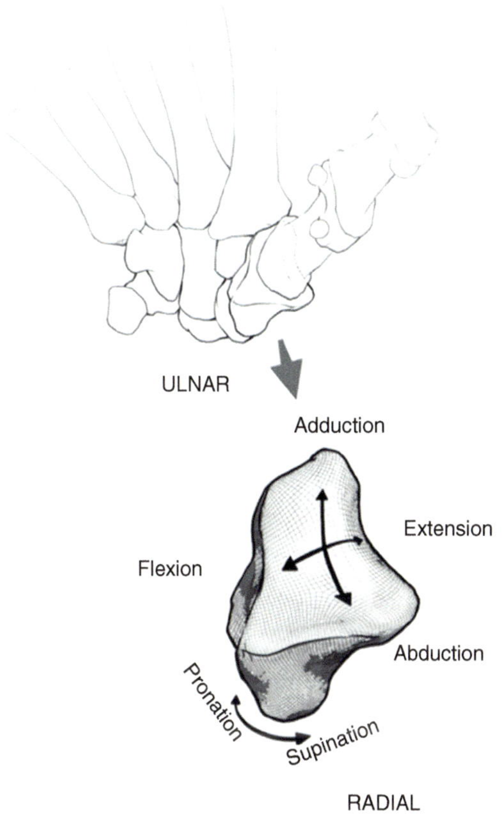


**Fig. 13.5** Arcs of motion about the trapezium. (Published with kind permission of S. Hegmann 2014. All Rights Reserved)

pinch, power grip, as well as precise touch. Even if the volar beak ligament is incompetent, the screw-home mechanism remains effective.

In considering the design for a proposed arthroplasty, there is an inherent tension between range of motion and stability, so the objectives must be carefully considered and matched to patients' needs.

## Pathomechanics of Disease

Pathology of the CMC joint is a function of both anatomy and pathophysiology. Ligamentous laxity of the basal joint leads to abnormal joint contact forces and which can result in articular damage; this becomes a self-reinforcing cycle.

Recent studies have demonstrated no differences between the architecture of CMC joints of men and women (when corrected for sex-related size differences), but have noted that when the CMC joint becomes plagued with osteoarthritis, its architecture changes in a number of possible disparate ways [5, 6, 68]. The "saddle" configuration preserves convexity in the volar-dorsal plane and concavity in the radioulnar plane, while the "dish" morphology demonstrates eburnation of the entire trapezial articular surface (with extensive rimming osteophytes) and is associated with a more severe Eaton stage [58, 59]. "Cirque" morphology, which demonstrates a concave volar slope and variably sized volar osteophytes at the metacarpal beak articulation, often shows minimal scaphoid or trapezoidal wear.

These may be distinct pathways, with the normal saddle shape progressing to either a "saddle" end-stage pattern, or progressively to a "dish" (concentric wear) or "cirque" (eccentric wear) pattern. Alternatively, the normal physiologic shape may degrade first to a "cirque" pattern and finally to a "dish" [59].

## Prosthetic Designs

Thumb CMC prostheses are conceptually categorized into a number of groups: total joint arthroplasty, hemiarthroplasty, and interposition arthroplasty [69]. Within each, there are a variety of shapes, materials, and fixation strategies, but all pursue the same overall goal: a thumb CMC joint that successfully balances mobility with stability. Many prosthetic implants have showed initial promise, but disappointing longer-term results (or unable to be replicated); many devices have been removed from the market.

## Total Joint Arthroplasty

With separate trapezial and metacarpal components, these implants have a good potential to replicate the native biomechanics of the CMC joint and possible improved strength compared with less anatomic configurations. These are

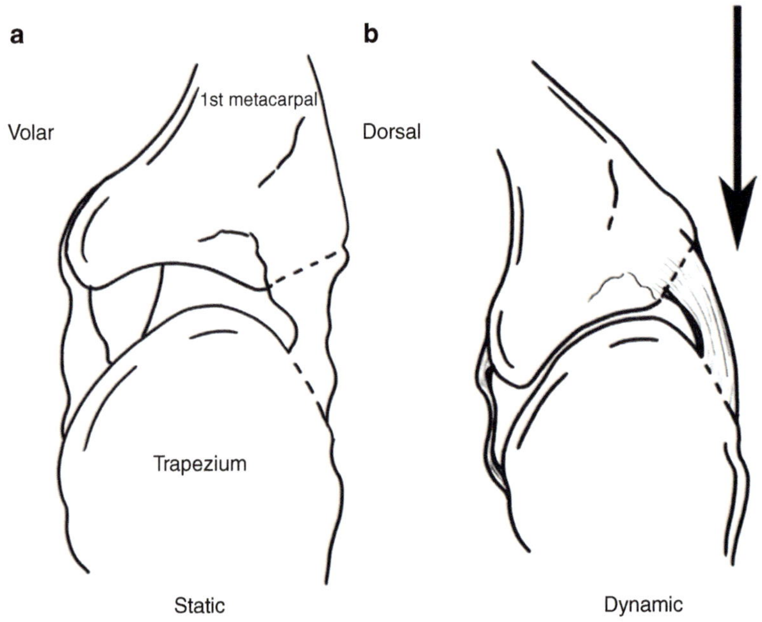


**Fig. 13.6** Dynamic force couple. (**a**) The trapeziometacarpal (TM) joint in the static resting position. The volar beak of the thumb metacarpal is disengaged from its recess in the trapezium, the TM joint space is large, and both the volar beak ligament and the dorsal ligament complex are lax. (**b**) The dynamic TM position of power pinch or power grip with screw-home torque rotation, in which the dorsal ligament complex tightens, the volar beak ligament becomes even more lax, the TM joint is compressed, and the volar beak of the thumb metacarpal is compressed into its recess in the trapezium. This forms a dynamic force couple that changes the TM joint from incongruity and laxity to congruity and rigid stability. (From: Edmunds [67] (with permission))

typically ball-and-socket designs, with the metacarpal stem articulating with the trapezial socket. Constrained (linked) implants are more stable, but have a higher risk of loosening, as there are considerably higher stresses placed on the bone-implant interface.

Notable total CMC joint implants include the de la Caffiniere prosthesis, a cemented ball-and-socket design that is likely the most commonly used (Fig. 13.7b). There has been considerably study of this prosthesis, and it has enjoyed better outcomes when performed for indications of pain and instability, rather than stiffness [26, 70, 71]. However, some series have found unacceptably high rates of loosening (approximately 40%), with both cemented and noncemented options [72]. Other total joint implants include the Elektra prosthesis, which has been fairly well-studied, although has very high failure rates from non-design surgeons [26, 73]. The Braun-Cutter prosthesis (SBI/Avanta Orthopaedics, San Diego, CA) is a cemented ball-and-socket design, although with limited results; this maybe reliable for use in elderly, low-demand patients [26]. The Avanta CMC prosthesis (Stryker, Mahwah, NJ) is a resurfacing articulation that aims to replicate the anatomy of the saddle joint, with cemented cobalt-chrome (CoCr) pegged trapezial and UHMWPE metacarpal components [26, 74]. There are many other similar designs, but none with results that demonstrate consistent safety, efficacy, and freedom from loosening/revision (Table 13.2); total joint arthroplasty has mostly fallen out of favor in the United States [26].

## Hemiarthroplasty

Hemiarthroplasty prosthesis designs are separated into anatomic and non-anatomic designs and are made in a variety of materials. The NuGrip (formerly PyroHemiSphere, Integra LifeSciences, Plainsboro Township, NJ) is a partial trapezial resurfacing design, with a stem in the metacarpal,

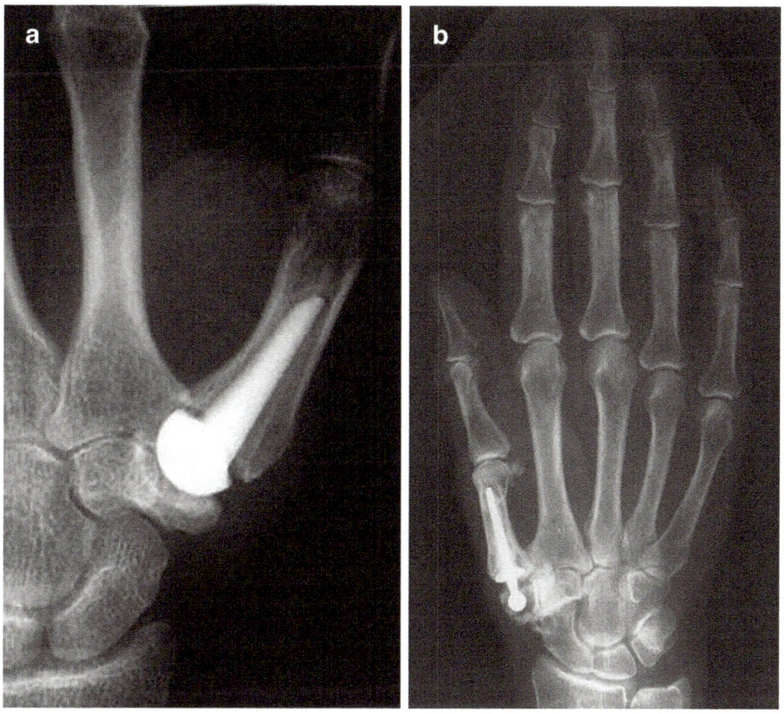


**Fig. 13.7** (**a**) A pyrolytic carbon hemiarthroplasty seen on posteroanterior radiograph at 17 months postoperatively. (From: Martinez de Aragon et al. [75] (with permission)). (**b**) Posteroanterior radiograph of de la Caffiniere prosthesis at 15 years postoperatively revealing loosening of both cup and stem with dislocation. Note the vertical position of the metal ring of the cup and dislocation of the components. Despite the radiographic appearance, this patient had excellent clinical and subjective scores. (From: van Capelle et al. [76] (with permission))

which articulates with the reamed surface of the trapezium (Fig. 13.7a) [26, 69]. These hemiarthroplasty configurations are inherently less constrained than total joint arthroplasties, which may improve the rate of trapezial component loosening with less stress and the bone-implant interface. However, the lesser constraint at the CMC articulation may require ligamentous stability, and several series have been plagued by metacarpal subluxation [69]. The Swanson titanium condylar hemiarthroplasty demonstrated excellent results by the design surgeon group, although these were not able to be reproduced (Vitale). Other examples include the PyroCarbon Saddle (Integra LifeSciences, Plainsboro Township, NJ) and CMI Carpometacarpal Implant (Wright/Tornier, Memphis, TN) (Table 13.2).

## Interposition Arthroplasty

Interposition arthroplasty designs seek to maintain trapezial height with a synthetic spacer, following either a partial or total trapezial resection. Unconstrained designs following partial resection include Pyrocardan (Wright/Tornier, Memphis, TN), a biconcave pyrocarbon spacer inserted into the CMC joint after minimal resection. Constrained designs following partial trapezial resection include Artelon (SMI, Morristown, NJ), a T-shaped biodegradable spacer intended to work as both an interposition spacer and an augment to the dorsal capsule, to prevent dorsoradial subluxation of the metacarpal (Fig. 13.8). Despite the theoretical benefits of this design, longer-term results have shown that patients treated with an Artelon were less satisfied and had lower grip strength than those treated with LRTI [69, 77]. Other interposition prostheses include the PyroDisk (Integra LifeSciences, Plainsboro Township, NJ), a biconcave disk with a central hole to permit stabilization; follow-up remains short, and the results have not been shown to be convincingly better than the alternatives (LRTI, etc.; Table 13.2) [69].

Interpositional arthroplasty designs may also be total trapezial replacements, made of varied material such as silicone (Swanson, Wright/Tornier, Memphis, TN), metallic (TrapEZX, Extremity Medical, Parsippany, NJ), and pyrocar-

**Table 13.2** Review of thumb CMC implants and outcomes

| Prosthesis | No. of implants | Mean follow-up (mo) | Implant survival at last follow-up (%) | Complications | Study |
|---|---|---|---|---|---|
| Elektra | 39 | 48 | 56 | Loosening | Klahn et al. 2013 [84] |
| ARPE | 65 | 60 | 94 | 5 Nonfunctional; radiologic cup subsidence in 16% | Martin-Ferrero 2014 [85] |
| Artelon | 32 | | 63 | 37% Explantation | Blount et al. 2013 [86] |
| BioPro | 143 | 72 | 94 | 6 Revisions | Pritchett et al. 2012 [87] |
| Ivory prosthesis | 22 | 67 | 95 | 1 Revision because of polythene wear and instability | Goubau et al. 2013 [88] |
| Arex615R | 68 | 36 | 87 | 8 Implants removed due to foreign body reaction | Semere et al. 2013 [89] |
| MA1A | 74 | 6 | 100 | 6 De Quervain, 1 aseptic loosening | Jager et al. 2013 [90] |
| Moje arthroplasty | 12 | 50 | 58 | All patients had loosening | Kaszap et al. 2012 [91] |
| Pi2 | 18 | 20 | 94 | 6 Implants revised | Maru et al. 2012 [79] |
| Pyrocarbon spacer | 70 | 24 | 91 | 6 Dislocations | Szalay et al. 2013 [92] |
| PyroDisk | 19 | 68 | 90 | 2 Patients had symptomatic instability | Barrera-Ochoa et al. 2014 [93] |
| Suture-button suspensionplasty | 21 | 34 | 100 | CRPS and index metacarpal fracture in same patient | Yao and Song 2013 [94] |

*CRPS* complex regional pain syndrome
From: Baker et al. [74] (with permission)

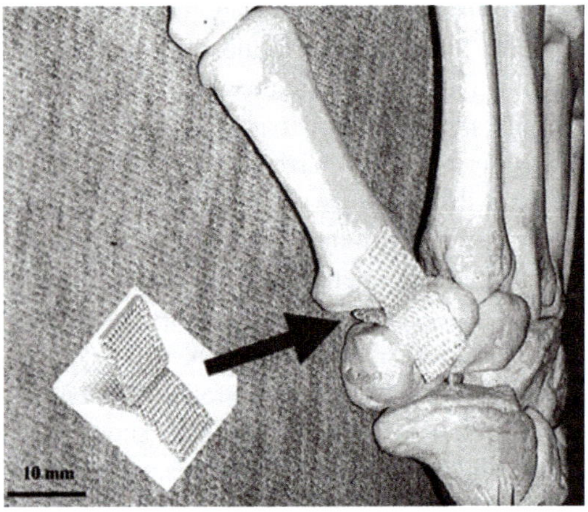


**Fig. 13.8** Artelon spacer in the trapeziometacarpal joint in a model. (From: Nilsson et al. [78] (with permission))

bon (Pi2, Wright/Tornier, Memphis, TN). These may not be traditionally stabilized (although some have include suture attachment points), but act as a mobile spacer. The various designs have had a number of serious issues, including silicone synovitis (Swanson) and secondary instability, and have generally had poorer results when compared with non-implant reconstructive procedures (Table 13.2) [69, 72].

## Prosthetic Materials and Fixation

### Materials

Thumb CMC implants are made from a variety of materials, including cobalt-chrome (CoCr), titanium, pyrocarbon, silicone, and synthetic hydrocarbons, each with a particular set of advantages and disadvantages. An ideal implant material should have excellent biocompatibility, integration with the host bone, wear characteristics (including boundary lubrication and surface degradation), and similar mechanical properties to the cortical bone. Although metallic designs (especially CoCr) are extremely strong and make for robust implants, they are many times stiffer and stronger than cortical bone, and this modulus mismatch may contribute to local stress concentration, implant loosening, and subsidence. Pyrolytic carbon, a synthetic material formed by the pyrolysis of hydrogen gas, has a stiffness similar to cortical bone and may better recapitulate the native biomechanical properties of the thumb CMC joint [72, 79]. Additionally, pyrocarbon has excellent boundary lubrication characteristics, derived from the surface adherence of phospholipids. Although the use of pyrocarbon implants have been supported by good evidence elsewhere in the hand, this has not yet been borne out for thumb CMC use [80–82].

Silicone was the original arthroplasty material used by Swanson, but its use has been curtailed sharply by the development of silicone synovitis, radiographic osteolysis, and frequent need for revision surgery [69]. Hydrocarbon materials, such as ultrahigh molecular weight polyethylene (UHMWPE), Gore-Tex (polytetrafluoroethylene [PTFE], Gore, Flagstaff, AZ), and Artelon (polycaprolactone-based polyurethanurea) have been designed with controllable degradation and mechanical properties. UHMWPE finds particular use in bearing surfaces (especially coupled with metal), while Gore-Tex and Artelon have found more limited applications as spacers, limited by significant synovitis, foreign body reactions, and osteolysis [16, 25, 69].

## Fixation

Prostheses may be cemented, may be cementless, or may have no bony fixation. Cemented designs allow for immediate range of motion and weight bearing, while cementless designs may allow for less bony resection, strong bone-implant interface (with either ingrowth or ongrowth surfaces, hydroxyapatite coating, and/or screw fixation), and a shorter operative time. The interpositional designs may either be free-floating (i.e., Swanson), or constrained (i.e., Artelon), which has the theoretical advantage of enhanced stability and decreased prosthetic instability [25, 69]. Any of the designs may be combined with soft tissue procedures to enhance ligamentous stability and may use other implants such as suture anchors, suture buttons, or staples.

## Conclusion

Thumb CMC arthroplasty aims to recreate the balance of the stability and mobility found in the native joint, which provides improved function and pain control. The current gold standard for surgical management is trapeziectomy, with or without LRTI or suspensionplasty, which provides reliable pain relief and return of strength. Any new arthroplasty technique must improve upon these proven methods in order to justify the increased risk and cost. Many prosthetic implants have been designed, but none have been able to successfully improve upon (or even replicate) the results of the classic procedures. However, there is a paucity of randomized controlled trials to compare outcomes between the different interventions, or even high-quality prospective studies examining different techniques.

## References

1. Moran SL, Berger RA. Biomechanics and hand trauma: what you need. Hand Clin. 2003;19(1):17–31. https://doi.org/10.1016/S0749-0712(02)00130-0.
2. Sodha S, Ring D, Zurakowski D, Jupiter JB. Prevalence of osteoarthrosis of the trapeziometacarpal joint. J Bone Joint Surg Am. 2005;87(12 I):2614–8. https://doi.org/10.2106/JBJS.E.00104.
3. Kalichman L, Hernández-Molina G. Hand osteoarthritis: an epidemiological perspective. Semin Arthritis Rheum. 2010;39(6):465–76. https://doi.org/10.1016/j.semarthrit.2009.03.001.
4. Haara MM, Heliövaara M, Kröger H, et al. Osteoarthritis in the carpometacarpal joint of the thumb. Prevalence and associations with disability and mortality. J Bone Joint Surg Am. 2004;86(7):1452–7. https://doi.org/10.2106/00004623-200407000-00013.
5. Schneider MTY, Zhang J, Crisco JJ, et al. Men and women have similarly shaped carpometacarpal joint bones. J Biomech. 2015;48(12):3420–6. https://

www.sciencedirect.com/science/article/abs/pii/S0021929015003206. Accessed 5 Mar 2017.
6. Halilaj E, Moore DC, Laidlaw DH, et al. The morphology of the thumb carpometacarpal joint does not differ between men and women, but changes with aging and early osteoarthritis. J Biomech. 2014;47(11):2709–14. https://doi.org/10.1016/j.jbiomech.2014.05.005.
7. Weiss A-PC, Goodman AD. Thumb basal joint arthritis. J Am Acad Orthop Surg. 2018;26(16):562–71. https://doi.org/10.5435/JAAOS-D-17-00374.
8. Choa RM, Parvizi N, Giele HP. A prospective case-control study to compare the sensitivity and specificity of the grind and traction-shift (subluxation-relocation) clinical tests in osteoarthritis of the thumb carpometacarpal joint. J Hand Surg Eur Vol. 2014;39(3):282–5. https://doi.org/10.1177/1753193413508714.
9. Ladd AL, Crisco JJ, Hagert E, Rose J, Weiss A-PC. The 2014 ABJS Nicolas Andry award: the puzzle of the thumb: mobility, stability, and demands in opposition. Clin Orthop Relat Res. 2014;472(12):3605–22. https://doi.org/10.1007/s11999-014-3901-6.
10. Eaton RG, Glickel SZ. Trapeziometacarpal osteoarthritis. Staging as a rationale for treatment. Hand Clin. 1987;3(4):455–71. http://www.ncbi.nlm.nih.gov/pubmed/3693416. Accessed 2 Mar 2017.
11. Ladd AL, Messana JM, Berger AJ, Weiss A-PC. Correlation of clinical disease severity to radiographic thumb osteoarthritis index. J Hand Surg Am. 2015;40(3):474–82. https://doi.org/10.1016/j.jhsa.2014.11.021.
12. Berger AJ, Momeni A, Ladd AL. Intra- and interobserver reliability of the Eaton classification for trapeziometacarpal arthritis: a systematic review. Clin Orthop Relat Res. 2014;472(4):1155–9. https://doi.org/10.1007/s11999-013-3208-z.
13. Hoffler CE, Matzon JL, Lutsky KF, Kim N, Beredjiklian PK. Radiographic stage does not correlate with symptom severity in thumb basilar joint osteoarthritis. J Am Acad Orthop Surg. 2015;23(12):778–82. https://doi.org/10.5435/JAAOS-D-15-00329.
14. Wolf JM, Delaronde S. Current trends in nonoperative and operative treatment of trapeziometacarpal osteoarthritis: a survey of US hand surgeons. J Hand Surg Am. 2012;37(1):77–82. https://doi.org/10.1016/j.jhsa.2011.10.010.
15. Bertozzi L, Valdes K, Vanti C, Negrini S, Pillastrini P, Villafañe JH. Investigation of the effect of conservative interventions in thumb carpometacarpal osteoarthritis: systematic review and meta-analysis. Disabil Rehabil. 2015;37(22):2025–43. https://doi.org/10.3109/09638288.2014.996299.
16. Wajon A, Vinycomb T, Carr E, Edmunds I, Ada L. Surgery for thumb (trapeziometacarpal joint) osteoarthritis. In: Wajon A, editor. Cochrane database of systematic reviews. Chichester, UK: John Wiley & Sons, Ltd; 2015. p. CD004631. https://doi.org/10.1002/14651858.CD004631.pub4.
17. Spaans AJ, van Minnen LP, Kon M, Schuurman AH, Schreuders AR (Ton), Vermeulen GM. Conservative treatment of thumb base osteoarthritis: a systematic review. J Hand Surg Am. 2015;40(1):16–21.e6. https://doi.org/10.1016/j.jhsa.2014.08.047.
18. Day CS, Gelberman R, Patel AA, Vogt MT, Ditsios K, Boyer MI. Basal joint osteoarthritis of the thumb: a prospective trial of steroid injection and splinting. J Hand Surg Am. 2004;29(2):247–51. https://doi.org/10.1016/j.jhsa.2003.12.002.
19. Monfort J, Rotés-Sala D, Segalés N, et al. Comparative efficacy of intra-articular hyaluronic acid and corticoid injections in osteoarthritis of the first carpometacarpal joint: results of a 6-month single-masked randomized study. Joint Bone Spine. 2015;82(2):116–21. https://doi.org/10.1016/j.jbspin.2014.08.008.
20. Heyworth BE, Lee JH, Kim PD, Lipton CB, Strauch RJ, Rosenwasser MP. Hylan versus corticosteroid versus placebo for treatment of basal joint arthritis: a prospective, randomized, double-blinded clinical trial. J Hand Surg Am. 2008;33(1):40–8. https://doi.org/10.1016/j.jhsa.2007.10.009.
21. Meenagh GK, Patton J, Kynes C, Wright GD. A randomised controlled trial of intra-articular corticosteroid injection of the carpometacarpal joint of the thumb in osteoarthritis. Ann Rheum Dis. 2004;63(10):1260 LP–1263. http://ard.bmj.com/content/63/10/1260.abstract.
22. Fowler A, Swindells MG, Burke FD. Intra-articular corticosteroid injections to manage trapeziometacarpal osteoarthritis—a systematic review. Hand. 2015;10(4):583–92. https://doi.org/10.1007/s11552-015-9778-3.
23. Gervis WH. Excision of the trapezium for osteoarthritis of the trapezio-metacarpal joint. J Bone Joint Surg Br. 1949;31-B(4):537–9. https://doi.org/10.1302/0301-620X.31B4.537.
24. Gangopadhyay S, McKenna H, Burke FD, Davis TRC. Five- to 18-year follow-up for treatment of trapeziometacarpal osteoarthritis: a prospective comparison of excision, tendon interposition, and ligament reconstruction and tendon interposition. J Hand Surg Am. 2012;37(3):411–7. https://doi.org/10.1016/j.jhsa.2011.11.027.
25. Vermeulen GM, Slijper H, Feitz R, Hovius SER, Moojen TM, Selles RW. Surgical management of primary thumb carpometacarpal osteoarthritis: a systematic review. J Hand Surg Am. 2011;36(1):157–69. https://doi.org/10.1016/j.jhsa.2010.10.028.
26. Huang K, Hollevoet N, Giddins G. Thumb carpometacarpal joint total arthroplasty: a systematic review. J Hand Surg Eur Vol. 2015;40(4):338–50. https://doi.org/10.1177/1753193414563243.
27. Martou G, Veltri K, Thoma A. Surgical treatment of osteoarthritis of the carpometacarpal joint of the thumb: a systematic review. Plast Reconstr Surg. 2004;114(2):421–32. https://doi.org/10.1097/01.PRS.0000131989.86319.B1.
28. Froimson AI. Tendon arthroplasty of trapeziometacarpal joint. Clin Orthop Relat Res. 1974;102:276. https://doi.org/10.1097/00003086-197407000-00038.
29. Eaton RG, Littler JW. Ligament reconstruction for the painful thumb carpometacarpal joint. J Bone

Joint Surg Am Vol. 1973;55(8):1655–66. https://doi.org/10.2106/00004623-197355080-00010.
30. Burton RI, Pellegrini VD. Surgical management of basal joint arthritis of the thumb. Part II. Ligament reconstruction with tendon interposition arthroplast. J Hand Surg Am. 1986;11(3):324–32. https://doi.org/10.1016/S0363-5023(86)80137-X.
31. DelSignore JL, Accardi KZ. Suture suspension arthroplasty technique for basal joint arthritis reconstruction. Tech Hand Up Extrem Surg. 2009;13(4):166–72. https://doi.org/10.1097/BTH.0b013e3181b4c388.
32. Putnam MD, Rattay R, Wentorf F. Biomechanical test of three methods to treat thumb CMC arthritis. J Wrist Surg. 2014;3(2):107–13. https://doi.org/10.1055/s-0034-1372518.
33. Takagi T, Weiss A-PC. Suture suspension arthroplasty with trapeziectomy for thumb carpometacarpal arthritis using a wide-awake approach. Tech Hand Up Extrem Surg. 2019;1 https://doi.org/10.1097/bth.0000000000000265.
34. Desai MJ, Brogan DM, Richard MJ, Mithani SK, Leversedge FJ, Ruch DS. Biomechanical comparison of suture-button suspensionplasty and LRTI for basilar thumb arthritis. Hand. 2016;11(4):438–43. https://doi.org/10.1177/1558944716643119.
35. Yao J, Zlotolow DA, Murdock R, Christian M. Suture button compared with K-wire fixation for maintenance of posttrapeziectomy space height in a cadaver model of lateral pinch. J Hand Surg Am. 2010;35(12):2061–5. https://doi.org/10.1016/J.JHSA.2010.09.007.
36. Avant KR, Nydick JA, White BD, Vaccaro L, Hess AV, Stone JD. Basal joint osteoarthritis of the thumb: comparison of suture button versus abductor pollicis longus suspensionplasty. Hand. 2015;10(1):80–4. https://doi.org/10.1007/s11552-014-9653-7.
37. Song Y, Cox CA, Yao J. Suture button suspension following trapeziectomy in a cadaver model. Hand (N Y). 2013;8(2):195–200. https://doi.org/10.1007/s11552-012-9473-6.
38. Kapoutsis DV, Dardas A, Day CS. Carpometacarpal and scaphotrapeziotrapezoid arthritis: arthroscopy, arthroplasty, and arthrodesis. J Hand Surg Am. 2011;36(2):354–66. https://doi.org/10.1016/j.jhsa.2010.11.047.
39. Logli AL, Twu J, Bear BJ, Lindquist JR, Schoenfeldt TL, Korcek KJ. Arthroscopic partial trapeziectomy with soft tissue interposition for symptomatic trapeziometacarpal arthritis: 6-month and 5-year minimum follow-up. J Hand Surg Am. 2018;43(4):384.e1–7. https://doi.org/10.1016/j.jhsa.2017.10.016.
40. Adams JE, Steinmann SP, Culp RW. Bone-preserving arthroscopic options for treatment of thumb basilar joint arthritis. Hand Clin. 2011;27(3):355–9. https://doi.org/10.1016/j.hcl.2011.05.005.
41. Parker WL, Linscheid RL, Amadio PC. Long-term outcomes of first metacarpal extension osteotomy in the treatment of carpal-metacarpal osteoarthritis. J Hand Surg Am. 2008;33(10):1737–43. https://doi.org/10.1016/j.jhsa.2008.08.003.
42. Chou FH, Irrgang JJ, Goitz RJ. Long-term follow-up of first metacarpal extension osteotomy for early CMC arthritis. Hand. 2014;9(4):478–83. https://doi.org/10.1007/s11552-014-9632-z.
43. Hartigan BJ, Stern PJ, Kiefhaber TR. Thumb carpometacarpal osteoarthritis: arthrodesis compared with ligament reconstruction and tendon interposition. J Bone Joint Surg Am. 2001;83-A(10):1470–8. http://jbjs.org/content/83/10/1470.abstract. Accessed 10 Apr 2016.
44. Vermeulen GM, Brink SM, Slijper H, et al. Trapeziometacarpal arthrodesis or trapeziectomy with ligament reconstruction in primary trapeziometacarpal osteoarthritis. J Bone Joint Surg Am. 2014;96(9):726–33. https://doi.org/10.2106/JBJS.L.01344.
45. Ganhewa AD, Wu R, Chae MP, et al. Failure rates of base of thumb arthritis surgery: a systematic review. J Hand Surg Am. 2019; https://doi.org/10.1016/j.jhsa.2019.05.003.
46. Leversedge FJ. Anatomy and pathomechanics of the thumb. Hand Clin. 2008;24(3):219–29.
47. Bettinger PC, Linscheid RL, Berger RA, Cooney WP, An K-N. An anatomic study of the stabilizing ligaments of the trapezium and trapeziometacarpal joint. J Hand Surg Am. 1999;24(4):786–98.
48. Bettinger PC, Berger RA. Functional ligamentous anatomy of the trapezium and trapeziometacarpal joint (gross and arthroscopic). Hand Clin. 2001;17(2):151–68.
49. Kuczynski K. Carpometacarpal joint of the human thumb. Plast Reconstr Surg. 1975;56(2):229. https://doi.org/10.1097/00006534-197508000-00060.
50. Edmunds JO. Current concepts of the anatomy of the thumb trapeziometacarpal joint. J Hand Surg Am. 2011;36(1):170–82. https://doi.org/10.1016/j.jhsa.2010.10.029.
51. Lin JD, Karl JW, Strauch RJ. Trapeziometacarpal joint stability: the evolving importance of the dorsal ligaments. Clin Orthop Relat Res. 2014;472(4):1138–45. https://doi.org/10.1007/s11999-013-2879-9.
52. Ladd AL, Lee J, Hagert E. Macroscopic and microscopic analysis of the thumb carpometacarpal ligaments: a cadaveric study of ligament anatomy and histology. J Bone Joint Surg Am. 2012;94(16):1468–77. https://doi.org/10.2106/JBJS.K.00329.
53. Bettinger PC, Smutz WP, Linscheid RL, Cooney WP, An KN. Material properties of the and trapeziometacarpal ligaments. J Hand Surg Am. 2000;25(6):1085–95. https://doi.org/10.1053/jhsu.2000.18487.
54. Gamble JG, Mochizuki C, Rinsky LA. Trapeziometacarpal abnormalities in Ehlers-Danlos syndrome. J Hand Surg Am. 1989;14(1):89–94. https://doi.org/10.1016/0363-5023(89)90064-6.
55. Jónsson H, Valtýsdóttir ST, Kjartansson Ó, Brekkan Á. Hypermobility associated with osteoarthritis of the thumb base: a clinical and radiological subset of hand osteoarthritis. Ann Rheum Dis. 1996;55(8):540–3. https://doi.org/10.1136/ard.55.8.540.
56. Wolf JM, Scher DL, Etchill EW, et al. Relationship of relaxin hormone and thumb carpometacarpal joint

arthritis. Clin Orthop Relat Res. 2014;472(4):1130–7. https://doi.org/10.1007/s11999-013-2960-4.
57. Clifton KB, Rodner C, Wolf JM. Detection of relaxin receptor in the dorsoradial ligament, synovium, and articular cartilage of the trapeziometacarpal joint. J Orthop Res. 2014;32(8):1061–7. https://doi.org/10.1002/jor.22640.
58. Lee AT, Williams AA, Lee J, Cheng R, Lindsey DP, Ladd AL. Trapezium trabecular morphology in carpometacarpal arthritis. J Hand Surg Am. 2013;38(2):309–15. https://doi.org/10.1016/j.jhsa.2012.10.038.
59. Ladd AL, Weiss A-PC, Crisco JJ, et al. The thumb carpometacarpal joint: anatomy, hormones, and biomechanics. Instr Course Lect. 2013;62:165–79. http://www.ncbi.nlm.nih.gov/pubmed/23395023. Accessed 8 Jan 2017.
60. Pellegrini VD, Olcott CW, Hollenberg G. Contact patterns in the trapeziometacarpal joint: the role of the palmar beak ligament. J Hand Surg Am. 1993;18(2):238–44. https://doi.org/10.1016/0363-5023(93)90354-6.
61. Ateshian GA, Ark JW, Rosenwasser MP, Pawluk RJ, Soslowsky LJ, Mow VC. Contact areas in the thumb carpometacarpal joint. J Orthop Res. 1995;13(3):450–8. https://doi.org/10.1002/jor.1100130320.
62. Koff MF, Ugwonali OF, Strauch RJ, Rosenwasser MP, Ateshian GA, Mow VC. Sequential wear patterns of the articular cartilage of the thumb carpometacarpal joint in osteoarthritis. J Hand Surg Am. 2003;28(4):597–604. https://doi.org/10.1016/S0363-5023(03)00145-X.
63. Cooney WP, Chao EYS. Biomechanical analysis of static forces in the thumb during hand function. J Bone Joint Surg - Am Vol. 1977;59(1):27–36. https://doi.org/10.2106/00004623-197759010-00004.
64. Cooney WP, Lucca MJ, Chao EY, Linscheid RL. The kinesiology of the thumb trapeziometacarpal joint. J Bone Joint Surg - Am Vol. 1981;63:1371–81. www.jbjs.org. Accessed 29 Oct 2019.
65. Coughlan MJ, Bourdillon A, Crisco JJ, Kenney D, Weiss A-P, Ladd AL. Reduction in cylindrical grasp strength is associated with early thumb carpometacarpal osteoarthritis. Clin Orthop Relat Res. 2017;475(2):522–8. https://doi.org/10.1007/s11999-016-5151-2.
66. Luria S, Waitayawinyu T, Nemechek N, Huber P, Tencer AF, Trumble TE. Biomechanic analysis of trapeziectomy, ligament reconstruction with tendon interposition, and tie-in trapezium implant arthroplasty for thumb carpometacarpal arthritis: a cadaver study. J Hand Surg Am. 2007;32(5):697–706. https://doi.org/10.1016/J.JHSA.2007.02.025.
67. Edmunds JO. Traumatic dislocations and instability of the trapeziometacarpal joint of the thumb. Hand Clin. 2006;22(3):365–92. https://doi.org/10.1016/j.hcl.2006.05.001.
68. Shih JG, Mainprize JG, Binhammer PA. Comparison of computed tomography articular surface geometry of male versus female thumb carpometacarpal joints. Hand. 2017:155894471668852. https://doi.org/10.1177/1558944716688528.
69. Vitale MA, Taylor F, Ross M, Moran SL. Trapezium prosthetic arthroplasty (silicone, Artelon, metal, and pyrocarbon). Hand Clin. 2013;29(1):37–55. https://doi.org/10.1016/j.hcl.2012.08.020.
70. Johnston P, Getgood A, Larson D, Chojnowski AJ, Chakrabarti AJ, Chapman PG. De la Caffinière thumb trapeziometacarpal joint arthroplasty: 16-26 year follow-up. J Hand Surg Eur Vol. 2012;37(7):621–4. https://doi.org/10.1177/1753193411433226.
71. Chakrabarti AJ, Robinson AHN, Gallagher P. De la Caffinière thumb carpometacarpal replacements: 93 cases at 6 to 16 years follow-up. J Hand Surg Eur Vol. 1997;22(6):695–8. https://doi.org/10.1016/S0266-7681(97)80427-5.
72. Srnec JJ, Wagner ER, Rizzo M. Implant arthroplasty for proximal interphalangeal, metacarpophalangeal, and trapeziometacarpal joint degeneration. J Hand Surg Am. 2017;42(10):817–25. https://doi.org/10.1016/j.jhsa.2017.07.030.
73. Krukhaug Y, Lie SA, Havelin LI, Furnes O, Hove LM, Hallan G. The results of 479 thumb carpometacarpal joint replacements reported in the Norwegian Arthroplasty Register. J Hand Surg Eur Vol. 2014;39(8):819–25. https://doi.org/10.1177/1753193413513988.
74. Baker RHJ, Al-Shukri J, Davis TRC. Evidence-based medicine: thumb basal joint arthritis. Plast Reconstr Surg. 2017;139(1):256e–66e. https://doi.org/10.1097/PRS.0000000000002858.
75. de Aragon JSM, Moran SL, Rizzo M, Reggin KB, Beckenbaugh RD. Early outcomes of pyrolytic carbon hemiarthroplasty for the treatment of trapezial-metacarpal arthritis. J Hand Surg Am. 2009;34(2):205–12. https://doi.org/10.1016/j.jhsa.2008.10.018.
76. van Cappelle HGJ, Elzenga P, van Horn JR. Long-term results and loosening analysis of de la Caffinière replacements of the trapeziometacarpal joint. J Hand Surg Am. 1999;24(3):476–82. https://doi.org/10.1053/jhsu.1999.0476.
77. Jörheim M, Isaxon I, Flondell M, Kalén P, Atroshi I. Short-term outcomes of trapeziometacarpal Artelon implant compared with tendon suspension interposition arthroplasty for osteoarthritis: a matched cohort study. J Hand Surg Am. 2009;34(8):1381–7. https://doi.org/10.1016/j.jhsa.2009.04.016.
78. Nilsson A, Liljensten E, Bergström C, Sollerman C. Results from a degradable TMC joint Spacer (Artelon) compared with tendon arthroplasty. J Hand Surg Am. 2005;30(2):380–9. https://doi.org/10.1016/j.jhsa.2004.12.001.
79. Maru M, Jettoo P, Tourret L, Jones M, Irwin L. Thumb carpometacarpal osteoarthritis: trapeziectomy versus pyrocarbon interposition implant (Pi2) arthroplasty. J Hand Surg Eur Vol. 2012;37(7):617–20. https://doi.org/10.1177/1753193411433176.

80. Daecke W, Kaszap B, Martini AK, Hagena FW, Rieck B, Jung M. A prospective, randomized comparison of 3 types of proximal interphalangeal joint arthroplasty. J Hand Surg Am. 2012;37(9):1770–1779.e3. https://doi.org/10.1016/j.jhsa.2012.06.006.
81. Reissner L, Schindele S, Hensler S, Marks M, Herren DB. Ten year follow-up of pyrocarbon implants for proximal interphalangeal joint replacement. J Hand Surg Eur Vol. 2014;39(6):582–6. https://doi.org/10.1177/1753193413511922.
82. Adams J, Ryall C, Pandyan A, et al. Proximal interphalangeal joint replacement in patients with arthritis of the hand: a meta-analysis. J Bone Joint Surg Br. 2012;94(10):1305–12. https://doi.org/10.1302/0301-620X.94B10.29035.
83. Tomaino MM. Thumb basilar joint arthritis. In: Green DP, Hotchkiss RN, Pederson WC, Wolfe SW, editors. Green's operative hand surgery. 5th ed. New York: Churchill Livingstone; 2005. p. 461–85.
84. Klahn A, Nygaard M, Gvozdenovic R. Elektra-prothese: prospektive langzeitbeobachtung. Handchirurgie Scan. 2013;2(01):33–4.
85. Martin-Ferrero M. Ten-year long-term results of total joint arthroplasties with ARPE implant in the treatment of trapeziometacarpal osteoarthritis. J Hand Surg Eur. 2014;39:826–32.
86. Blount AL, Armstrong SD, Yuan F, Burgess SD. Porous polyurethaneurea (Artelon) joint spacer compared to trapezium resection and ligament reconstruction. J Hand Surg. 2013;38(9):1741–5.
87. Pritchett JW, Habryl LS. A promising thumb basal joint hemiarthroplasty for treatment of trapeziometacarpal osteoarthritis. Clin Orthop Relat Res. 2012;470:2756–63.
88. Goubau JF, Goorens CK, Van Hoonacker P, Berghs B, Kerckhove D, Scheerlinck T. Clinical and radiological outcomes of the Ivory arthroplasty for trapeziometacarpal joint osteoarthritis with a minimum of 5 years of follow-up: a prospective single-centre cohort study. J Hand Surg Eur Vol. 2013;38(8):866–74.
89. Semere A, Forli A, Corcella D, Mesquida V, Loret MG, Moutet F. Foreign body reaction in osteoarthritis of the trapeziometacarpal joint treated by trapezectomy and interposition of a L-polylactic acid "anchovy"(Arex® 615R). A series of eight cases. Chir Main. 2013;32(3):161–8.
90. Jager T, Barbary S, Dap F, Dautel G. Evaluation of postoperative pain and early functional results in the treatment of carpometacarpal joint arthritis. Comparative prospective study of trapeziectomy vs. MAIA (®) prosthesis in 74 female patients. Chir Main. 2013;32(2):55–62.
91. Kaszap B, Daecke W, Jung M. High frequency failure of the Moje thumb carpometacarpal joint arthroplasty. J Hand Surg Eur Vol. 2012;37(7):610–6.
92. Szalay G, Meyer C, Scheufens T, Schnettler R, Christ R, Schleicher I. Pyrocarbon spacer as a trapezium replacement for arthritis of the trapeziometacarpal joint; a follow-up study of 60 cases. Acta Orthop Belg. 2013;79(6):648–54.
93. Barrera-Ochoa S, Vidal-Tarrason N, Correa-Vázquez E, Reverte-Vinaixa MM, Font-Segura J, Mir-Bullo X. Pyrocarbon interposition (PyroDisk) implant for trapeziometacarpal osteoarthritis: minimum 5-year follow-up. J Hand Surg. 2014;39(11):2150–60.
94. Yao J, Song Y. Suture-button suspensionplasty for thumb carpometacarpal arthritis: a minimum 2-year follow-up. J Hand Surg. 2013;38(6):1161–5.

# 14 Primary Carpometacarpophalangeal Joint Arthroplasty

Anton Borgers, Matthias Vanhees, and Frederik Verstreken

## Introduction

Osteoarthritis of the thumb base is a common condition in the general population, affecting up to 75% of women over 70 years of age [1]. Postmenopausal women are particularly affected, with a radiographic prevalence of 33%. A quarter of patients also shows radiographic signs of scapho-trapezio-trapezoidal (STT) osteoarthritis [2]. Only one in three patients affected will actually complain of basal thumb pain [3]. The majority of people will not seek medical attention because they remain asymptomatic or learn to cope with some degree of disability.

**Supplementary Information** The online version of this chapter (https://doi.org/10.1007/978-3-030-68880-6_14) contains supplementary material, which is available to authorized users.

A. Borgers
Orthopedic Department, AZ Monica Hospital, Antwerp, Belgium

Orthopedic Department, AZ Turnhout Hospital, Turnhout, Belgium
e-mail: Anton.borgers@azturnhout.be

M. Vanhees · F. Verstreken (✉)
Orthopedic Department, AZ Monica Hospital, Antwerp, Belgium

Orthopedic Department, Antwerp University Hospital, Edegem, Belgium
e-mail: matthias.vanhees@azmonica.be; frederik.verstreken@azmonica.be

The first phase of management is conservative, including immobilization, anti-inflammatory drugs, physiotherapy, or intra-articular injections. The use of night splinting for 1 year has shown to result in a significant improvement in pain [4]. The current evidence on the use of injection therapy is equivocal. Corticosteroid injections demonstrated a more positive effect on medium-term pain scores compared to hyaluronic acid injections [4]. Multimodal treatment, combining an intra-articular corticosteroid injection and splinting, has a long-lasting effect on pain in up to 80% of patients with Eaton stage 1 osteoarthritis [5]. Khan showed that in cases with more advanced degeneration (Eaton stages 3–4), the effect duration of a single corticosteroid injection decreases [6]. Manual therapy, combined with therapeutic exercises, has shown short- to medium-term improvements on pain scores [7]. In general, nonoperative treatment has demonstrated to postpone or avoid surgery in 70% of cases [8].

When conservative treatments fail, surgery may be indicated. A wide range of procedures has been described for the surgical management of thumb base osteoarthritis. In selected cases, symptomatic early-stage osteoarthritis can be managed with joint-sparing surgery. Denervation of the CMC joint has been described as a measure to relieve pain with less morbidity and rehabilitation. This technique is rarely considered, but some authors have published favorable results in


G. J. W. King, M. Rizzo (eds.), *Arthroplasty of the Upper Extremity*, https://doi.org/10.1007/978-3-030-68880-6_14

small case series. Lifchez et al. demonstrated 75% pain improvement in 11 of 12 cases; Loréa reported excellent pain relief in 12 out of 14 patients [9, 10].

Minimally invasive arthroscopic techniques are gaining popularity in the treatment of small joint problems of the hand. In the CMC joint, arthroscopy is being used for articular debridement and synovectomy, capsular shrinkage, removal of loose bodies, and partial or complete resection of the trapezium [11]. A series of 18 patients undergoing arthroscopic partial trapeziectomy with capsular shrinkage and temporary pinning demonstrated functional improvements and a significant increase in tip and key pinch strength at 7-year follow-up [12]. No further surgery was needed in this small series of patients, despite advanced osteoarthritis in some cases. Arthroscopic treatment techniques are further advancing and might play a more important role in the treatment of CMC osteoarthritis in the future.

Metacarpal abduction-extension osteotomy, as described by Wilson, was developed to unload the palmar joint area of the CMC joint during pinch [13]. A 9.9-year follow-up of 13 patients after metacarpal osteotomy demonstrated ten patients (77%) being satisfied or very satisfied with a mean VAS pain score of 2 [14]. Ligamentous stabilization procedures (Eaton-Littler) are available to provide pain relief and functional improvement. Ligamentous stabilization surgery aims to reconstruct the attenuated volar beak ligament (palmar oblique ligament) that causes subluxation of the CMC joint in early OA. Goubau et al. modified the classic Wilson osteotomy by combining it with a trapezial opening wedge osteotomy and ligamentous stabilization [15]. While indications are limited, these procedures are mainly reserved for younger patients, as they do not compromise further procedures when needed.

Arthrodesis has primarily been proposed in younger patients and manual workers, where loading of the thumb is essential. It provides a final solution when fusion is obtained, but there is a relatively high risk of non-union (8–21%), and it requires a long period of immobilization [16]. Although it is a reliable procedure for power grip, the absence of a mobile CMC joint can hinder during dexterous tasks in daily living, and the procedure can cause secondary degenerative changes at the neighboring STT joint over time.

Gervis first described the trapeziectomy procedure in 1949 [17]. In order to improve outcome, many alterations and additions have been made to the original stand-alone excision of the trapezial bone. The most common ones are the interposition of tendon or synthetic spacers, often in combination with ligamentous stabilization (Burton-Pellegrini [18], Weilby [19], Delsignore [20]). Over recent years the use of suture-button suspension following trapeziectomy is gaining popularity, in order to minimize donor morbidity of tendon grafts and prevent shortening of the thumb ray [21].

Trapeziectomy with ligament reconstruction and tendon interposition (LRTI) is currently considered to be the gold standard, and good long-term outcome results have been reported [22–24]. However, the recovery time can be long, and a significant number of patients remain unsatisfied, complaining of residual pain, esthetic concerns, and loss of mobility and pinch strength [25]. This has led to a continuous quest for alternative procedures, including total joint replacement [26]. Considering its success in orthopedics as a whole, and specifically in hip and knee replacements, many attempts have been made to match these results for the thumb base [27].

Since its introduction by De la Caffinière in 1974, the CMC total joint replacement has become the treatment of choice in some parts of Europe over these last decades [28]. Many implant designs that were developed and used have been abandoned because of poor results and unacceptable failure rates. Nevertheless, more recent reports of larger series with good outcome and longer-term survival rates became available for other implants, to support this treatment option. This chapter will provide a guide on clinical and surgical decision-making, with a focus on implants that have stood the test of time, are supported by a minimum of 5 years of clinical follow-up, and are currently still available on the market.

## Patient Selection

Signs and symptoms of thumb base osteoarthritis include pain, loss of functionality, and decreased grip strength. Patients typically complain of radial-sided wrist pain and fatigue over the thenar mass. Key and tip pinch and power grip are painful, leading to a marked disability during activities of daily living and manual labor. The classic "shoulder sign" refers to swelling that may occur over the thumb base secondary to inflammation, osteophyte formation, and dorsal subluxation of the metacarpal.

Clinical examination reveals tenderness over the CMC joint line with palpation. Axial loading and circumduction (grinding or crank test) will often provoke pain and crepitus. The neighboring MCP and STT joints are carefully examined for local tenderness, as pathology here will affect the choice of surgical treatment. The STT joint is palpated about 1 cm proximal to the CMC joint line and just distal to the scaphoid tubercle.

Longstanding dorsal subluxation of the CMC joint leads to adduction of the first metacarpal and contracture of the first webspace. Secondary metacarpophalangeal (MCP) hyperextension due to progressive volar plate attenuation and increased pull of the extensor muscles leads to the so-called Z-deformity of the thumb and is associated with decreased pinch strength [29]. The MCP joint needs to be carefully checked for range of motion and hyperextension deformity, which can be flexible and correctable, or become a fixed extension contracture in chronic disease. This is a prognostic factor for poor functional outcome and will impact further decision-making. Stabilization with capsulodesis or arthrodesis has been suggested for MCP hyperextension beyond 35° when symptomatic or causing functional impairment [29, 30]. A significant decrease in MCP joint hyperextension has been demonstrated following total joint replacement, often obviating the need for further stabilization (Fig. 14.1). In a reported study of 96 arthroplasties, Toffoli specifically looked at the impact on MCP joint deformity. In cases where MCP hyperextension was limited to less than 30°, no residual hyperextension was present in 72% of cases, and 80% of correctable Z-deformities were completely corrected [31]. In contrast, following trapeziectomy, an increase of MCP hyperextension is anticipated and soft tissue procedures to address this tend to stretch over time [32]. Robles-Molina found an MCP hyperextension of 3.5° and 17.8° following total joint replacement versus LRTI, respectively [33]. For fixed extension contractures or when degenerative changes are present at the MCP joint, an arthrodesis of the joint in a functional position is the preferred treatment option.

## Medical Imaging

The standard radiographic workup should include a posteroanterior (PA) and lateral view of the thumb and CMC joint (Kapandji views) and a Robert's view (shoulder flexion and internal rotation, and forearm hyperpronation) to obtain a true AP view of the CMC and STT joint [34] (Fig. 14.2). Stress views (PA view with thumbs pressed together) can be used when CMC insta-

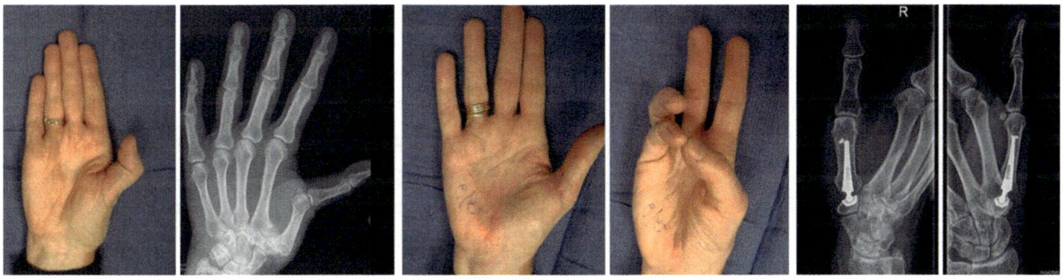


Fig. 14.1 Preoperative MCP hyperextension of 45° with marked subluxation of the thumb CMC joint, volar MCP capsulodesis was performed combined with total joint replacement

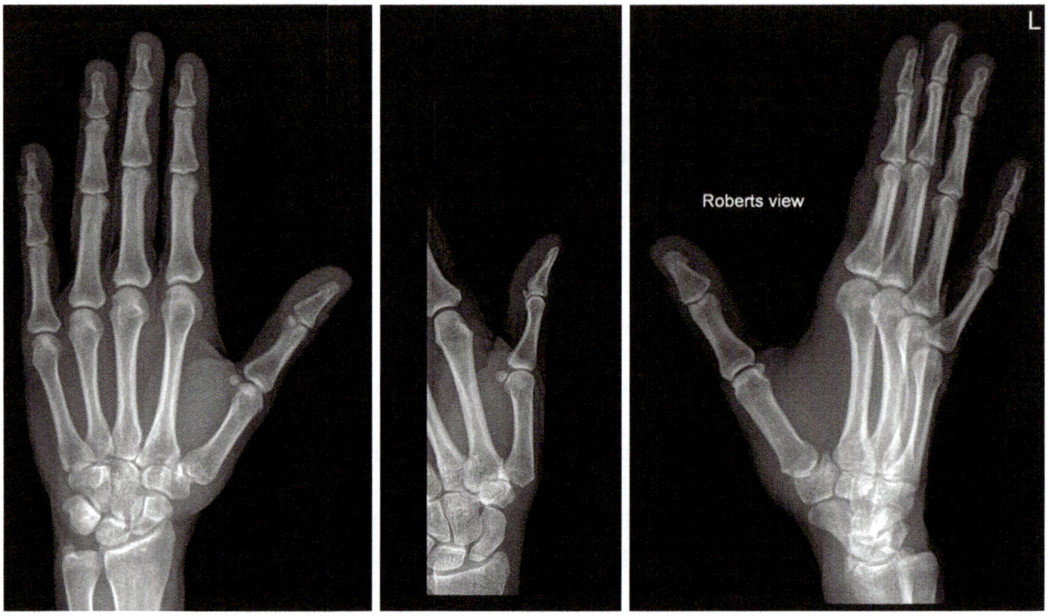


**Fig. 14.2** Preoperative radiographic workup with Kapandji PA and lateral views and Robert's view

bility is suspected, especially in younger patients [35]. Radiographs should be assessed for joint space narrowing, loose bodies, osteophyte formation, joint congruency, and bone cyst formation. The trapezium is checked for general bone stock, looking closely at the height, depth, and width. A dysplastic shape of the trapezium might influence treatment options and should be noted at this point. Early degenerative changes may be undetectable on plain radiographs, whereas CT scan will show joint space narrowing of the volar corner of the CMC joint [36]. When prosthetic replacement of the joint is indicated, and there is doubt about the bone quality or the size of the trapezium to accommodate a standard-sized cup (9 mm diameter in most implants), a CT scan can also aid in planning. MRI is rarely indicated but can assist in the diagnosis in younger patients or when a discrepancy is present between the clinical signs and radiographs.

## Staging

Two descriptive radiological staging systems have been proposed, one by Eaton-Littler in 1973, modified by Glickel in 1987 (Table 14.1), and one by Dell in 1978 (Table 14.2) [37, 38]. Both are useful for guiding treatment and for research purposes, but the correlation with intraoperative findings or patient complaints is limited [39].

**Table 14.1** The four stages of the Eaton-Littler (modified by Glickel 1987) classification

| Stage | Description |
|---|---|
| I | Subtle carpometacarpal joint space widening |
| II | Slight carpometacarpal joint space narrowing, sclerosis, and cystic changes with osteophytes or loose bodies <2 mm |
| III | Advanced carpometacarpal joint space narrowing, sclerosis, and cystic changes with osteophytes or loose bodies >2 mm |
| IV | Arthritic changes in the carpometacarpal joint as in stage III with scaphotrapezial arthritis |

Ladd et al. introduced the thumb osteoarthritis (ThOA) index as a measurable alternative or addition to the Eaton classification [39]. The ThOA index is measured on a single Robert's view radiograph and is based on the width and height of the trapezium. It has shown a better correlation with intraoperative findings and eburnation of the trapezial bone. Further validation of the ThOA index and correlation with patient-reported outcome measures is needed.

## Indications and Contraindications (Table 14.3)

When considering CMC joint arthroplasty, the typical patients are elderly women with limited forceful activities in daily life, Eaton stage 2–3 osteoarthritis on radiographs, who have failed a course of conservative treatment. Total joint arthroplasty (TJA) is rarely indicated in younger patients with heavier daily activities, and when there is an indication, they need to be well instructed about the risk of failure and revision surgery. As with any prosthetic implant, components will wear out faster with increased loading. However, these patients may benefit more from the improved recovery of strength and function after total joint arthroplasty.

Insufficient bone stock due to severe osteoporosis or eburnation of the trapezium needs to be considered, as it may impede stable impaction of the components. Concomitant asymptomatic osteoarthritis of the STT joint is considered a relative contraindication for CMC arthroplasty. In symptomatic pantrapezial osteoarthritis, trapeziectomy is the better option as it addresses both degenerative joint surfaces. Generalized joint laxity is no formal contraindication, but in hyperlax patients, extra caution is warranted to minimize the risk of prosthetic dislocation. In this patient population, the use of more constrained or dual-mobility implants should be considered.

**Table 14.2** Dell classification of thumb OA (1978)

| Stage | Radiological description |
|---|---|
| I | Joint narrowing or subchondral sclerosis but neither subluxation nor osteophyte formation |
| II | Small osteophyte at the ulnar border of the distal articular surface of the trapezium, increased density of the subchondral bone. Subluxation <1/3 of metacarpal surface |
| III | Prominent osteophyte at the ulnar border of the trapezium. Metacarpal subluxated radially and dorsally ⩾ 1/3 of its base |
| IV | Complete loss of joint space. Frequent subchondral cysts |

## Implant Types

Over the past decades, several implants have been designed. Currently available implants can be categorized into three large groups based on their principal design type: interposition arthroplasty, hemiarthroplasty (HA), and total joint arthroplasty (TJA) [26].

### Interposition Arthroplasty

Interposition arthroplasty is the insertion of a nonabsorbable synthetic implant between the partially recessed articular surfaces of the trapezium and metacarpal base. Different shapes of implants and materials are available (spherical, saddle joint, biconcave). These implants are not fixed but act as spacers to preserve the length of the thumb while preserving motion. Mixed outcome results have been published following interposition of soft synthetic spacers (RegJoint®, Artelon®). These implants show high failure rates mainly due to osteolysis, collapse, and foreign body reactions [40–43]. The PyroDisk® (Ascension Orthopedics Inc., Austin, TX, USA) is a biconcave pyrocarbon disc interposed between the partially recessed trapezium and the first metacarpal (Fig. 14.3). Smeraglia et al. have published good clinical outcomes using this implant with a 94% survival rate after a minimum follow-up of 8 years [44]. There are no other data available that confirm these long-term results. Oh et al. conducted a retrospective study comparing

**Table 14.3** Indications and contraindications for CMC arthroplasty

| Indications | Contraindications | Relative contraindications |
|---|---|---|
| Eaton-Littler stage II–III OA | Symptomatic STT OA | Asymptomatic STT OA |
| | Insufficient bone quality | Age younger than 50 |
| | Insufficient trapezium size | Heavy manual labor |
| | Infection | Dysplastic trapezium |
| | | Metal hypersensitivity |

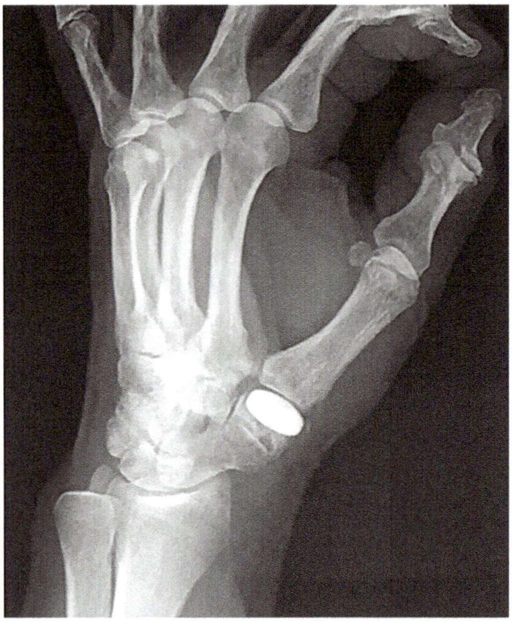

Fig. 14.3 Postoperative radiograph PyroDisk® interposition arthroplasty

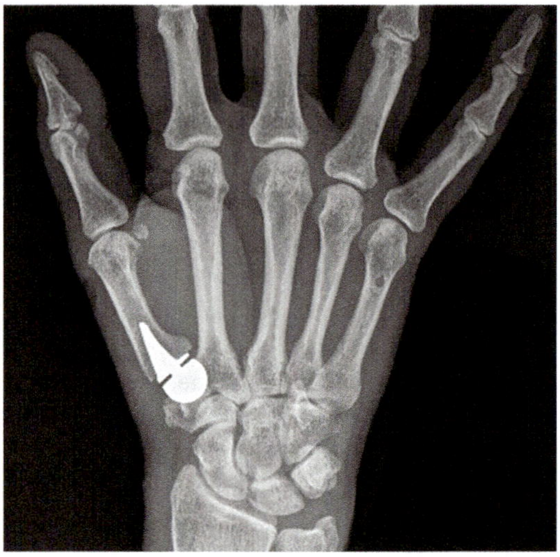

Fig. 14.4 Postoperative radiograph of the BioPro® Modular Thumb implant

LRTI to the PyroDisk® implant with a minimum of 2-year follow-up. These authors reported similar objective and subjective outcomes. Pinch strength was significantly higher in the PyroDisk® group. Although there were some radiographic changes around the implants, no revision surgery was needed [45].

## Hemiarthroplasty

In hemiarthroplasty (HA) only the metacarpal base is replaced to articulate with a partially recessed trapezium. The trapezial resection can be either concave or convex, depending on the corresponding shape of the prosthesis. The hemiarthroplasty was introduced to minimize thumb ray collapse after total or partial trapeziectomy. Swanson silicone hemiarthroplasty implants were first introduced in the 1970s [46]. After initial satisfying results with these implants, long-term complications were reported. Instability and silicone synovitis led to a high revision rate, and this implant was abandoned [47]. Subsequent hemiarthroplasty implants were made of titanium, pyrocarbon, or cobalt-chrome and have shown promising short- to mid-term results [48–50]. The available evidence beyond 5 years, however, is limited, and good outcome reported by the inventors has not always shown to be reproducible. In contrast to the excellent survival rate reported by Pritchett et al. using the BioPro® Modular Thumb implant (BioPro, Port Huron, MI, USA), others have reported a 50% failure rate using this implant [51, 52] (Fig. 14.4).

NuGrip® (Ascension Orthopedics Inc., Austin, TX, USA) is a PyroCarbon hemiarthroplasty implant with a spherical head that articulates with a concavely recessed trapezium (Fig. 14.5). A small series of ten patients with 9.5 months mean follow-up was published. Within this short follow-up, 30% had revision surgery due to implant instability [53].

Persistent pain, loosening of the metacarpal stem, and subsidence through the trapezium are among the biggest concerns in hemiarthroplasty. To address the problem of instability and in search of a more anatomical, saddle-shaped implant, the Stablyx® Arthroplasty System (Skeletal Dynamics, LLC, Miami, FL) was developed. It is commercially available since 2013, but only a small series of 12 patients with a follow-up of 2 years has been published [54].

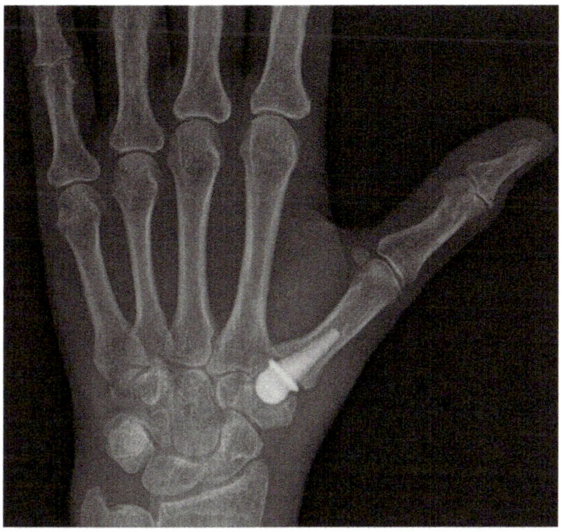


**Fig. 14.5** Postoperative radiograph of the NuGrip® PyroCarbon hemiarthroplasty

## Total Joint Arthroplasty

In total joint arthroplasty (TJA), both the trapezial and metacarpal sides of the CMC joint are replaced with a prosthetic implant. A ball-and-socket implant replaces the native saddle joint, allowing for a greater arc of motion in all directions while eliminating translation.

The latest generation of implants has evolved to an uncemented cup and stem with a metal-on-polyethylene (PE) ball-and-socket articulation (Fig. 14.6).

The metacarpal stem preparation and implant insertion rarely cause problems, but the alignment of the stem has an important impact on the ROM and stability of the implant. The stem shape can be anatomical (slightly curved) or non-anatomical (straight). Modern implants use a modular neck system with an adaptable neck angle and length to ensure optimal congruency and stability. The trapezial component consists of a conical or hemispherical cup. Precise positioning and fixation of the cup into the trapezium is the most critical step in the procedure and is achieved through either impaction of a press-fit implant or screwing in of a threaded cup. To ensure initial stability and improve bony ingrowth, most available cups are coated with porous titanium and/or hydroxyapatite.

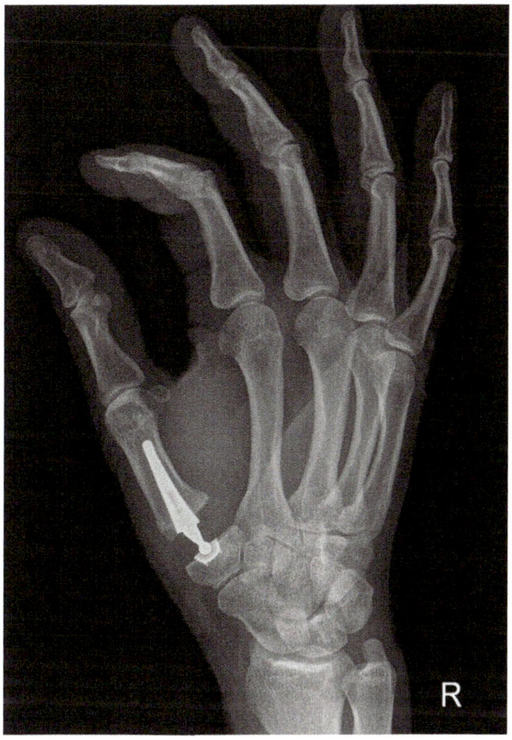


**Fig. 14.6** Postoperative radiograph of the Arpe total joint arthroplasty

### Complications

The most common complication after CMC arthroplasty is dislocation, which is mostly attributed to technical errors when it occurs in the early postoperative period. The main reasons are wrong positioning and orientation of the cup or insufficient osteophyte removal (Fig. 14.7). Late dislocations are usually caused by advanced polyethylene wear or trauma.

A trapezial fracture with secondary cup loosening or dislocation of the prosthesis can occur early following a perioperative iatrogenic fracture or technical error. Certain types of implants, using a screw cup and metal-on-metal articulation, demonstrated a high incidence of early cup loosening attributed to metallosis (3–47% with the Elektra® metal-on-metal TJA) [55, 56].

Persistent pain after CMC replacement can have multiple reasons such as low-grade infection, instability, bony impingement, loosening, metal hypersensitivity, or symptomatic STT osteoarthritis. Goubau et al. reported a high inci-

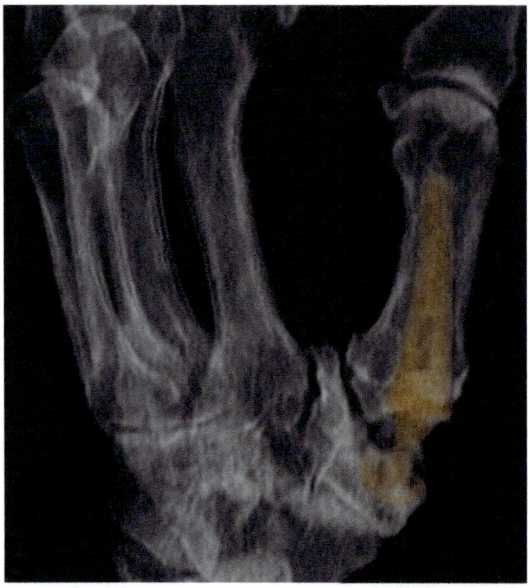

**Fig. 14.7** 3D reconstruction image of an insufficiently removed ulnar osteophyte leading to impingement and instability

dence of De Quervain tendinopathy as a complication of joint replacement, but found no relation to the potential lengthening of the thumb ray as was previously suggested [57]. Some authors therefor suggest to routinely combine a prophylactic release of the first extensor compartment with total joint arthroplasty [33].

## Reported Outcomes

Many authors have published case series using different implants evaluated by a variety of objective and patient-reported outcome measures making a comparison between implants and surgical techniques challenging [58–60].

Non-randomized trials comparing total joint arthroplasty to trapeziectomy with LRTI demonstrated that TJA had some significant advantages. Robles-Molina et al. found in a retrospective comparative study with a mean 4.8 year follow-up that patients following Arpe® prosthesis (Zimmer Biomet, Warsaw, IN, USA) had a significantly higher pinch strength (11.8 kg vs 8.4 kg) and greater arc of motion. The Kapandji opposition score was marginally higher in the TJA group versus the LRTI group (9.5 vs. 9.0). More important was the decreased retropulsion found in 40% of LRTI cases. An increase in preoperative MCP hyperextension was observed following LRTI, but no significant change was observed in the Arpe® group. There was no difference in QuickDASH scores or VAS pain scores between the two groups. But reoperation rates were higher in the TJA group, 9.7% versus 5.9% [33]. Reoperations in the Arpe® group were needed for three dislocated implants, and two patients in the LRTI group underwent subsequent surgery for MCP hyperextension.

A prospective comparative trial conducted by Cebrian-Gomez et al. using the Ivory® prosthesis (Stryker, Memometal, Bruz, France) with a minimum follow-up of 2 years (mean 4 years) also showed higher pinch strength and better abduction. These authors found a significant difference in QuickDASH score and VAS pain score in favor of the Ivory® group. Furthermore, in the prosthesis group, 93% of patients would have the same surgery again, compared to 79% of patients in the LRTI group. Three revision procedures were reported in the Ivory® group, and none in the LRTI group. Patients with TJA returned significantly faster to daily activities and work [61]. Ulrich-Vinther et al. confirmed these favorable clinical outcomes in a 1-year follow-up study [62]. Patients reached significantly better strength and range of motion at a faster rate in comparison to LRTI. There was one revision for early loosening of a cup. However, these authors used the Elektra® prosthesis (Small Bone Innovations International, Péronnas, France) which has shown to develop catastrophic failure rates due to cup loosening [55, 56].

The only randomized controlled trial comparing trapeziectomy and LRTI to TJA was recently published. Thorkildsen et al. demonstrated a significantly better recovery of range of motion (Kapandji score) and strength values in the first 6 months following TJA, but found no significant difference in strength and QuickDASH or Kapandji score after 12–24 months. Abduction and extension remained significantly better after 2 years in the arthroplasty group. Unfortunately, owing to the use of the Elektra® metal-on-metal prosthesis, five cups had to be revised in the first year because of loosening [63].

Long-term survival rates depend on the type of implant and the length of follow-up. Generally, the uncemented, metal-on-PE, ball-and-socket arthroplasties that are still on the market (Maïa®, Arpe®, and Ivory®) have shown favorable long-term results (Table 14.4).

Two studies were published with patients treated with the Ivory® implant with a minimum follow-up of 10 years and demonstrated survival rates of, respectively, 85 and 95%. Vissers et al. published their results in 24 patients. Two patients showed loosening of the cup [64]. Tchurukdichian et al. reported a 5.5% revision rate mainly due to dislocation or trapezial fracture. A 7.3% dislocation rate was found in 110 arthroplasties, leading to implant removal in four cases and one cup revision; three implants could be reduced in a closed manner. After 10 years 88% of patients remained satisfied or very satisfied [65].

**Table 14.4** Results of available long-term follow-up studies on primary CMC arthroplasty

| | *n* | Implant | Mean follow-up (months) | Survival rate % | Mechanism of failure | RR % |
|---|---|---|---|---|---|---|
| *Interposition arthroplasty* | | | | | | |
| Smeraglia et al. 2020 [44] | 46 | Pyrodisk | 113 | 94 | Painful instability | 6.5 |
| *Hemiarthroplasty* | | | | | | |
| Krukhaug et al. 2014 (NAR) [47] | 326 | Swanson silastic | 120 | 89 | Dislocation (18)<br>Pain | 10 |
| Krukhaug et al. 2014 (NAR) [47] | 71 | Swanson titanium | 120 | 94 | Pain | 5.6 |
| Phaltankar et al. 2002 [48] | 18 | Swanson titanium | 34 | 94 | Dislocation loosening | 5.3 |
| Pritchett et al. 2012* [51] | 143 | BioPro Modular Thumb | 72.1 | 94 | 4 stem loosening<br>2 subluxations | 4.2 |
| Florez et al. 2018 * [54] | 12 | Stablyx Arthroplasty System | 24 | 100 | None | 0 |
| De Aragon et al. 2009 [49] | 54 | PyroCarbon Ascension MCP | 22 | 80 | Loosening dislocation | 27.8 |
| *Total joint arthroplasty* | | | | | | |
| Vissers et al. 2019 [64] | 26 | Ivory | 130 | 82 | PE wear | 15 |
| Tchurukdichian et al. 2020 * [65] | 110 | Ivory | 120 | 95 | Traumatic dislocation, trapezial fracture | 7.3 |
| Martin-Ferrero 2014 [67] | 65 | Arpe | 120 | 93.9 | Dislocation, cup loosening | 7.7 |
| Dumartinet-Gibaud et al. 2020 [68] | 80 | Arpe | 138 | 85 | Cup loosening, dislocation, instability | 26.2 |
| Cootjans et al. 2017 [66] | 166 | Arpe | 80 | 95 | Dislocation, PE wear | 3 |
| Benaiss et al. 2011 [86] | 61 | Rubis II | 143 | 84 | Dislocation | 11.5 |
| Dehl et al. 2017 [87] | 115 | Rubis II | 120 | 89 | Dislocation, loosening | 4.3 |
| Toffoli et al. 2017 [31] | 96 | Maïa | 76.5 | 93 | Cup loosening | 8.3 |
| Krukhaug et al. 2014 (NAR) [47] | 29 | Elektra | 60 | 90 | Dislocation, instability, cup loosening | 6.9 |
| Semere et al. 2015 [88] | 64 | Roseland | 150 | 91 | Cup loosening, subsidence | 9.4 |
| Johnston et al. 2012 [69] | 39 | De la Caffinière | 192 | 73.9<br>26 (radiographic) | Cup loosening, pain | 26 |
| Tchurukdichian et al. 2019 [82] | 200 | Moovis (dual mobility) | 48.2 | 97 | 1 dislocation | 0.5 |

*RR* revision rate
* indicates publications co-authored by the designer of the implant/device

The Arpe® total joint arthroplasty also demonstrated good medium- to long-term survival rates. Cootjans et al. published a 5-year survival rate of 96% in a series of 166 prostheses [66]. Martin-Ferrero reported a 93.9% survival rate at 10 years of follow-up, with the main complication being dislocation [67]. Dumartinet-Gibaud et al. published a survival rate of 85% and 80% at 10 and 15 years, respectively. These authors, however, reported a high rate of early failures caused by surgical technical errors, confirming the steep learning curve of TJA. When excluding the first 30 cases, survival rates were 92% and 85% at 10 and 15 years, respectively. They observed a steady decline in implant survival beyond 15 years, independent of age, manual labor, and surgical approach. The mean time to revision was 212 months [68].

The "De la Caffinière"® cemented total joint arthroplasty has the longest published follow-up of 39 implants but is no longer commercially available. The survival rate at 26 years, with failure defined as "revision or removal of the implant," was 74%. When failure was considered as "at risk" (signs of radiographic loosening), survival dropped to 26% [69]. This high loosening rate is probably one of the reasons of why cement fixation has been abandoned and replaced by porous-coated implants.

## Authors' Preferred Technique

The patient is installed in a supine position with the hand on a hand table. The surgery is generally performed under locoregional nerve block with an upper arm tourniquet, but in selected patients, we have also used WALANT anesthesia. It has the advantage that implant stability and active ROM can be tested during the procedure. Following preparation of the arm in the usual sterile manner, thumb length is marked, and preoperative range of motion of the CMC and MCP joints is checked.

### Approach

Multiple approaches to the basal thumb joint have been described and are commonly used. The authors prefer to use a dorso-radial approach, as it allows optimal visualization of the CMC joint. It is also their preferred approach for resection of the trapezium, so that at any point during the procedure, the treatment plan can be adapted if needed.

A 3-centimeter incision is made starting over the proximal aspect of the first metacarpal, further extended in proximal direction over the anatomical snuffbox, centered between the extensor pollicis longus and extensor pollicis brevis tendon (Fig. 14.8). Subcutaneous veins and sensory branches of the radial nerve are identified and retracted. The fascia is incised, and the radial artery is identified at the level of the scaphotrapezial joint, running from proximal volar to distal dorsal. Using blunt dissection, the artery is mobilized and retracted dorsally. This allows for a safe longitudinal incision of the CMC joint capsule. The capsule is released of the base of the first metacarpal in a T-shape, leaving two flaps for later reinsertion and closure. The capsule is further released of the trapezium, to fully expose the saddle joint and the dorsal and volar horns of the trapezium. With the use of an oscillating saw, a minimal (2–3 mm) resection of the base of the first metacarpal is performed. The cut is made perpendicular to the long axis of the metacarpal and parallel to the joint surface, directed about 10° distally to remove the osteophytes at the volar beak. Alternatively, the volar osteophytes can be removed with a rongeur. Next, a minimal trapezial cut is made just below or level with the lowest central point of the concave saddle joint in order to remove the horns of

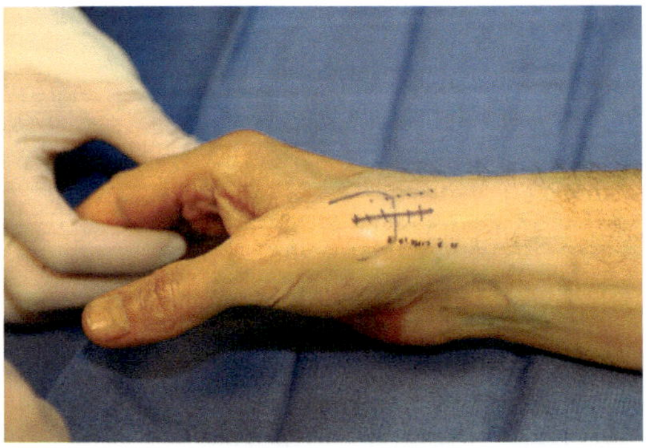

**Fig. 14.8** A 3-centimeter incision is marked, centered over the CMC joint for the dorso-radial approach

the trapezial bone (Fig. 14.9). It is important to remove all osteophytes and loose bodies, particularly on the medial side of the trapezium between the first and second metacarpal. Failing to do so will lead to impingement with the first metacarpal and increase the risk of dorsal dislocation of the prosthesis with thumb adduction-opposition. The direction of the trapezial cut should be in the "plane of the trapezium." The direction of the STT joint or proximal articular surface of the trapezium can be used as a reference (Fig. 14.10).

## Metacarpal Stem

The metacarpal medullary canal is prepared with broaches of increasing size, until a press fit with rota-

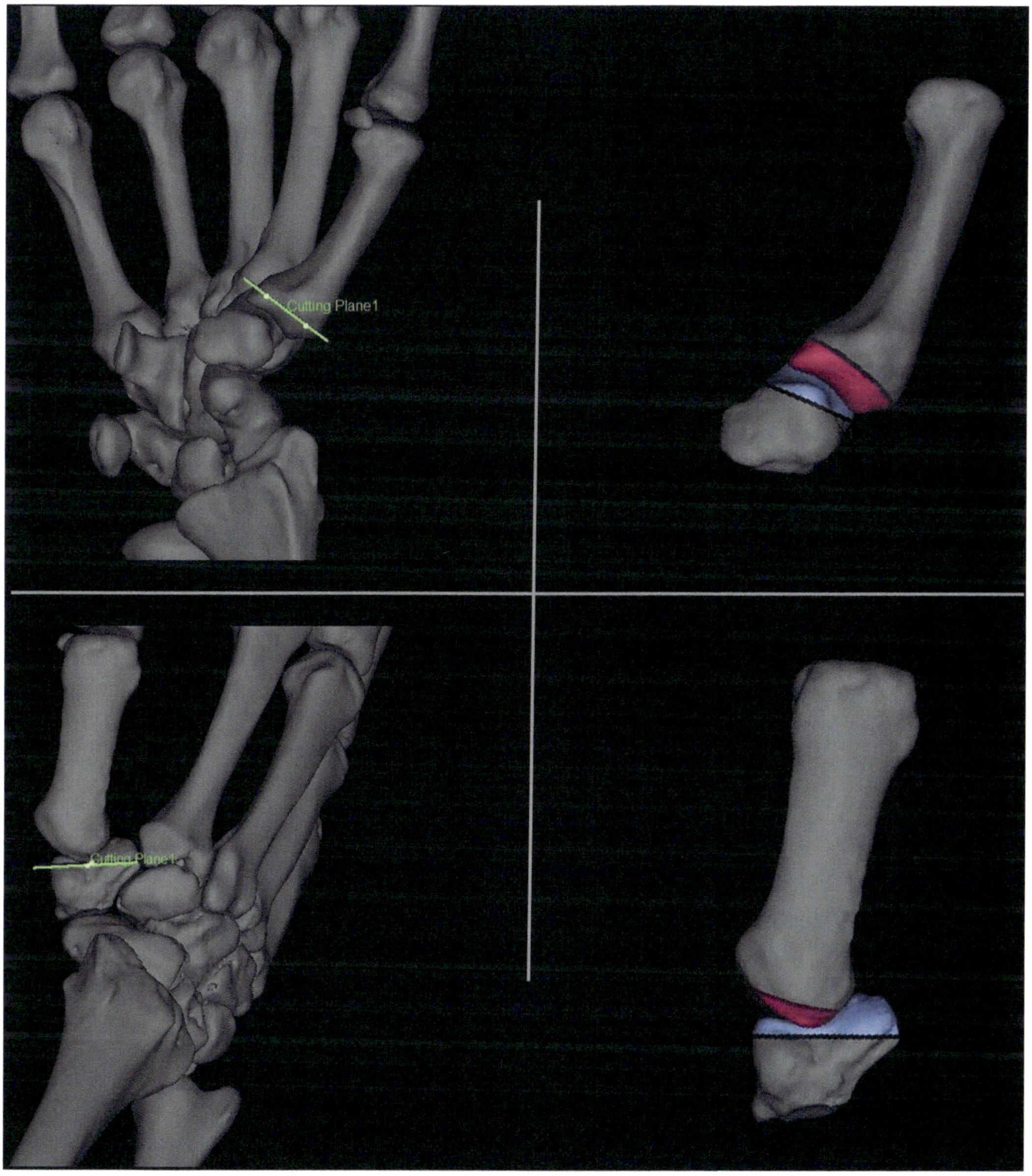


**Fig. 14.9** 3D reconstructed image showing ideal direction of cutting planes

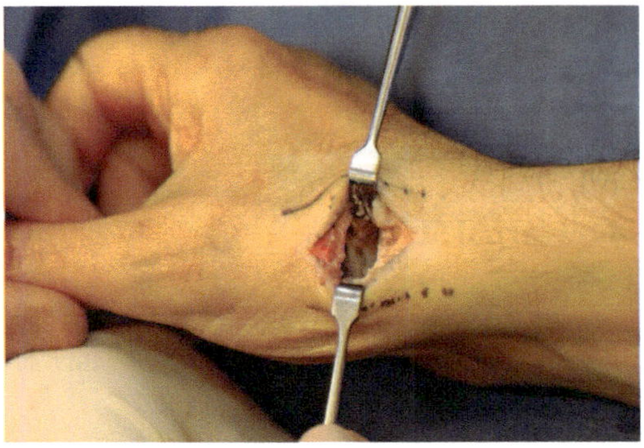

Fig. 14.10 Intraoperative image of articular gap after bone resection

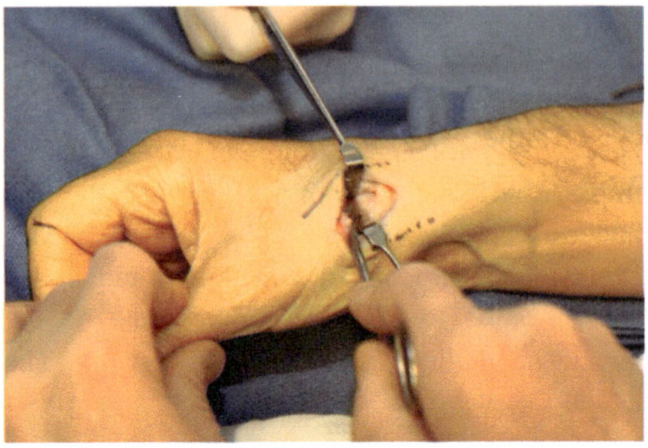

Fig. 14.11 Marking the center of the trapezium with a hemostat

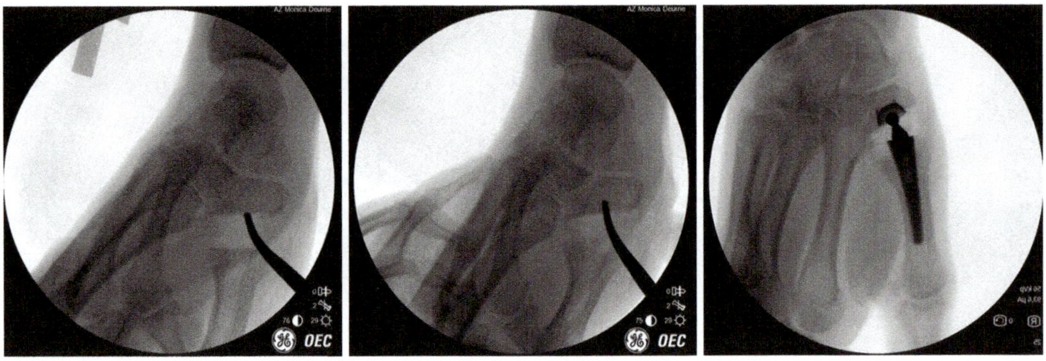


Fig. 14.12 Intraoperative fluoroscopic control of central cup positioning

tional stability is achieved. Cortical contact is not essential to prevent subsidence of the stem [70]. The size of the final implant will therefore be more dependent on bone quality than on the size of the intramedullary canal. At this point, a trial stem of the appropriate size is inserted, flush with the metacarpal base.

## Trapezial Cup

Precise cup positioning is the most technically demanding step in total joint arthroplasty, given the size and position of the trapezium and the non-anatomical shape of the cup.

The center of the trapezial surface is marked using a sharp instrument (awl or mosquito) (Fig. 14.11). Osteophyte formation on the trapezium can be misleading, so the correct position of the entry point is checked under fluoroscopy on AP and lateral views

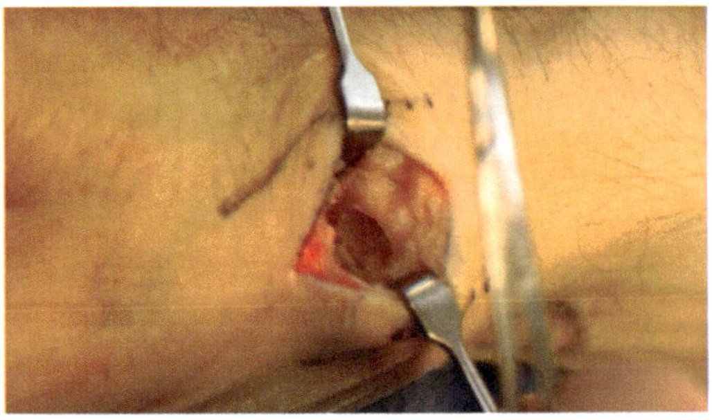

Fig. 14.13 Reaming of the trapezium, demonstrating the small margin for error

(Fig. 14.12). Ideally, this central point on the trapezium should be in line with the central axis of the first metacarpal when positioned in a neutral position (30° abducted and extended in relation to the axis of the second metacarpal). Subsequently, the trapezium is reamed down to the appropriate size cup with a shaped rasp (Fig. 14.13). When the subchondral bone is very sclerotic, the use of high-speed burr can be helpful in the initial preparation of the trapezium. It is essential to have good access to the trapezium at this stage of the procedure, and further release of the first metacarpal base may be indicated to obtain this. The cup needs to be positioned well centered in the trapezium to allow not only stable impaction of the final implant but also for biomechanical reasons. Eccentric positioning of the cup may lead to impingement and instability of the final prosthesis. The definitive cup is impacted using the instrumentation provided by the manufacturer.

If a trapezial fracture should occur during surgery or if the trapezial bone quality is deemed insufficient for stable implant insertion, the treatment plan needs to be adapted, and conversion to a trapeziectomy with ligament reconstruction and tendon interposition can be performed. Failing to recognize this complication will most likely lead to early cup loosening, secondary displacement, and instability.

### Head and Neck

Modern implants have the choice between a straight and offset modular neck in different lengths with 2 mm increments. After the cup is placed in the correct position, different neck lengths can be tested for trial reduction, checking stability, and range of motion (Fig. 14.14). The authors prefer an offset neck over the straight neck for two reasons. Our own experience when using 3D preoperative planning of the procedure confirmed that an offset neck provides a better reconstruction of normal anatomy and alignment, and it has been shown to decrease neck-cup impingement [71]. After confirmation of stability and range of motion of the joint replacement with longitudinal traction, maximal retropulsion, abduction, and opposition, the definitive metacarpal component and head and neck component are implanted (Fig. 14.15). If needed, the insertion depth of the metacarpal stem can be adjusted, to obtain the correct tension. The dorsal capsule is closed primarily or reattached to the metacarpal base using a looped nonabsorbable suture around the metacarpal stem (Fig. 14.16).

## Aftercare

The thumb is placed in a padded splint or cast for 2 weeks, leaving the thumb interphalangeal joint free to prevent tendon adhesions. At 2 weeks postoperatively, a removable thumb splint is fit-

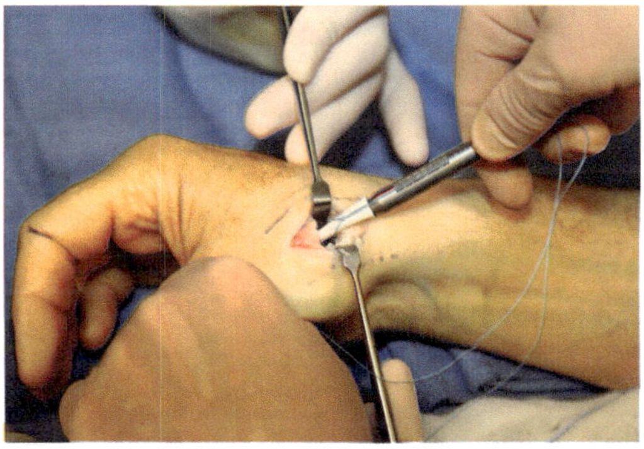

**Fig. 14.15** Insertion of the definitive stem with looped suture for capsule reattachment

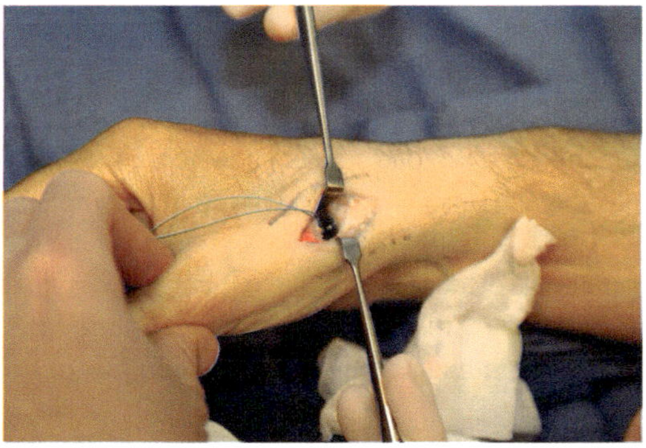

**Fig. 14.14** Reduction of the ball-and-socket articulation

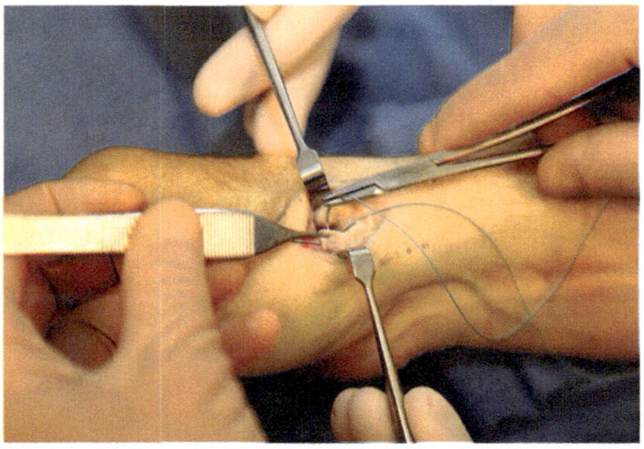

**Fig. 14.16** Primary closure of the capsule

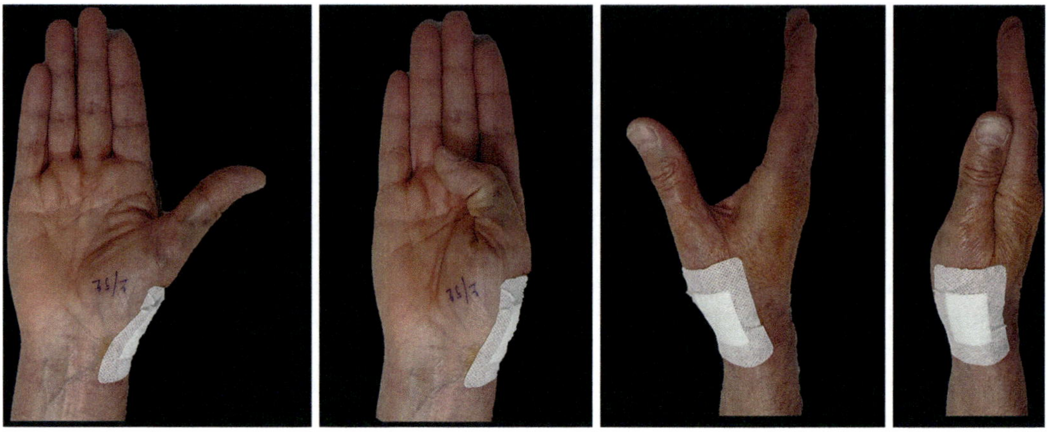

**Fig. 14.17** Typical patient at 2 weeks after TJA, demonstrating a near normal range of motion with minimal pain

**Table 14.5** Tips and tricks in total joint arthroplasty

| |
|---|
| Sufficient release of the first metacarpal to allow unrestricted access to the trapezium |
| Minimal bone resection of the trapezium, to keep enough bone stock for stable impaction of the trapezial cup |
| Complete resection of all osteophytes around the CMC joint to prevent impingement and instability |
| Use fluoroscopy to confirm the correct starting point for reaming of the trapezium |
| Correct positioning and orientation of the cup to prevent instability |
| Confirmation of unrestricted range of motion and complete stability with different head and neck components, before implantation of the final components |
| Stable fixation of the capsule to increase stability and allow early return to function |

ted, and rehabilitation is started with gentle active range of motion exercises (Fig. 14.17). At 6 weeks postoperatively, the splint can be discarded, and passive range of motion exercises can be started to further increase mobility if needed. Return to normal daily activities is allowed at this stage, although patients are advised to refrain from heavy loading of the thumb for 3 months (Table 14.5).

## Discussion

Many procedures have been suggested for the surgical treatment of CMC osteoarthritis, and all have their inherent advantages and disadvantages. Studies that have compared different treatment options were not able to prove superiority of one treatment option [23, 24, 33, 45, 60–63, 72, 73]. This complicates decision-making, and final treatment will depend on specific patient factors and surgeon preferences.

Based on the available literature, there are limited arguments for interposition arthroplasty or hemiarthroplasty, given the lack of qualitative long-term follow-up data. Implant arthroplasty with the PyroDisk could be a potential alternative, but more comparative studies to LRTI and TJA are needed to determine its place in the treatment of CMC osteoarthritis [44, 45, 74]. Data concerning modern TJA is more compelling, with favorable clinical outcome and long-term survival rates (Table 14.4).

As mentioned earlier, TJA leads to a faster recovery, improved function, and better restoration of thumb alignment and cosmesis (Fig. 14.18). In comparison to the gold standard, the significantly faster convalescence and better strength are most noticeable in the first year following TJA. Beyond 1 year, an increased range of motion and pinch strength will remain, compared to LRTI [33, 61, 63]. These potential benefits need to be discussed with the patient and weighed against the increased cost of implant arthroplasty and the significantly higher risk of complications (Table 14.6).

A recent and detailed systematic review compared pooled failure rates of trapeziectomy to failure rates of all implants published in the lit-

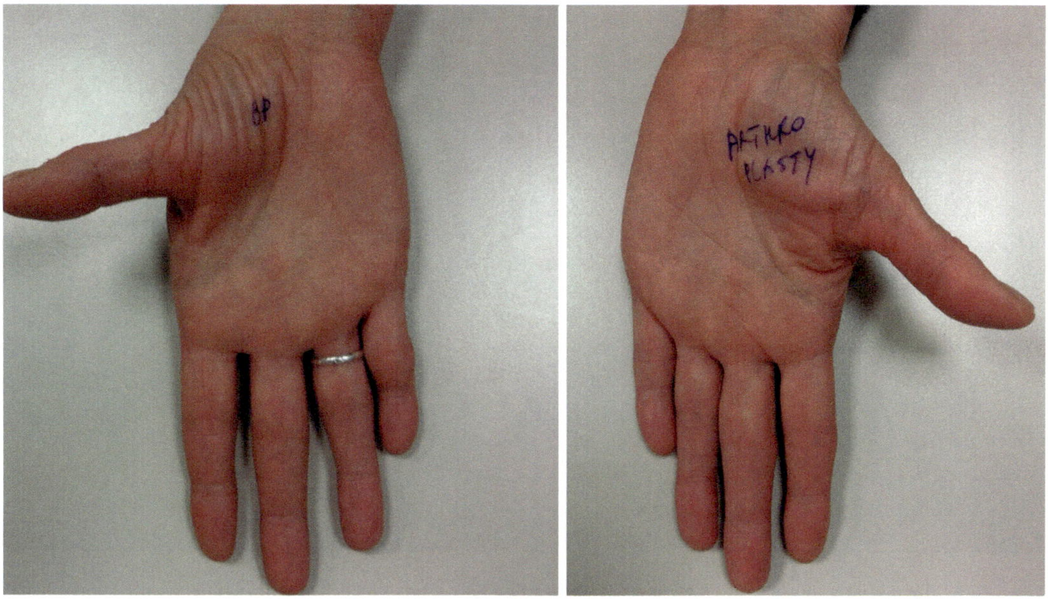


**Fig. 14.18** Clinical postoperative image of a patient who underwent an LRTI (left photo) and total joint arthroplasty (right photo), note the better restoration of thumb length and cosmesis

**Table 14.6** Why (not) consider CMC total joint replacement?

| Advantages | Disadvantages |
|---|---|
| Less painful | More expensive implant |
| Earlier return of function | Technically demanding [68] |
| Better key and tip pinch strength | Learning curve (30 cases) |
| Greater arc of motion | Higher complication rate: Dislocation, loosening |
| Better restoration of thumb length and cosmesis | Long-term survival uncertain |
| Stabilizes MCP hyperextension deformity | |
| Good medium- to long-term results | |
| Conversion to trapeziectomy possible | |

erature [59]. These data demonstrated an overall higher revision rate per patient-year for all implant arthroplasties compared to trapeziectomy. TJA had a more favorable revision rate compared to interposition and hemiarthroplasty. The criterion for failure was not related to patient outcome, but defined by the fact that revision surgery had been performed. This criterion is open for debate as it may have influenced the conclusion. Revision options following arthroplasty are straightforward and will often consist of implant removal and trapeziectomy, with an outcome comparable to primary trapeziectomy [75, 76], whereas revision options following trapeziectomy are limited, have an unpredictable outcome, and are therefore less commonly performed. The difference in revision rates between implant types could be attributed to errors in surgical technique or implant design flaws, as some implants have been shown to have high early failure rates.

Total joint arthroplasty is a technically demanding procedure, and errors will lead to complications and poor outcome (Fig. 14.19). One of the more critical steps in the procedure is the precise and stable positioning of the trapezial component. Guidelines on ideal cup orientation are limited. Lussiez et al. reported up to 22% of cup mispositioning on postoperative radiographs when using the second metacarpal as a reference [77]. Brauns et al. investigated the effect of cup orientation on the stability of the total joint prosthesis. These authors demonstrated that an orientation parallel to the proximal articular surface of the trapezium (PAST) is a reliable and reproducible method. Neutral positioning of the cup allows for a physiological range of motion of the joint and minimizes the risk of dislocation. Of all

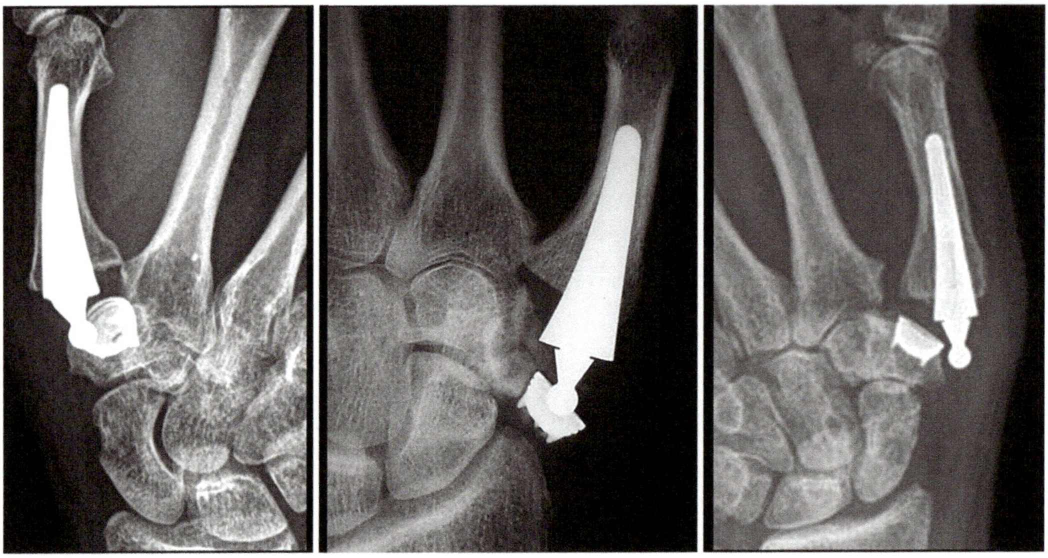

**Fig. 14.19** Total joint arthroplasty is a technically demanding procedure, and errors will lead to complications

movements, thumb adduction and opposition carry the highest risk for dislocation of the head in dorsal direction, and this risk increases with dorsal inclination of the cup [71, 78]. Current implant designs are essentially non-anatomical, transforming a biconcave saddle joint into a ball-and-socket joint [79]. This has proven to be a successful design but introduces some inherent problems, such as possible instability, fixation issues of the trapezial component, and limited revision options. There is a clear trend in orthopedic arthroplasty toward resurfacing designs, aiming to restore normal anatomy and biomechanics through limited bony resection and ligament balancing. Although attempts have been made to mimic this approach for CMC arthroplasty, the results have not yet been successful. Some specific problems that complicate this approach for the CMC joint are the high load and complex biomechanics, the relatively small size of the trapezium, marked osteophyte formation, ligament wear, and joint deformity [80].

Dislocation, cup loosening, and polyethylene wear are among the biggest concerns with total joint replacement. A newer generation of total joint implants tries to address these problems through the use of a dual-mobility interface. This concept has since long been used in hip arthroplasty and has some potential advantages. Due to the larger head size, the distance to prosthetic dislocation is increased. It decreases stress and wear on the trapezial implant because loads are shared between the two articulations. The combination of the small and big articulation results in a greater arc of motion [81]. The first reported 4-year outcome of the Moovis® (Stryker) dual-mobility implant shows a 97% survival with 0.5% dislocation [82]. It remains to be seen if the theoretical advantages will translate into better clinical outcome and longer survival. Concerns about increased polyethylene wear in dual-mobility have not been confirmed with the latest design and PE quality in hip arthroplasty [83, 84]. Another factor to consider is the metal composition of the trapezial cup. Titanium has traditionally been used here for its biocompatibility. In the dual-mobility concept, the inner aspect of the cup becomes a bearing surface and titanium may be less effective due to poor wear characteristics. One of the newer designs on the market, the Touch® prosthesis (KeriMedical, Geneva, Switzerland), has therefore replaced titanium for stainless steel in cup production. Polyethylene wear of the cup liner is occasionally seen in patients with longer follow-up, specifically when performing heavy activities. It can cause pain and instability and eventually accelerate loosening of the components. Advances in polyethylene cross-linking, diffusion of vitamin E, and addition of nanomaterials are potential ways to reinforce PE and reduce wear in future implants [85].

As many designs had to be retracted because of high failure rates, the widespread use of national registries would be of great benefit to closely monitor outcome. Not only could it allow for early tracking of failures; it would also facilitate the collection of reliable long-term outcome data on a large number of patients, as has been proven successful for hip and knee arthroplasty follow-up in some countries.

## Conclusion

No surgical procedure has been shown to be overall superior, and high-quality outcome research is lacking. Resection of the trapezium, often combined with interposition and ligament reconstruction, has traditionally been the most commonly performed procedure and has the lowest complication rate and cost. Nevertheless, TJA has become a valid treatment option. It allows for a shorter rehabilitation time, and there is evidence that it leads to a better functional recovery, range of motion, and strength. Medium- to long-term studies demonstrate good functional results and survival rates of a selected group of implants. However, longevity beyond 15 years is to be determined. Patient and implant selection together with a flawless surgical technique are paramount to achieve the best possible results. When salvage is necessary because of complications, the conversion to trapeziectomy is possible with an outcome similar to primary resection of the trapezium. New implant designs try to address some of the current disadvantages of CMC arthroplasties, but further research and longer follow-up are needed.

## References


1. Sodha S, Ring D, Zurakowski D, Jupiter JB. Prevalence of osteoarthritis of the trapeziometacarpal joint. J Bone Joint Surg. 2005;87:12.
2. Becker SJE, Briet JP, Hageman MGJS, Ring D. Death, taxes, and Trapeziometacarpal Arthrosis. Clin Orthop Relat Res. 2013;471(12):3738–44.
3. Armstrong AL, Hunter JB, Davis TRC. The prevalence of degenerative arthritis of the base of the thumb in post-menopausal women. J Hand Surg. 1994;19(3):340–1.
4. Riley N, Vella-Baldacchino M, Thurley N, Hopewell S, Carr AJ, Dean BJF. Injection therapy for base of thumb osteoarthritis: a systematic review and meta-analysis. BMJ Open. 2019;9:e027507.
5. Day CS, Gelberman R, Patel AA, Vogt MT, Ditsios K, Boyer MI. Basal joint osteoarthritis of the thumb: a prospective trial of steroid injection and splinting. J Hand Surg. 2004;29(2):247–51.
6. Khan M, Waseem M, Raza A, Derham D. Quantitative assessment of improvement with single corticosteroid injection in thumb CMC joint osteoarthritis? Open Orthop J. 2009;3(1):48–51.
7. Villafañe JH, Valdes K, Pedersini P, Berjano P. Thumb carpometacarpal osteoarthritis: a musculoskeletal physiotherapy perspective. J Bodyw Mov Ther. 2019;23(4):908–12.
8. AJ-DJM B. Reduction in the need for operation after conservative treatment of osteoarthritis of the first carpometacarpal joint: a seven year prospective study. Scand J Plast Reconstr Surg Hand Surg. 2001;35(4):415–7.
9. Tuffaha SH, Quan A, Hashemi S, Parikh P, O'Brien-Coon DM, Broyles JM, et al. Selective thumb carpometacarpal joint denervation for painful arthritis: clinical outcomes and cadaveric study. J Hand Surg. 2019;44(1):64.e1–8.
10. Loréa PD. First carpometacarpal joint denervation: anatomy and surgical technique. Tech Hand Upper Extrem Surg. 2003;7(1):26–31.
11. Wong CW Yee, Ho P Cheong. Arthroscopic management of thumb carpometacarpal joint arthritis. Hand Clin . W.B. Saunders. 2017. Vol 33 p. 795–812.
12. Hofmeister EP, Leak RS, Culp RW, Osterman AL. Arthroscopic hemitrapeziectomy for first carpometacarpal arthritis: results at 7-year follow-up. Hand. 2009;4(1):24–8.
13. Hobby JL, Lyall HA, Meggitt BF. First metacarpal osteotomy for trapeziometacarpal osteoarthritis. J Bone Joint Surg Series B. 1998;80(3):508–12.
14. Chou FH, Irrgang JJ, Goitz RJ. Long-term follow-up of first metacarpal extension osteotomy for early CMC arthritis. Hand. 2014;9(4):478–83.
15. Goubau JF, Ackerman P, Kerckhove D, van Hoonacker P, Berghs B. Addition–subtraction osteotomy with ligamentoplasty for symptomatic trapezial dysplasia with metacarpal instability. J Hand Surg Eur Vol. 2012;37(2):138–44.
16. Rizzo M, Moran SL, Shin AY. Long-term outcomes of trapeziometacarpal arthrodesis in the management of trapeziometacarpal arthritis. J Hand Surg Am. 2009;34(1):20–6.

17. Gervis WH. Excision of the trapezium for osteoarthritis of the trapeziometacarpal joint. J Bone Joint Surg. 1949;31-B(4):537–9.
18. Burton RI, Pellegrini VD. Surgical management of basal joint arthritis of the thumb. Part II. Ligament reconstruction with tendon interposition arthroplasty. J Hand Surg Am. 1986;11(3):324–32.
19. Weilby A. Tendon interposition arthroplasty of the first carpo-metacarpal joint. J Hand Surg Br. 1988;13(4):421–5.
20. DelSignore JL, Accardi KZ. Suture suspension arthroplasty technique for basal joint arthritis reconstruction. Tech Hand Up Extrem Surg. 2009;13(4):166–72.
21. DeGeorge BR, Chawla SS, Elhassan BT, Kakar S. Basilar thumb arthritis: the utility of suture-button suspensionplasty. Hand. 2019;14(1):66–72.
22. Avisar E, Elvey M, Wasrbrout Z, Aghasi M. Long-term follow-up of trapeziectomy with abductor pollicis longus tendon interposition arthroplasty for osteoarthritis of the thumb carpometacarpal joint. J Orthop. 2013;10(2):59–64.
23. Vermeulen GM, Slijper H, Feitz R, Hovius SER, Moojen TM, Selles RW. Surgical management of primary thumb carpometacarpal osteoarthritis: a systematic review. J Hand Surg. 2011;36(1):157–69.
24. Vandenberghe L, Degreef I, Didden K, Fiews S, de Smet L. Long term outcome of trapeziectomy with ligament reconstruction/tendon interposition versus thumb basal joint prosthesis. J Hand Surg Eur Vol. 2013;38(8):839–43.
25. Spekreijse KR, Vermeulen GM, Kedilioglu MA, Slijper HP, Feitz R, Hovius SE, et al. The effect of a bone tunnel during ligament reconstruction for trapeziometacarpal osteoarthritis: a 5-year follow-up. J Hand Surg. 2015;40(11):2214–22.
26. Lerebours A, Marin F, Bouvier S, Egles C, Rassineux A, Masquelet AC. Trends in trapeziometacarpal implant design: a systematic survey based on patents and administrative databases. J Hand Surg. 2020;45:223–38.
27. Learmonth ID, Young C, Rorabeck C. The operation of the century: total hip replacement. Lancet. Elsevier. 2007;370:1508–19.
28. de La Caffiniere JY, Aucouturier P. Trapeziometacarpal arthroplasty by total prosthesis. Hand. 1979;11(1):41–6.
29. Degeorge B, Dagneaux L, Andrin J, Lazerges C, Coulet B, Chammas M. Do trapeziometacarpal prosthesis provide better metacarpophalangeal stability than trapeziectomy and ligamentoplasty? Orthop Traumatol Surg Res. 2018;104(7):1095–100.
30. Poulter RJ, Davis TRC. Management of hyperextension of the metacarpophalangeal joint in association with trapeziometacarpal joint osteoarthritis. J Hand Surg Eur Vol. 2011;36(4):280–4.
31. Toffoli A, Teissier JMAÏA. Trapeziometacarpal joint arthroplasty: clinical and radiological outcomes of 80 patients with more than 6 years of follow-up. J Hand Surg. 2017;42(10):838.e1–8.
32. Miller NJK, Davis TRC. Palmar plate capsulodesis for thumb metacarpophalangeal joint hyperextension in association with trapeziometacarpal osteoarthritis. J Hand Surg Eur Vol. 2014;39(3):272–5.
33. Robles-Molina MJ, López-Caba F, Gómez-Sánchez RC, Cárdenas-Grande E, Pajares-López M, Hernández-Cortés P. Trapeziectomy with ligament reconstruction and tendon interposition versus a trapeziometacarpal prosthesis for the treatment of thumb basal joint osteoarthritis. Orthopedics. 2017;40(4):e681–6.
34. Robert M. The classic: radiography of the trapeziometacarpal joint. Degenerative changes of this joint. Clin Orthop Relat Res. 2014;472(4):1095–6.
35. Wolf JM, Oren TW, Ferguson B, Williams A, Petersen B. The carpometacarpal stress view radiograph in the evaluation of trapeziometacarpal joint laxity. J Hand Surg Am. 2009;34(8):1402–6.
36. Saltzherr MS, van Neck JW, Muradin GSR, Ouwendijk R, Luime JJ, Coert JH, et al. Computed tomography for the detection of thumb base osteoarthritis: comparison with digital radiography. Skelet Radiol. 2013;42(5):715–21.
37. Eaton R, Glickel S. Trapeziometacarpal osteoarthritis. Staging as a rationale for treatment. Hand Clin. 1987 [cited 2020 Apr 17];3(4):455–71.
38. Dell PC, Brushart TM, Smith RJ. Treatment of trapeziometacarpal arthritis: results of resection arthroplasty. J Hand Surg. 1978;3(3):243–9.
39. Ladd AL, Messana JM, Berger AJ, A-PC W. Correlation of clinical disease severity to radiographic thumb osteoarthritis index. J Hand Surg Am. 2015;40(3):474–82.
40. Kennedy AM, Barker J, Estfan R, Packer GJ. The use of the RegJoint™ implant for base of thumb osteoarthritis: results with a minimum follow-up of 2 years. Hand Surg Rehabil. 2020;39(1):53–8.
41. Vitale MA, Taylor F, Ross M, Moran SL. Trapezium prosthetic arthroplasty (silicone, artelon, metal, and pyrocarbon). Hand Clin. 2013;29(1):37–55.
42. Clarke S, Hagberg W, Kaufmann RA, Grand A, Wollstein R. Complications with the use of Artelon in thumb CMC joint arthritis. Hand. 2011;6:282–6.
43. van Royen K, Kestens B, van Laere S, Goubau J, Goorens C. Short-term results after total trapeziectomy with a poly-L/D-Lactide spacer. J Wrist Surg. 2018;07(05):394–8.
44. Smeraglia F, Barrera-Ochoa S, Mendez-Sanchez G, Basso MA, Balato G, Mir-Bullo X. Partial trapeziectomy and pyrocarbon interpositional arthroplasty for trapeziometacarpal osteoarthritis: minimum 8-year follow-up. J Hand Surg Eur Vol. 2020;175319342090680:27.
45. Oh W-T, Chun Y-M, Koh I-H, Shin J-K, Choi Y-R, Kang H-J. Tendon versus pyrocarbon interpositional arthroplasty in the treatment of trapeziometacarpal osteoarthritis. Biomed Res Int. 2019;2019:1–10.
46. Swanson AB. Disabling arthritis at the base of the thumb: treatment by resection of the trapezium and

flexible (silicone) implant arthroplasty. J Bone Joint Surg Am. 1972;54(3):456–71.
47. Krukhaug Y, Lie SA, Havelin LI, Furnes O, Hove LM, Hallan G. The results of 479 thumb carpometacarpal joint replacements reported in the Norwegian Arthroplasty Register. J Hand Surg Eur Vol. 2014;39(8):819–25.
48. Phaltankar PM, Magnussen PA. Hemiarthroplasty for trapeziometacarpal arthritis - A useful alternative? J Hand Surg Br. 2003;28B(1):80–5.
49. de Aragon JSM, Moran SL, Rizzo M, Reggin KB, Beckenbaugh RD. Early outcomes of pyrolytic carbon hemiarthroplasty for the treatment of trapezial-metacarpal arthritis. J Hand Surg Am. 2009;34(2):205–12.
50. Caudwell M, Bayne G, Page RS. Anatomic pyrocarbon hemiarthroplasty for thumb carpometacarpal osteoarthritis in patients under 65 years: mid term results. J Hand Surg (Asian-Pac Volume). 2018;23(04):469–73.
51. Pritchett JW, Habryl LS. A promising thumb basal joint hemiarthroplasty for treatment of trapeziometacarpal osteoarthritis. Clin Orthop Relat Res. 2012;470(10):2756–63.
52. Marinello PG, Shreve M, Evans PJ. Outcomes of a cementless thumb basal joint hemiarthroplasty for the treatment of trapeziometacarpal osteoarthritis. Oral Presentation at AAHS Annual Meeting. 2016.
53. Van RJ, Kimmenade D, Bullens PH, Raven EE. Short term results of the Ascension® Nugrip™ Cmc implant for thumb carpometacarpal osteoarthritis. Internet J Orthop Surg. 2014;22(1):1–7.
54. Florez GB, Rubio F. Carpometacarpal hemiarthroplasty. Oper Tech Orthop. 2018;28(1):43–8.
55. Klahn A, Nygaard M, Gvozdenovic R, Boeckstyns MEH. Elektra prosthesis for trapeziometacarpal osteoarthritis: a follow-up of 39 consecutive cases. J Hand Surg Eur Vol. 2012;37(7):605–9.
56. Thorkildsen RD, Johansson CB, Hogmalm J, Johansson PH, Røkkum M. Early cup loosening after metal-on-metal total joint replacement of the trapeziometacarpal joint: a retrieval study. J Hand Surg. 2020;45(3):213–22.
57. Goubau J, Goubau L, Goorens C, van Hoonacker P, Kerckhove D, Vanmierlo B, et al. De Quervain tenosynovitis following trapeziometacarpal ball-and-socket joint replacement. J Wrist Surg. 2015;04(01):035–42.
58. Giddins G. Functional outcomes after surgery for thumb carpometacarpal joint arthritis. J Hand Surg Eur Vol. 2020;45(1):64–70.
59. Ganhewa AD, Wu R, Chae MP, Tobin V, Miller GS, Smith JA, et al. Failure rates of base of thumb arthritis surgery: a systematic review. J Hand Surg. 2019;44(9):728–741.e10.
60. Huang K, Hollevoet N, Giddins G. Thumb carpometacarpal joint total arthroplasty: a systematic review. J Hand Surg Eur Vol. 2015;40(4):338–50.
61. Cebrian-Gomez R, Lizaur-Utrilla A, Sebastia-Forcada E, Lopez-Prats FA. Outcomes of cementless joint prosthesis versus tendon interposition for trapeziometacarpal osteoarthritis: a prospective study. J Hand Surg Eur Vol. 2019;44(2):151–8.
62. Ulrich-Vinther M, Puggaard H, Lange B. Prospective 1-year follow-up study comparing joint prosthesis with tendon interposition arthroplasty in treatment of trapeziometacarpal osteoarthritis. J Hand Surg. 2008;33(8):1369–77.
63. Thorkildsen RD, Røkkum M. Trapeziectomy with LRTI or joint replacement for CMC1 arthritis, a randomized controlled trial. J Plast Surg Hand Surg. 2019;53(6):361–9.
64. Vissers G, Goorens CK, Vanmierlo B, Bonte F, Mermuys K, Fils JF, et al. Ivory arthroplasty for trapeziometacarpal osteoarthritis: 10-year follow-up. J Hand Surg Eur Vol. 2019;44(2):138–45.
65. Tchurukdichian A, Guillier D, Moris V, See LA, Macheboeuf Y. Results of 110 IVORY® prostheses for trapeziometacarpal osteoarthritis with a minimum follow-up of 10 years. J Hand Surg Eur Vol. 2020;0(0):1–7.
66. Cootjans K, Vanhaecke J, Dezillie M, Barth J, Pottel H, Stockmans F. Joint survival analysis and clinical outcome of total joint arthroplasties with the ARPE implant in the treatment of trapeziometacarpal osteoarthritis with a minimal follow-up of 5 years. J Hand Surg. 2017;42(8):630–8.
67. Martin-Ferrero M. Ten-year long-term results of total joint arthroplasties with ARPE® implant in the treatment of trapeziometacarpal osteoarthritis. J Hand Surg Eur Vol. 2014;39(8):826–32.
68. Dumartinet-Gibaud R, Bigorre N, Raimbeau G, Jeudy J, saint Cast Y. Arpe total joint arthroplasty for trapeziometacarpal osteoarthritis: 80 thumbs in 63 patients with a minimum of 10 years follow-up. J Hand Surg Eur Vol. 2020;0(0):1–5.
69. Johnston P, Getgood A, Larson D, Chojnowski AJ, Chakrabarti AJ, Chapman PG. De la Caffinière thumb trapeziometacarpal joint arthroplasty: 16-26 year follow-up. J Hand Surg Eur Vol. 2012;37(7):621–4.
70. Duerinckx J, Perelli S, Caekebeke P. Short report letter: cortical contact is unnecessary to prevent stem subsidence in cementless trapeziometacarpal arthroplasty. J Hand Surg Eur Vol. 2018;43(1):98–9.
71. Brauns A, Caekebeke P, Duerinckx J. The effect of cup orientation on stability of trapeziometacarpal total joint arthroplasty: a biomechanical cadaver study. J Hand Surg Eur Vol. 2019;44(7):708–13.
72. Yuan F, Aliu O, Chung KC, Mahmoudi E. Evidence-based practice in the surgical treatment of thumb carpometacarpal joint arthritis. J Hand Surg. 2017;42(2):104–112.e1.
73. Jager T, Barbary S, Dap F, Dautel G. Analyse de la douleur postopératoire et des résultats fonctionnels précoces dans le traitement de la rhizarthrose. Étude prospective comparative de 74 patientes trapézectomie-interposition vs prothèse MAIA®. Chir Main. 2013;32(2):55–62.
74. Barrera-Ochoa S, Vidal-Tarrason N, Correa-Vázquez E, Reverte-Vinaixa MM, Font-Segura J, Mir-Bullo X. Pyrocarbon interposition (PyroDisk) implant for

trapeziometacarpal osteoarthritis: minimum 5-year follow-up. J Hand Surg Am. 2014;39(11):2150–60.
75. Lenoir H, Erbland A, Lumens D, Coulet B, Chammas M. Trapeziectomy and ligament reconstruction tendon interposition after failed trapeziometacarpal joint replacement. Hand Surg Rehabil. 2016;35(1):21–6.
76. Kaszap B, Daecke W, Jung M. Outcome comparison of primary trapeziectomy versus secondary trapeziectomy following failed total trapeziometacarpal joint replacement. J Hand Surg. 2013;38(5):863–871.e3.
77. Lussiez B, Atlan F. Analyse radiologique de deux types de cupules de prothèse trapézo-métacarpienne. À propos de 50 cas Chirurgie de la Main. 2012;31(6):395.
78. Duerinckx J, Caekebeke P. Trapezium anatomy as a radiographic reference for optimal cup orientation in total trapeziometacarpal joint arthroplasty. J Hand Surg Eur Vol. 2016;41(9):939–43.
79. D'Agostino P, Dourthe B, Kerkhof F, Vereecke EE, Stockmans F. Impact of osteoarthritis and total joint arthroplasty on the kinematics of the trapeziometacarpal joint: a Pilot study. J Hand Surg. 2018;43(4):382.e1–382.e10.
80. D'Agostino P, Dourthe B, Kerkhof F, Harry Van Lenthe G, Stockmans F, Vereecke EE. In vivo biomechanical behavior of the trapeziometacarpal joint in healthy and osteoarthritic subjects. Clin Biomech. 2017;49:119–27.
81. Lussiez B. Prothèses trapézométacarpiennes à double mobilité – principes biomécaniques. Chir Main. 2015;34(6):388–9.
82. Tchurukdichian A, Gerenton B, Moris V, See LA, Stivala A, Guillier D. Outcomes of double-mobility prosthesis in Trapeziometacarpal joint arthritis with a minimal 3 years of follow-up: an advantage for implant stability. Hand. 2019;0(0):1–7.
83. di Laura A, Hothi H, Battisti C, Cerquiglini A, Henckel J, Skinner J, et al. Wear of dual-mobility cups: a review article. Int Orthop. 2017;41(3):625–33.
84. Boyer B, Neri T, Geringer J, di Iorio A, Philippot R, Farizon F. Long-term wear of dual mobility total hip replacement cups: explant study. Int Orthop. 2018;42(1):41–7.
85. Yousef S. Polymer nanocomposite artificial joints. In: Carbon nanotubes - current progress of their polymer composites: IntechOpen, London, UK; 2016. p. 253–73.
86. Benaiss S, Dunaud J-L, Gueriat F, Henry L, Hornstein S, Laterzaleroy C, et al. La prothèse trapézo-métacarpienne rubis 2 : résultats à plus de dix ans à propos de 61 implantations. Chir Main. 2011;30(6):435.
87. Dehl M, Chelli M, Lippmann S, Benaissa S, Rotari V, Moughabghab M. Results of 115 Rubis II reverse thumb carpometacarpal joint prostheses with a mean follow-up of 10 years. J Hand Surg Eur Vol. 2017;42(6):592–8.
88. Semere A, Vuillerme N, Corcella D, Forli A, Moutet F. Results with the Roseland® HAC trapeziometacarpal prosthesis after more than 10 years. Chir Main. 2015;34(2):59–66.

# 15 Revision/Failed Carpometacarpophalangeal Joint Arthroplasty

Maria Yan, Nicole Zelenski, Samyd S. Bustos, Doga Kuruoglu, and Steven L. Moran

## Introduction

Thumb carpometacarpal (CMC) arthroplasty is the preferred treatment for thumb CMC arthritis. It is the third most common hand surgical procedure performed in the United States, with carpal tunnel release and trigger finger release being more common [1]. The overall goal of thumb CMC arthroplasty is to resolve pain and preserve function. There are several procedures that have been described for the treatment of thumb CMC arthritis including arthrodesis, trapeziectomy with or without soft tissue interposition and ligamentous reconstruction, suspension arthroplasty, and CMC prosthetic replacement [2–6]. Despite all the options, soft tissue arthroplasty, consisting of trapeziectomy with ligament reconstruction and tendon interposition (LRTI), is the most common procedure performed for the treatment CMC arthritis in the United States [7].

Primary soft tissue arthroplasty of the first CMC joint is generally well-tolerated, has few complications, and offers reliable pain relief; however a small percentage of patients have persistent pain or develop recurrent symptoms during the course of follow-up [8]. Conservative treatment, such as splinting and steroid injections, can be successful in many of these cases; however, revision surgery may be indicated in cases of persistent pain or limited thumb function. Overall, the incidence of reoperation following primary CMC surgery has been reported between 2.5% and 5% [8–10]. Mattilia examined 1142 trapeziometacarpal arthroplasties and found that young patients (defined as age less than <55 years) had an increased risk for revision surgery [8].

In general, failure of CMC arthroplasty can be broken into three broad categories: *(1) failure to address underlying pathology, (2) mechanical failure of surgery or implant, and (3) iatrogenic pain caused by surgery*. Mechanical failures such as nonunions in cases of CMC fusion, impingement, or subsidence of the metacarpal and prosthetic implant loosening typically have superior outcomes following revision surgery when com-

M. Yan · S. S. Bustos · D. Kuruoglu
Division of Plastic and Reconstructive Surgery, Mayo Clinic, Rochester, MN, USA
e-mail: Yan.maria@mayo.edu; Bustos.Samyd@mayo.edu; Kuruoglu.doga@mayo.edu

N. Zelenski
Department of Orthopedic Surgery, Mayo Clinic, Rochester, MN, USA

S. L. Moran (✉)
Division of Plastic and Reconstructive Surgery, Mayo Clinic, Rochester, MN, USA

Department of Orthopedic Surgery, Mayo Clinic, Rochester, MN, USA
e-mail: Moran.steven@mayo.edu


G. J. W. King, M. Rizzo (eds.), *Arthroplasty of the Upper Extremity*,
https://doi.org/10.1007/978-3-030-68880-6_15

pared to iatrogenic nerve-based complications [11]. The most common cause of secondary surgery is reported to be metacarpal subsidence causing pain due to contact between the metacarpal and scaphoid [8]. Other less common reasons for revision surgery include neuritis of the superficial branch of the radial nerve, incomplete trapeziectomy, and untreated scaphotrapezoidal arthritis [10].

While these situations are uncommon, the management of these patients can be complicated by previous surgical scarring and prolonged patient disability. Several studies have described various revision techniques which include re-excision arthroplasty with and without soft tissue interposition, ligament reconstruction, and fusion. This chapter will focus on identifying the cause of persistent pain and its surgical management.

## Evaluation and Diagnosis

### Clinical Evaluation

In cases of continuing pain after first CMC arthroplasty, a systematic diagnostic plan should be followed. Pain within the first 3–6 months after the primary surgery should be considered residual surgical pain and treated with conservative measurements such as activity modification and splinting. If the pain persists for more than 6 months, then further investigation should be performed in order to assure the best outcome. Technical errors of the primary arthroplasty and other causes of thumb pain should first be ruled out [10]. Understanding the etiology of failure is imperative for successful treatment; however this can be difficult to identify with scarring and altered postsurgical anatomy; thus we follow the steps outlined below to avoid misdiagnosis [11].

#### History and Physical Exam

Physical examination should include thumb range of motion and grip and pinch strength. One should rule out thumb metacarpophalangeal (MCP) joint hyperextension, deformity, and ongoing painful instability. A positive grind test can indicate painful subsidence of the metacarpal. Careful palpation of the space between the base of the first and second metacarpal bones as well as STT joint should be performed to rule out a painful remaining osteophyte on the second metacarpal base, STT arthritis in cases of prosthetic arthroplasty, or untreated scaphoid-trapezoid arthritis in cases of trapeziectomy. *Other etiologies for basilar thumb pain such as de Quervain's synovitis, stenosing tenosynovitis of the thumb (trigger thumb), and FCR tendinitis should be ruled out.*

Mechanical symptoms indicating failure of CMC arthroplasty often present as a deep pain, grinding, or feeling of instability with pinch or grip. Patients can present with subsidence as well as instability of the base of the metacarpal. A patient with symptomatic subsidence demonstrates evidence of radiographic subsidence as well as point tenderness at the base of the thumb that is worse with gripping and pinching. Stability of ligament reconstruction can be evaluated by examining the thumb CMC joint location to the lateral edge of the scaphoid, and whether it remains stable, or can be easily displaced or subluxated with gentle force (Fig. 15.1).

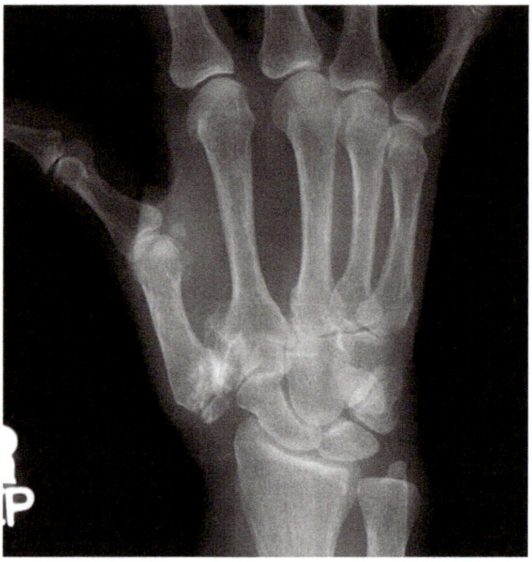

**Fig. 15.1** AP radiograph of a 68-year-old female, who has undergone previous hemi-trapeziectomy and tendon interposition. She presents with symptomatic subsidence with pain at base of the metacarpal on exam. The patient also suffered from symptomatic MP hyperextension which produced pain during key pinch at the base of the metacarpal and the MP joint

Symptomatic pinch or grasp weakness can also be the result of failure to correct MCP hyperextension deformity (Fig. 15.1). Patients should be evaluated for MCP joint hyperextension or degenerative changes to ensure this is not the reason for continuing symptoms. Diagnostic injections can aid in identifying this as a pain generator in these complex patients.

Overconstraint of the base of the metacarpal can present as an abduction contracture of the first web space and results in an inability of the palm and thumb to lie flat on the exam table. It may lead to impingement of the base of the first metacarpal with the trapezoid or second metacarpal, and tenderness is often elicited with palpation over these areas. Overconstraint can result following suspensionplasty procedures using tendon or suture suspension techniques.

Finally, neurogenic pain can result from injury to scaring to either the branches of the superficial branch of the radial nerve (SBRN) or the terminal branches of the lateral antebrachial cutaneous nerve (LABC). Pain is often described as diffuse and burning, but may present as a discrete neuroma within or near the scar. Patients are often hypersensitive to touch. A Tinel's sign may be elicited over the neuroma. For these cases we find that proximal selective nerve blocks of either the LABC and/ or the SBRN can help to identify the nerve injured and suggest if surgical exploration is required [12].

### Radiological Findings

Radiographs can aid in identifying subsidence, scaphotrapezoidal arthritis, MCP joint arthrosis, or STT arthritis. Radiographs will also identify evidence of prosthetic implant failure, subluxation, or metallosis. Radiographs should include posteroanterior, lateral, and oblique views of the thumb and wrist. Focused thumb CMC joint visualization should be achieved with the true anteroposterior or Robert's view, which consists of placing the forearm in maximal pronation with the dorsum of the thumb rested on the X-ray cassette [13]. Other views include the true lateral or Bett's view which allows for a visualization of all trapezial articulations without overlap [14]. This requires positioning the forearm in a neutral position, with the thumb abducted and an ulnar deviation of the wrist. An ulnar deviation and thumb abduction view can also be used to assess for STT pathology [15].

A basalar joint stress view can be performed to assess for dynamic instability. This is a posteroanterior view that can be obtained by asking the patient to press his thumbs together. This view is excellent for assessment of subluxation of the thumb CMC joint prior to index surgery, but can also asses for residual instability or dynamic implant subluxation as causes of persistent pain [13, 16]. In order to assess metacarpal subsidence, the pinch lateral view is recommended. The patient is asked to press the thumb against a flexed index finger and the beam of the machine centered over the CMC joint [16, 17].

While radiographs have been the main imaging technique for the diagnosis and assessment ongoing CMC pain after arthroplasty, additional imaging modalities can be used. Computed tomography (CT) scans can be helpful in detecting residual fragments of trapezium or osteophytes leading to impingement. CT scans can be particularly valuable in cases of pain following pyrocarbon implantation where small trapezial fractures can be obscured by the implant itself (Fig. 15.2). Bone Scans can help distinguish bone and joint pain from neurogenic or scar-related pain, but we find selective nerve injections more valuable.

## Causes of Failure

### Retained Trapezium

In Cooney's study of 154 CMC arthroplasty procedures, the retained trapezium, as seen in cases of hemitrapeziectomy and arthroscopic trapeziectomy, was a noted risk factor for recurrent pain. Because the trapezium articulates with five surrounding bones, persistent pain generators can exist between the retained trapezium and the scaphoid, trapezoid, index metacarpal, or thumb metacarpal. Removal of the remaining trapezium was shown by Cooney and to resolve pain and improve function (Fig. 15.3). Other options could certainly include interposition arthroplasty and trapezial denervation [18].

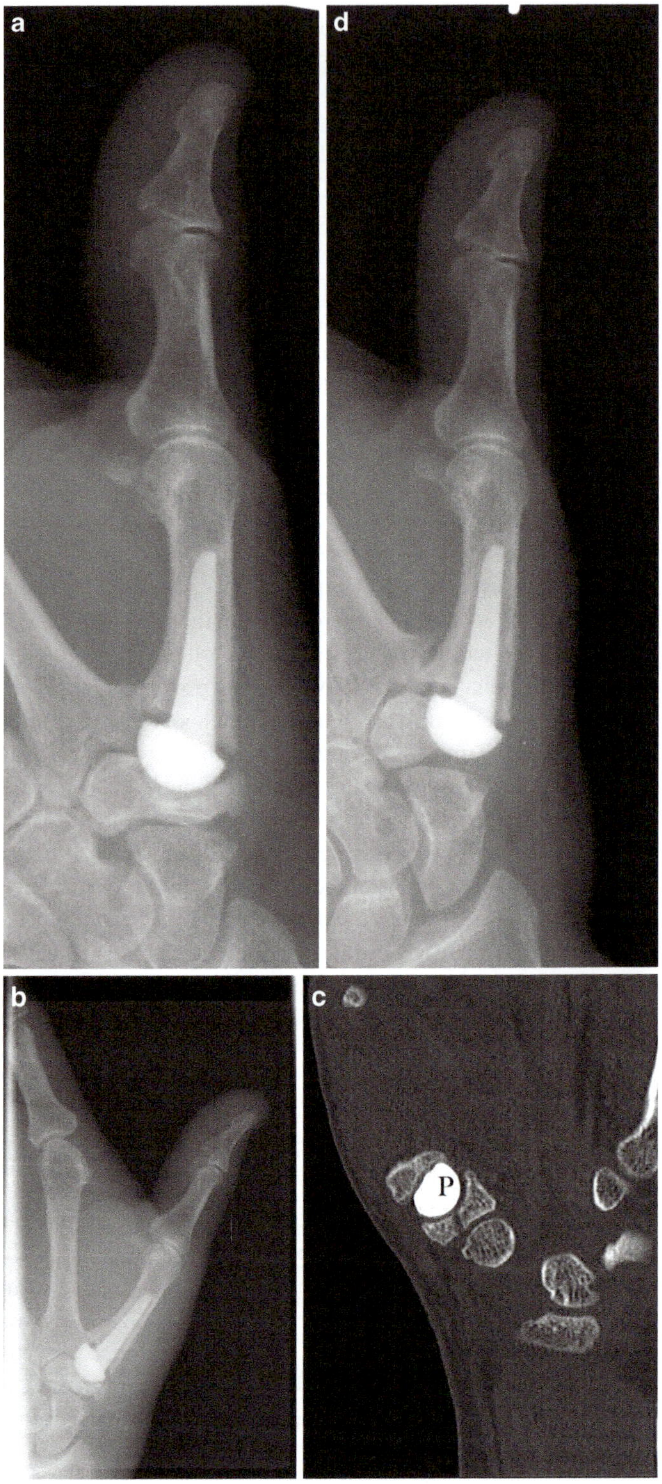


**Fig. 15.2** A 65-year-old female who had pyrocarbon hemiarthroplasty of thumb 3 years prior to CMC arthritis (**a**). Patient presents with pain at the base of her thumb following a fall. Plain radiographs do not reveal significant change from prior radiographs (**b**); however CT scan shows a fracture of the trapezium accounting for patient's pain (**c**). Patient was revised to trapeziectomy, and pyrocarbon now articulates painlessly with scaphoid. Patient returned to full function (**d**)

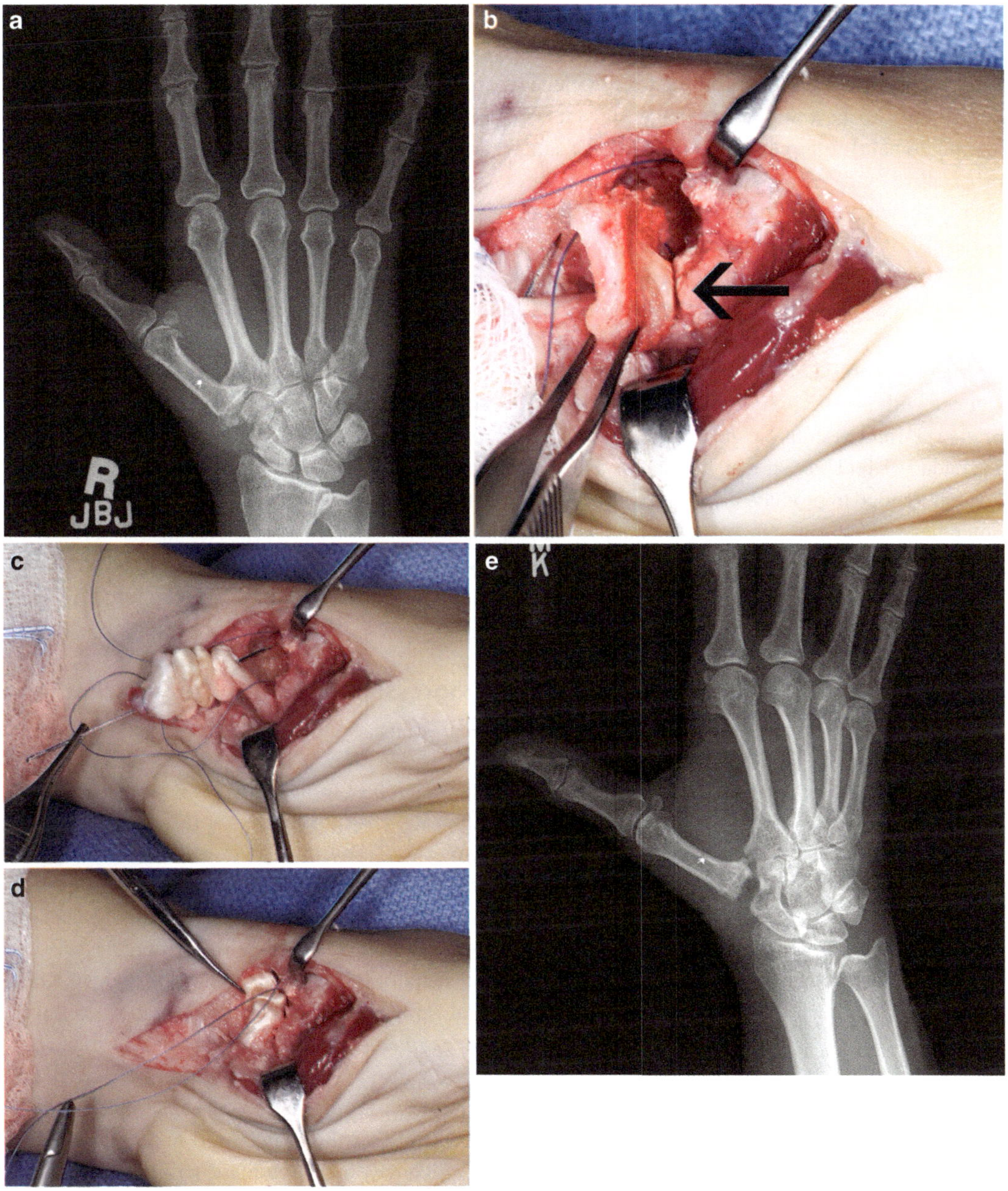


**Fig. 15.3** Images of a retained trapezium in a patient with persistent thumb pain following trapeziectomy. AP radiograph showing opacity site of trapezial resection (**a**). Figure (**b**) shows retained proximal trapezium (arrow) which is removed. The remaining portion of the flexor carpi radialus is used to perform an LRTI (**c** and **d**). AP radiograph (**e**) showing radiographic improvement with clinical restoration of thumb motion

## Subsidence

Some researchers have reported metacarpal subsidence as the most common complication after trapeziectomy [9]. It can occur vertically or dorso-radially with impingement of the adjacent scaphoid, second metacarpal base, or trapezoid [19]. Subsidence to some degree occurs after the majority of CMC arthroplasty procedures if a prosthetic replacement is not used [20]; however subsidence does not always produce pain, and radiographic subsidence in the absence of clinical symptomatology is not an indication for revision. Pain with associated metacarpal-scaphoid/

trapezoid impingement or secondary metacarpal scaphoid arthritis is a cause for revision.

There is little high-level comparative evidence describing the best way to manage subsidence leading to painful impingement [21–23]. To date, prospective and retrospective studies have not clearly shown a benefit of any revision procedure in terms of providing superior function, pain relief, grip strength, or any outcome measure when comparing to isolated trapeziectomy [20, 23–32].

Many surgeons have suggested managing subsidence with an alternative suspension technique or newer interosseous suspension sutures [33]. Secondary LRTI, as shown by Sadhu and colleagues, tended to produce worse patient-reported outcomes when compared to primary arthroplasty [34]. Several techniques have been described besides the classic LRTI which may be used to suspend or stabilize the metacarpal, and these would include the use of the ECRL or a slip of the APL tendon [35]. An argument could also be made for the use of acellular dermal matrix or another form of interposition material to fill the trapezial void and prevent further metacarpal subsidence [22]. For recalcitrant cases, Jones and colleagues have also demonstrated the use of a pyrocarbon CMC implant placed into the remaining metacarpal and articulated against the distal scaphoid to resolve symptoms of subsidence (Fig. 15.2) [36].

## Missed Arthritis

Peritrapezial arthritis can cause residual pain after CMC arthroplasty [37]. In the setting of trapeziectomy, failure to address scaphotrapezoid arthritis at the time of surgery can cause lingering pain, and this articulation should always be evaluated prior to (and during) the index operation [38]. This joint is often hard to isolate on exam and should be evaluated preoperatively with ulnar deviation and thumb abduction views as well as examined visually at every trapeziectomy procedure [15, 37]. The presence of scaphotrapezoid arthritis is a contraindication for CMC implant arthroplasty as this surgery will not address this joint and arthritis here may be a cause of lingering symptoms or pain after implant arthroplasty. A large series of second-generation implant arthroplasty for trapeziometacarpal arthritis indicated STT arthritis to be the most common cause for revision [6].

Insufficient resection of the trapezium or residual osteophytes may also result in lingering pain in these patients which can be corrected by a completion of excision. In Cooney's [9] study, 3 out of 17 revisions were caused by residual arthritis after primary hemi-resection of trapezium with soft tissue arthroplasty. Exploration of recess between the first and second metacarpal base at the initial and revision surgery is recommended. In both Cooney's and Megerle's studies, the authors noted osteophytes at the metacarpal base to be a cause of ongoing pain and should be removed during the revision procedure [9, 10].

## Progression of Arthritis in Adjacent Joints

Progression of arthritis happens most commonly after trapeziometacarpal arthrodesis, but may also occur following prosthetic arthroplasty (Fig. 15.4). Fusion of the thumb CMC joint may accelerate the natural progress of the degenerative osteoarthritis and result in arthritis between the scaphoid, trapezium, and trapezoid. In Rizzo et al.'s [39] retrospective study on the 126 thumb trapeziometacarpal arthrodesis with a mean follow-up of 11.2 years, the authors reported that radiographic progression of scaphotrapeziotrapezoid (STT) arthritis occurred in 39 cases (31%) in which 8 were symptomatic (6%) and 2 required additional surgery. In another study with follow-up averaging almost 8 years, Damen et al. noted that the radiographic progression to STT arthritis occurred more quickly in the fused thumbs compared to non-operated contralateral thumbs [40]. Other studies show lower rates of peritrapezial arthritis and may be the result of shorter follow-up [41, 42]. Patients should be counseled on the potential development of peritrapezial arthritis which may require subsequent surgical intervention if one is considering

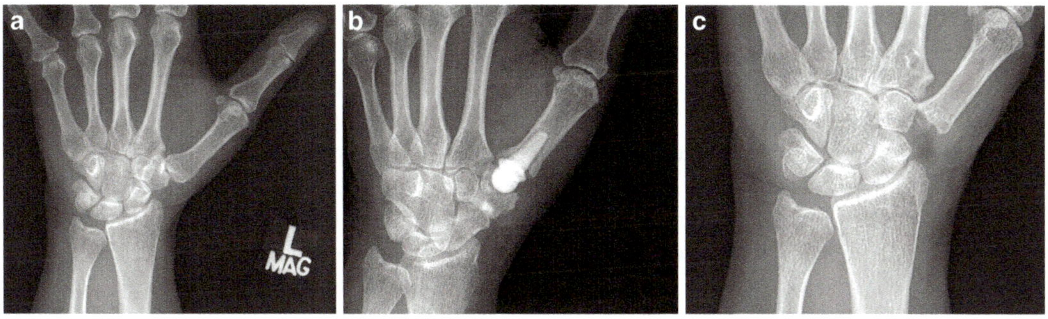


**Fig. 15.4** Images of a 63-year-old active female with CMC arthritis, as seen in AP radiograph (**a**). Patient was treated with second-generation pyrocarbon implant with good restoration of motion and strength. At 18 months patient started complaining of pain palmarly at the base of STT joint. Postoperative radiographs at 2 years after placement of pyrolytic carbon implant show evidence of scaphotrapezial arthritis (**b**). Patient was converted to trapeziectomy with Thompson suspensionplasty with resolution of symptoms (**c**)

trapeziometacarpal fusion as salvage for failed primary CMC arthroplasty.

## Neuritis and Complex Regional Pain Syndrome (CRPS)

SBRN and lateral antebrachial cutaneous nerve (LABCN) injury with the development of secondary neuritis are two of the most common complications following CMC arthroplasty (Megerle 2011). During the standard approach to the first CMC joint, the superficial sensory branch of the radial nerve (SBRN) is encountered and should be identified and protected by raising thick skin flaps containing the nerve. Symptoms should be managed nonoperatively for at least 6 months following the initial procedure with desensitization therapy prior to considering operative intervention. Neurolysis or repair can be performed of the SBRN or LABCN. In severe cases, targeted muscle reinnervation (TMR) or regenerative peripheral nerve interfaces (RPNI) may play a role in the treatment of this condition.

CRPS is an autonomic sensory dysfunction disorder and may result in the presence or absence of nerve injury. It is characterized by pain, swelling, limited range of motion, vasomotor instability, skin changes, and patchy bone demineralization [43]. It can be the result of direct nerve injury or due to a sympathetic response to the surgery. One should ensure the pain is not be generated by a nerve injury prior to attributing the pain to CRPS. Selective nerve blocks can often identify nerve injuries. When nerve injury and compression have been excluded, treatment of CRPS should include patient education, and a multidisciplinary team approach and revision surgery should be avoided [44].

## MCP Hyperextension

Failure to address hyperextension of greater than 30–40° can result in pain and weakness after MCP arthroplasty [45, 46]. Hyperextension of the MCP should ideally be evaluated before surgery and addressed during the index procedure. Unaddressed hyperextension after MCP arthroplasty can result in adduction deformity of the metacarpal and lead to impingement. Residual pinch or grasp weakness is a clue that MCP hyperextension has not been addressed. It may be hard to differentiate if MCP hyperextension is a cause of failure or a natural progression of metacarpal collapse; regardless of the cause, it has been noted to be present in over 10% of patients requiring CMC arthroplasty revision [47].

## Special Considerations in the Setting of Implant Arthroplasty

Prosthetic CMC arthroplasty has had a problematic history. Early metal implant designs, used primarily in Europe, had a high incidence of aseptic cup loosening, metallosis, and dislocation resulting in unacceptably high rates of implant removal [48–51]. Newer designs which have avoided metal on metal articulations have shown more promise with failure rates running between 4% and 11% [52–54]. Most cases of failed prosthetic CMC arthroplasty can be converted to a trapeziectomy with removal of the trapezial component with the trapezium and in some cases removal of the metacarpal stem [55].

Within the United States and in Europe, the use of hemiarthroplasty with metal or pyrocarbon has gained popularity over the last two decades. Despite the newer materials and implant design, these hemiarthroplasties still have complication rates which are higher than primary trapeziectomy with or without suspensionplasty [6]. Subluxation is the most common complication that may be encountered after hemi-implant arthroplasty and is the primary cause of implant failure. In series of 54 thumb CMC joints treated with pyrolytic carbon hemiarthroplasty, de Aragon reported that 10 out of 15 failed cases were due to metacarpal subluxation or dislocation [56]. The authors attributed the high rate of subluxation to the creation of a shallow trapezial cup.

In cases of hemiarthroplasty, adequate metacarpal base resection, use of larger implants, centralized cup placement within the trapezium, and strong capsuloligamentous reconstruction are key to prevent postoperative instability and dorsal subluxation [56, 57]. Maintaining the implant's position during the early capsular healing phase can be facilitated with absorbable interosseous sutures or a Kirschner wire [24, 56, 57].

Symptomatic subluxation rates have decreased with use of a second-generation pyrocarbon implants. In a large series of 47 patients who underwent CMC implant arthroplasty, only 3.5% needed revision for instability. In this series the most common reason for revision or implant removal was the development of STT arthritis. Interestingly, the rates of subsidence were similar between implant arthroplasty and trapeziectomy with suspensionplasty (13%) [58]. While much less common, infection, aseptic loosening, and trapezial fracture have also been described as rare complications of CMC hemiarthroplasty. These complications may warrant implant removal and conversion to complete trapeziectomy [56].

## Treatment

If a patient presents with symptoms following primary CMC arthroplasty and they have failed conservative treatment, secondary surgery or revision arthroplasty should be considered if underlying pathology can be identified. Diagnostic accuracy is crucial for a successful revision surgery. Complications that can be overcome with a revision surgery are typically mechanical, including metacarpal subsidence, subluxation, implant failure, and ongoing arthritis. Patient expectations should be tempered prior to revision [34].

There are several surgical techniques for revision CMC arthroplasty; no technique has been proven to be superior. Revision surgery should be individualized based on the origin of failure in the primary surgery addressing all sites of pathology [59]. Ultimately, the aim is to relieve pain, reestablish movement, regain grip, and recuperate overall hand function [60]. Papatheodorou et al. [59] described three components of the revision procedure for failed thumb CMC arthroplasty: *(1) preserving the space flanked by the metacarpal and scaphoid, (2) identifying and addressing any underlying scaphotrapezoid joint arthritis, and (3) treating MCP hyperextension.*

## Revision Interposition Arthroplasty With or Without Suspension

Mechanical pain or the presence of painful crepitation on physical examination can be overcome by soft tissue revision arthroplasty [9]. In cases of subsidence of the thumb base and MCP joint hyperextension, a repeat suspension with or without soft tissue interposition and MCP fusion can produce successful outcomes [8]. Patients who additionally have findings of substantial instability on exam should also undergo ligament reconstruction [59].

For revision procedures, our preference is to utilize a dorsal exposure to the CMC joint. A longitudinal incision is made extending from the midshaft of the thumb metacarpal across the line of the first dorsal compartment to the radial styloid. Care is taken to identify and protect superficial cutaneous nerves. The SPRN is identified, and a neurolysis is performed if the nerve is encased in scar tissue as this may be the cause of neuropathic pain. The deep branch of the radial artery and the tendon of the APL are identified and mobilized. The interval between the APL and EPB is used to enter the joint. Localization of surgery site can be identified with the aid of fluoroscopy if necessary. Once the site of the CMC joint resection is reached, the cavity of the previous trapeziectomy or tendon interposition is examined to search for fluid or evidence of synovitis. We assess external and internal tendon structure integrity and identify displacement of previously placed autologous or alloplastic interpositions. The space between the base of the first and second metacarpal bone should be meticulously inspected and palpated to identify residual bone fragments. We then systematically remove any remaining trapezium, the ulnar "toe" of the first metacarpal, and any osteophyte at the base of the second metacarpal. Finally, the scaphotrapezoid junction is assessed for evidence of arthrosis, and if present the proximal 2–3 mm of the trapezoid are excised sharply with an osteotome (Fig. 15.5). At this point the surgeon must decide if they wish to proceed with soft tissue interposition or repeat suspension. If there was symptomatic preoperative instability, we would recommend repeat suspension.

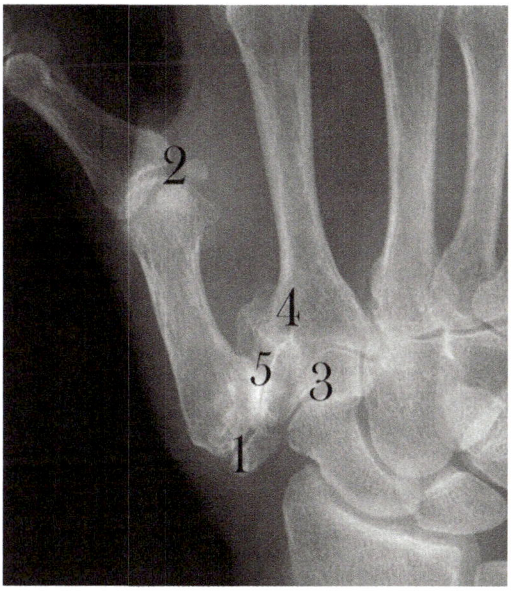

**Fig. 15.5** Areas which can result in ongoing mechanical pain and impingement following CMC surgery can include (1) retained trapezium, (2) MP joint hyperextension or MP arthritis, (3) trapezial or trapezoidal arthritis, (4) osteophytes at second metacarpal base, (5) first metacarpal base. All areas should be evaluated at time of revision

There are several techniques used for primary CMC suspensionplasty that can also be used for revision suspension [10]. The remaining intact portion of the FCR tendon can still be used for secondary surgery after failed LRTI [61]. However if the tendon is not available, then ECRL, APL, or extensor carpi radialis brevis (ECRB) can be utilized (Fig. 15.6). The abductor pollicis longus (APL) has been reported to be a fast and reliable technique with minimal donor site morbidity (Fig. 15.7). Our preference is to use one of the slips of the APL to perform a suspensionplasty modified from Thompson [62]. A distally based slip of the APL is passed through the first metacarpal base from dorsal radial to volar and ulnar [11]. The tendon is then passed through an oblique tunnel in the second metacarpal shaft form volar radial to the dorsum of the metacarpal at the ECRL insertion at the base of the second metacarpal. Here the APL tendon slip is placed on tension, suspending the metacarpal base. The tendon is either anchored with a bone anchor or weaved into the insertion of the ECRL tendon. If the surgeon desires, additional tendon can be placed into the void left by the resected trapezium.

Another option is to harvest a portion of the ECRL and position the tendon volarly between the first and the second metacarpals and sewn

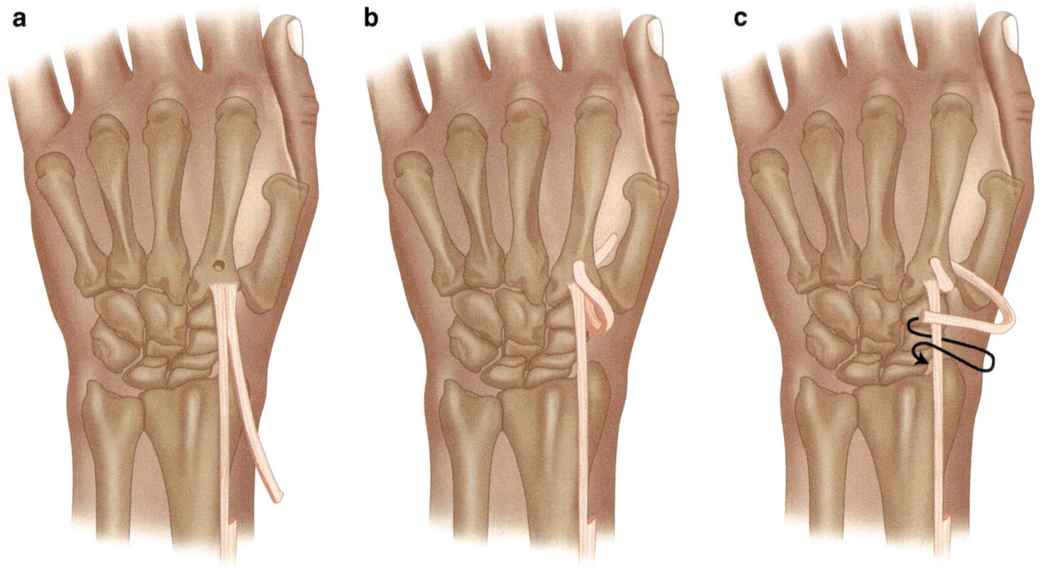


**Fig. 15.6** Artist rendition of the ECRL being used as an interposition graft and suspensionplasty for management of failed primary CMC arthroplasty. (**a**) The radial half to one third of the ECRL may be passed through a drill hole in the base of the second metacarpal. (**b**) The tendon is passed through the base of the first metacarpal. (**c**) The tendon can then be placed as an interpositional spacer into the space left by the trapezium or passed around the APL and back to the ECRL insertion to suspend the metacarpal. (Copyright Mayo Clinic)

back onto itself. Kakinoki et al. [63] reported a successful case of secondary suspension arthroplasty with ligament reconstruction between the first and second metacarpals in an active young patient that developed impingement after failed ligament reconstruction and tendon interposition.

If there are no suitable local tendons available, suspensionplasty with a free triceps tendon-olecranon bone graft can be considered. The thumb base is excavated taking care to leave a cortical rim intact. An olecranon bone plug is placed into the cavity. Next, an interference fixation is performed using a screw. A hole is drilled at the base of the second metacarpal, and the triceps tendon graft is passed through it, and then it is woven through itself to act as a spacer between the index and thumb metacarpal bases. The authors reported satisfactory outcomes with low donor site morbidity [64]. Alternatives to tendon include the use of suture suspension between the first and second metacarpal can also be performed; this construct can be reinforcement with a tendon-based suspensionplasty if there is remaining instability after revision LRTI [35].

Alternatives to suspension can include simple hematoma distraction arthroplasty or the placement of an interposition spacer between the metacarpal and the scaphoid. Acellular dermal matrix can be folded to supplement the previous interposition in order to add volume and support (Fig. 15.7). Drill holes in the trapezoid can be used to pass sutures from the trapezoid to the base of the metacarpal over the tendon suspension to hold the interposition inside this space occupied previously by the trapezium [65]. Alternatives to acellular dermal matrix could include allograft tendon of tensor fascia lata. Soft tissue interposition could also be added to augment any of the suspension procedures mentioned above.

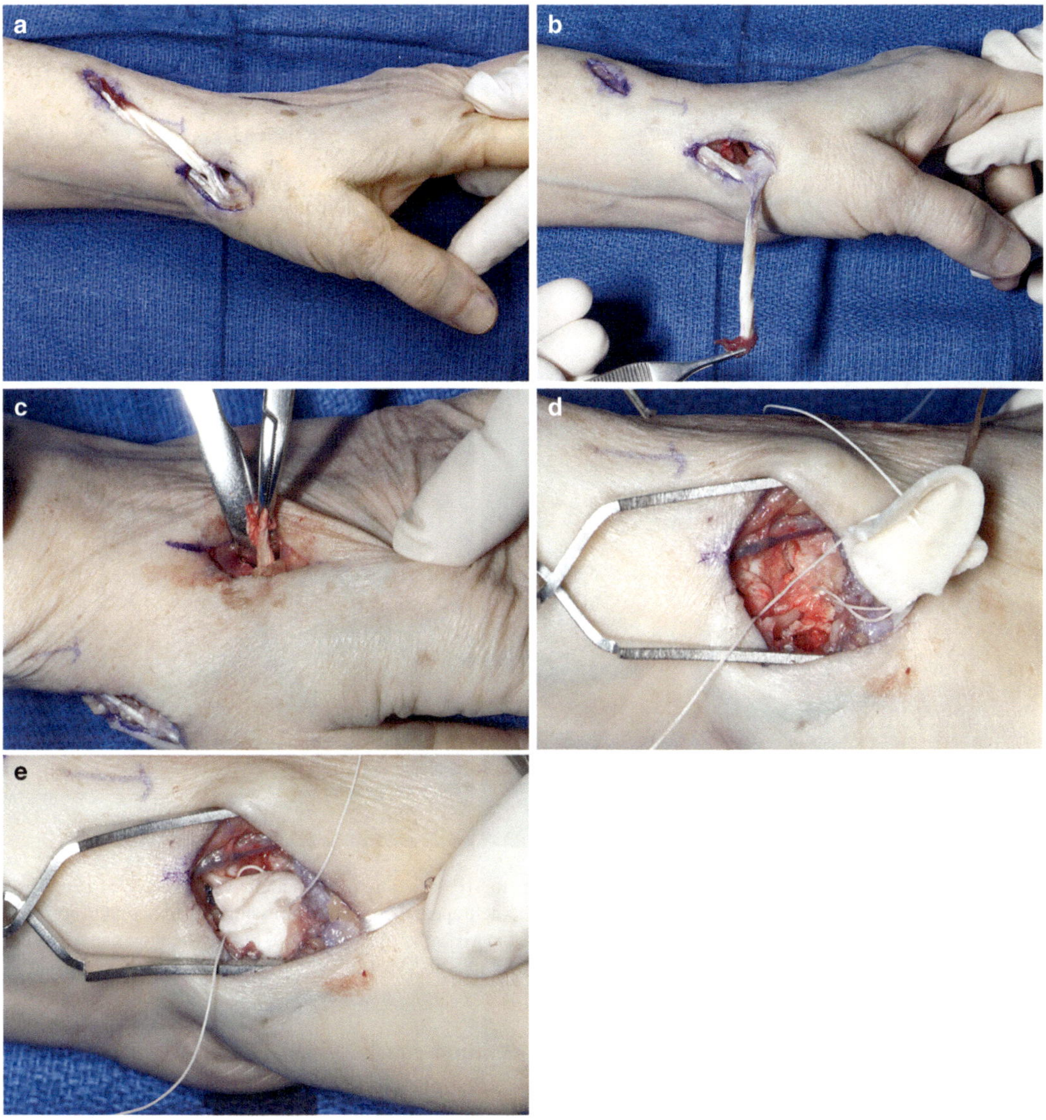


**Fig. 15.7** The modified Thompson suspensionplasty is similar to the ECRL tendon procedure described in Fig. 15.6; however a strip of the APL (**a**, **b**) is passed through the first metacarpal base and then through the second metacarpal base (**c**) to suspend the first metacarpal. In this case, additional acellular dermis was sewn into the space left by the trapezial void to provide additional soft tissue to prevent subsidence (**d**, **e**)

## Revision of Prosthetic CMC Arthroplasty

As implant arthroplasty continues to gain in popularity, revision procedures will become more common [6]. Causes of failure can include recurrent/persistent pain, dislocation, loosening, and infection. In rare cases, dislocation may be amenable to closed reduction and immobilization; however trapezial fracture, erosion, or gross implant failure typically requires removal of the implant (if possible) and conversion to a complete trapeziectomy and ligament interposition or suspensionplasty.

### Implant Salvage

If implant subluxation is identified with no other causes of failure, the previous implant can be removed, and a round bur can be used to deepen the trapezial cup allowing for appropriate

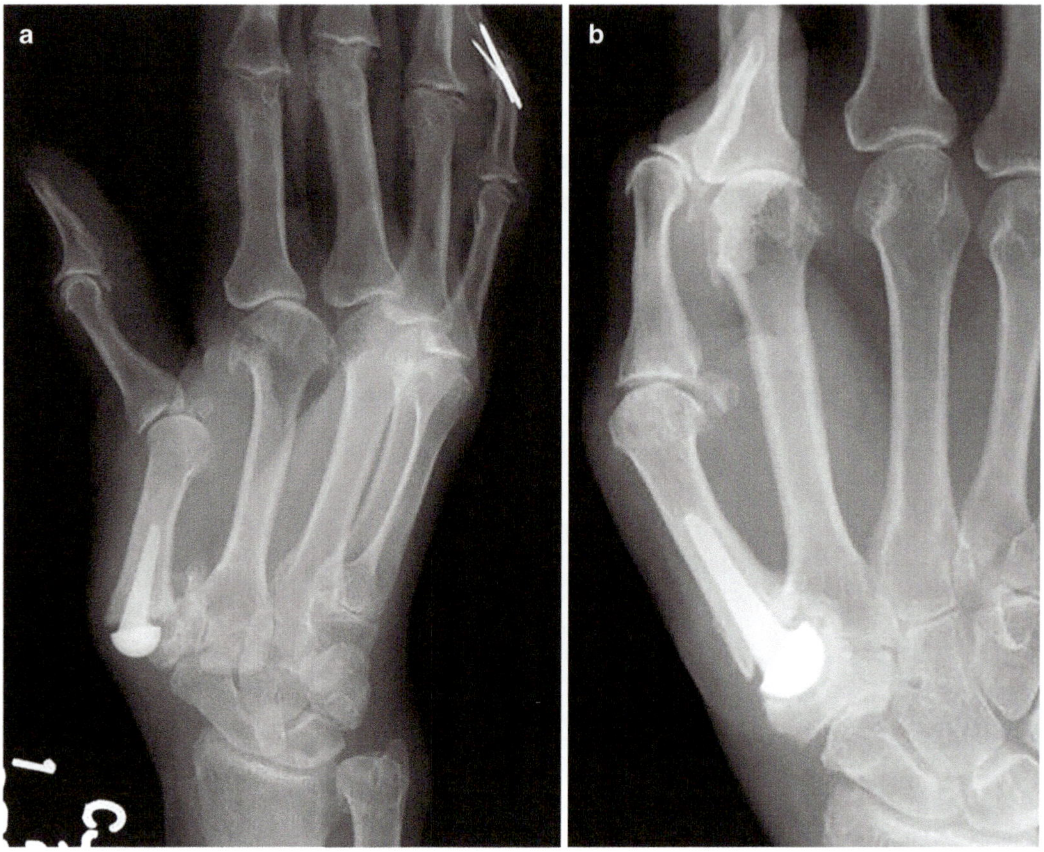


Fig. 15.8 (a) AP radiograph showing a dislocation of a first-generation pyrocarbon CMC hemiarthroplasty with associated hyperextension of thumb MP. Failure to address thumb MP hyperextension may have contributed to MP dislocation. The patient was salvaged by deepening the trapezial cup and addressing MP hyperextension with an MP volar plate plication. Figure (b) shows an AP radiographs at 1 year following revision surgery

implant position and stability (Fig. 15.8). Once appropriate contouring is done, K-wires are used to drill holes on both the dorsal metacarpal base and the trapezium. The implant is replaced, and then a heavy absorbable suture is based in a figure-of-eight suture pattern through the drill holes. The suture is tied with the thumb metacarpal in flexion. This suture is helpful in preventing can repeat subluxation and dislocation in the early postoperative period. Capsular flaps are then sutured back over the prosthesis. If the capsule is deficient, a slip of the APL can be used to reinforce the joint capsule. Postoperative immobilization should be continued for 4–6 weeks.

If STT arthritis has developed in the presence of a well-seated hemiarthroplasty, consideration can be given to selective interposition arthroplasty of the STT joint. We perform this procedure through a dorsal approach with mobilization of the radial artery to expose the scaphotrapezial joint. The capsule is opened, and the proximal joint surface of the trapezium is removed and replaced with acellular dermis or fascia lata. The capsule is then repaired, and the thumb is immobilized for 2 weeks. Alternatively the trapezium may be removed for pyrocarbon hemiarthroplasty, and the pyrocarbon proximal component can articulate on the scaphoid (Fig. 15.2).

## Revise to LRTI

One option for a failed implant arthroplasty is to remove the implant through the original incision and plicate and invaginate the capsule or the tendon of the APL into the cavity left by the removed implant [66, 67]. Any of the revision LRTI techniques listed above can also be used to salvage and suspend the remaining metacarpal once the implant has been removed. K-wires can be used to augment suspension by being passed from the first to second metacarpal to stabilize the base of the first metacarpal for 4–6 weeks. If there is persistent adduction contracture of the first metacarpal after removal of the implant, the fascia over the muscle and attachment of the adductors to the first metacarpal should be divided [60]. Additionally, MP joint hyperextension should be addressed if present [66, 67].

## **Fusion Thumb to Index** (Fig. 15.9)

Thumb-index metacarpal arthrodesis aims to provide a painless, stable first metacarpal base in recalcitrant cases but has the disadvantages of decreased range of motion, shortening of the affected thumb, and difficulty achieving union requiring prolonged immobilization. Despite this, arthrodesis maintains the osseous foundation of thumb and may be beneficial for patients with a high-demand job such as laborers [68].

An incision is made between the thumb and index metacarpal/carpometacarpal joint. Care is taken to preserve sensory branches of the radial nerve, and the radial artery is identified, retracted, and protected. Dissection is carried down to the interval of the intermetacarpal space and the previous trapeziectomy site. If a previous interposition and suspensionplasty was performed, it is resected to expose the base of the first metacarpal.

An incision on the dorsal ulnar border of the thumb metacarpal is made in order to expose the index finger-trapezoid metacarpal space. The entire trapezoid and the index finger CMC joint are exposed, as well as the base of the thumb. Once the bone ends are clearly visualized, the trapezoid, radial aspect of the index metacarpal, and the base of the thumb metacarpal are prepared. A good contour is required to match the space, like a portion of a "cup and cone". Meticulous debridement with a curette followed by perforation through the subchondral bone is to expose a well-prepared fusion surface of about 70 or 80% of the cancellous bone. It is important to maintain a few islands of cortical bone to minimize subsidence. Supplemental iliac crest or distal radius bone graft can be used at the surgeon's discretion.

The thumb is positioned in a position of pronation and abduction, and K-wires are placed into the thumb metacarpal across the fusion site. The position of the thumb is checked for acceptable radial and palmar abduction. If bone stock is poor, K-wires can be used for definitive fixation. If bone stack is of good quality and the fusion site is large enough, screws, staples, or small miniplates can be used for fixation. Passive thumb movements are reassessed to assure thumb tip to finger pinch is still possible. The thumb is immobilized in a thumb spica splint or cast until bony union is achieved (usually 8 weeks).

## Outcomes

Outcomes of revision surgery for CMC arthroplasty are conflicting. Most of the evidence comes from small retrospective case series. Conolly et al. [60] reported a relatively low success rate after revision arthroplasty. They reviewed 17 patients with failed CMC arthroplasty, of which12 were primary silastic implant arthroplasty; they reported good results in 53% patients, fair results in 18%, and poor results in 29% [60]. They found a high rate of failure of revision surgeries for failed implant arthroplasty. Additionally, three of four patients with symptomatic impingement after LRTI were treated with a silastic implant and did poorly [60].

Papatheodorou et al. [59] had a higher rate of success. They reported on 32 patients who underwent soft tissue interposition and distracting pinning with or without ligament reconstruction after failed CMC arthroplasty. Good outcomes were reported in 84.4% patients and fair results in 15.6%. Pain was decreased in all patients and strength increased. Cooney et al. [9] also reported good results. They reviewed 17 arthroplasties

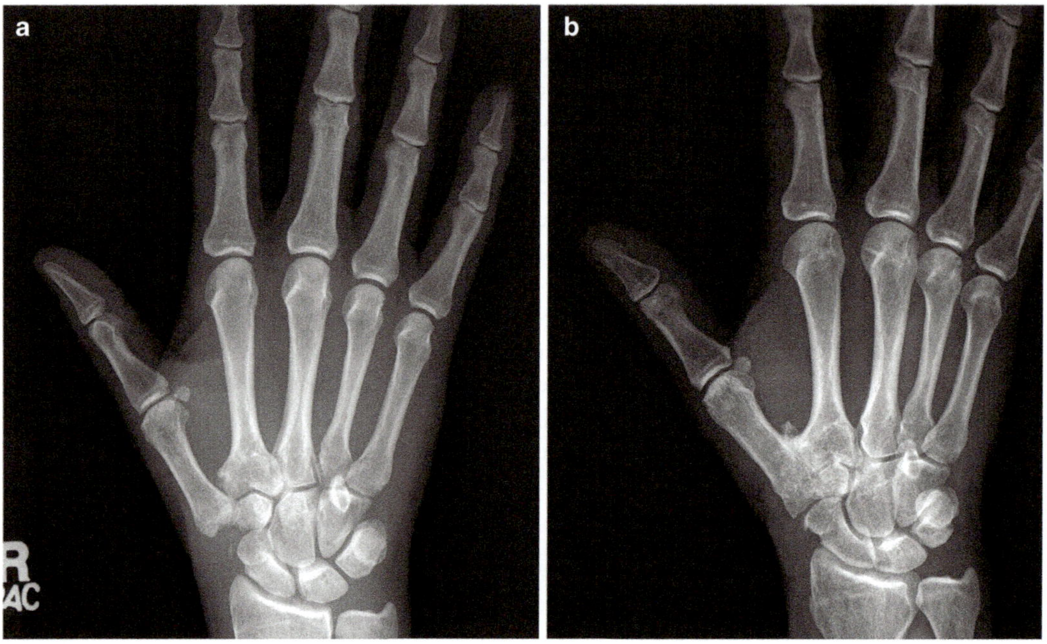


**Fig. 15.9** AP radiograph of a 50-year-old laborer with a failed prosthetic arthroplasty which was converted to trapeziectomy (**a**). Patient complained of ongoing pain and weakness with pinch. To provide stronger pinch, which was not provided by trapeziectomy alone, the patient underwent a fusion of the first metacarpal to second metacarpal base to relieve pain and resort pinch. Figure (**b**) shows AP radiograph of successful arthrodesis

requiring revision due to mechanical pain in 15 patients and reported good results in 76% revision surgeries, fair results in 12%, and poor results in 12%. The authors excluded patients with neuropathic pain in their paper.

Renfree et al. [64] studied 15 patients who underwent revision for continued pain after CMC arthroplasty. Overall, 75% of patients reported better function and capability of carrying out activities of daily living; however, half of patients continued to complain of moderate or severe thumb and hand weakness. Each patient had an average of 4.5 procedures with an overall rate of complication of 27% [64].

Mattilia has the largest series reporting 65 revisions in 50 patients out of a cohort of 1142 patients. According to the Connolly-Rath score, 54% of patients felt they achieved fair functional results, while only 8% had good and 10% had poor results. Regardless of these outcomes, most patients reported they had benefited from their revision surgery [8].

The salvage of prosthetic arthroplasty appears to be more favorable. Kaszap and colleagues reported on 15 patients who had failed prosthetic arthroplasty. A variety of prosthesis were used including in the study, including the de la Caffiniére (Howmedica, Inc., Newbury, UK), Elektra with screwed CoCr cup (Stryker Inc., Kalamazoo, MI, USA), Elektra with PE cup (Stryker, Inc.), and the Moje Acamo (Moje, Inc., Petersberg, Germany) device. A matched paired analysis was performed between patients who had undergone salvage of prosthetic arthroplasty to patients undergoing a primary trapeziectomy. Following removal of the trapezium and prosthesis, range of motion, Kapandji score, pain score, and DASH (Disabilities of the Arm, Shoulder, and Hand) score did not differ considerably from patients undergoing primary trapeziectomy. In particular, the results of strength testing were not significantly different between groups. This study suggests that secondary trapeziectomy, after failed trapeziometacarpal joint replacement arthroplasty, can do as well as those undergoing primary trapeziectomy [69].

Soft tissue revision arthroplasty has a higher success rates when the surgeon is treating ongoing mechanical pain. Treatment of neurogenic pain after peripheral nerve damage is challenging and is associated with a poor prognosis [64]. In a series of 16 patients, 4 patients with neuropathy of the SBRN were treated with neurolysis, and all continued to have poor results [10].

In general, the literature shows that the majority of patients benefit from revision surgery when mechanical etiology can be addressed; however, patients should be advised that improvement of symptoms is variable [10, 34]. With careful diagnosis of the cause of recurring pain, reasonable function and pain relief can be achieved. It appears that better results may be achieved in those with prosthetic replacement if converted to a trapeziectomy. Although generally only one revision is required, repeat revision surgeries are not uncommon and do not negatively affect outcome [8, 9].

## References


1. Van Heest AE, Kallemeier P. Thumb carpal metacarpal arthritis. J Am Acad Orthop Surg. Published online 2008. https://doi.org/10.5435/00124635-200803000-00005.
2. Gervis WH. Excision of th trapezium for osteoarthritis of the trapezio-metacarpal joint. Postgrad Med J. Published online 1948. https://doi.org/10.1136/pgmj.24.271.262.
3. Vadstrup LS, Schou L, Boeckstyns MEH. Basal joint osteoarthritis of the thumb treated with weilby arthroplasty: a prospective study on the early postoperative course of 106 consecutive cases. J Hand Surg Eur Vol. Published online 2009. https://doi.org/10.1177/1753193409105084.
4. Yao J. Suture-button suspensionplasty for the treatment of thumb carpometacarpal joint arthritis. Hand Clin. Published online 2012. https://doi.org/10.1016/j.hcl.2012.08.013.
5. Manrique OJ, Rajesh A, Asaad M, et al. Surgical outcomes after abdominoperineal resection with Sacrectomy and soft tissue reconstruction: lessons learned. J Reconstr Microsurg. 2020;36(1):064–72. https://doi.org/10.1055/s-0039-1697629.
6. Vitale MA, Taylor F, Ross M, Moran SL. Trapezium prosthetic arthroplasty (silicone, artelon, metal, and pyrocarbon). Hand Clin. Published online 2013. https://doi.org/10.1016/j.hcl.2012.08.020.
7. Garcia-Elias M, Tandioy-Delgado FA. Modified technique for basilar thumb osteoarthritis. J Hand Surg Am. Published online 2014. https://doi.org/10.1016/j.jhsa.2013.11.024.
8. Mattila S, Waris E. Revision of trapeziometacarpal arthroplasty: risk factors, procedures and outcomes. Acta Orthop. 2019;90(4):389–93. https://doi.org/10.1080/17453674.2019.1599253.
9. Cooney WP, Leddy TP, Larson DR. Revision of thumb trapeziometacarpal arthroplasty. J Hand Surg Am. Published online 2006. https://doi.org/10.1016/j.jhsa.2005.10.018.
10. Megerle K, Grouls S, Germann G, Kloeters O, Hellmich S. Revision surgery after trapeziometacarpal arthroplasty Arch Orthop Trauma Surg. Published online 2011. https://doi.org/10.1007/s00402-010-1128-x.
11. Hess DE, Drace P, Franco MJ, Chhabra AB. Failed thumb carpometacarpal arthroplasty: common etiologies and surgical options for revision. J Hand Surg Am. Published online 2018. https://doi.org/10.1016/j.jhsa.2018.03.052.
12. Mackinnon SE, Dellon AL. The overlap pattern of the lateral antebrachial cutaneous nerve and the superficial branch of the radial nerve. J Hand Surg Am. Published online 1985. https://doi.org/10.1016/S0363-5023(85)80076-9.
13. Clancey GJ. Radiograph assessment of the basal thumb joint. Orthop Nurs. Published online 1989. https://doi.org/10.1097/00006416-198907000-00021.
14. Patel TJ, Beredjiklian PK, Matzon JL. Trapeziometacarpal joint arthritis. Curr Rev Musculoskelet Med. Published online 2013. https://doi.org/10.1007/s12178-012-9147-6.
15. Degeorge BR, Pulos N, Shin AY. Obtaining a reliable scaphotrapeziotrapezoid radiograph: pronation, ulnar deviation, and thumb abduction. Tech Hand Up Extrem Surg. Published online 2018. https://doi.org/10.1097/BTH.0000000000000199.
16. Barron OA, Eaton RG. Save the trapezium: double interposition arthroplasty for the treatment of stage IV disease of the basal joint. J Hand Surg Am. Published online 1998. https://doi.org/10.1016/S0363-5023(98)80114-7.
17. Melville DM, Taljanovic MS, Scalcione LR, et al. Imaging and management of thumb carpometacarpal joint osteoarthritis. Skeletal Radiol. Published online 2015. https://doi.org/10.1007/s00256-014-1997-0.
18. Tuffaha SH, Quan A, Hashemi S, et al. Selective thumb carpometacarpal joint denervation for painful arthritis: clinical outcomes and cadaveric study. J Hand Surg Am. Published online. 2019; https://doi.org/10.1016/j.jhsa.2018.04.030.
19. Duncan SFM. Reoperative. Hand Surg. 2012; https://doi.org/10.1007/978-1-4614-2373-7.
20. Gangopadhyay S, McKenna H, Burke FD, Davis TRC. Five- to 18-year follow-up for treatment of trapeziometacarpal osteoarthritis: a prospective comparison of excision, tendon interposition, and ligament reconstruction and tendon interposition. J

Hand Surg Am. Published online 2012. https://doi.org/10.1016/j.jhsa.2011.11.027.
21. Kadiyala RK, Gelberman RH, Kwon B. Basal joint arthrosis: radiographic assessment of the trapezial space before and after ligament reconstruction and tendon interposition arthroplasty. J Hand Surg (British Eur Vol). Published online 1996. https://doi.org/10.1016/S0266-7681(96)80093-3.
22. Downing ND, Davis TRC. Trapezial space height after trapeziectomy: mechanism of formation and benefits. J Hand Surg Am. 2001;26(5):862–8. https://doi.org/10.1053/jhsu.2001.27761.
23. Field J, Buchanan D. To suspend or not to suspend: a randomised single blind trial of simple trapeziectomy versus trapeziectomy and flexor carpi radialis suspension. J Hand Surg Eur Vol. Published online 2007. https://doi.org/10.1016/j.jhsb.2007.02.005.
24. Bakri K, Moran SL. Thumb carpometacarpal arthritis. Plast Reconstr Surg. 2015;135(2):508–20. https://doi.org/10.1097/PRS.0000000000000916.
25. Davis TRC, Brady O, Dias JJ. Excision of the trapezium for osteoarthritis of the trapeziometacarpal joint: a study of the benefit of ligament reconstruction or tendon interposition. J Hand Surg Am. Published online 2004. https://doi.org/10.1016/j.jhsa.2004.06.017.
26. Kriegs-Au G, Petje G, Fojtl E, Ganger R, Zachs I. Ligament reconstruction with or without tendon interposition to treat primary thumb carpometacarpal osteoarthritis: a prospective randomized study. J Bone Jt Surg - Ser A. Published online 2004. https://doi.org/10.2106/00004623-200402000-00001.
27. Salem H, Davis TRC. Six year outcome excision of the trapezium for trapeziometacarpal joint osteoarthritis: is it improved by ligament reconstruction and temporary Kirschner wire insertion? J Hand Surg Eur Vol. Published online 2012. https://doi.org/10.1177/1753193411414516.
28. Davis TRC, Pace A. Trapeziectomy for trapeziometacarpal joint osteoarthritis: is ligament reconstruction and temporary stabilisation of the pseudarthrosis with a Kirschner wire important? J Hand Surg Eur Vol. Published online 2009. https://doi.org/10.1177/1753193408098483.
29. De Smet L, Sioen W, Spaepen D, van Ransbeeck H. Treatment of basal joint arthritis of the thumb: trapeziectomy with or without tendon interposition/ligament reconstruction. Hand Surg. Published online 2004. https://doi.org/10.1142/S0218810404001942.
30. Tägel M, Kopylov P. Swanson versus APL arthroplasty in the treatment of osteoarthritis of the trapeziometacarpal joint: a prospective and randomized study in 26 patients. J Hand Surg Am. Published online 2002. https://doi.org/10.1054/jhsb.2002.0836.
31. Belcher HJCR, Nicholl JE. A comparison of trapeziectomy with and without ligament reconstruction and tendon interposition. J Hand Surg Am. Published online 2000. https://doi.org/10.1054/jhsb.2000.0431.
32. Davis TRC, Brady O, Barton NJ, Lunn PG, Burke FD. Trapeziectomy alone, with tendon interposition or with ligament reconstruction?: a randomized prospective study. J Hand Surg Eur Vol. Published online 1997. https://doi.org/10.1016/S0266-7681(97)80426-3.
33. Song Y, Cox CA, Yao J. Suture button suspension following trapeziectomy in a cadaver model. Hand. Published online 2013. https://doi.org/10.1007/s11552-012-9473-6.
34. Sadhu A, Calfee RP, Guthrie A, Wall LB. Revision ligament reconstruction tendon interposition for trapeziometacarpal arthritis: a case-control investigation. J Hand Surg Am. 2016;41(12):1114–21. https://doi.org/10.1016/j.jhsa.2016.09.005.
35. Jones DB, Rhee PC, Shin AY, Kakar S. Salvage options for flexor carpi radialis tendon disruption during ligament reconstruction and tendon interposition or suspension arthroplasty of the trapeziometacarpal joint. J Hand Surg Am. Published online 2013. https://doi.org/10.1016/j.jhsa.2013.06.014.
36. Sonoda LA, Jones NF. Failed suture button suspensionplasty of the thumb carpometacarpal joint salvaged using pyrocarbon arthroplasty. J Hand Surg Am. Published online 2017. https://doi.org/10.1016/j.jhsa.2017.03.017.
37. Irwin AS, Maffulli N, Chesney RB. Scapho-trapezoid arthritis. A cause of residual pain after arthroplasty of the trapezio-metacarpal joint. J Hand Surg Am. Published online 1995. https://doi.org/10.1016/S0266-7681(05)80092-0.
38. Tomaino MM, Vogt M, Weiser R. Scaphotrapezoid arthritis: prevalence in thumbs undergoing trapezium excision arthroplasty and efficacy of proximal trapezoid excision. J Hand Surg Am. Published online 1999. https://doi.org/10.1053/jhsu.1999.1220.
39. Rizzo M, Moran SL, Shin AY. Long-term outcomes of trapeziometacarpal arthrodesis in the management of trapeziometacarpal arthritis. J Hand Surg Am. Published online 2009. https://doi.org/10.1016/j.jhsa.2008.09.022.
40. Damen A, Dijkstra T, Van der Lei B, Den Dunnen WFA, Robinson PH. Long-term results of arthrodesis of the carpometacarpal joint of the thumb. Scand J Plast Reconstr Surg Hand Surg. Published online 2001. https://doi.org/10.1080/028443101317149372.
41. Carroll RE, Hill NA. Arthrodesis of the carpometacarpal joint of the thumb. J Bone Joint Surg Br. Published online 1973. https://doi.org/10.1302/0301-620x.55b2.292.
42. Ishida O, Ikuta Y. Trapeziometacarpal joint arthrodesis for the treatment of arthrosis. Scand J Plast Reconstr Surg Hand Surg. Published online 2000. https://doi.org/10.1080/02844310050159828.
43. Bruehl S. An update on the pathophysiology of complex regional pain syndrome. Anesthesiology. Published online 2010. https://doi.org/10.1097/ALN.0b013e3181e3db38.
44. Perez RS, Zollinger PE, Dijkstra PU, et al. Evidence based guidelines for complex regional pain syndrome type 1. BMC Neurol. Published online 2010. https://doi.org/10.1186/1471-2377-10-20.
45. Armbruster EJ, Tan V. Carpometacarpal joint disease: addressing the metacarpophalangeal joint defor-

mity. Hand Clin. Published online 2008. https://doi.org/10.1016/j.hcl.2008.03.013.
46. Poulter RJ, Davis TRC. Management of hyperextension of the metacarpophalangeal joint in association with trapeziometacarpal joint osteoarthritis. J Hand Surg Eur Vol. Published online 2011. https://doi.org/10.1177/1753193411400359.
47. Munns JJ, Matthias RC, Zarezadeh A, et al. Outcomes of revisions for failed trapeziometacarpal joint arthritis surgery. J Hand Surg Am. Published online 2019. https://doi.org/10.1016/j.jhsa.2018.10.025.
48. Søndergaard L, Konradsen L, Rechnagel K. Long–term follow–up of the cemented caffinière prosthesis for trapezio–metacarpal arthroplasty. J Hand Surg (British Eur Vol. Published online 1991. https://doi.org/10.1016/0266-7681(91)90019-K.
49. de la Caffiniere JY, Aucouturier P. Trapezio-metacarpal arthroplasty by total prosthesis. Hand. Published online 1979. https://doi.org/10.1016/S0072-968X(79)80007-8.
50. Hansen TB, Homilius M. Failed total carpometacarpal joint prosthesis of the thumb: results after resection arthroplasty. J Plast Surg Hand Surg. Published online 2010. https://doi.org/10.3109/02844311.2010.483126.
51. Kaszap B, Daecke W, Jung M. High frequency failure of the Moje thumb carpometacarpal joint arthroplasty. J Hand Surg Eur Vol. Published online 2012. https://doi.org/10.1177/1753193412454252.
52. Badia A, Sambandam SN. Total joint arthroplasty in the treatment of advanced stages of thumb carpometacarpal joint osteoarthritis. J Hand Surg Am. Published online 2006. https://doi.org/10.1016/j.jhsa.2006.08.008.
53. Bricout M, Rezzouk J. Complications and failures of the trapeziometacarpal Maia® prosthesis: a series of 156 cases. Hand Surg Rehabil. Published online 2016. https://doi.org/10.1016/j.hansur.2016.02.005.
54. Cootjans K, Vanhaecke J, Dezillie M, Barth J, Pottel H, Stockmans F. Joint survival analysis and clinical outcome of total joint arthroplasties with the ARPE implant in the treatment of trapeziometacarpal osteoarthritis with a minimal follow-up of 5 years. J Hand Surg Am. Published online 2017. https://doi.org/10.1016/j.jhsa.2017.05.007.
55. Froschauer SM, Holzbauer M, Hager D, Schnelzer R, Kwasny O, Duscher D. Elektra prosthesis versus resection-suspension arthroplasty for thumb carpometacarpal osteoarthritis: a long-term cohort study. J Hand Surg Eur Vol. Published online 2020. https://doi.org/10.1177/1753193419873230.
56. de Aragon JSM, Moran SL, Rizzo M, Reggin KB, Beckenbaugh RD. Early outcomes of pyrolytic carbon hemiarthroplasty for the treatment of trapezial-metacarpal arthritis. J Hand Surg Am. Published online 2009. https://doi.org/10.1016/j.jhsa.2008.10.018.
57. Swanson AB, Swanson G de G, Watermeier JJ. Trapezium implant arthroplasty: long-term evaluation of 150 cases. J Hand Surg Am. Published online 1981. https://doi.org/10.1016/S0363-5023(81)80165-7.
58. Vitale M, Hsu C, Rizzo M, Moran S. Pyrolytic carbon arthroplasty versus suspensionplasty for trapezial-metacarpal arthritis. J Wrist Surg. Published online 2016. https://doi.org/10.1055/s-0036-1593735.
59. Papatheodorou LK, Winston JD, Bielicka DL, Rogozinski BJ, Lourie GM, Sotereanos DG. Revision of the failed thumb carpometacarpal arthroplasty. J Hand Surg Am. Published online 2017. https://doi.org/10.1016/j.jhsa.2017.07.015.
60. Conolly WB, Rath S. Revision procedures for complications of surgery for osteoarthritis of the carpometacarpal joint of the thumb. J Hand Surg Am. 1993;18(4):533–9. https://doi.org/10.1016/0266-7681(93)90166-D.
61. Eaton RG, Littler JW. Ligament reconstruction for the painful thumb carpometacarpal joint. J Bone Jt Surg - Ser A. Published online 1973. https://doi.org/10.2106/00004623-197355080-00010.
62. Diao E. Trapezio-metacarpal arthritis: trapezium excision and ligament reconstruction not including the LRTI arthroplasty. Hand Clin. Published online 2001;17(2):223–36.
63. Kakinoki R, Hashimoto K, Tanaka H, Akagi M. Suspension arthroplasty combined with ligament reconstruction of the thumb carpometacarpal joint to salvage two failed arthroplasties: a case report. J Orthop Case Rep. 2017;7(1):50–3. https://doi.org/10.13107/jocr.2250-0685.684.
64. Renfree KJ, Dell PC. Functional outcome following salvage of failed trapeziometacarpal joint arthroplasty. J Hand Surg Am. Published online 2002. https://doi.org/10.1054/jhsb.2001.0648.
65. Kokkalis ZT, Zanaros G, Weiser RW, Sotereanos DG. Trapezium resection with suspension and interposition arthroplasty using acellular dermal allograft for thumb carpometacarpal arthritis. J Hand Surg Am. Published online 2009. https://doi.org/10.1016/j.jhsa.2009.03.001.
66. Weilby A. Tendon interposition arthroplast of the first carpo-metacarpal joint. J Hand Surg Am. Published online 1988. https://doi.org/10.1016/0266-7681(88)90171-4.
67. Weilby A, Søndorf J. Results following removal of silicone trapezium metacarpal implants. J Hand Surg Am. 1978;3(2):154–6. https://doi.org/10.1016/S0363-5023(78)80064-1.
68. Shah A, Ellis RD. Thumb-index metacarpal arthrodesis for stabilization of the flail thumb. J Hand Surg Am. Published online 1994. https://doi.org/10.1016/0363-5023(94)90060-4.
69. Kaszap B, Daecke W, Jung M. Outcome comparison of primary trapeziectomy versus secondary trapeziectomy following failed total trapeziometacarpal joint replacement. J Hand Surg Am. Published online 2013. https://doi.org/10.1016/j.jhsa.2013.01.030.

# Part VI

# Metacarpophalangeal Joint Arthroplasty

# 16 Design Considerations for Metacarpophalangeal Joint Arthroplasty

Robert D. Beckenbaugh, William F. Ogilvie, and Jerome Klawitter

## Introduction

The metacarpophalangeal (MCP) joint is the ball and socket, diarthrodial (synovial) joint connecting the metacarpal and proximal phalangeal bones of the hand. The head of the metacarpal bone has a convex, generally spherical shape, and the base of the proximal phalanx has a shallow concave surface that mates with the metacarpal head. The MCP joint allows for three motions: flexion-extension, abduction-adduction (radial-ulnar), and pronation-supination (rotational). MCP joint stability, alignment, and motion are achieved by the combined actions of the shape of the articular surfaces of the bones, the joint capsule, ligaments, muscles, and tendons. The ball and socket shape of the articular surfaces resists subluxation and dislocation and allows for flexion-extension, abduction-adduction, and pronation-supination motion. The joint capsule, the collateral ligaments, the palmar ligaments, and the extensor hood form the MCP capsuloligamentous system that maintains joint alignment and resists joint subluxation and dislocation. The extrinsic muscles of the forearm act through the flexor and extensor tendons and together with the intrinsic muscles of the hand to form the MCP musculotendinous system that provides motion and power to the fingers.

R. D. Beckenbaugh (Deceased)
Department of Orthopedic Surgery, Mayo Clinic, Rochester, MN, USA

W. F. Ogilvie
Ensemble Orthopedics, LLC, Austin, TX, USA
e-mail: wogilvie@ensembleortho.com

J. Klawitter (✉)
Smith & Nephew, Austin, TX, USA
e-mail: jerry.klawitter@smith-nephew.com


G. J. W. King, M. Rizzo (eds.), *Arthroplasty of the Upper Extremity*,
https://doi.org/10.1007/978-3-030-68880-6_16

## Clinical Need

Hand surgeons attempt to relieve pain, correct deformity, restore function, and enhance the appearance of the metacarpophalangeal (MCP) joint in the diseased or injured hand. MCP joint pain, deformity, and dysfunction can result from rheumatoid arthritis, osteoarthritis, and post-traumatic conditions.

### Rheumatoid Arthritis

Rheumatoid arthritis of the MCP joint is a chronic, often progressive inflammatory disease where the earliest symptoms of pain and swelling are due to intra-articular synovitis. The synovitis may progress and lead to changes of the bone, cartilage, and the capsuloligamentous and musculotendinous systems of the MCP joint resulting in loss of hand function and deformity of the digits. Ulnar deformity of the digits can result from destruction of the joint capsule and ligaments, exaggeration of the ulnar shift of the flexor tendons, intrinsic muscle contractures, and collapse of the wrist with its associated radial deviation of the metacarpals. A volar subluxation deformity with eventual dislocation of the MCP joint may occur in rheumatoid patients if the palmar force exerted by the flexor tendons, when largely unopposed by ulnarly dislocated extensor tendons, overpowers the weakened capsular structures. Disease progression can also result in flexure contractures and rotation deformities of the MCP joint. Instability and misalignment of the other digits of the rheumatoid hand can further contribute to MCP joint deformity. Patients with rheumatoid arthritis often suffer a progressive loss of hand strength in addition to the disease-related deformities.

### Osteoarthritis

Osteoarthritis causes degenerative changes to and loss of joint cartilage that results in pain due to bone-on-bone contact at the articular surface of the MCP joint. Often the bone, joint capsule, ligaments, tendons, and muscles of the osteoarthritic MCP joint are near normal. Patients with osteoarthritis have digits with few deformities and the potential for near normal motion and strength. Limitations in hand function caused by osteoarthritis are most often due to the pain associated with joint motion.

### Post-Traumatic Arthritis

Post-traumatic arthritis results from a MCP joint arthrosis caused by injury. Post-traumatic arthritis of the MCP is like osteoarthritis of the MCP joint in that patients with post-traumatic arthritis often have the potential for near normal motion and strength but are functionally limited by the pain associated with joint motion.

## MCP Joint Arthroplasty

Surgical treatment for MCP joint pain and dysfunction is most often performed on patients with rheumatoid arthritis and includes synovectomy, soft tissue releases, arthrodesis, soft tissue arthroplasty, and joint replacement arthroplasty using a variety of prostheses. In cases where more conservative treatments have failed, relief of pain and restoration of function often require arthrodesis (fusion) or joint arthroplasty. Arthrodesis, while effective in eliminating pain, does not allow for joint motion and is functionally limiting. While resection arthroplasty and soft tissue arthroplasty remain surgical options, joint replacement arthroplasty using a prosthetic implant is considered more desirable [1]. MCP joint arthroplasty using a prosthetic joint replacement can be divided into three distinct procedures.

### Bone Surgery Procedure

The bone surgery procedure is when the prosthetic device is placed in the MCP joint. An osteotomy is performed to remove the diseased or damaged articular surfaces of the metacarpal and phalangeal bones and to provide sufficient space for the intra-bone portion of the MCP prosthesis. Removal of the ends of the bone requires care and precision so that the resulting cut surface of the bone mates accurately to the implant device. In addition to the osteotomy, the medullary cavity of the metacarpal and phalangeal bones is usually prepared, using a rotary burr or broach, to conform to the size and shape of the implant intramedullary stem.

### Soft Tissue Procedure

A soft tissue procedure is usually performed at the time of joint arthroplasty to reconstruct the capsuloligamentous and musculotendinous system. Reconstruction of the soft tissues helps restore proper joint alignment and joint stability after MCP arthroplasty using a prosthetic implant. This is especially true in cases involving rheumatoid arthritis where the joint aligning and stabilizing soft tissues are damaged.

An additional soft tissue reconstructive procedure may be required at some time after joint arthroplasty. This additional soft tissue procedure is performed to correct recurring deformity usually associated with the presence or progression of rheumatoid arthritis.

## Postoperative Care and Rehabilitation

Postoperative care and rehabilitation consisting of wound management, splinting, and exercise under the supervision of a hand therapist is performed after implantation of MCP joint replacement prostheses. Splinting and exercise programs will vary from patient to patient, as well as among different physicians. Regardless of patient or physician, however, a supervised postoperative therapy regime is essential in achieving successful results after replacement arthroplasty of the MCP joint. The postoperative care and rehabilitation portion of MCP arthroplasty lasts for a period of 12 weeks or more.

## Literature Review

A review of the medical literature describing MCP arthroplasty using a prosthesis provides a clear picture of the outcomes surgeons intend to achieve from the procedure and the complications encountered during treatment. The desired outcomes of MCP joint arthroplasty are (1) relief of pain, (2) improvement in hand function, (3) reduction or correction of finger deformity, (4) improvement in the appearance of the hand, and (5) obtaining a long-term result. In like manner, the complications encountered during MCP joint arthroplasty are (1) implant fracture, (2) adverse implant wear, (3) implant site infection, (4) adverse bone changes (fracture, resorption, cyst formation), (5) implant migration, (6) foreign body reaction, and (7) implant revision.

## MCP Joint Prostheses

Prostheses of many different designs have been implanted in the MCP joint. A variety of hinged (constrained) prostheses, single-piece flexible silicone rubber prostheses, and two-piece semi-constrained prostheses have been tried. Essentially all the various MCP implants reported in the literature rely on intramedullary stems, both with and without use of bone cement, to achieve prosthetic fixation.

### Hinged MCP Prostheses

Brannon and Klein implanted the first prosthesis into the MCP joint in 1953 [2]. The Brannon-Klein prosthesis is a hinged metal implant that saw very limited use. Numerous additional hinged MCP prostheses, including the Flatt [3], Steffee [4], Schultz [5], Nicolle [6, 7], KY Alumina [8, 9], and Isoelastic [10] prostheses, followed the pioneering work or Brannon and Klein. The Brannon-Klein and Flatt prostheses were fixed hinge, uni-axis implants that constrained motion to only flexion-extension. The fixed hinge, uni-axis designs evolved to two-part, snap-fit, linked implants, such as the Steffee and Schultz prostheses, which allowed for multi-axis motion with limits to the extent of flexion-extension, abduction-adduction, and pronation-supination. Fixed hinge, uni-axis and multi-axis, semi-constrained, hinge joint MCP prostheses are reported to have numerous shortcomings, as summarized below, and are no longer in use today:

1. Bone resorption resulting in implant subsidence, angular migration, cortical perforation, and implant loosening [2–4, 7, 10]
2. Frequent fractures occurring at the stem, axle, and the hinge portion of the prostheses [3–5]
3. Fracture of the metacarpal and phalangeal bones following surgery [10]
4. Peri-articular, hypertrophic bone formation resulting in reduced joint motion [5]
5. Recurrent deformities including ulnar deviation, subluxation and dislocation, and pronation and supination of the digits [2–5, 7, 10]
6. Infections and problematic healing [3, 7, 10]
7. Stiffness and limited joint motion [2, 5, 7, 9, 10]
8. Amputation [3]

### Flexible Silicone Rubber MCP Prostheses

The failure of hinged prostheses led to the use of medical-grade silicone rubber material to produce flexible MCP prostheses. The Swanson prosthesis was the first flexible silicone device to be implanted in the MCP joint. In general, flexible silicone MCP prostheses are one-piece devices having intramedullary stems to maintain alignment and an inter-bone spacer portion that prevents the ends of the bones from contacting each other. Separating the end of the bone with an inter-bone silicone material is intended to eliminate bone-to-bone contact and relieve pain. Four flexible silicone MCP joint prostheses are commercially available and in clinical use today in the Unites States. They are the following:

1. Swanson MCP joint replacement, produced by Wright Medical Technology
2. Stryker Silicone MCP joint replacement, produced by Stryker Orthopedics
3. NeuFlex® MCP joint replacement, produced by DePuy Synthes
4. Integra® Silicone MCP joint replacement, produced by Integra LifeSciences

#### Swanson Flexible Silicone MCP Prostheses

Development of the Swanson flexible silicone MCP prosthesis began in 1962 [11], and the first use was reported in 1966 [12]. Swanson describes flexible silicone MCP implants as dynamic spacers that maintain the internal alignment and spacing of the joint while acting as a mold to support the surrounding capsuloligamentous system [13–15]. The Swanson flexible silicone MCP is a cement-free prosthesis where MCP joint stability is said to be achieved by means of intramedullary stems, surgical reconstruction of the capsuloligamentous and musculotendinous systems, and encapsulation of the implant by dense fibrous tissue. The intramedullary stems of silicone MCP prostheses are reported to move freely (piston) within the medullary cavity increasing range of motion and prolonging implant life by reducing the stresses concentrations [16, 17]. In 1975 the medical-grade silicone material used to produce the original Swanson flexible silicone MCP prosthesis was replaced with a "high-performance (HP)" silicone elastomer intended to improve wear resistance and resistance to tear propagation. In 1986 another silicone material designated "HP 100" was introduced to further enhance wear and tear resistance [18]. Titanium grommets were introduced in 1987 to protect the silicone implants from abrasion and tearing resulting from contact with sharp bony edges [11].

#### Stryker Flexible Silicone MCP Prosthesis

The Stryker flexible silicone MCP prosthesis is a one-piece, cement-free, silicone elastomer implant having as its design origin the Niebauer Silicone-Dacron prosthesis first reported by Niebauer in 1968 [19]. The Niebauer prosthesis has a rectangular inter-bony hinge that is made of a silicone elastomer reinforced with Dacron cloth. Use of the Niebauer Silicone-Dacron prosthesis has been discontinued due to problems of high fracture rate and bone resorption [1, 20]. In the mid-1980s, the Sutter Corporation refined the design of the original Niebauer prosthesis resulting in an all silicone prosthesis that retained the hinge design of the Niebauer prosthesis. The Sutter MCP prosthesis is now being produced by Stryker and will hereafter be referred to as the Stryker silicone MCP prosthesis. The Stryker silicone MCP prosthesis differs from the Swanson silicone MCP prosthesis in two ways: (1) the intra-bone spacer portion of the Stryker silicone prosthesis is rectangular providing broad, flat surfaces to mate with ends (osteotomized surfaces) of the metacarpal and the proximal phalanx, and (2) the center of rotation of the Stryker silicone prosthesis is located in a more palmar position than that of the Swanson silicone MCP implant, thus increasing the extension moment and reducing the flexion moment as compared to the Swanson implant [21]. The stems of the Stryker silicone MCP prosthesis are smooth and have rectangular cross-sections that allow for a pistoning motion within the medullary cavity similar to the Swanson silicone MCP prosthesis. Two stem configurations are available, a straight stem and a stem having a pre-flex angle of 30°. The 30°pre-flex design is intended to approximate the anatomic position of the hand in the relaxed position reducing stress in the hinge during full flexion.

### NeuFlex® Silicone MCP Prosthesis

The NeuFlex® silicone MCP prosthesis is a one-piece, cement-free, flexible silicone implant with an inter-bone hinge portion like the Stryker silicone MCP prosthesis. The stems of the NeuFlex prosthesis are in 30 degrees of flexion mimicking the position of the MCP joint in the resting position.

### Integra® Silicone MCP Prosthesis

The Integra® silicone MCP prosthesis is a one-piece, cement-free, flexible silicone implant with an inter-bone hinge portion similar to the Stryker and NeuFlex® silicone MCP prostheses. The stems of the Integra prosthesis are in 30 degrees of flexion when the device is unloaded mimicking the position of the MCP joint in the resting position. The geometry of the inter-bone hinge portion and the intramedullary stems is the same as the Integra® PyC total MCP joint replacement so both can be used interchangeably. Design of the Integra® PyC total MCP prosthesis will be discussed in detail later in the chapter.

## Outcomes of Flexible Silicone MCP Prostheses

### Joint Pain

Assessment of preoperative and postoperative pain is often complicated in MCP joint arthroplasty because many of the patients have multiple joint disease and are on chronic anti-inflammatory or analgesic medications both prior to and after surgery. Additionally, assessment of pain is a subjective determination, and different methods are often used for the assessment making comparisons of result difficult. Mannerfelt et al. followed 144 Swanson implants in 50 rheumatoid arthritis patients for an average of 30 months (range 18–42 months) [22]. Preoperatively 36 patients had pain: 10 mild pain, 19 moderate pain, and 7 severe pain. Postoperatively 44 patients were pain-free, and 6 patients had mild pain. Blair et al. followed 115 Swanson implants in 28 patients for an average of 54 months and reported 71% have experienced significant pain relief [3]. Vahvanen and Viljakka report mild pain postoperatively in 16% of 32 patients with an average follow-up of 44.5 months (range 12–120 months) [23]. Kirschenbaum et al. report that one-third of 27 patients treated with 144 Swanson silicone MCP replacements had pain preoperatively and all of these patients were relieved of pain following surgery [24]. Olsen et al. followed 16 rheumatoid arthritis patients having 60 Swanson implants for an average of 7 years postoperatively (5–10 years range) and report pain relief was acceptable in 8 of the 16 patients [25]. Gellman et al. followed 901 Swanson implants placed in 264 patients for an average of 8 years and reported average preoperative pain of 2.9 on a scale of 0–10, with a score of 10 equaling as much pain as possible. Average postoperative pain decreased to a level of one. Nine percent of Gellman's patients had slightly increased pain postoperatively, 20% indicated their pain had slightly decreased, and 71% report improvement from their preoperative level of pain [26]. Hansraj et al. followed 170 Swanson implants for an average of 5.2 years (2–10 years range) and reported postoperative pain was found to be severe in 4% of the joints, moderate in 3%, slight in 39%, and not present in 54% [27]. Simmen and Gschwend et al. followed 207 Swanson implants for an average of 56 months and reported 87% with no pain, 12% light pain, and 1% moderate pain [28]. Poulenus et al. followed 88 implants for an average of 108 months and reported 99% were pain-free [29].

### MCP Joint Motion

Limited joint motion is an indication for MCP joint arthroplasty, and one of the goals of MCP joint arthroplasty is to (1) increase the arc of motion and (2) reduce extension deficit, i.e., relocate the arc of motion from a nonfunctional position to a more functional position. Table 16.1 summarizes MCP joint motion data from 14 publications reporting on a total of 2935 Swanson silicone prostheses with mean follow-up times ranging from 30 to 116 months. The data in Table 16.1 demonstrate that MCP arthroplasty

**Table 16.1** Range of motion for Swanson flexible silicone MCP prostheses

| Author | Number N of joints | Mean follow-up (mos.) | Preop active arc of motion (°) | Postop active arc of motion (°) | Preop extension deficit (°) | Postop extension deficit (°) |
|---|---|---|---|---|---|---|
| Kirschenbaum [24] | 144 | 102 | 27 | 44 | 63 | 16 |
| Gellman [26] | 901 | 96 | 40 | 50 | 50 | 10 |
| Hansraj [27] | 170 | 62 | 38 | 27 | 45 | 28 |
| Blair [3] | 115 | 54 | 26 | 43 | 60 | 13 |
| Bieber [30] | 210 | 63 | 17 | 39 | 56 | 22 |
| Swanson [17] | 170 | 70 | 46 | 38 | 26 | 6 |
| Beckenbaugh [31] | 186 | 32 | – | 38 | – | 10 |
| Vahvanen [23] | 107 | 44 | – | 34 | – | 7 |
| Wilson [32] | 185 | 116 | – | 29 | – | 21 |
| Fleming [33] | 339 | 66 | – | 47 | – | – |
| Simmen [28] | 207 | 56 | 37 | 32 | 36 | 13 |
| Rothwell [34] | 92 | 30 | 34 | 35 | 46 | 16 |
| Sollerman [35] | 21 | 54 | – | 42 | – | 11 |
| Poulenus [29] | 88 | 108 | – | 32 | – | 15 |
| Total | 2935 | | | | | |

using the Swanson flexible silicone prosthesis is more effective in reducing the extension lag than in increasing the arc of motion.

## MCP Joint Deformity

Blair et al. followed 115 Swanson flexible silicone prostheses implanted in 28 patients for an average of 54 months and reported 43% had recurrence of preoperative ulnar deformity and 27% ended up with a pronation deformity [3]. Ferlic et al. followed 162 Swanson flexible silicone prostheses implanted in 44 patients for an average of 38 months and reported 9% of the patients had a recurrent ulnar deformity ranging from 25° to 44° [36]. Kay et al. report that of the 31 of 34 patients having a preoperative ulnar deviation deformity, 13 (42%) were completely or moderately improved after MCP arthroplasty using a Swanson prosthesis and 18 (58%) were unchanged [37]. Wilson et al. followed 375 Swanson implants placed in 77 patients for 115.2 months and reported 43% had a recurrence of ulnar drift greater than 20° [32]. Kischenbaum et al. followed 144 Swanson prostheses implanted in 27 patients for 102 months and reported that preoperative ulnar drift averaging 28° was reduced to 7° postoperatively [24]. Bieber et al. report that for 210 Swanson prostheses implanted in 46 patients for an average of 63 months, the ulnar drift deformity was reduced from 25° preoperatively to 12° postoperatively [30]. Kay et al. report 94% of patients had preoperatively MCP joint subluxation, and 62.5% of these patients were improved after MCP joint arthroplasty with a Swanson prostheses [37]. Blair et al. report 28% of digits with Swanson prostheses had persistent extensor tendon subluxation or dislocation [3]. Wilson et al. report 17% postoperative MCP joint subluxation after MCP joint arthroplasty using a Swanson prosthesis [32]. Beckenbaugh et al. report 11.3% of 403 digits with Swanson prostheses had postoperative recurrent deformities including ulnar drift, subluxation, and digit rotation [31]. Rothwell et al. followed 92 Swanson implants for an average of approximately 30 months and reported a change in ulnar deformity from a preoperative value of 33° to 4° postoperatively [34]. Sollerman [35] et al. report a postoperative ulnar drift of 10° after a mean follow-up period of 54 months, and Poulenus [29] et al. report ulnar deformity of 11° for 88 Swanson implants followed for an average of 108 months. Poulenus [29] also report 7% of the Swanson implanted had dislocated. Simmen and Gschwend followed 207 Swanson implants for an average of 56 months and reported 11% persistent palmar subluxations, 82.6% of patients with ulnar deformity less than 10°, 16.4% with less than 30°, and 1% more than 30° [28].

### Hand Strength and Function

Blair et al. conducted hand strength and hand functional testing on 28 patients having 115 MCP arthroplasties using Swanson prostheses [3]. Functional tests included objective measurements of key-pinch and grip strength and a determination of the activities of daily living using a patient questionnaire rating the ability to perform 22 tasks. There was no significant objective measurement demonstrating improvement in key-pinch, grip strength, or activities of daily living following MCP joint arthroplasty using Swanson prostheses. However, when asked subjectively to rate satisfaction with hand function using a 5-point scale, 68% of Blair's patients felt their hand function was much improved. Fleming et al. report 79% of patients treated with Swanson prostheses felt subjectively better, 15% felt little improvement and 6% felt a decrease in function [33]. Olsen et al. report only 45% of patient's treated with Swanson prostheses regarded their hand function as better than before the operation and that his clinic has abandoned use of the Swanson silicone prosthesis [25]. Mannerfelt and Andersson report no significant gain in patient gross hand power and pinch strength following MCP joint arthroplasty using Swanson silicone prostheses, while, subjectively, 58% of patients thought they had an excellent functional result, 38% judged themselves improved, and 4% considered their condition unchanged [22]. Kay et al. report that a subjective assessment of daily activities by patients resulted in an 84% satisfactory rating and a 16% limited function rating [37]. Gellman et al. report that although most patients have no measurable increase in strength, most subjectively think their function is improved [26]. Bieber et al. report no change in objective determinations of grip and pinch strength for 210 digits with Swanson silicone MCP joint arthroplasties placed in 46 patients [30]. However, Bieber's patients' subjective impression of function, rated on a scale from zero to five, improved from the preoperative average of 1.9 to a postoperative average of 3.9. Beckenbaugh et al. report 42% of patients believed their hands were stronger after silicone MCP joint arthroplasty, whereas 26% believed their hands were weaker [31]. Beckenbaugh goes on to report that 60% of patients felt function was improved, 26% felt function was unchanged, and 14% felt function was worse. Rothwell et al. followed 92 Swanson implants for approximately 30 months, used the Baltimore Test of Upper Extremity Function (UEFT) to evaluate function after MCP joint arthroplasty, and reported a preoperative score of 71 (range 15–92) and a postoperative score of 90 (47–96). A UEFT score of 90 is considered a "functional" score showing capability to conduct a wide variety of day-to-day functions [34].

### Patient Satisfaction

Olsen report that 56% of patients reviewed after MCP arthroplasty with Swanson silicone prostheses were not satisfied with the result [25]. Vahvanen and Viljakka report 11% of patients judged the result after MCP arthroplasty with a Swanson prostheses as unacceptable [23]. Fleming et al. report 91% of patients interviewed were satisfied with the results of Swanson silicone MCP joint arthroplasty and 85% stated they would undergo the same surgery again [33]. Kirschenbaum et al. report a long-term study in which all 27 patients followed were satisfied with the function and appearance of their hand following MCP joint arthroplasty with Swanson silicone prostheses [24]. Beckenbaugh et al. report that 60% of patients believed the appearance of their hands improved and 72% believed that their hands improved generally [31]. Sixty-six percent of Beckenbaugh patients stated they would undergo the operation again, 20% said they would not, and 14% were undecided. Blair et al. report patient satisfaction after Swanson silicone MCP joint arthroplasty was high, stating that "Despite limited active motion of the metacarpophalangeal joint, a high rate of recurrence of finger deformity, and little measurable change in function of the hand, our patients remained satisfied with this procedure: they were pleased with the pain relief, and with the improvement in appearance of the hand, and 86 per cent of them stated that they would undergo the surgery again" [3].

## Implant Fracture

Fractures of Swanson silicone prostheses have been reported in several publications. Table 16.2 below presents the number of fractured implants as a percentage of the total number of implants in each of several 14 publications, representing 2804 implants with mean follow-up ranging from 30 to 102 months. Hagert et al. [12] report a detailed investigation of mechanical damage to 62 Swanson silicone prostheses implanted for periods ranging from 9 months to 5.5 years postoperatively and identified 3 types of damage to the implants: (1) surface damage, (2) cracking or fragmentation of the implant midsection, and (3) stem fracture. Hagert et al. report 4.8% of implants showed surface damage, 13.5% had cracking and fragmentation of the midsection, and 10.6% had fractured. The fracture rates for reported Swanson silicone prostheses and summarized in Table 16.2 range from 0% to a probable rate of 84%.

## Infection

Blair [3] et al. report an infection in three (2.6%) patients having Swanson silicone MCP joint arthroplasty requiring one amputation and removal of one prosthesis. Fleming et al. [33] report an infection rate of 0.03% for Swanson silicone MCP implants, Ferlic et al. [36] report an infection rate of 1.2%, Mannerfelt et al. [22] report an infection rate of 0.7%, Beckenbaugh et al. [31] report an infection rate of 0.6%, Bieber et al. [30] report an infection rate of 0.9%, Jensen et al. [38] report an infection rate of 2.7%, Maurer et al. [39] report an infection rate of 3.6% ,and Wilson et al. [32] report an infection rate of 1.3%

## Bone Changes

Blair et al. report cortical bone erosion about the stems of Swanson silicone MCP prostheses in 41% of implants and hypertrophic bone formation in 35% of implants [3]. Hagert et al. report that in areas where Swanson prostheses are in contact with bone, erosion was found in the metacarpal bone in 25% of joints studies, in the proximal phalanx in 22%, and in both bones in 53% [12]. Hypertrophic bone formation in the form of a bony spur located at the volar end of the metacarpal bone occurred in 64% of the joints Hagert studied [12]. Olsen and Sonne-Holm report bony erosions were found in the proximal phalanx in 17.6% of digits with Swanson silicone MCP prostheses [25]. Kay et al. followed nine patients having Swanson silicone MCP prostheses for a period of 5 years postoperatively and reported erosion of the radial aspect of the cortex of the shaft of the metacarpals, particularly the index, was seen in several

**Table 16.2** Fracture of Swanson prostheses

| Author | Number *N* patients | Follow-up (mos.) | Fractures confirmed | Fractures probable | Fractures confirmed + probable |
|---|---|---|---|---|---|
| Blair [3] | 115 | 54 | 21% | | 21% |
| Swanson [17] | 170 | 70 | 3% | | 3% |
| Ferlic [36] | 162 | 38 | 9% | | 9% |
| Olsen [25] | 60 | 84 | 18% | | 18% |
| Mannerfelt [22] | 144 | 30 | 3% | | 3% |
| Kay [37] | 34 | 60 | 50% | 32% | 84% |
| Vahvanen [23] | 107 | 44 | 4% | 10% | 14% |
| Gellman [26] | 901 | 96 | 14% | | 14% |
| Kirschenbaum [24] | 144 | 102 | 10% | | 10% |
| Hansraj [27] | 170 | 62 | 7% | | 7% |
| Hagert [12] | 62 | 42 | 11% | | 11% |
| Bieber [30] | 210 | 63 | 0% | | 0% |
| Fleming [33] | 339 | 55 | 4% | | 4% |
| Beckenbaugh [31] | 186 | 30 | 17% | 10% | 27% |
| Averages | 2804 | | | | |

cases [37]. Vahvanen and Viljakka report osteolysis and bone loss around the stem and hinge portion of Swanson MCP prostheses in 24% of the cases studied and bone overgrowth at the hinge in 9% of cases [23]. Wilson et al. report 14% of patients treated with Swanson silicone MCP prostheses had cortical erosions due to stem impingement [32]. Kirschenbaum et al. report some degree of collapse of the metacarpophalangeal joint spaces, and erosion of the metacarpals and phalanges was observed on last follow-up in all 144 arthroplasties studied [24]. Hansraj et al. report that 8% of digits with Swanson silicone MCP prostheses showed bone resorption adjacent to the implant and 48% of implants showed sclerosis [27]. Beckenbaugh et al. report excessive bone resorption or hypertrophic bone spur formation in 55% of MCP joints treated with silicone prostheses [31].

## Soft Tissue Reactions

Hirakawa et al. report billions of silicone particles, most of which are smaller than 1 μm, are present adjacent to failed silicone implants, and may be associated with inflammation and bone resorption [40]. Hansraj et al. followed 170 Swanson silicone MCP prostheses for an average of 5.2 years and reported severe synovitis was seen in 7% of MCP joints, moderate synovitis in 25%, slight synovitis is 17%, and no synovitis in 51% [27]. Post-implant synovitis is manifested as recurrent pain, synovial thickening, erythema around the joint, painful limitation of movement, and/or non-tender axillary lymphadenopathy. Synovial reactions to silicone particles in patients with rheumatoid arthritis are well recognized [31, 36, 41–43]. Lymphadenopathy associated with failed silicone implants has also been reported [41, 44–47]. However, silicone synovitis is rarely documented histologically after arthroplasty of the MCP joint with use of a silicone prosthesis, suggesting that silicone synovitis after joint arthroplasty using a silicone prosthesis is uncommon [3, 23–25, 37]. Wanivenhaus et al. studied 126 silicone prostheses, 49% of which were MCP implants, for an average follow-up of 116 months (SD 54.8 months) [48]. A radiographically intact osseous bed was found in 41% of the patients. The remaining 59% of implants showed varying degrees of destruction of the implant osseous bed. Osteolysis and bone cyst formation was reported in the implant osseous bed, and cyst formation was additionally reported in bones at a distance from the implant site. Histological examination in 11 cases revealed silicone particles surrounded by foreign-body giant cells that appeared like the tissue reaction seen with polyethylene wear debris. Fourteen percent of patients with silicone implants in situ for 1–3 years were found to have massive osseous bed lysis, and 55% massive osseous bed lysis was seen after more than 5 years' time in situ. Wanivenhaus et al. report no cases of silicone synovitis or lymphadenopathy and state that synovitis observed after implantation of silicone implants develops based on the primary disease – rheumatoid arthritis. Wanivenhaus et al. conclude that silicone wear particles lead to histiocyte reactions that result in lysis of the implant bone bed and the development of cysts in adjoining bone. They recommend that silicone implants be used only in cases where no alternative exists.

## Revisions

Gellman et al. report 6% of 901 Swanson silicone prostheses followed for an average of 96 months were revised due to fracture and 1% were revised due to infection [26]. Wilson et al. report 1.06% of Swanson silicone implants were revised with a replacement and 1.9% were removed but not replaced [32]. Hansraj et al. report 6.5% of Swanson silicone implants were revised during an average 5.2 year follow-up period and a survivorship rate of 90% at 10 years using Kaplan and Meier actuarial methods [27].

Literature describing outcomes for other flexible silicone MCP prostheses is more limited than for the Swanson MCP prosthesis. Bass et al. report on 168 Stryker MCP prostheses implanted in 34 patients and followed for an average of 27 months [18]. Twenty percent of the implants were shown to have fractured during the follow-up period and 45% followed for more than 3 years were found to have fractured. At the final follow-up examination, the average ulnar drift for non-fractured implants was 11° and in the fractured implants was 23°. Bass et al. report there was no correlation between implant fracture and patient satisfaction and that 80% of the patients said they would undergo the procedure again. However, Bass et al. stated that due to the high implant fracture incidence, they have abandoned use of the Stryker silicone MCP prosthesis. McArthur and Milner report a short-term randomized comparison of 41 Stryker MCP prostheses and 31 Swanson silicone MCP prostheses evaluated at period of 6 months and 12 months postoperatively [21]. They report no implant fractures were observed in either group. In the Swanson group, an increase in the arc of motion from 29° preoperatively to 36° was found at the 12-month follow-up assessment, and in the Stryker group, there was no significant difference between the arc of motion pre- and postoperatively. The extension deficit was reduced by 24° at the 12-month follow-up for the Swanson prosthesis and 16° at 12 months for the Stryker prosthesis. There was no significant difference in the preoperative grip strength between the Swanson and the Stryker groups. At 12 months the mean grip strength for the Swanson group had increase from a mean of 3.0 kgf to a significantly improved 6.0 kgf. The Stryker prosthesis increase from 4.5 kgf preoperatively to 6.5 kgf at 12 months, but the difference was not significant. Each group made a subjective assessment of pain, function, and aesthetic outcomes using a 5-point linear analog scale. The patients rated pain as reduced and function as improved and were very happy with the aesthetic result, and there was no difference between the two groups. Delaney et al. reported results of a double-blind clinical trial comparing Swanson and NeuFlex flexible silicone MCP joint replacements [49]. There were 37 implants in the Swanson group and 40 in the NeuFlex group. Assessments of range of movement, grip strength, and hand function were undertaken preoperatively and up to 2 years following implantation. There were no differences between the two groups in respect to arc of metacarpophalangeal joint motion, ulnar deviation, grip strength, or the SODA function test at follow-up. There was a significant difference in flexion, with mean active flexion values of 59° for Swanson implants compared to and 72° for NeuFlex implants. Escott et al. report results of a randomized prospective clinical trial comparing motion and function of Swanson and NeuFlex flexible silicone MCP joint replacements [50]. A total of 33 patients who had rheumatoid arthritis underwent primary MCP arthroplasty of all 4 fingers in 40 hands; 20 received Swanson implants, and 20 received NeuFlex implants. The primary outcome was active MCP flexion with secondary outcomes of active MCP extension, arc of motion, ulnar drift, grip strength, and assessment using the Michigan Hand Questionnaire. The two groups were not significantly different by individual digit for active MCP extension, ulnar drift, and composite flexion. Functional outcomes did not differ between groups. Active MCP flexion was significantly greater with NeuFlex implants compared with Swanson implants. Patients with Swanson implants reported higher Michigan Hand Questionnaire scores in the function and aesthetics. Boe et al. report long-term outcomes for 325 consecutive silicone MCP arthroplasties (type of silicone implant not reported) [51]. At a mean follow-up of 7.2 years, silicone MCP arthroplasty resulted in significant improvement in postoperative pain and arc of motion with no improvement in grip strength. Over the 14-year study period, 44 implants (13.5%) required revision surgery. The authors conclude silicone arthroplasty is a reliable option for improvement of pain, range of motion, and short-term ulnar drift with low revision rate. The authors counsel, however, that patients should he informed long-term implant fracture and progressive recurrence of deformity are expected and the risk appears to be substantial for osteoarthritis and post-traumatic patients.

### Summary: Flexible Silicone MCP Prostheses

MCP joint arthroplasty using flexible silicone MCP prostheses has been reported to relieve pain, improve the appearance of the hand, and reduce extension deficit. Flexible silicone MCP prostheses also are reported to result in a high rate of recurrence of deformity, a high fracture rate, adverse bone changes, and little measurable change in function of the hand. Limiting features are the following:

1. Flexible silicone MCP prostheses are interpositional spacers that do not restore the kinematics or joint biomechanics of the MCP joint.
2. Flexible silicone MCP prostheses are indicated for elderly patients who have gross deformity, but they are questionable for implantation in younger patients, who have a high grip strength and who have a further life expectancy.
3. Silicone wear debris results in histiocytic reaction leading to osteolysis and bone cyst formation.

Beevers and Seedhom [52] authored a review of the clinical results of past and current MCP prostheses and arrived at several conclusions which are worth re-stating:

1. "Flexible prostheses cannot transmit high forces, and are only reliable in rheumatoid hands with little grip strength. If they are placed in rheumatoid hands or osteoarthritic hands with high (normal) grip strength, fracture is more likely."
2. "Some silicone rubber or hinged prostheses may be considered to be satisfactory in elderly patients who have gross deformity, but they are certainly inadequate for implantation in younger patients, who have a high grip strength and who have a further life expectancy of 50 or more years, since fracture will occur very quickly after implantation. These patients who may have less advanced rheumatoid disease or post-traumatic OA will benefit from a surface replacement prosthesis which will restore the anatomy of the joint. It is important that ligaments and muscles surrounding the joint are still functional to provide joint stability."
3. "Surgical intervention is often deferred until the hand is grossly deformed. Often the structure of the MP joint is so badly affected at the time of operation that only a salvage procedure can be carried out to restore at best a small measure of function and improve appearance. If surgical intervention could be offered at an earlier stage of the arthritis, an MP surface prosthesis that more accurately restores the anatomy of the joint could be used. The natural biomechanics of the MP joint would then be restored and the large forces could be transmitted without fracture, allowing normal function."

## Semi-constrained, Two-Component MCP Prostheses

Two-component, semi-constrained MCP joint prostheses consist of individual, non-linked, metacarpal and proximal phalangeal components that utilize intramedullary stems for fixation. They typically are anatomic joint surface replacements that allow for a full range of unrestricted physiologic joint motion. Review of the literature identified four two-part, non-linked, total MCP joint prostheses: (1) WEL MCP prosthesis, (2) the digital joint operative arthroplasty (DJOA) MCP prosthesis, (3) the Stryker SR MCP prosthesis, and (4) the Integra® PyroCarbon (PyC) MCP prosthesis.

### WEL MCP Prosthesis

The WEL MCP prosthesis has a stainless steel metacarpal component with a spherical head and a fluted stem that is press-fit into the medullary bone bed after metacarpal osteotomy. The phalangeal component is similarly made of stainless steel and is press-fit into the phalangeal bone. The phalangeal component has a cup shaped, high-density polyethylene, articulating surface which is contoured to mate with the head of the metacarpal component. The literature reports use of one WEL MCP prosthesis in one patient. In September 1976, Welsh implanted one WEL MCP in the ring finger of a 17-year-old girl suffering from juvenile rheumatoid arthritis [53]. He published a case report in 1982 that reports the joint was stable and pain-free 4 years postoperatively. No other report of use of a WEL MCP prosthesis has been found.

## Digital Joint Operative Arthroplasty (DJOA) Prosthesis

The DJOA prosthesis consists of a stainless steel metacarpal component having a grooved stem portion coated with polyethylene. The articular surface of the metacarpal component is cylindrical with a circumferential protrusion at the center. The phalangeal component is made of polyethylene with an articular surface designed to mate with the stainless steel metacarpal head. Although the two components are not linked together, the protrusion on the metacarpal head engages a mating slot on the phalangeal component that restricts abduction-adduction and pronation-supination motion [54]. The DJOA prosthesis is to be implanted without bone cement and relies on a press fit for initial fixation. Rittmeister et al. [55] report on 19 DJOA prostheses implanted in 9 patients and followed for an average of 66 months. Postoperatively, the DJOA implants resulted in an extension deficit of 15° and an arc of motion of 29°. No patients subjectively scored the outcomes as "good," 11 scored "fair," and 8 scored "poor." Radiographic assessment showed that all 19 DJOA prostheses were subluxed. Ulnar deformities recurred in all patients. Migration of the proximal and distal tips in the radial direction occurred in eight joints and was associated with peri-prosthetic thinning of the cortical bone. All 19 DJOA implants migrated along the longitudinal axis of the finger. Longitudinal migration averaged 5 mm, ranging from 2 to 15 mm, and resulted in implant subsidence to such an extent that it restricted joint motion.

## Stryker SR MCP Prosthesis

The Stryker SR MCP is a semi-constrained implant designed for minimal resection of the effected MCP joint and preservation of the collateral ligaments. The proximal component is made from cobalt chrome, the distal component is made from polyethylene, and the implant is intended to be implanted with bone cement. The SR MCP implant is available for sale in the United States as a humanitarian use device. Humanitarian use is for conditions or diseases which typically affect fewer than 4000 people in the United States per year.

## Pyrolytic Carbon MCP Prosthesis

The pyrolytic carbon MCP prosthesis is a two-component device consisting of a pyrolytic carbon coating on a graphite substrate. The metacarpal component has a ball-shaped articular head and a stem with a rectangular cross section that is press-fit into the metacarpal bone bed after metacarpal osteotomy. The phalangeal component has a cup-shaped articular surface to mate with the ball-shaped metacarpal head, and a stem of rectangular cross section that is press-fit into the bone bed of the proximal phalanx. Cook et al. report the results of animal studies [56], Beckenbaugh reported preliminary favorable results from a clinical trial of a first-generation PyC total joint replacement design [57], and Cook et al. reported an 11.7 years long follow-up [58] of clinical trial outcomes. The first-generation PyC total MCP joint replacement served as the basis for a second-generation design described later in the chapter.

## Summary: Semi-constrained, Two-Component MCP Prostheses

Semi-constrained, two-component MCP prostheses have been found to relieve pain, enhance cosmetic appearance, and reestablish functional strength and joint motion. To perform these functions, semi-constrained, two-component MCP prostheses must have the following attributes:

1. Prosthesis should establish normal MCP joint geometry – size and shape – and maintain alignment of the articular surfaces and bones.
2. Prosthesis should possess sufficient strength and durability (wear and fatigue resistance) to withstand biomechanical forces of the normal MCP joint.
3. Prosthesis should achieve stable, long-term fixation.
4. Prosthesis should require minimal bone resection to preserve and maintain the joint capsuloligamentous and musculotendinous systems of the MCP joint.
5. Prosthesis should be made of a material that is biochemically and biomechanically compatible with bone and soft tissues.

## Biomechanics of the MCP Joint

Knowledge of biomechanics of the hand and MCP joint is essential for design of a joint replacement that will withstand forces acting on the implant. Osteoarthritic and post-traumatic joint arthroplasty patients have the potential for normal hand function, and a total MCP joint replacement must withstand the magnitude and direction of joint forces active in the normal healthy hand.

The MCP joint of the hand is a non-weight-bearing joint. Napier [59] and Landsmeer [60] divided the essential activities of the hand into the functions of power grasp and precision handling by means of pinch. The forces produced during high strength grasp and pinch hand functions result from isometric contractions of the extrinsic muscles of the forearm. The literature was reviewed to determine (1) grasp and pinch strength for normal and diseased hands; (2) the magnitude and direction of the MCP joint reaction force (JRF) resulting from the isometric functions of grasp and pinch; and (3) the JRF acting at the MCP joint during dynamic motion of the fingers.

## Hand Strength

Swanson [61] et al. investigated grasp and pulp pinch strengths for a normal population of 50 males and 50 females. Swanson results are presented in Table 16.3.

Walker [62] reported grasp and pulp pinch strengths for a normal population of males and females. Walker results are presented in Table 16.4.

Chao [63] et al. reported the grasp strength and tip and pulp pinch strengths for a population of 40 normal subjects (18 males and 22 females). Chao results are presented in Table 16.5.

**Table 16.3** Normal isometric hand strength measures – Swanson results

| Swanson hand strength | | | | |
|---|---|---|---|---|
| Function | Finger | Male (N) | Female (N) | F/M (%) |
| Pulp pinch | Index | 52 | 35 | 67% |
| Grasp | | 466 | 241 | 52% |
| | | | Average | 60% |

**Table 16.4** Normal isometric hand strength measures – Walker results

| Walker hand strength | | | | |
|---|---|---|---|---|
| Function | Finger | Male (N) | Female (N) | F/M (%) |
| Pulp pinch | Index | 73.5 | 55.5 | 76% |
| | Long | 65 | 48.8 | 75% |
| | Ring | 46.7 | 34 | 73% |
| | Little | 37.2 | 25.1 | 67% |
| Grasp | | 153.2 | 79.4 | 52% |
| | | | Average | 69% |

Weightman [64] report pinch strength for a group of 11 normal females for each of 5 different finger postures having MCP joint flexion angles ranging from 20° to 52°. Weightman results are presented in Table 16.6.

Boatwright [65] et al. report grasp strengths for a normal population of males and females divided into groups of less than and greater than 60 years of age. Boatwright results are presented in Table 16.7.

Josty [66] et al. report grasp strength for a normal population of males having different occupations. Josty results are presented in Table 16.8.

Swanson [61], Walker [62], and Chao [63] also report pinch strength for individual fingers. These data are summarized in Table 16.9.

The data presented in the series of tables above show grasp and pinch strength of the normal female hand to be approximately 60–70% that of the normal male hand. The first six tables indicate that for the normal male and female hand, the strength of the index and long fingers are essentially the same while the strengths of the ring and little fingers are about 67% and 47%, respectively, that of the index finger.

In addition to the strength of normal hands, several investigators report on the strength of diseased hands. Linscheid [67] reports the pinch strength of the diseased hand to range from 5 to 20 N, Hagert [68] reports the diseased hand to have a pinch strength of 20 N, and Walker [62] report the pulp pinch strength for the arthritic hand to be 13 N.

**Table 16.5** Normal isometric hand strength measures – Chao results

| Chao hand strength | | | | |
|---|---|---|---|---|
| Function | Finger | Male (N) | Female (N) | F/M (%) |
| Tip pinch | Index | 62.2 ± 9.8 | 46.7 ± 10.5 | 75% |
| | Long | 62.5 ± 18.8 | 45.1 ± 12.0 | 72% |
| Pulp pinch | Index | 63.7 ± 13.1 | 44.0 ± 8.9 | 69% |
| | Long | 61.6 ± 14.3 | 44.2 ± 8.9 | 72% |
| Grasp | | 363.1 ± 84.1 | 215.9 ± 60.8 | 59% |
| | | | Average | 70% |

**Table 16.6** Normal isometric hand strength measures – Weightman results

| Weightman hand strength | | |
|---|---|---|
| Function | MCP flexion° | Strength (N) |
| Index finger pinch postures | 15 | 35.8 |
| | 20 | 33.5 |
| | 29 | 34.8 |
| | 34 | 34.2 |
| | 52 | 34.3 |
| | Average | 34.5 |

**Table 16.7** Normal isometric hand strength measures – Boatwright results

| Boatwright hand strength | | | | |
|---|---|---|---|---|
| Function | Age | Male (N) | Female (N) | F/M (%) |
| Grasp | <60 years | 537 ± 91 | 332 ± 54 | 62% |
| | >60 years | 333 ± 98 | 207 ± 61 | 62% |
| | Average | 435 ± 95 | 269 ± 57 | 62% |

**Table 16.8** Normal isometric hand strength measures – Josty results

| Josty hand strength | | |
|---|---|---|
| Function | Profession | Male (N) |
| Grasp | Office worker | 446 |
| | Mechanic | 508 |
| | Farmer | 520 |
| | Average | 491 |

**Table 16.9** Normal isometric hand strength measures – summary results

| Summary pinch strength | | | | | |
|---|---|---|---|---|---|
| Investigator | Gender | Index | Long | Ring | Little |
| Swanson | Male | 100% | 104% | 71% | 43% |
| | Female | 100% | 105% | 69% | 47% |
| Walker | Male | 100% | 88% | 64% | 51% |
| | Female | 100% | 88% | 615 | 45% |
| Chao | Male | 100% | 97% | na | na |
| | Female | 100% | 100% | na | na |
| Average | Male | 100% | 96% | 68% | 47% |
| | Female | 100% | 98% | 65% | 46% |
| | M & F | 100% | 97% | 66% | 47% |

## Conclusions

1. Average grasp strength for normal male dominant hand = approximately 380 N.
2. Average pinch strength for the index finger of the normal male dominant hand = approximately 60 N.
3. Average grasp strength for normal female hand = approximately 60% of the strength of the normal male hand.
4. Average pinch strength for normal female hand = approximately 70% of the strength of the normal male hand.
5. Relative strength of the fingers for the normal male and female hand:
   index, 1.00; long, 1.00; ring, 0.67; and little, 0.47.
6. The pinch strength of the diseased arthritic hand has been observed to range from 5 to 20 N, which is about 10–30% of normal strength.

## MCP Joint Reaction Force

### Isometric Hand Function

Biomechanical analyses determining the magnitude and direction of the MCP JRF for the isometric hand function of pinch and grasp have been reported by Weightman [64], Chao [69], and Berme [70]. The biomechanical analyses are based on the shape of the bones and the structure and function of the tendons, ligaments, and muscles and apply to both the male and female hand. The bones of the MCP joint and the coordinate system used by Chao are shown in Fig. 16.1. For the sake of uniformity and comparison, the data reported by Berme and Weightman will be represented using Chao's coordinate system and nomenclature (Fig. 16.1).

Chao et al. report a three-dimensional force analysis for hand functions of pinch and grasp consisting of a multiple mechanical linkage of the bones of the hand and accounting for the active forces of tendons and muscles. The analyses apply a unit external load to the finger in a manner corresponding to a specific hand function. The resulting JRF is calculated as a dimensionless multiple of the unit external force. Chao's results are shown in Table 16.10.

Berme et al. [70] conducted a three-dimensional biomechanical analysis of the MCP joint of the index finger and combined the results with pinch function measurements made on four individuals to calculate JRFs. Although Berme did not define the pinching function as being a tip pinch or pulp pinch, an illustration presented in the text of his paper indicates a pulp pinch was used. Berme reported the magnitude of the external force applied to the index finger and calculated the components of the resulting JRF. For the sake of comparison, the JRFs reported by Berme were transformed from newtons (N) to a dimensionless multiple of a unit external applied force, and the results are shown in Table 16.11.

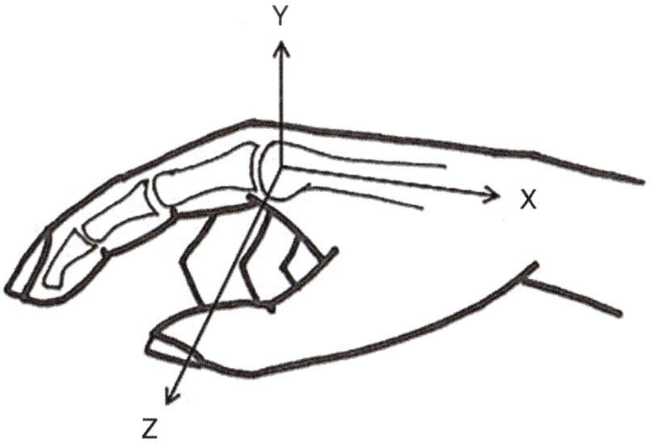


**Fig. 16.1** Coordinate system for hand measurements by Chao

**Table 16.10** MCP joint reaction force – Chao results

| Chao joint reaction force | | | | | |
|---|---|---|---|---|---|
| Dimensionless MCP joint reaction force: index finger | | | | | |
| | | Multiple of unit applied force | | | |
| Function | Flexion angle° | *X* | *Y* | *Z* | Resultant |
| Tip pinch | 48 | −3.5 ~ −3.9 | 2.1 ~ 2.3 | 0.1 ~ 0.2 | 4.3 |
| Pulp pinch | 48 | −4.0 ~ −4.6 | 2.2 ~ 2.4 | 0.1 ~ 0.1 | 4.9 |
| Grasp | 62 | −3.2 ~ −3.7 | 2.9 ~ 3.1 | 0.3 ~ 0.4 | 4.6 |

Weightman [64] conducted a two-dimensional biomechanical analysis to determine the MCP JRF resulting from five pinching postures, each pinching posture having a different MCP joint flexion angle. Weightman reported MCP JRFs as a dimensionless multiple of a unit external applied force, and the results are shown in Table 16.12.

As illustrated in the previous tables, biomechanical analyses conducted by Chao, Berme, and Weightman have determined the dimensionless MCP JRF for pinching function of the index

**Table 16.11** MCP joint reaction force – Berme results

| Berme joint reaction force | | | | | |
|---|---|---|---|---|---|
| Dimensionless joint reaction force: index finger pinch | | | | | |
| | | Multiple of unit applied force | | | |
| Flexion angle° | | *X* | *Y* | *Z* | Resultant |
| Subject 1 | 40 | 4.6 | 1.7 | 0 | 4.9 |
| Subject 2 | 60 | 4.9 | 5.6 | 0 | 7.4 |
| Subject 3 | 35 | 5.1 | 1.6 | 0 | 5.4 |
| Subject 4 | 35 | 2.8 | 2.9 | 0 | 4.1 |
| | Average | 4.3 | 3.1 | 0 | 5.5 |

**Table 16.12** MCP joint reaction force – Weightman results

| Weightman joint reaction force | | |
|---|---|---|
| Dimensionless joint reaction force index finger pinch | | |
| Posture | Flexion angle° | Resultant multiple of applied unit force |
| Posture 1 | 20 | 5.6 |
| Posture 2 | 52 | 4.8 |
| Posture 3 | 34 | 4.3 |
| Posture 4 | 29 | 3.9 |
| Posture 5 | 15 | 3.5 |
| | Average | 4.4 |

finger (male or female) to be relatively constant, having mean values of 4.3 (tip pinch) and 4.9 (pulp pinch), 5.5, and 4.4, respectively. The three-dimensional biomechanical analyses conducted by Chao and Berme demonstrate the JRF for pinching lies essentially in the X-Y (flexion-extension) plane. Weightman compared the results of his two-dimensional analysis with the three-dimensional analyses of Chao and Berme and concluded that pinching was accurately represented by a two-dimensional (flexion-extension) analysis. The results of Chao's analysis also demonstrate that the joint reaction force resulting from the grasp hand function lies essentially in the X-Y (flexion-extension) plane. The assumption that pinch and grasp are two-dimensional hand functions allows for a depiction of the magnitude and direction of the joint forces as is shown in Fig. 16.2.

Biomechanical analyses demonstrate that the primary components of the JRF acting at the MCP joint are (1) a normal force acting to push the metacarpal and phalangeal bones together and (2) a dorsovolar (shear) force acting to sublux the phalangeal bone in the volar (palmar) direction. The components of the joint force reported by Chao and Berme establish the direction of the JRF. A positive JRF angle, as shown in Fig. 16.2 indicates a dorsally directed force on the phalanx. Weightman's biomechanical analysis assumed the direction of the JRF to be 15° for one pinch posture and 20° for the other four pinching postures. Table 16.11 summarizes the MCP flexion angles and the corresponding JRF angles calculated from X-Y components of the JRFs reported by Chao and Berme. The JRF

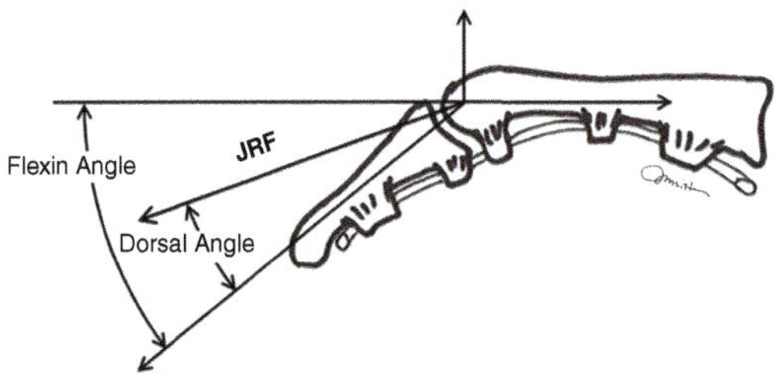


**Fig. 16.2** Two-dimensional representation of MCP joint reaction force

**Table 16.13** MCP joint reaction force angle – summary results

| Summary joint reaction force | | |
|---|---|---|
| Finger function | MCP flexion° | JRF angle° |
| Chao | | |
| Tip pinch | 48 | 17 |
| Pulp pinch | 48 | 20 |
| Grasp | 62 | 21 |
| Berme | | |
| Subject 1 | 40 | 20 |
| Subject 2 | 60 | 11 |
| Subject 3 | 35 | 18 |
| Subject 4 | 35 | 19 |
| Weightman | | |
| Pinch posture 1 | 20 | 15 |
| Pinch posture 2 | 52 | 20 |
| Pinch posture 3 | 34 | 20 |
| Pinch posture 4 | 29 | 20 |
| Pinch posture 5 | 15 | 20 |
| | Average | 18.4 |

angles reported by Weightman are also shown in Table 16.13.

The data demonstrate that the dorsal angle of the MCP JRF averages approximately 18.5° and is relatively constant for pinch and grasp hand functions with MCP joint flexion angles ranging from 15 to 62°. It is concluded from the biomechanical analyses presented above that MCP joint reaction forces for pinch and grasp hand functions (1) lie primarily in the flexion-extension plane; (2) are approximately five times that of the external force applied to the finger; and (3) are inclined to the phalanx at a constant dorsal angle of approximately 20°.

Dimensionless JRFs obtained from the biomechanical modeling for a specific hand function can be converted to JRFs expressed in newtons by multiplying the dimensionless JRF by the appropriate value of hand strength determined experimentally. Hand strength measurements, presented earlier in this literature review, show pinch strength for a healthy male index finger to be approximately 60 N. Combining the 60 N pinch strength with the five times dimensionless multiplier results in a JRF of approximately 300 N for the index finger of a healthy adult male hand.

**Table 16.14** MCP joint reaction force – Chao results

| Chao joint reaction force | | | | | |
|---|---|---|---|---|---|
| MCP joint reaction force magnitude: index finger | | | | | |
| | | Joint reaction force (N) | | | |
| Function | Flexion angle° | X | Y | Z | Resultant |
| Tip pinch | 48 | 175 ~ 196 | 104 ~ 116 | 7.7 ~ 8.7 | 204 ~ 228 |
| Pulp pinch | 48 | 199 ~ 228 | 107 ~ 121 | 3.8 ~ 5.8 | 226 ~ 258 |
| Grasp | 62 | 219 ~ 253 | 198 ~ 213 | 21 ~ 25 | 296 ~ 332 |

**Table 16.15** Estimates of maximum joint reaction forces

| Maximum joint reaction force magnitude | | | | |
|---|---|---|---|---|
| | Joint reaction force (N) | | | |
| Gender | Index | Long | Ring | Little |
| Healthy male | 350 | 350 | 232 | 163 |
| Healthy female | 245 | 245 | 162 | 114 |

A similar determination of the index finger JRF for the grasp cannot be made directly from grasp strengths measurements because grasp strength is the combined result of all the fingers of the hand. However, Chao [69] devised a method for measuring the contribution of individual fingers to the overall grasp strength and reported the index finger MCP JRF in newtons resulting from the grasp hand function as shown in Table 16.14. Table 16.14 also shows JRF data for tip pinch and pulp pinch functions. The JRF magnitudes shown are the values Chao recommends be used to provide strength requirements for prosthetic joint design and for development of bench test criteria to perform laboratory evaluations of artificial finger joint implant devices.

The JRFs recommended by Chao for determining strength requirements for finger joint implants give an upper range of 258 N for index finger pinch and a somewhat greater value of 332 N for grasp. The value of 258 N for pinch is less than, but in general agreement with, the 300 N value calculated from a compilation of literature values for healthy male index finger strength and dimensionless JRF magnitudes. Based on these data, the maximum JRF for the MCP joint of the index of the healthy adult male hand grasp was considered to be 350 N. The 350 N value for grasp JRF is somewhat greater than that recommended by Chao to provide the strength requirement for prosthetic joint design.

Establishing the maximum joint reaction force for the MCP joint for the index finger of the healthy adult male hand allows for estimation of the maximum MCP JRF for the other fingers of the healthy adult male and female hand. Estimation of the joint reaction forces for all MCP joints of the hand is based upon (1) the relative strength of the fingers with index, 1; long, 1; ring, 0.66; and little, 0.47 and (2) the female hand having 70% the strength of the male hand. Table 16.15 shows the maximum JRF estimated for the MCP joints for healthy male and female hands.

## Dynamic Hand Function

The maximum JRF at the MCP joint during isometric function of the hand is useful in determining the strength requirements for artificial joint replacements. JRF at the MCP joint during dynamic function of the hand is of interest in developing laboratory tests to evaluate wear of artificial joint replacements. During flexion and extension, Beevers and Seedhom [71] report there is only a small load acting on the MCP joint. Tamai et al. [72] report a compression force at the MCP joint of approximately 14 N when maintaining the joint in the neutral position with a balance of muscle forces and a compression force of approximately 20 N when maintaining the MCP joint at 45 degrees of flexion. Sibly and Unsworth [73] report fingers are lightly loaded when they move and estimate the normal forces at the MCP joint to be less than 10 N. Stoke [74] reported development of an MCP joint simulator which reproduced flexion-extension motion by means of cables which mimicked the flexor and extensor tendons and fixed and movable pulleys which mimicked the tendon sheaths and volar plate. The simulator resulted in a joint force having a magnitude of 10 N–15 N for flexion angles of 10–90°. In addition to the forces acting on the MCP during movement, Dumbleton [75] reported that the sliding velocity for the surfaces of the MCP joint can be as high as 200 mm/second.

## Conclusions

The literature reporting biomechanical evaluations of pinch and grasp hand functions was reviewed to determine the magnitude and direction of an MCP JRF suitable to establish the strength requirement for MCP joint implant design and testing. The most demanding hand function was found to be grasp. The JRF establishing the implant design criteria is characterized as follows:

1. MCP joint flexion for isometric grip function = 60°
2. Magnitude of MCP JRF for isometric grip function = 350 N
3. Direction of MCP JRF = 20° dorsal angle
4. Magnitude of MCP JRF for dynamic hand function = 20 N
5. Maximum sliding velocity for MCP joint = 200 mm/second

## Total MCP Joint Arthroplasty

Design and manufacture of a functional and durable total MCP joint arthroplasty is a complex and multifaceted problem involving anatomical, biocompatibility, biomechanical, and surgical considerations. From a functional perspective, mechanical design considerations address the joint range of motion, force transmission capabilities, and wear resistance of the components. Anatomical issues involve the sites of tendon and ligament insertion, centers of rotation, the size and shape of the articulating surfaces and intramedullary canals, and the need for a range of sizes to accommodate the vast majority of arthroplasty patients. Surgical considerations include the need of instrumentation to facilitate an accurate osteotomy, achieve minimal bone removal, preserve supporting soft tissues, and achieve accurate placement of the prosthesis.

Design of a second-generation PyC total MCP joint prosthesis will be used to illustrate the design principles and processes. The objective is to develop a prosthesis to replace diseased and damaged MCP joints to relieve pain and restore strength and motion. To meet this objective, a comprehensive product development and quality assurance program is used to develop a prosthesis that meets the anatomic, kinematic, and biomechanical needs of a functional and durable total MCP joint arthroplasty.

## PyC Total MCP Joint

Development of PyC MCP prostheses dates to the late 1970s. At that time, researchers at Tulane University were interested in the use of PyC as an orthopedic joint replacement because its successful history of use in artificial mechanical heart valves proved the material to be biocompatible, to have high strength, and to be fatigue and wear resistant. Also, at that time, Robert Beckenbaugh, MD, hand surgeon at the Mayo Clinic, was interested in improving outcomes of MCP joint arthroplasty. Dr. Beckenbaugh's interest in improving MCP joint arthroplasty resulted in design of a ball and socket total MCP joint arthroplasty made of PyC. Prototypes were produced and implanted in baboons in collaboration with Jerome Klawitter, PhD, at the Tulane University in 1977. Results from the animal study were favorable and demonstrated the potential for a total MCP joint arthroplasty made of PyC [56]. Based on the animal study, a clinical trial was initiated at the Mayo Clinic. Between 1979 and 1987, 151 PyC total MCP joint prostheses having the same design as used in the animal study were implanted in 53 patients. Of the 151 implants in 53 patients, 26 patients (71 implants) were available for review at an average of 11.7 years (range, 10.1–16.0 years) after implantation. Three patients (11 implants) were lost to follow-up, and 20 patients (51 functioning implants) died after the implant had been in situ for an average of 7.2 years, and 18 implants in 11 patients were revised. Results of the clinical trial demonstrate PyC is a biologically and biomechanically compatible, wear-resistant, and durable material for total metacarpophalangeal joint arthroplasty [58]. The PyC implants used in the animal study and clinical trial were produced by CarboMedics, Inc., Austin, TX. CarboMedics business was producing PyC heart valves, and it was not interested in developing PyC for orthopedic use and only produced enough PyC MCP prostheses to use in the clinical trial.

## Second-Generation PyC Total MCP Joint Arthroplasty

In 1996 Ascension Orthopedics, Inc., began a collaboration with Dr. Beckenbaugh to develop and commercialize a second-generation PyC MCP arthroplasty (SG PyC MCP). Clinical experience gained during clinical trial of the first-generation PyC MCP identified shortcomings in the design, and Ascension Orthopedics Inc., working with Dr. Beckenbaugh, refined the design resulting in the SG PyC MCP prosthesis. Development of the SG PyC MCP followed the principles of design control: (1) identify user needs, (2) conduct risk assessment, (3) establish design inputs, (4) conduct design process, (5) verify design outputs, and (6) validate that the device meets user needs. Figure 16.3 illustrates the shape of the first-generation PyC MCP and that of the SG PyC MCP implant. Table 16.16 gives dimensions of both implants. The SG PyC MCP is currently manufactured and distributed by Integra LifeSciences as the Integra® PyroCarbon MCP Total Joint.

The first-generation PyC MCP prosthesis used in the clinical trial and the SG PyC MCP are both two-part, unconstrained, ball and socket designs. Design refinements incorporated in the SG PyC MCP are based on anatomic, kinematic, biomechanical, device strength and durability, and surgical considerations. The design process combined past surgical and clinical experience,

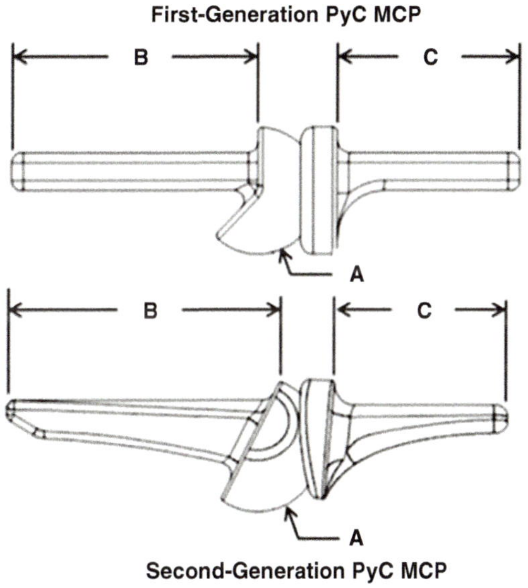


Fig. 16.3 Illustrations of the first-generation PyC MCP and SG PyC MCP

Table 16.16 Dimensions of the first-generation and SG PyC MCP prostheses

| Design | Size | A mm | B mm | C mm |
|---|---|---|---|---|
| | | Metacarpal head diameter | Metacarpal stem length | Phalangeal stem length |
| First-generation PyC MCP joint arthroplasty | Small | 8.2 | 25.0 | 17.8 |
| | Medium | 10.2 | 25.0 | 18.0 |
| | Large | 12.8 | 25.0 | 19.3 |
| Second-generation MCP joint arthroplasty | 5 | 9.8 | 16.5 | 14.1 |
| | 10 | 9.8 | 19.3 | 15.6 |
| | 20 | 11.3 | 23.0 | 16.7 |
| | 30 | 12.9 | 26.6 | 18.3 |
| | 40 | 14.6 | 30.2 | 21.2 |
| | 50 | 16.4 | 33.7 | 22.8 |

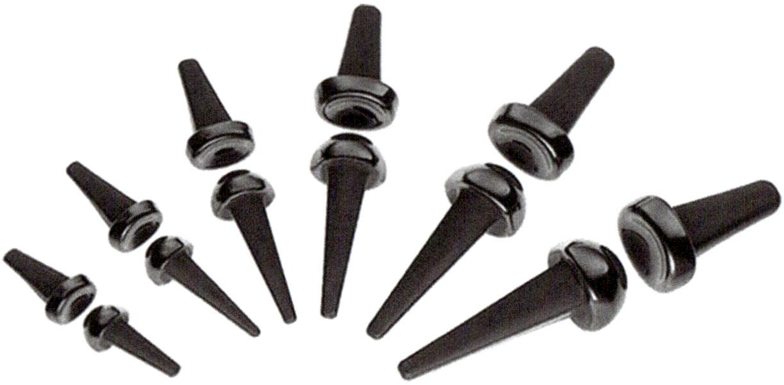

**Fig. 16.4** Six sizes of the SG PyC MCP prosthesis

published data describing structure and function of the hand and MCP joint, in vitro testing, and numerous cadaver laboratory sessions to assess form and function.

## Sizes

The SG PyC MCP is provided in six sizes as illustrated in Fig. 16.4. Six sizes were developed to allow surgeons the ability to accommodate a wide range of anatomical needs. Six sizes minimize the difference between adjacent sizes allowing for a more accurate anatomic fit. The number of sizes was based on past surgical experience and published data describing the size and shape of the human MCP joint. Table 16.17 shows dimensions of the MCP joint reported by Unsworth and Alexander [76].

## Preservation of Joint Ligaments

The articular surface of the SG PyC MCP metacarpal component terminates at a planar subarticular collar. In contrast, the metacarpal collar on the clinical trial design component consists of intersection planes. Intersection planes required the surgeon to create two accurate intersecting osteotomies to mate with those of the prosthesis resulting in a demanding surgical technique. The single, planar subarticular collar greatly simplifies the osteotomy. The subarticular collars are inclined to the long axis of the device at 118° degrees for the metacarpal component and 85° for the phalangeal component (Fig. 16.5). The inclined collars minimize resection at the dorsal aspect of the metacarpal neck and the palmar aspect of the proximal phalangeal neck preserving the insertion sites for the collateral and accessory ligaments as shown in Fig. 16.6. Additionally, relief planes are provided on the dorsal-ulnar and dorsal-radial aspects of the articular surface of the metacarpal component. The relief planes provide a free, non-interfering pathway for the collateral ligaments.

## Phalangeal Dorsal Prominence

A feature of the SG PyC MCP phalangeal component is a proximal rim that is inclined to the subarticular collar at 10° as shown in Fig. 16.7. Inclination of the proximal rim provides a dorsal prominence to resist palmar subluxation. In conjunction with the 85° inclination of the subarticular collar, the inclined proximal rim diminishes the bulk of the phalangeal component in the palmar location so as not to interfere with the path of the collateral or palmar ligaments.

## Spherical Center of Rotation and "Stem Offset"

The spherical center of the SG PyC MCP metacarpal component is offset from the long axis of the stem in the palmar direction to reestablish the anatomic center of rotation of the joint. Also, the location of the phalangeal component stem is similarly offset. As shown in Table 16.18, the stem offset increases with increasing implant size. The magnitude of stem offset was established by evaluating prototype designs for extension lag and hyperextension in the cadaver laboratory setting.

**Table 16.17** Dimension of the human MCP joint

| Position of medullary cavity with respect to metacarpal center of rotation, mm | | | | | | | | |
|---|---|---|---|---|---|---|---|---|
| | Sagittal plane | | | | Transverse plane | | | |
| | Metacarpal | | Proximal phalanx | | Metacarpal | | Proximal phalanx | |
| | Dorsal | | Dorsal | | Ulnar | | Ulnar | |
| Finger | Avg | SD | Avg | SD | Avg | SD | Avg | SD |
| Index | 2.18 | 0.97 | 0.89 | 1.23 | 0.55 | 1.91 | 0.16 | 1.02 |
| Long | 2.67 | 0.74 | 1.35 | 1.67 | 0.33 | 1.91 | 0.28 | 2.14 |
| Ring | 2.58 | 0.59 | 1.62 | 1.07 | 0.66 | 0.93 | 0.02 | 1.58 |
| Little | 2.46 | 0.44 | 0.90 | 1.35 | 0.16 | 1.48 | -0.14 | 0.59 |
| Radius of metacarpal head in the frontal and transverse plane, mm | | | | | | | | |
| | Male (36) | | | | Female (24) | | | |
| | Sagittal plane | | Transverse plane | | Sagittal plane | | Transverse plane | |
| Finger | Rf | SD | Rt | SD | Rf | SD | Rt | SD |
| Index | 8.20 | 0.67 | 7.02 | 0.54 | 7.57 | 0.99 | 6.96 | 0.61 |
| Long | 7.67 | 0.56 | 8.52 | 0.93 | 7.19 | 0.67 | 7.77 | 1.21 |
| Ring | 7.48 | 0.59 | 7.48 | 0.65 | 6.68 | 1.00 | 6.96 | 0.43 |
| Little | 7.00 | 0.52 | 7.28 | 1.30 | 6.01 | 0.86 | 6.15 | 0.43 |

| Width of metacarpal head, mm | | | | |
|---|---|---|---|---|
| | Male (36) | | Female (24) | |
| Finger | Wm | SD | Wf | SD |
| Index | 17.47 | 1.34 | 16.89 | 2.38 |
| Long | 17.35 | 1.27 | 15.82 | 1.88 |
| Ring | 14.95 | 1.27 | 13.69 | 1.20 |
| Little | 14.40 | 1.02 | 12.76 | 0.68 |
| | Male (36) | | Female (24) | |
| Finger | Lm | SD | Lf | SD |
| Metacarpal mean length, mm | | | | |
| Index | 70.4 | 2.1 | 67.0 | 4.5 |
| Long | 70.1 | 2.4 | 66.0 | 6.8 |
| Ring | 58.4 | 4.8 | 56.6 | 4.8 |
| Little | 55.9 | 2.0 | 53.1 | 4.3 |
| Proximal phalanx mean length, mm | | | | |
| Index | 43.7 | 2.0 | 42.4 | 2.3 |
| Long | 48.3 | 2.0 | 45.0 | 3.0 |
| Ring | 45.0 | 1.5 | 41.7 | 1.8 |
| Little | 36.0 | 1.3 | 33.5 | 1.8 |

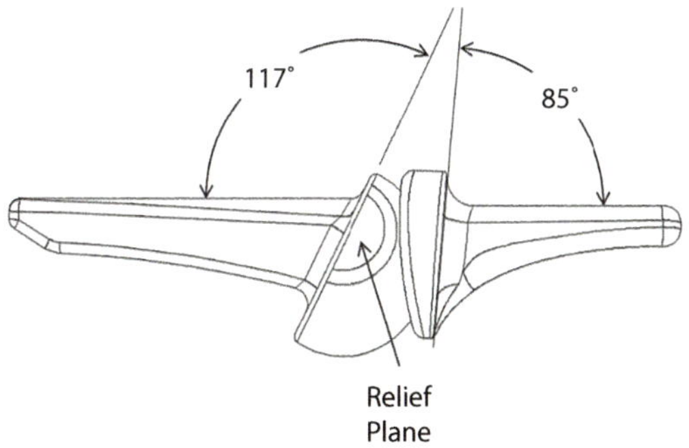


**Fig. 16.5** Planar subarticular collars

## Range of Motion

Accurate placement of the components of the SG PyC MCP is intended to result in a total joint arthroplasty which reestablishes functional kinematics. The range of motion for all sizes of the prosthesis is 20° of hyper extension, 90° of flexion, and ±15° of radial and ulnar motion as shown in Fig. 16.8.

## Fixation

Cement-free fixation of the SG PyC NCP is initially achieved by press-fit insertion. Implant

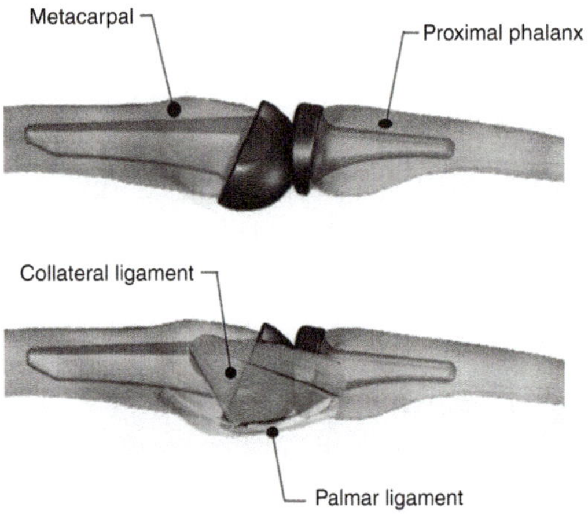


**Fig. 16.6** Preservation of ligament insertion sites

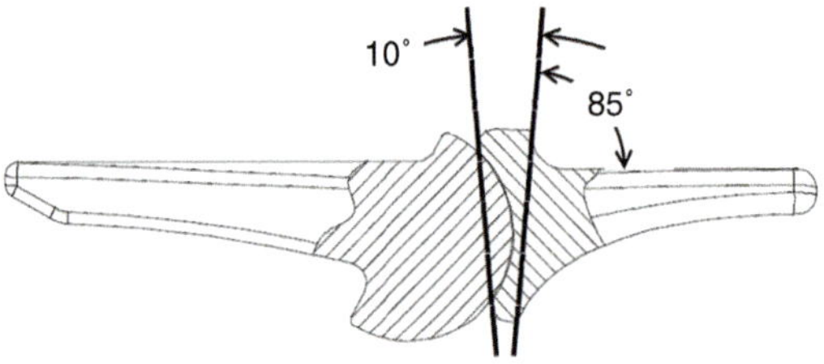


**Fig. 16.7** Dorsal prominence of the phalangeal component

**Table 16.18** SG PyC MCP stem offset values

| Size | Offset, mm |
|---|---|
| 5 | 0.2 |
| 10 | 0.2 |
| 20 | 0.4 |
| 30 | 0.5 |
| 40 | 0.6 |
| 50 | 0.7 |

stems are designed to conform to the anatomic shape of the intramedullary cavity [77, 78] and achieve a press fit by compaction of cancellous bone. The metacarpal stem has an inverted trapezoidal cross section with the wide base oriented toward the dorsal aspect of the canal. It tapers from a broad section at the subarticular collar to a narrow and short section at the stem tip designed to fill approximately one-half the length of the intramedullary canal. The phalangeal stem com-

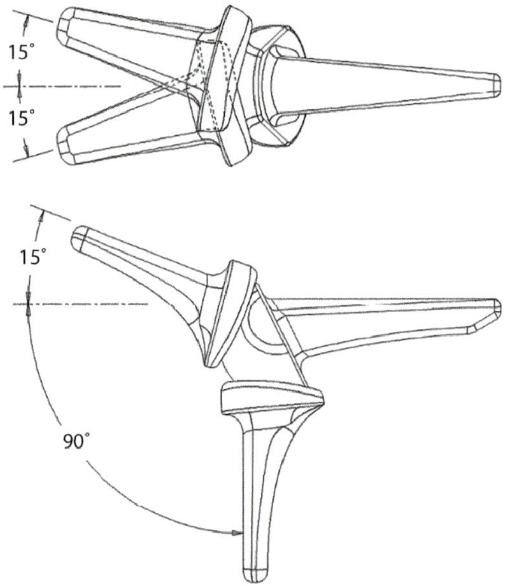


**Fig. 16.8** SG PyC MCP range of motion

ponent is trapezoidal in cross section with the wide base of the trapezoid oriented toward the palmar aspect of the canal. Like the metacarpal component, it tapers from a broad section at the subarticular collar to a narrow section at the stem tip intended to fill approximately one-half the length of the intramedullary canal of the proximal phalanx.

Animal studies demonstrate that long-term fixation of PyC implants is achieved by means of direct bone apposition or fixation including the presence of a thin, stable fibrous tissue membrane [79–82]. In the long-term follow-up of patients in the Mayo clinical trial, Cook [58] reports radiographic evaluation which showed a low rate of periprosthetic radiolucency and that the PyC implants had a rim of sclerotic bone indicative of osseointegration. Although subsidence was observed initially, it did not progress notably over time. Key factors are good alignment to minimize nonphysiological stresses and careful bone preparation to minimize thermal damage and voids within the press-fit cavity. When there is a paucity of cancellous bone, impact grafting should be used to achieve an initially stable press fit.

## PyroCarbon Material Processing and Properties

### Material Processing

Pyrolytic carbon is a name for a family of synthetic carbon materials produced by the thermal decomposition of a hydrocarbon gas such as methane, propane, acetylene, etc. The form of pyrolytic carbon used as a biomaterial is a high-density and isotropic form of pyrolytic carbon produced in a fluidized bed reaction chamber and is called PyroCarbon. The SG PyC MCP consists of a PyroCarbon layer encasing a precision-machined graphite substrate. The PyroCarbon layer is approximately 0.5 mm thick and is produced by levitating graphite substrates in a fluidized bed reaction chamber heated to 1400 °C. The bed, consisting of fine granules of a high temperature ceramic material such as zirconium oxide, is fluidized by a mixture of an inert gas and propane. Pyrolysis of propane occurs at high temperature producing carbon-free radicals that combine and deposit onto the graphite substrate forming a layer of PyroCarbon. Following the coating process, components are polished, cleaned, and inspected to ensure they meet specifications. A schematic illustrating the fluidized bed PyC deposition process is shown in Fig. 16.9.

### Material Properties

A considerable amount of research has been conducted to determine the physical and mechanical properties of PyroCarbon and the influence of the manufacturing conditions on properties. The properties of PyroCarbon reported in Table 16.19 are directly related to deposition process parameters such as reaction chamber temperature, total gas flow rate, hydrocarbon gas concentration, and fluidized bed surface area [83]. A detailed description of the coating process is given by More [83].

The elastic modulus of PyC (29.4 GPa) is similar to cortical bone (21 GPa) [84] and less than that of titanium (114 GPs) and CoCr alloy (200 GPa). A modulus of elasticity like that of

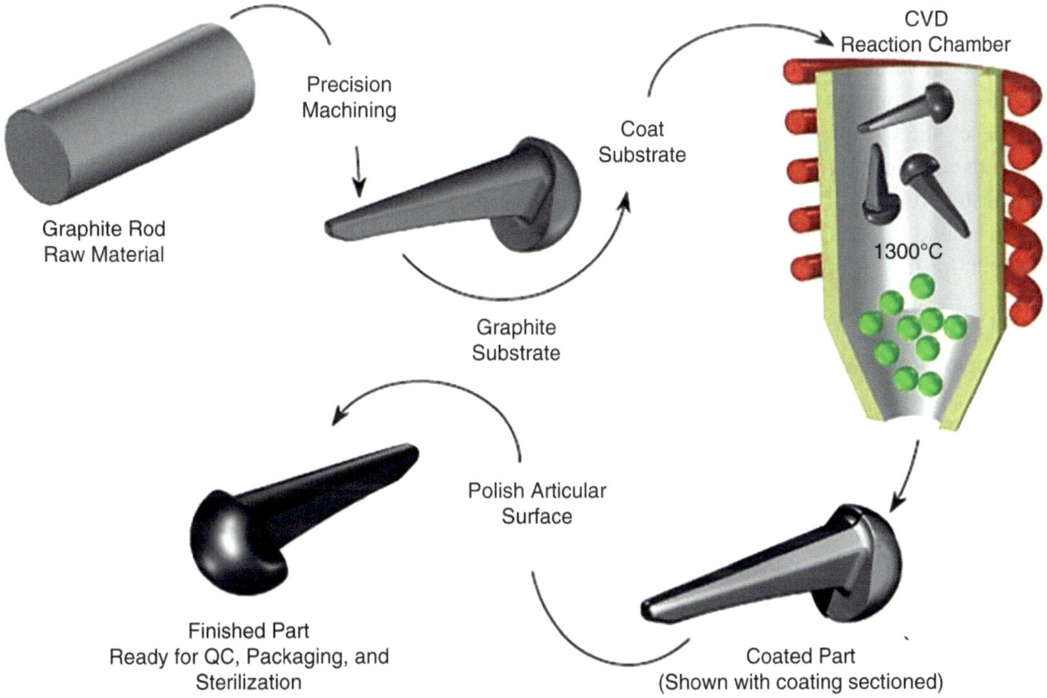


**Fig. 16.9** PyroCarbon manufacturing process

**Table 16.19** PyroCarbon material properties

| Property | Value |
|---|---|
| Flexural strength (MPa) | 493.7 ± 12 |
| Strain-to-failure (%) | 1.58 ± 0.03 |
| Young's modulus (GPa) | 29.4 ± 0.4 |
| Diamond pyramid hardness, 500 gm load | 235.9 ± 3.3 |
| Density (gm/cm$^3$) | 1.93 ± 0.01 |

bone contributes to biomechanical compatibility and reduces stress shielding [85]. Regarding surface finish, when removed from the coater, PyroCarbon parts have a microporous surface with a surface roughness of approximately Ra = 500 nm. The articulating surface of metacarpal and phalangeal components is polished to a mirror finish having a surface roughness of approximately Ra = 20 nm. The stem portion of each prosthesis retains the microporous finish to promote tissue adherence.

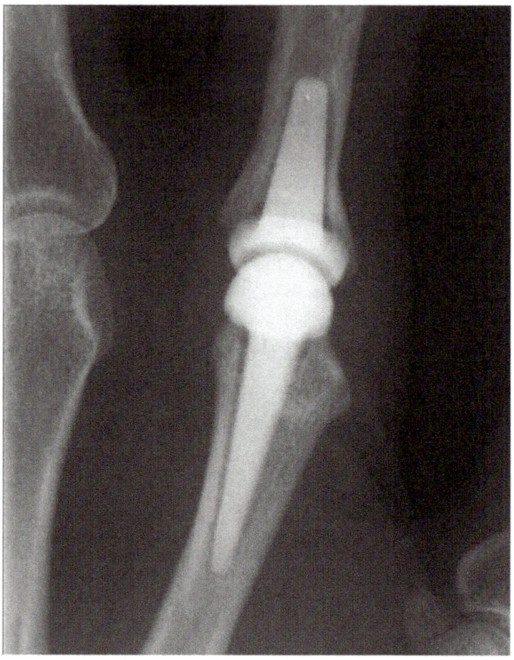

**Fig. 16.10** Radiographic image of the graphite substrate and the radiolucent PyC coating

## Radiographic Appearance

PyroCarbon is not readily visible on radiographs due to its poor X-ray absorption. A small amount (10 weight percent, approximately 1 atomic percent) of fine tungsten particles is added to the graphite substrate material when it is produced to make the implants visible radiographically. However, the 0.5-mm-thick coating of pure PyC remains radiolucent and appears as a lucent seam as illustrated in Fig. 16.10. Evaluation of a lucent seam around the stem as a sign of loosening must account for the lucent PyC coating.

## Strength and Fatigue

In vitro verification testing was conducted to evaluate three distinct characteristics of the SG PyC MCP: (1) load to failure strength testing, (2) cyclic fatigue endurance testing, and (3) cyclic wear testing. Strength and fatigue testing were conducted with specimens mounted and loaded to produce worst-case support and loading conditions as determined by MCP joint biomechanics. Figure 16.11 illustrates how load was applied to a metacarpal component. This support condition represents the MCP joint flexed at 60° with the joint reaction force acting at a 20° dorsal angle to the centerline of the proximal phalanx, the finger posture for maximum pinch and grip of the hand. Additionally, one-third of the proximal stem is left unsupported representing loss of proximal bone support. Similar worst-case conditions were used to test the phalangeal component.

The strength and fatigue performance requirement for the proximal and distal components is a minimum fracture strength of 80 lbf, representing the maximum biomechanical joint force for the male index finger. All sizes had to meet the strength requirement for male index finger since any size implant could be placed in any finger location. Strength tests were conducted on size 10, 30, and 50 metacarpal and phalangeal components. Cyclic endurance tests were carried out for ten million cycles with load varying from 8 to 80 lbf per cycle using the size 10 prosthesis. The summary of strength and fatigue test results shown in Table 16.20 demon-

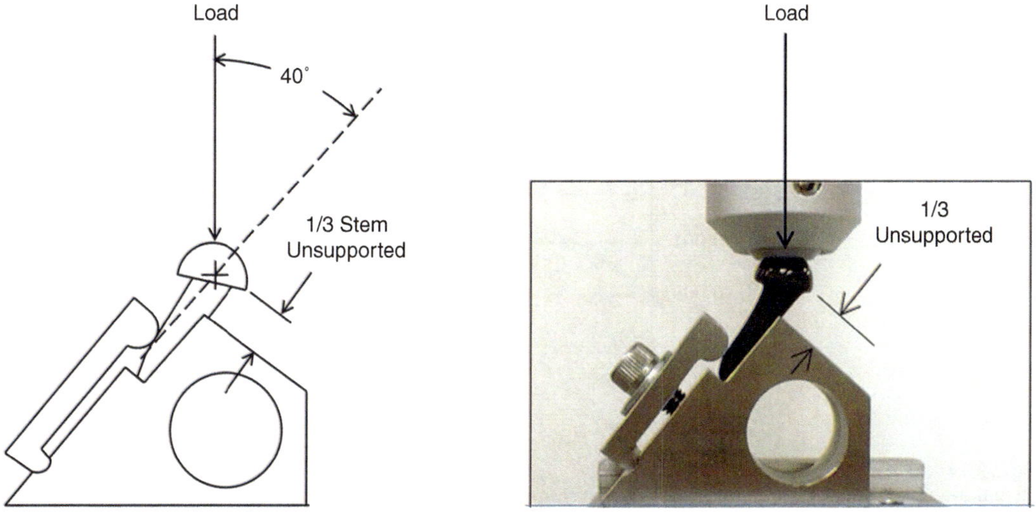


**Fig. 16.11** Metacarpal component mounted in fixture used for strength and fatigue testing

**Table 16.20** Summary of mechanical test results

| Test | Requirement | Size and component | Fracture load |
|---|---|---|---|
| Strength | 80 lbf minimum | 10 proximal | 279 ± 46 lbf |
| | | 30 proximal | 351 ± 56 lbf |
| | | 50 proximal | 454 ± 64 lbf |
| | | 10 distal | 186 ± 22 lbf |
| | | 30 distal | 234 ± 31 lbf |
| | | 50 distal | 353 ± 64 lbf |
| Cyclic fatigue | Survive ten million 8–80 lbf load cycles | 10 proximal<br>10 distal | No failure occurred |

strates that all sizes met the performance requirements.

## Wear Testing

Wear testing of the SG PyC MCP was conducted for ten million cycles in a joint simulator with sterilized bovine blood serum as a lubricant at room temperature with a load of 14 lbf and a motion of ±45°. CoCr alloy spherical head components coupled with UHMWPE cups were included as controls. Figure 16.12 shows the MCP joint wear test machine, and Fig. 16.13 shows the wear test results. No detectable wear was measured for the distal PyC component, and penetrating wear was observed with the UHMWPE component as expected.

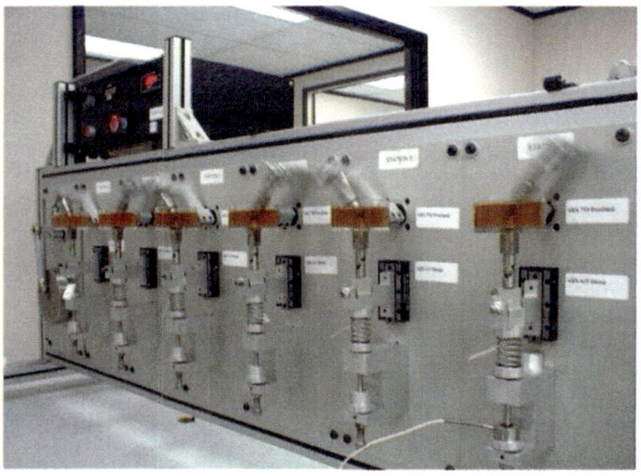

**Fig. 16.12** Station MCP joint wear test machine

## Surgical Instrumentation

Instrumentation was developed to achieve accurate surgical insertion of the SG PyC MCP. Transparent radiographic overlays are furnished to assist in determining appropriate implant. The instrumentation, shown in Fig. 16.14, includes an awl, a longitudinal axis alignment guide, cutting guides, intramedullary canal broaches, sizing trials and extractors, and implant impactors. During the surgical procedure, the cutting guide instrumentation aids in resection of the metacarpal and phalangeal bones at the appropriate angle, so the collar of the implant will mate accurately with the cut surface of the bone. Broaches compact medullary cancel-

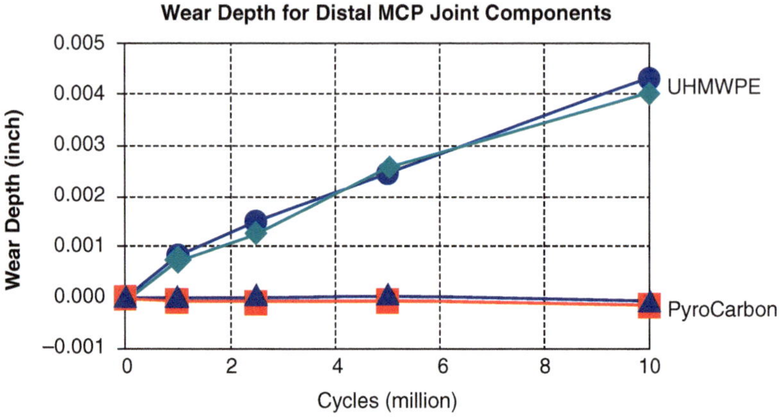


**Fig. 16.13** Wear test results

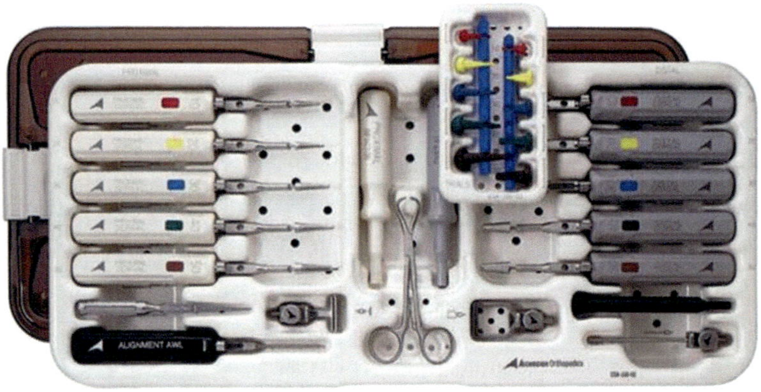


**Fig. 16.14** SG PyC MCP instrument system

lous bone resulting in a cavity smaller than the implant stem to achieve a tight press fit.

## Validation Testing

Validation of the SG PyC MCP was performed in the cadaver laboratory setting. Multiple surgeons used the surgical instrumentation to implant SG PyC MCP prostheses in large- and small-size male and female hands as described in the surgical technique. Results of the validation determined that the instrumentation met user needs for a total MCP joint arthroplasty. The SG PyC MCP prosthesis received CE Mark Certification in 1999 and FDA Premarket Approval (PMA) in 2001. Since the regulatory approval, company records show approximately 25,000 SG PyC MCP prostheses have been implanted. The SG PyC MCP is manufactured and distributed by Integra LifeSciences, Inc., as the Integra® PyC MCP Total Joint.

## Integra Silicone MCP Prosthesis

Following introduction and use of the SG PyC MCP, it was reported that occasionally during surgery it was found a total joint replacement was not indicated. Recognizing that a preoperative assessment to implant a total joint prosthesis may be questioned at time of surgery, it was decided to develop a single-piece flexible silicone prosthesis having the size same shape as the SG PyC MCP prosthesis. This allows for replacing the total joint prosthesis with a silicone prosthesis at any time during the surgical procedure. The instrumentation developed for the SG PyC MCP prosthesis works equally well for the silicone prosthesis. Development of the silicone MCP

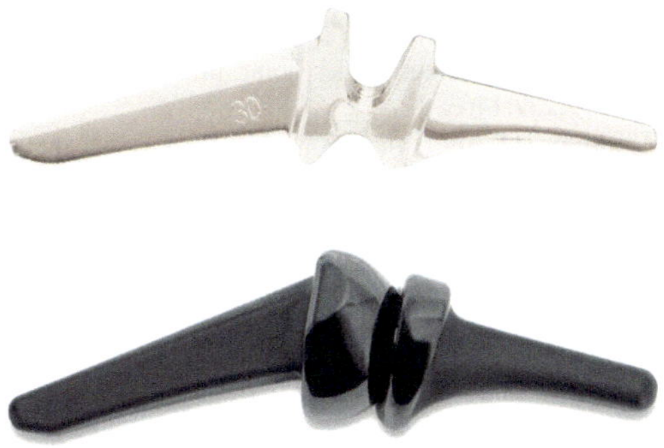

**Fig. 16.15** Comparison of the Integra® Silicone MCP to the Integra® PyC MCP total joint

prosthesis used finite element analysis to optimize the design and strength and fatigue testing to ensure durability [86]. The silicone MCP received regulatory clearance in 2002 and is now manufactured and distributed as the Integra® Silicone MCP. Figure 16.15 shows a comparison of the Integra® Silicone MCP to the Integra® PyC MCP Total Joint.

## References


1. Beckenbaugh R, Linscheid R, Arthroplasty in the hand and wrist, Operative hand surgery, ed. by Green D, 3rd edition, New York, NY: Churchill Livingstone, 1988.
2. Brannon EW, Klein G. Experiences with a finger-joint prosthesis. J Bone Joint Surg. 1959;41A(I):87–102.
3. Blair WF, Shurr DG, Buckwalter JA. Metacarpophalangeal joint arthroplasty with a metallic hinged prosthesis. Clin Orthop Relat Res. 1984;184:157–63.
4. Steffee AD, Beckenbaugh RD, Lincheid RL, Dobyns JH. The development, technique, and early clinical results of the total joint replacement for the metacarpophalangeal joint of the fingers. Orthopedics. 1981;4(2):175–80.
5. Adams BD, Blair WF, Schurr DG. Schultz metacarpophalangeal arthroplasty: a long-term follow-up study. J Hand Surg. 1990;15A(4):641–5.
6. Griffiths RW, Nicolle FV. Three years' experience of metacarpophalangeal joint replacement in the rheumatoid hand. Hand. 1975;7(3):275–83.
7. Varma SK, Milward TM. The Nicolle finger joint prosthesis: a reappraisal. J Hand Surg. 1991;13A(2):187–90.
8. Doi K, Kuwata N, Kawai S. Alumina ceramic finger implants: a preliminary biomaterial and clinical evaluation. J Hand Surg. 1984;9A(5):740–9.
9. Minami M, Yamazaki J, Kato S, Ishii S. Alumina ceramic prosthesis arthroplasty of the metacarpophalangeal joint in the rheumatoid hand: a 2-4-year follow-up study. J Arthroplasty. 1988;3(2):157–66.
10. Vermeiren JAH, Dapper MML, Schoonhoven LA, Merx PWJ. Isoelastic arthroplasty of the metacarpophalangeal joints in rheumatoid arthritis: a preliminary report. J Hand Surg. 1994;19A(2):319–24.
11. Swanson AB, de Groot-Swanson G, Ishikawa H. Use of grommets for flexible implant resection arthroplasty of the metacarpophalangeal joint. Clin Orthop Relat Res. 1997;(342):22–33.
12. Hagert CG, Eike O, Olsson NM, Ashcan W, Moving A. Metacarpophalangeal joint implants. Scand J Plast Reconstr Surg. 1975;9:147–57.
13. Swanson AB. Flexible implant arthroplasty for arthritic finger joints: rationale, technique, and results of treatment. J Bone Joint Surg. 1972;54A:435–55.
14. Swanson AB. Flexible implant arthroplasty in the hand and extremities. St. Louis: CV Mosby; 1973.
15. Swanson AB, de Groot-Swanson G, Leonard J. Postoperative rehabilitation programs in flexible implant arthroplasty of the digits. In: Hunter J, Schneider L, Mackin E, Callahan A, editors. Rehabilitation in the hand. 4th ed. St. Louis: CV Mosby; 1995. p. 1351–75.
16. Beevers RD, Seedhom BB. Metacarpophalangeal joint prostheses. A review of the clinical results of past and current designs. J Hand Surg. 1995;20B:125–36.
17. Swanson AB. Silicone rubber implants for replacement of arthritic or destroyed joints of the hand. Clin Orthop Relat Res. 1997;(342):4–10.
18. Bass RL, Stern PJ, Nairus JG. High implant fracture incidence with Sutter silicone metacarpophalangeal joint arthroplasty. J Hand Surg. 1996;21A(5):813–8.
19. Niebauer JJ, Shaw JL, Doren WW. The silicone-Dacron hinge prosthesis: design, evaluation and application. J Bone Joint Surg. 1968;50A:634.
20. Goldner JL, Gould JS, Urbaniak JR, McCollum DE. Metacarpophalangeal joint arthroplasty with silicone-Dacron prostheses (Niebauer type): six and a half years' experience. J Hand Surg Am. 1977;2(3):200–11.
21. McArthur PA, Milner RH. A prosoective randomizes comparison of Sutter and Swanson Silastic spacers. J Hand Surg. 1998;23-B(5):574–7.
22. Mannerfelt L, Andersson K. Silastic arthroplasty of the metacarpophalangeal joints in rheumatoid arthritis. J Bone Joint Surg. 1975;57-A(4):484–9.
23. Vahvanen V, Viljakka T. Silicone rubber implant arthroplasty of the metacarpophalangeal joint in rheumatoid arthritis: a follow-up of 32 patients. J Hand Surg. 1986;11A(3):333–9.
24. Kirschenbaum D, Schneider LH, Adams DC, Cody RP. Arthroplasty of the metacarpophalangeal joints with use of silicone implants in patients who have rheumatoid arthritis. J Bone Joint Surg. 1993;75-A(1):3–12.

25. Olsen I, Gebuhr P, Sonne-Holm S. Silastic arthroplasty in rheumatoid MCP-joints. Acta Orthop Scand. 1994;65(4):430–1.
26. Gellman H, Stetson W, Brumfield RH, Costigan W, Kuschner SH. Silastic metacarpophalangeal joint arthroplasty in patients with rheumatoid arthritis. Clin Orthop Relat Res. 1997;(342):16–21.
27. Hansraj KK, Ashworth CR, Ebramzadeh E, Todd AO, Griffin MD, Ashley EM, Cardilli AM. Swanson metacarpophalangeal joint arthroplasty in patients with rheumatoid arthritis. Clin Orthop Relat Res. 1997;(342):11–5.
28. Simmen BR, Gschwend N. Swanson silicone rubber interpositional arthroplasty of the wrist and of the metacarpophalangeal joints in rheumatoid arthritis. Acta Orthop Belg. 1988;54(2):196.
29. Poulenus L, Simonetta C, Egloff DV. Long-term results from metacarpophalangeal arthroplasty. Ann Chir Main. 1983;2(2):160.
30. Bieber EJ, Weiland AJ, Volenec-Dowling S. Silicone implant arthroplasty of the metacarpophalangeal joint for rheumatoid arthritis. J Bone Joint Surg. 68-A(2):206–9.
31. Beckenbaugh RD, Dobyns JH, Linscheid RL, Bryan RS. Review and analysis of silicone- metacarpophalangeal implants. J Bone Joint Surg. 1976;58A:483–7.
32. Wilson YG, Sykes PJ, Niranjan NS. Long-term follow-up of Swanson's Silastic arthroplasty for the metacarpophalangeal joints in rheumatoid arthritis. J Hand Surg. 1993;18B(1):81–91.
33. Fleming SG, Hay EL. Metacarpophalangeal joint arthroplasty eleven-year follow-up study. J Hand Surg. 1984;9-8(3):300–2.
34. Rothwell AG, Greig KJ, O'Neill JB. Hand function following Silastic arthroplasty of the metacarpophalangeal joints in the rheumatoid hand. J Hand Surg. Feb 1997;22B(1):90.
35. Sollerman CJ, Geiger M. Polyurethane versus silicone for endoprosthetic replacement of the metacarpophalangeal joints in rheumatoid arthritis. Scand J Plast Reconstr Surg Hand Surg. 1996;30:145–50.
36. Ferlic DC, Clayton ML, Holloway M. Complications of silicone implant surgery in the metacarpophalangeal joint. J Bone Joint Surg. 1975;57-A(7):991–4.
37. Kay AGL, Jeffs JV, Scott JT. Experience with Silastic prostheses in the rheumatoid hand. Ann Rheum Dis. 1978;27:255–8.
38. Jensen CM, Boeckstyns MEH, Kristiansen B. Silastic arthroplasty in rheumatoid MCP-joints. Acta Orthop Scand. 1986;57:138–40.
39. Maurer RJ, Ranawat CS, MacCormack RR, Inglis AE, Straub LR. Long-term follow-up for the Swanson MP arthroplasty for rheumatoid arthritis. J Hand Surg. 1990;15A(5):810–1.
40. Hirakawa K, Bauer TW, Culver JE, Wilde AH. Isolation and quantitation of debris particles around failed silicone orthopedics implants. J Hand Surg. 1996;21A(5):819–27.
41. Christie AJ, Weinberger KA, Detrich M. Silicone lymphadenopathy and synovitis complications of silicone elastomer finger joint prosthesis. JAMA. 1977;237:1463–4.
42. Ekfors TO, Arc HM, Maki J, Aho AJ. Cystic osteolysis induced by silicone prosthesis. Arch Pathol Lab Med. 1984;108:225–7.
43. Gordon M, Bulloch PG. Synovial and osseous inflammation in failed silicone prosthesis. J Bone Joint Surg. 1975;57A:991–3.
44. Bernstein SA, Strickland RW, Lazarus E. Axillary lymphadenopathy due to Swanson implant. J Rheumatol. 1993;20:1066–9.
45. Kircher T. Silicone lymphadenopathy: a complication of silicone elastomer finger joint prosthesis. Hum Pathol. 1980;11:240–4.
46. Murakata LA, Rangwala AF. Silicone lymphadenopathy with concomitant malignant lymphoma. J Rheumatol. 1989;16:1480–3.
47. Paplanus SH, Payne CM. Axillary lymphadenopathy 17 years after digital silicone implants: study with x-ray analysis. J Hand Surg. 1988;13A:411–2.
48. Wanivenhaus A, Lintner F, Wurnig C, Missaghi-Schinzl M. Long-term reaction of the osseous bed around silicone implants. Arch Orthop Trauma Surg. 1991;110:146–50.
49. Delaney R, Trail IA, Nuttall D. A comparative study of outcomes study of outcome between the NeuFlex and Swanson metacarpophalangeal joint replacements. J Hand Surg Br. 2005;30(1):3–7.
50. Escott BG, Kara R, Judd M, et al. NeuFlex and Swanson metacarpophalangeal implants for rheumatoid arthritis: prospective randomized, controlled clinical trial. J Hand Surg Am. 2010;35(1):44–51.
51. Boe C, Wagner E, Rizzo M. Long-term outcomes of silicone, metacarpophalangeal arthroplasty: a longitudinal analysis of 325 cases. J Hand Surg Eur Vol. 2018;43(10):1076–82.
52. Beevers DJ, Seedhom BB. Metacarpophalangeal joint prostheses, a review of the clinical results past and current. J Hand Surg. 1995;20B(2):125–36.
53. Welsh RP, Hastings DE, White R. Resurfacing arthroplasty for the metacarpophalangeal joint. Acta Orthop Belg. 1982;48(6):924–7.
54. Condamine JL, Benoit JY, Comtet JJ, Aubriot JH. Proposed digital arthroplasty, critical study of the preliminary results. Arthoplatie Digitale. 1988;7(4):282–97.
55. Rittmeister M, Porsch M, Starker M, Kerschbaumer F. Metacarpophalangeal joint arthroplasty in rheumatoid arthritis: results of Swanson implants and digital joint operative arthroplasty. Arch Orthop Trauma Surg. 1999;119:190–4.
56. Cook SD, Beckenbaugh RD, Weinstein AM, Klawitter JJ. Pyrolite carbon implants in the metacarpophalangeal joints of baboons. Orthopedics. 1983;6(8):952–61.
57. Beckenbaugh RD. Preliminary experience with a noncemented nonconstrained total joint arthroplasty for the metacarpophalangeal joints. Orthopedics. 1983;6(3):962–5.

58. Cook SD, Beckenbaugh RD, Redondo J, Popich LS, Klawitter JJ, Linscheid RL. Long term follow-up of pyrolytic carbon implants in the metacarpophalangeal joint. J Bone Joint Surg. 1999;81-A(5):635–48.
59. Napier JR. The prehensile movements of the hand. J Bone Joint Surg. 1956;34B(4):286–92.
60. Landsmeer JMF. Power grip and precision handling. Ann Rheum Dis. 1962;21:164.
61. Swanson AB, Matev IB, deGroot G, The strength of the hand, Bull Prosthet Res. 1970 Fall;XIII:1.
62. Walker E. Clinical evaluation of finger joints. In: Human joints and their artificial replacements. Springfield: C.C. Thomas; 1977. p. 348–51.
63. Chao, et al. Chapter 5: Hand strength functional assessment and its clinical application. In: Biomech of the hand; 1989.
64. Weightman B, Amis AA. Finger joint force predictions related to design of joint replacements. J Biomed Eng. 1982;4:197–205.
65. Boatright JR, Kiebzak GM, O'Neil DM, et al. Measurement of thumb abduction strength: normative data and a comparison with grip and pinch strength. J Hand Surg. 1997;22A(5):843–8.
66. Josty IC, Tyler MPH, Sewell PC, Roberts NH. Grip and pinch strength variations in different types of work. J Hand Surg. 1977;22B(2):266.
67. Linscheid RL, Dobyns JH. Total joint arthroplasty - the hand. Mayo Clin Proc. 1979;54:516–26.
68. Hagert CG. Advances in hand surgery: finger joint implants. Surg Annu. 1978;10:253–75.
69. Chao, et al. Chapter 3 Muscle and joint forces in the hand. In: Biomech of the hand; 1989. Teanneck, NJ: World Scientific Publishion.
70. Berme JP, Purves WK. A biomechanical analysis of the metacarpophalangeal joint. J Biomech. 1977;10:409–12.
71. Beevers DJ, Seedhom BB. Design of a non-constrained, non- cemented, modular metacarpophalangeal. Proc Inst Mech Eng H. 1995;209:185–95.
72. Tamie K, et al. Three-dimensional geometric analysis of the metacarpophalangeal joint. J Hand Surg. 1998;13A(4):521–9.
73. Sibly F, Unsworth A. Wear of cross-linked polyethylene against itself: a material suitable for surface replacement of the finger joint. J Biomed Eng. 1991;13:217–20.
74. Stoke SM, Unsworth A, Viva C, Haslock I. A finger function simulator and the laboratory testing of Swanson prostheses. Proc Inst Mech Eng H. 1990;204:233–40.
75. Dumbleton JH. Tribology of natural and artificial joints, Chapter 3. Amsterdam: Elsevier Scientific Publishing Co.; 1981. p. 52.
76. Unsworth A, Alexander WJ. Dimensions of the metacarpo-phalangeal joint with particular reference to joint prostheses. Mech Eng. 1979;8(2):75–80.
77. Lazar G, Schulter-Ellis FP. Intramedullary structure of human metacarpals. J Hand Surg Am. 1980;5(5):477–81.
78. Schulter-Ellis FP, Lazar GT. Internal morphology of human phalanges. J Hand Surg Am. 1984;9(4):490–5.
79. Anderson RC, et al. An evaluation of skeletal attachment to LTI pyrolytic carbon, porous titanium, and carbon-coated porous titanium implants. Clin Orthop Relat Res. 1984;182:242–57.
80. Cook SD, et al. Quantitative histologic evaluation of LTI carbon, carbon-coated aluminum oxide and uncoated aluminum oxide dental implants. J Biomed Mater Res. 1983;17(3):519–38.
81. Kent JN, et al. A clinical comparison of LTI carbon, alumina, and carbon-coated alumina blade-type implants in baboons. J Biomed Mater Res. 1982;16(6):887–99.
82. Thomas KA, et al. The effect of surface treatments on the interface mechanics of LTI pyrolytic carbon implants. J Biomed Mater Res. 1985;19(2):145–59.
83. More RB, Haubold AD, Bokros JC. Pyrolytic carbon for long-term medical implants. In: Biomaterials science: Elsevier Inc., Academic Press; 2013. p. 209–22.
84. Rho JY, Ashman RB, Turner CH. Young's modulus of trabecular and cortical bone material: ultrasonic and microtensile measurements. J Biomech. 1993;26(2):111–9.
85. Huiskes R, Weinans H, van Rietbergen B. The relationship between stress shielding and bone resorption around total hip stems and the effects of flexible materials. Clin Orthop Relat Res. 1992;274:124–34.
86. Podnos E, et al. FEA analysis of silicone MCP implant. J Biomech. 2006;39(7):1217–26.

# Primary MCP Arthroplasty

# 17

Marco Rizzo and Peter M. Murray

## Introduction

A pain-free, stable, and mobile metacarpophalangeal (MCP) joint is important for good hand function. The MCP joint is most commonly afflicted by inflammatory arthritis, but post-traumatic arthritis and osteoarthritis are also common and can lead to substantial pain and dysfunction. Conservative treatments include activity modification, splinting, topical and oral anti-inflammatory medications, and steroid injections. Surgery is considered for chronic pain, deformity, and loss of function in patients who fail conservative measures.

The most common surgical options for the arthritic MCP joint include arthroplasty and arthrodesis. While successful arthrodesis can be pain relieving and is the preferred surgical treatment for the thumb MCP joint arthritis, it is less desirable in the fingers. In addition to the loss of flexion and extension of the joint, the inability to abduct and adduct the digits can result in diminished hand function, especially when more than one digit is fused.

Silicone MCP arthroplasty, introduced by Swanson in 1962, has remained the gold standard in surgical management of MCP arthritis, especially in patients with rheumatoid arthritis [1]. However, over the last two to three decades, the introduction of surface gliding implants has become an alternative to the traditional silicone implants. The primary choices in the United States include pyrocarbon (Integra Life Sciences, Austin, TX) and the metal-plastic surface replacement arthroplasty (Stryker, New Jersey). These implants have favorable material properties compared to silicone. However, they are modular and non-constrained and require more competent soft tissues to maintain joint stability.

The aim of this chapter is to review the indications, technique, and outcomes of primary MCP arthroplasty in the surgical management of MCP joint arthritis.

## Silastic MCP Arthroplasty

### Design Characteristics

Silicone MCP arthroplasty has been utilized for nearly 60 years. Introduced initially by Swanson,

**Supplementary Information** The online version of this chapter (https://doi.org/10.1007/978-3-030-68880-6_17) contains supplementary material, which is available to authorized users.

M. Rizzo (✉)
Department of Orthopedic Surgery, Division of Hand Surgery, Mayo Clinic, Rochester, MN, USA
e-mail: Rizzo.marco@mayo.edu

P. M. Murray
Department of Orthopedic Surgery, Mayo Clinic, Jacksonville, FL, USA
e-mail: murray.peter@mayo.edu


G. J. W. King, M. Rizzo (eds.), *Arthroplasty of the Upper Extremity*,
https://doi.org/10.1007/978-3-030-68880-6_17

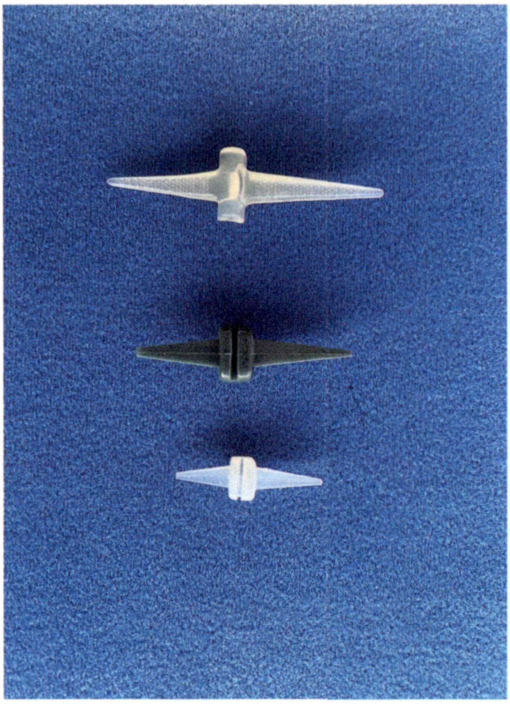

**Fig. 17.1** The silicone MCP implants. The Swanson implant (top), the Stryker silastic implants (middle), and the Integra silastic implant (bottom)

they are one-piece intramedullary stemmed implants that provide some inherent stability and have a flexible hinge that allows for motion [1–3]. Numerous variations on the original design are available, but the general design features are similar (Fig. 17.1) [4–7].

Following implantation, a new joint capsule forms around the implant by means of encapsulation [8]. Excessive implant fixation or cementing has been shown to limit the longevity of this implant [3]. In fact, a small amount of pistoning and micromotion is advantageous, offloading the implant to ultimately improve survival. Like all implants, competent bone and soft-tissue joint stabilizers will share the load and improve stability and ultimately survival.

Short-term and some long-term subjective and objective results have been encouraging. Unfortunately, silastic implants have not been as durable long term, and component fracture and recurrent deformity have been observed. In addition, the debris associated with implant wear may create an inflammatory response, and even lymphadenopathy in some cases, resulting in silicone synovitis and further bone and joint destruction [9, 10].

## Indications/Contraindications

Silicone arthroplasty is indicated for both inflammatory and noninflammatory arthritis of the MCP joint. While some of the newer modular implants are considered for noninflammatory arthritis, silicone remains the implant of choice in the management of inflammatory arthritis for most surgeons. Even with the success of disease-modifying antirheumatic drugs (DMARDs), many cases of MCP arthritis remain inflammatory in etiology. Thus, silastic implants continue to be a mainstay in the management of MCP arthritis.

Contraindications for silastic MCP arthroplasty include patients with incompetent musculature, insufficient bone stock, loss of neuromuscular function, and infection.

## **Technique** (Fig. 17.2)

Silastic MCP arthroplasty is performed from a dorsal approach. In cases of multiple digits, a transverse skin incision over the MCP joints can be utilized. Alternatively a longitudinal skin incision(s) over the MCP joints may be performed. In nonrheumatoid patients, I prefer a tendon splitting approach to the joint, which is a similar technique to that described in the latter section focused on modular MCP implants.

In cases of inflammatory arthritis, we prefer an approach that splits the radial sagittal band. This allows for tightening of the sagittal band for extensor tendon centralization. The dorsal capsule is split longitudinally to reveal the joint. The bone cuts are then made, beginning first with the metacarpal head resection. These cuts are made perpendicular to the axis of the metacarpal or with a slight radial inclination in the coronal plane to counteract the tendency for recurrent ulnar drift. In the sagittal plane, the cuts are gen-

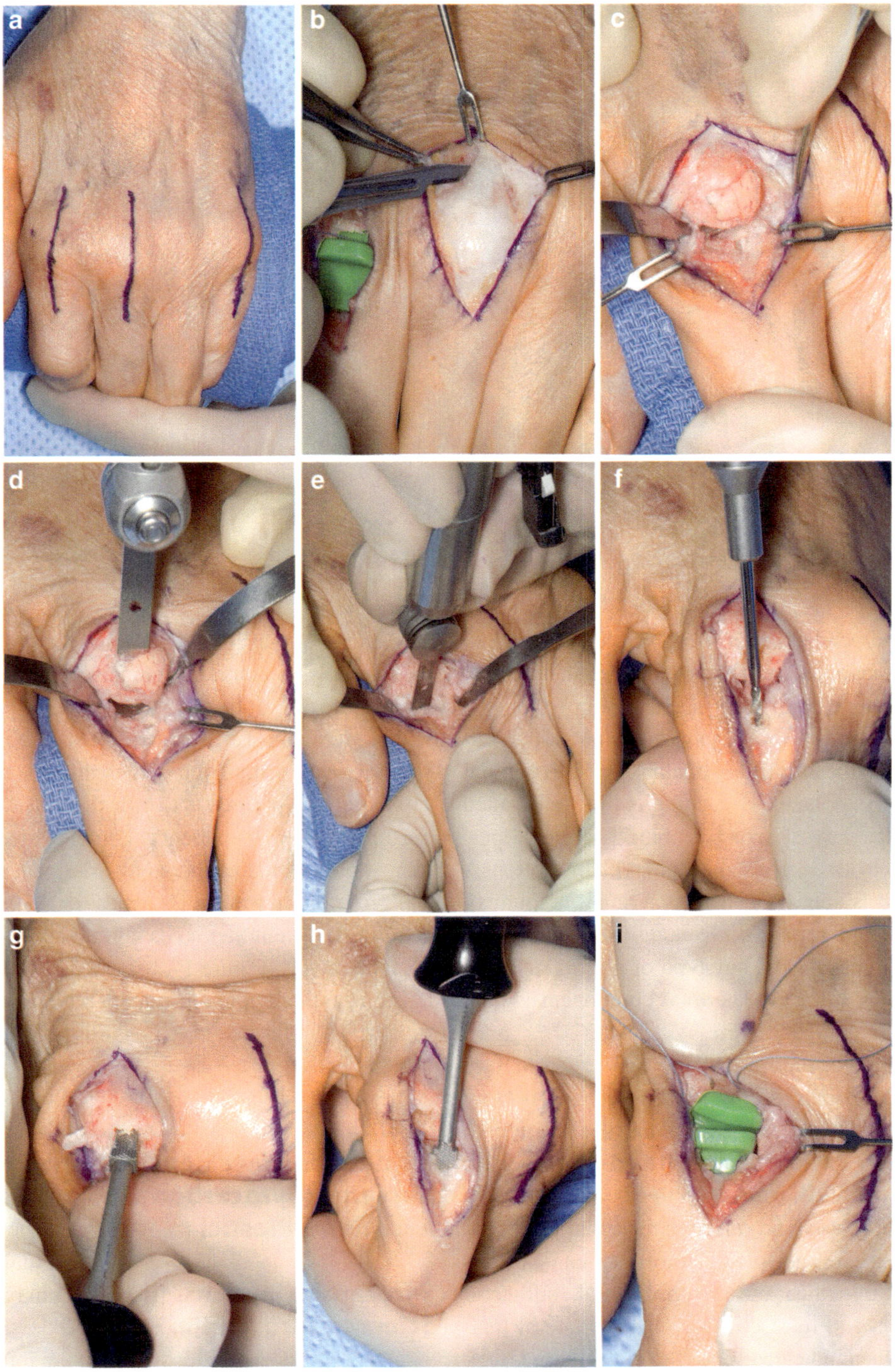


**Fig. 17.2** Illustration of a case example silicone implants. (**a**) A longitudinal individual incisions or a single transverse incision (multiple digits) can be utilized. (**b**) The joint is exposed by dividing the radial sagittal band (seen on middle finger in this figure), and (**c**) the joint is exposed via a longitudinal incision of the capsule. The volar soft tissues are released. (**d**) The metacarpal cut is made with a transverse cut perpendicular to the axis of the shaft. (**e**) The proximal phalanx is also cut perpendicular to its axis, typically resecting a minimum amount to allow for access to the canal and correct erosive deformities. (**f**) A side-cutting burr can be utilized to help enlarge the canal, especially in patients with sclerotic bone. (**g, h**) Broaching up to the largest size and best fit is performed. (**i**) Trialing is completed and stability confirmed through the arc of motion. (**j**) The final implants are inserted, and (**k**) soft-tissue balancing can be then performed with collateral ligament suturing, followed by extensor tendon centralization

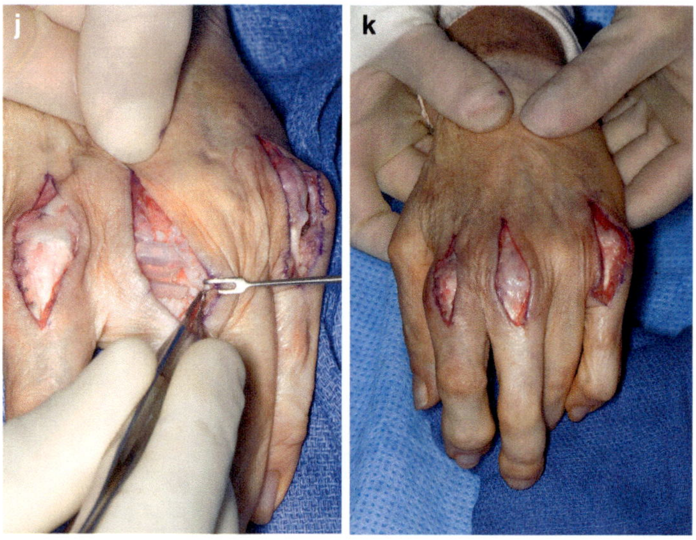


**Fig. 17.2** (continued)

erally perpendicular, or slightly volarly angled, to the metacarpal axis. The proximal phalangeal cut is then made with care taken to simply remove 2–3 mm of the bone, again with the cut perpendicular to the axis of the phalanx on both coronal and sagittal planes. Broaching is then performed up to the largest size possible. Trialing is performed to assess for stability as well as motion. A good fit is such that there is a small amount of pistoning of implant with enough separation with the implant to avoid any type of impingement of the boney surfaces. The final component is then inserted.

This procedure in patients with inflammatory arthritis is often as much soft tissue as it is bony in nature. In patients with volar subluxation of the carpus, a volar plate and soft-tissue release can be helpful in maintaining the alignment of the arthroplasty and resisting recurrent joint subluxation. Coronal plane deformity can be corrected by plication of the radial collateral ligament and release of the ulnar collateral ligament when indicated. Both flexion and ulnar drift can be improved with an ulnar intrinsic release and even cross intrinsic transfers. Extensor tendon centralization can be achieved with tightening of the radial sagittal band and (when indicated) release of the ulnar sagittal band.

Postoperatively, the MCP joint is immobilized for 4 weeks in neutral alignment and extension allowing for IP motion. Alternatively, for patients with severe ulnar drift, an extension outrigger splint can be employed which allows passive extension and permits active flexion. At 4 weeks postoperatively, the patient can then graduate to a removable splint, and therapy working on motion and progression toward activities for daily living is initiated. Strengthening is initiated at 3 months postoperatively. Figure 17.3 and Video 17.1 highlights a case example of a patient who underwent successful silastic MCP arthroplasty for osteoarthritis.

## Modular Surface Replacement Implants (Pyrocarbon and Metal-Plastic)

### Pyrocarbon Implants (Integra Life Sciences, Inc., Austin, TX, USA)

Pyrocarbon is a unique material that makes us a two- to three-dimensional carbon matrix. It was initially introduced and has been utilized in replacement of heart valves for many years [11]. It is formed via pyrolysis of hydrocarbon gas,

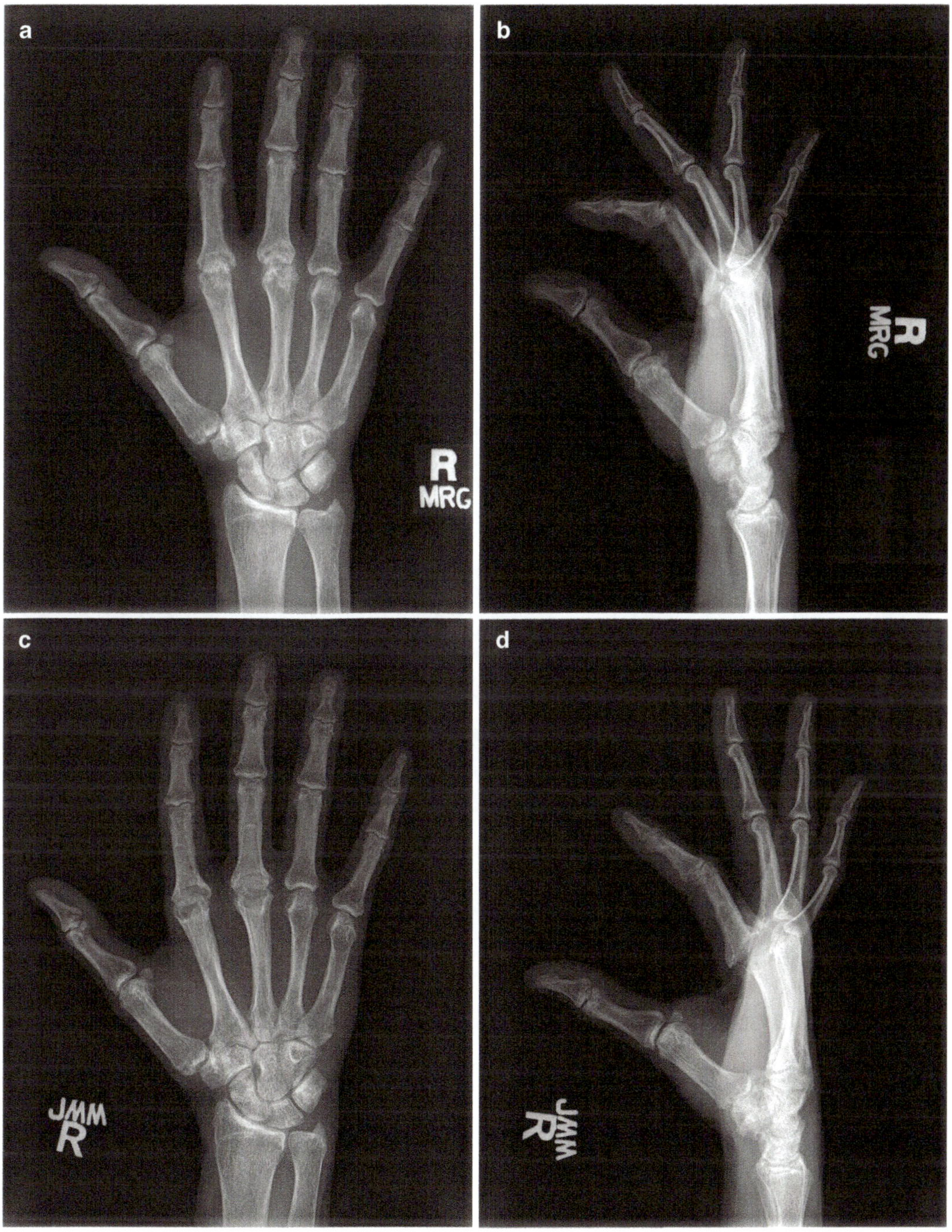


Fig. 17.3 A 68-year-old female with pain and (**a, b**) advanced arthritis of the index and long finger MCP joints. (**c, d**) PA and lateral radiographs at 4 years postsurgery demonstrate some subsidence, but overall stable joints

whereby graphite is heated to 1300 degrees Celsius. The process results in a material with mechanical properties that fall between graphite and diamond.

With an elastic modulus very similar to the cortical bone, it serves as an excellent load-sharing device, minimizing stress-shielding. Pyrocarbon implants also exhibit exceptional

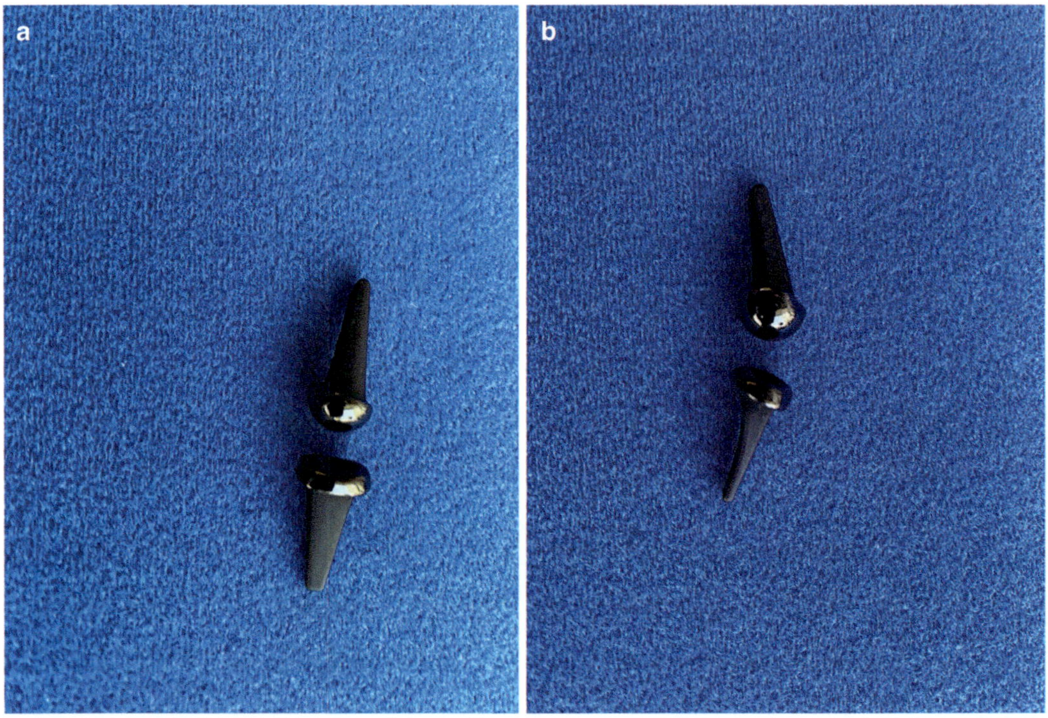


**Fig. 17.4** The pyrocarbon implant. (**a**) View from the side and (**b**) view from above

wear characteristics, with minimal particular debris on repetitive cyclic loading. In addition, as it is biologically inert, the little particulate debris that these implants create is less likely to generate the immune-mediated responses that can be seen with silicone and polyethylene particles. Unfortunately, the stems of these implants have little/no osseous ingrowth and depend primarily on appositional growth of the bone around the implant to help provide stability. Animal studies have also demonstrated that, when compared to cobalt chrome, pyrocarbon can be a favorable "cartilage-friendly" articular surface [12]. In a hip hemiarthroplasty canine model, pyrocarbon yielded no inflammatory response and generated less surface cracks and promoted more fibrocartilage regeneration against its exposed articulation than cobalt chrome, suggesting that there is a role for it as a hemiarthroplasty.

Pyrocarbon was initially studied for application in small joint replacement in 1979 [13]. The original design has been modified from its inception. The current design is a polished pyrocarbon ball and socket joint anatomically and kinematically simulating the native MCP, maintaining its center of rotation and arc of curvature. The intramedullary stems are smooth, tungsten-coated pyrocarbon intramedullary stems (Fig. 17.4).

## Metal-Plastic (SRA) Implants (Stryker Inc., Kalamazoo, MI, USA)

The SRA implant design is a cobalt-chrome-polyethylene implant with porous coated, titanium metacarpal component and all-polyethylene phalangeal component. (Fig. 17.5) Originally designed by Dr. Ronald Linscheid, it predates the pyrocarbon implant. Like the pyrocarbon implant, it is a ball-socket design better mimicking the anatomy and kinematics of the native MCP joint than silastic implants. The metacarpal head design is such that it has an offset, and narrows from dorsal to palmar, that helps provide stability with MCP flexion and laxity with extension. In addition, differentiating it from pyrocarbon, there

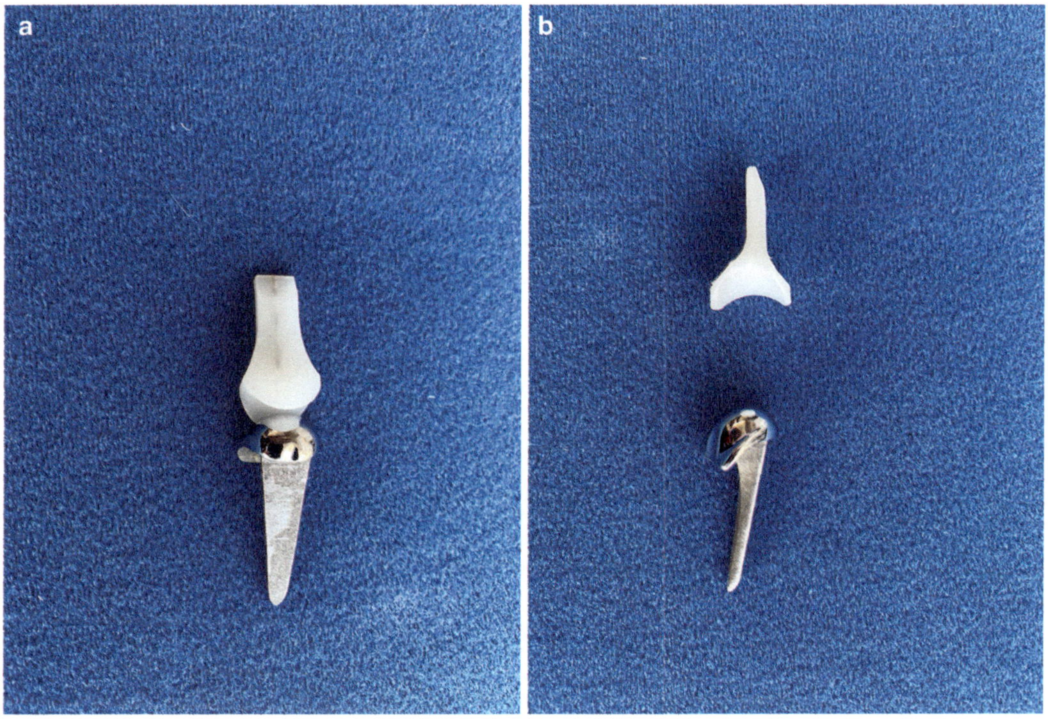


**Fig. 17.5** The SRA implant. (**a**) View from the above and (**b**) view from the side

are radial-ulnar flares aimed at providing coronal plane stability, resisting the tendency for radial and ulnar drift of the digits. The proximal component titanium stem has flares that resist rotation and allow for ease of insertion. The distal component is all-polyethylene and requires cementing for fixation. The proximal component can be press fit or cemented. As a result, medullary canal bone-implant fixation is far superior with the SRA implant when compared to pyrocarbon implants.

Though it lacks the favorable material properties and wear characteristics of pyrocarbon, the polyethylene-metal articulation is reliable and has stood the test of time in joint arthroplasty. Advances in cross-linking of polyethylene have minimized the wear debris. While titanium's elastic modulus is further from that of cortical bone than pyrocarbon, it is a reliable load-sharing material and good at minimizing stress-shielding.

The use or need for cementing can be helpful for fixation to the bone but poses challenges in removing these implants. Resection of cemented components invites bone loss during removal.

## Indications/Contraindications

The indications for surface gliding implants like pyrocarbon and SRA arthroplasty are similar to silicone and include osteoarthritis and post-traumatic and inflammatory arthritis. Given the less constrained design, it demands more soft-tissue competence for stability. As many patients with osteoarthritis have better soft-tissue stabilizers, the surface gliding implants are an excellent option for managing arthritis in this patient population. Figure 17.6 illustrates a case example of patient with osteoarthritis who underwent pyrocarbon MCP arthroplasty for middle finger MCP arthritis. Figure 17.7 illustrates a case example of a patient who underwent SRA arthroplasty.

However, most patients who present with MCP arthritis have inflammatory arthritis. These patients tend to have poorer soft-tissue compe-

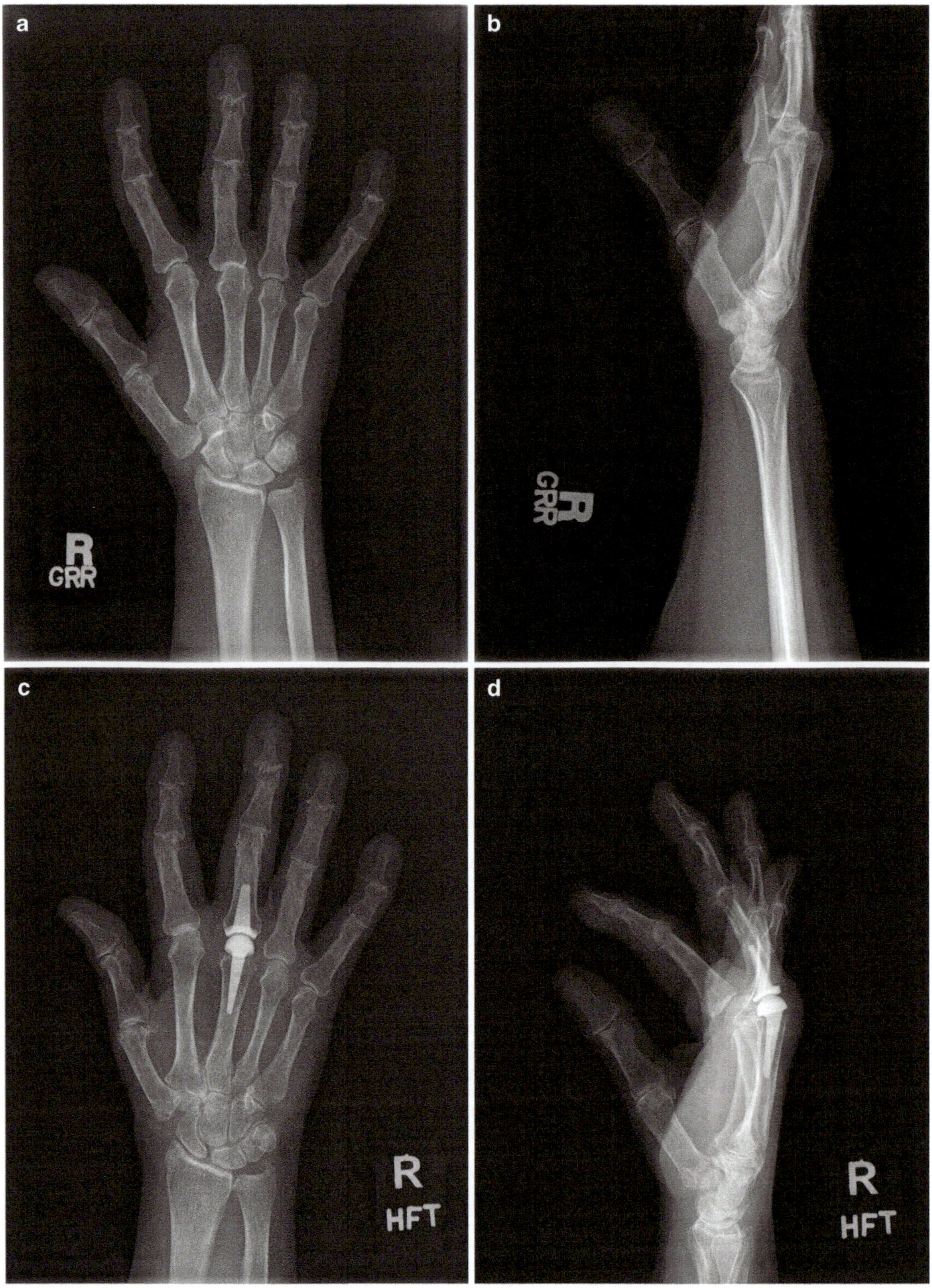


**Fig. 17.6** A 73-year-old female with significant (**a**, **b**) arthritis of her long MCP joint. She underwent (**c, d**) pyrocarbon MCP arthroplasty. Intraoperatively, she was lax at the radial collateral ligament

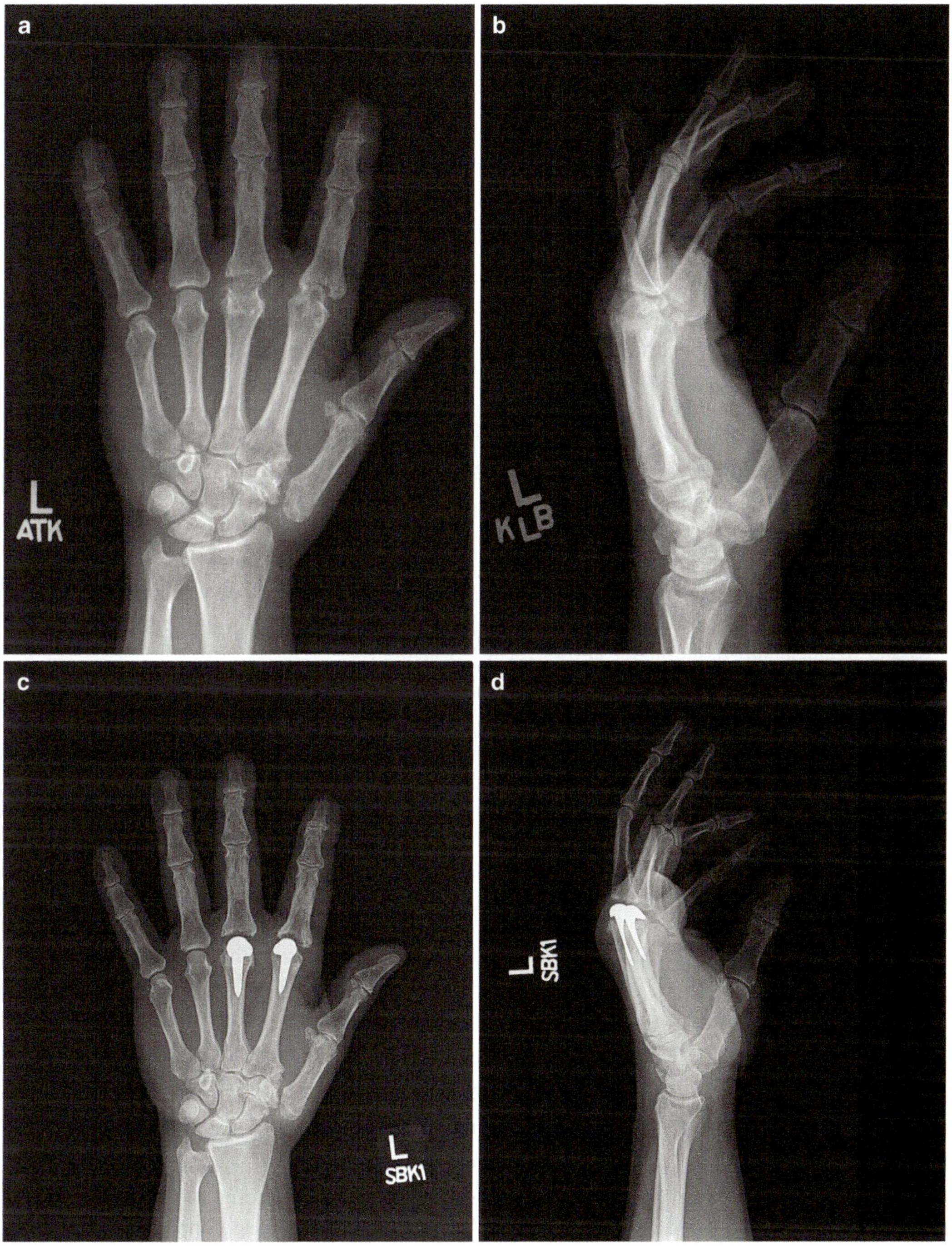


**Fig. 17.7** (**a, b**) A 70-year-old male with advanced arthritis of the index and long finger MCP joints. He underwent SRA MCP arthroplasty. (**c, d**) Radiographs at 6 months postoperative demonstrated stable implants

tence and are vulnerable to recurrent deformity, dislocation, and instability. In these patients, the role of unconstrained surface gliding MCP implants is less clear. Patients with mild and/or well-controlled inflammatory arthritis are likely to be better candidates.

Contraindications to pyrocarbon and SRA implants include patients with poorly controlled inflammatory arthritis, significant deformities, ongoing or history of infection (relative), muscle incompetence, neurologic compromise, poor bone stock/quality, incompetent soft tissues, and unrealistic expectations.

Preoperative radiographs are critical in helping determine the feasibility of surface gliding implants. Patients with subluxation and frank dislocation of the MCP joints, as seen in cases of severe inflammatory arthropathy, are less likely candidates for the pyrocarbon or SRA joints. Further, chronic instability invites bone loss over the dorsal proximal phalanx, and the significant bone loss makes any implant arthroplasty a challenge, let alone less constrained prostheses. Also, significant ulnar drift of the MCP joints is linked to radial collateral ligament and sagittal band insufficiency which can undermine the success of gliding implants. Less severe or more subtle bone loss and ligament/soft-tissue laxity allows for a greater feasibility of surface gliding implants.

Due to its attractive biologic properties and its favorable wear characteristics, a novel indication for the use of pyrocarbon MCP arthroplasty lies in the setting of acute/subacute trauma. In these cases, it can serve as both a total joint replacement and a hemiarthroplasty. In fact, even in the setting of arthrosis, pyrocarbon hemiarthroplasty has been shown to be an effective option at a variety of joints including the wrist, shoulder, and thumb base as well as the finger [14–20].

## Technique

The surgical approaches for insertion are similar to silicone implants, and a dorsal (for single and multiple digits) or transverse (for multiple digits) incision can be utilized. In patients with inflammatory arthritis, the radial sagittal band is released to expose the joint capsule which is then split longitudinally to reveal the joint. This allows for plication and centralization of the extensor tendons at closure. For osteoarthritic patients, a tendon splitting approach is appropriate, which can simply be re-approximated/repaired following implant placement. The MCP joint is then flexed and the metacarpal head exposed. At the dorsal one-third point of the metacarpal head, a k-wire can be used to confirm the start point for broaching. It is inserted longitudinally down the canal of the metacarpal and confirmed to be appropriately positioned with fluoroscopy. This also helps identify the start point for the alignment and cutting guide of the metacarpal.

With the pyrocarbon system, a cutting guide is placed and the distal metacarpal cut is made. The guide is then removed and the rest of the cut is made freehand. Clinically, this is an oblique cut that removes the entire metacarpal head while preserving the collateral ligaments. For the SRA implant, the metacarpal cut is made in a similar manner as that for silicone – simply perpendicular, or slightly radially inclined, to the coronal plane axis of the metacarpal at the bone-cartilage interface. Care should be made to protect the collateral ligament origin with the metacarpal head resection.

Resection of the metacarpal head allows for exposure of the proximal phalanx articular surface and the volar plate. A volar plate contracture release can then be performed, if indicated. For both the metal-plastic and pyrocarbon implant systems, the proximal phalangeal cut is perpendicular to the axis of the phalanx. This can be done freehand with the SRA technique. For the pyrocarbon system, an alignment/cutting guide is inserted in the canal at the dorsal third junction. A k-wire, followed by fluoroscopic evaluation, helps confirm the appropriate placement of the alignment guide. The cut at the proximal phalanx begins with the guide in place and is completed freehand after removal of the intramedullary guide.

After making the bone cuts, broaching is performed up to the largest size that fits the canals. The use of side-cutting burrs can be helpful in preparing the canals to maximize fit, especially in patients with thick cortices or healthier bone. The implant can then be trialed and the range of motion of the joint assessed. Stability can also be assessed in both coronal and sagittal planes. When indicated, adjustments to the soft tissues, such as tightening of collateral ligaments

(Fig. 17.6 and Videos 17.2 and 17.3) and further volar release, can then be performed, and the joint can be re-trialed in preparation for the permanent insertion.

If the joint is not stable enough following trialing with the surface gliding trials, the pyrocarbon system has silicone trials that match the bony cuts as a fallback option. The SRA implant manufacturer also has silicone implants that could be used if the surface gliding implants are no longer feasible. Following placement of the final components, the motion and stability are reassessed. Soft-tissue balancing is then completed and the extensor tendon repaired or centralized.

Rehabilitation protocols vary based on the diagnosis and severity of deformity and disease. In patients with rheumatoid arthritis, the first 3–4 weeks following surgery, a forearm-based splint immobilizing the MCP joints in extension, while allowing IP motion, is utilized. Thereafter, a low profile static splint is made for the patient, and a short-arc MCP motion protocol is initiated that increases the motion weekly or biweekly over the subsequent 4–6 weeks. At approximately 2–3 months post-surgery, the patient may begin strengthening.

Patients with osteoarthritis and those with more reliable soft-tissue stabilizers are able to progress with therapy sooner. Depending on joint stability and the status of the collateral ligaments, protected early motion can begin within 2 weeks. If collateral ligament tightening or soft-tissue balancing was necessary, then a longer period of immobilization (closer to that of patients with inflammatory arthritis) should be utilized.

## Results in the Literature

### Silicone

As it has been utilized the most between implant choices over the last 60 years, there is a broad experience with silastic implants for MCP joint reconstruction. Chung et al. examined the role of surgical intervention (n = 70 patients) when prospectively compared to medical management (n = 93 patients) for the treatment of rheumatoid arthritis with severe ulnar drift with and without extensor lag [21]. The groups matched nicely with respect to age, gender, race, education, and deformity. At 1-year follow-up, subjective and objective outcomes were improved in the surgically treated cohort. They concluded that while nonoperative treatment did not deteriorate over the 1-year follow-up period, surgery afforded deformity correction and improved function.

The silicone implant is very successful at early and intermediate follow-up with regard to pain, improvement in motion, and correction of extensor lag and coronal malalignment [4, 22–29]. Unfortunately, long-term outcomes show disappointingly high rate of implant fracture and recurrence of deformity [13–15]. Despite these complications, the rate of revision is surprisingly low for these implants, suggesting that implant failure does not equate to a universally poor outcome [3, 10, 13, 15, 16].

In the setting of rheumatoid and inflammatory arthritis, several large series have been reported with sizeable numbers and relatively longer-term follow-up. Goldfarb and Stern published their experience with 208 joints treated with silastic MCP implants with a 14-year average follow-up period [30]. Their findings demonstrated short-term improvements in alignment and MCP motion, with the mean arc of motion improving from 30 degrees (preoperatively) to 46 degrees postoperatively. However, over time the motion improvements decreased back down to 36 degrees at final follow-up. In a similar manner, the extension deficit improved significantly early postoperatively – from 57 degrees preoperatively to 11 degrees immediately postoperatively – and worsened slightly over time to 23 degrees at final follow-up. Ulnar drift similarly worsened over time from a near-neutral alignment to an average of 16 degrees. Implant fractures were also common, with 63% of implants broken, and implant fracture was associated with increased ulnar drift ($p < 0.001$). Subjectively, at final follow-up, only 38% of the hands were satisfied with their function and only 27% of the hands were pain-free. The authors concluded that long-term outcomes of silicone MCP arthroplasty for rheumatoid arthritis are associated with early good results that worsen over time. Trail et al. reviewed the outcomes of 1336 implants in 381 patients treated with silastic MCP arthroplasty over a 17-year period [31]. Their implant fracture's rate of 67% at final follow-up was similar to that of Goldfarb and Stern. However, the overall revision surgery rate was less than 6%. Adjunct procedures that improved survival included soft-tissue balancing, crossed intrinsic transfer, and realignment of the wrist. The use of grommets did not protect implants from fracture.

We examined our experience of 325 joints over a 14-year period with an average 7-year follow-up period [32]. The 5-, 10-, and 15-year survival-free from revision rates were 98%, 95%, and 95%, respectively. Radiographically, the outcomes were not as favorable, and the 5-, 10-, and 15-year survival rates free from radiographic implant fracture were 93%, 58%, and 35%, respectively. This appears to correlate with recurrent ulnar drift as the 5-, 10-, and 15-year survival rates free from coronal plane deformity of greater than 10 degrees were 81%, 37%, and 17%, respectively. Clinically, significant improvements in their postoperative pain levels and MCP arc of motion were experienced. We concluded that pain relief and functional improvement are reliable, but silicone MCP arthroplasty carries a high fracture rate over time, which correlates with recurrent ulnar drift.

## Surface Replacement Arthroplasty (SRA)

The metal-plastic SRA is an established alternative to silicone for MCP reconstruction. Unfortunately, little has been published with respect to its use. As it was designed by Dr. Linscheid, we have had considerable experience with this implant at our institution, more for inflammatory than noninflammatory arthritis.

Claxton et al. reviewed the Mayo Clinic experience with the use of SRA implants for rheumatoid arthritis [33]. Eighty fingers in 27 patients underwent treatment with the SRA implant with a 9.5-year average follow-up period (minimum of 2 years). Pain relief, grip strength, and arc of motion were significantly improved. Thirteen fingers (16%) underwent revision and 29 (36%) needed reoperation. Kaplan-Meier analysis for survivorship at 1 , 5 , 10 , and 20 years was 100%, 95%, 85%, and 69%, respectively. Analysis for reoperations demonstrated 1-, 5-, 10-, and 20-year survival free from reoperation to be 89%, 80%, 65%, and 46%, respectively. Complications were not uncommon and included functional instability with and without joint subluxation occurring in 31% of digits. Less common complications included delayed wound healing, tendon or ligament rupture, ligament laxity, heterotopic bone, and synovitis. While the outcomes are worrisome to some degree, it may be more related to the diagnosis than the implant. The use of non-constrained implants in the setting of inflammatory arthritis carries greater risk of failures due to the poorer soft-tissue constraints in these patients.

With respect to the use of SRA in noninflammatory arthritis, there are no published reports to date. Our experience has been submitted and is awaiting review. It consists of 18 digits in 15 patients with an average 6.9-year follow-up period. Pain relief and functional improvement have been predictable, but the overall patient satisfaction rate is 72%. Unfortunately, three digits have necessitated revision surgery, and the Kaplan-Meier analysis for 2-, 5-, 10-, and 15-year survivorship was 89%, 89%, 76%, and 76% respectively. Five joints have required reoperation, and the most common indication for reoperation was stiffness. The KM analysis for reoperations at 2, 5, 10, and 15 years was 72%, 72%, 62%, and 62%, respectively.

## Pyrocarbon

There have been numerous publications examining outcomes of pyrocarbon MCP arthroplasty [34–40]. Cook et al. were the first to publish their results and examined 71 MCP pyrocarbon arthroplasties in 26 patients at an average 12-year follow-up period [41]. Inflammatory arthritis was the most common diagnosis treated in the authors' experience. Kaplan-Meier analysis demonstrated an 82% 5-year and 81% 10-year survivorship, with a predicted 2% annual failure rate. Clinically, pain relief was generally excellent and MCP joint arc of motion improved 16 degrees. The patients achieved a more extended posture with an overall improved hand function. Radiographic outcomes (in 53 of 71 fingers) noted that 94% maintained MCP joint reduction. While there was a trend toward recurrent ulnar drift over time, at the most recent follow-up, the recurrent ulnar drift was not worse than preoperative measurements. The authors concluded that pyrocarbon arthroplasty was a viable option in the management of MCP joint arthritis.

Subsequent series have also reported encouraging outcomes, especially in treating patients with osteoarthritis. Parker et al. also examined a large series of 130 MCP primary pyrocarbon arthroplasties, of which 116 were available for radiographic analysis, with an average 17-month follow-up period [35]. Most of the patients had rheumatoid arthritis (96 joints) versus 20 joints with osteoarthritis. At this early follow-up, the authors noted a 99% survivorship and generally excellent clinical results and pain relief. Patient satisfaction was also greater than 90%. The overall complication rates were 6% minor and 9% major among the cohorts, with more in the RA group that included two cases of hand dysfunction and recurrent ulnar drift requiring repeat soft-tissue balancing, one patient with dislocation, and one case of stiffness that underwent manipulation under anesthesia. The OA group had two "major" complications: one extensor tendon disruption and another for persistent pain that required implant removal. Radiographically, the OA group had generally stable overall radiographic appearance. However, in inflammatory arthritis patients, the radiographic analysis was more worrisome. While most were not revised because the patient was asymptomatic, there was a 14% dislocation rate. In addition, nearly all (95%) had increased radiolucent seam, 55% had axial subsidence, and 45% were noted to have periprosthetic erosions.

Kopylov et al. reported their results with the use of pyrocarbon in patients with rheumatoid arthritis in 14 patients (40 fingers) [34]. The minimum follow-up period was 3 years. Clinically, all patients had pain relief and improved clinical outcomes and motion. Complications were noted in two joints: one patient was revised secondary to excessive loosening.

The results of pyrocarbon MCP arthroplasty have been promising for osteoarthritis. Wall and Stern examined 11 cases with a minimum 2-year follow-up (average 4 years) [38]. Range of motion was improved and pain relief was excellent, but grip strength did not improve. Patient outcome measures were generally excellent. All patients were able to return to their preoperative employment. Complications included one finger with extensor tendon subluxation, and another was revised to arthrodesis secondary to persistent pain. Radiographically, while there was an average 3 millimeter subsidence, no implant migration, fracture, or dislocation was experienced. They concluded that pyrocarbon MCP arthroplasty was a good surgical option for patients with osteoarthritis.

Nunez and Citron reported a short-term experience with the use of pyrocarbon MCP joints in patients with osteoarthritis [11]. In seven patients with ten MCP joints and an average follow-up of 2.2 years (range 1–4 years), they noted pain scores improved significantly. Radiographically, there was no evidence of implant failure or loosening. Overall, there were excellent patient satisfaction scores. The authors concluded that pyrocarbon MCP arthroplasty is a promising solution for osteoarthritis. In a larger series, Simpson-White and Chojnowski reviewed 18 fingers in 10 patients treated with pyrocarbon MCP arthroplasty for osteoarthritis, with an average follow-up period of approximately 5 years [38]. Pain scores and Quick DASH measures were all improved, with all but one patient being satisfied. Range of motion also improved. One case was revised to a silicone MCP implant due to negatively affected pinch. Radiographically, the authors also appreciated radiographic subsidence of the implants (and of some components up to 5 mm), but no dislocations or overt loosening. Similar to Walls and Stern, the authors concluded that pyrocarbon implants are a good option for the management of MCP joint OA.

In the largest published report to date, Dickson and colleagues examined outcomes of 51 fingers in 36 patients treated for osteoarthritis, with a minimum 5-year follow-up period (average 103 months) [37]. The authors noted that pain scores improved significantly postoperatively. The average VAS (1–10) final pain score was 0.9 (range 0–7). In addition, MCP range of motion averaged 54 degrees (range 20–80), and the final grip strength was 25 kg (range 11–45). The final Quick DASH and Patient Evaluation Measures (PEM) averaged 28.9 (range 0–56.8) and 26.5 (range 10–54), respectively. The overall implant survivorship was 88% at 10 years. The most common complication was dislocation, which occurred in three joints. They were treated as follows: one was stable following closed reduction, one was revised to silicone, and the third was "up-sized" to larger components. One patient had subluxation of the MCP joint, which was corrected with upsizing the implant. One case of CRPS was noted. There were two "late" complications of stiffness, which underwent manipulation and percutaneous soft-tissue release. One patient sustained a prosthetic stem fracture and another had aseptic loosening. Both of these cases were revised to silicone arthroplasty. Interestingly, all the implant revisions were performed within the first 18 months following surgery, and the authors attributed it to a learning curve and felt that this was a reflection more of "technical issues" rather than inherent problems with the implant. They concluded that, in nonrheumatoid patients, pyrocarbon MCP arthroplasty provides good pain relief, function, motion, and satisfaction.

Due to its material properties, durability, biomechanical characteristics, and features, pyrocarbon has been considered and utilized as a hemiarthroplasty. This has been described in the treatment of thumb CMC and finger proximal interphalangeal joint arthritis [17, 19, 42]. This has also been applied to the severely damaged MCP in the setting of trauma. Houdek et al. reviewed outcome of pyrocarbon MCP arthroplasty or hemiarthroplasty in the setting of trauma with a table saw and non-reconstructable cartilage loss, with a 4-year average follow-up interval [15]. Ten fingers in seven patients were treated that underwent MCP arthroplasty in the acute setting. Four patients were treated with a total MCP arthroplasty and six underwent hemiarthroplasty. At final follow-up, the mean MCP arc of motion was 56 degrees (range 30–70). Overall pain relief was excellent and there were no revision surgeries. No cases of infection occurred and the implants maintained stable position radiographically. There was a 50% reoperation rate for tenolysis, which is not that unexpected, given the fact that these patients had concomitant tendon injuries. The authors concluded that pyrocarbon can be viable option in the management of acute intra-articular trauma with resultant non-repairable cartilage injury.

## Discussion

Patient selection is very important when deciding the optimal choice of implant. Most surgeons consider silicone to be the gold standard in the management of MCP arthritis, especially in cases of inflammatory arthritis. The lack of competent soft-tissue stabilizers invites recurrent deformity, subluxation, and instability. When considering surface gliding implants in the setting of inflammatory arthritis, these non-constrained implants should be reserved for patients with mild involvement and well-controlled disease. However, in the setting of osteoarthritis and stable post-traumatic arthritis, the surface gliding implants are an excellent alternative to silicone. When comparing the SRA and pyrocarbon, the literature reflects a larger experience with pyrocarbon. This may be due to the need for cementing with the SRA implant.

Good surgical technique is critical to help insure optimal outcomes with these implants. In the setting of inflammatory arthritis, it is very important to understand the "soft-tissue" balancing and stabilization are as (if not more) important than the bony procedure. This includes ligament balancing, volar capsule release, centralization of the extensor tendons, and (when indicated) intrinsic release/transfer.

With the surface replacement implants, protection of the collateral ligaments and preservation of bone stock are critical. Identification of the bone-cartilage interface along the dorsal distal metacarpal will serve as starting point for the bone cuts just distal to the collateral ligament origin. However, this may be altered by the arthritis, and care needs to be taken in removing the osteophytes prior to making this determination as it may result in excessive bone resection. Release of the volar plate and soft tissues may also be necessary when utilizing the surface replacement implants, especially if there is a component of preoperative subluxation. This maneuver helps ensure placement of the appropriate-sized implant and will help facilitate stability of the joint. Distally, only 2–3 millimeters of bone resection off the proximal phalanx is necessary. Removal of too much can negatively affect stability and compromise the collaterals, which insert on the volar aspect of the proximal phalanx. We encourage removal of all articular cartilage as this could result in recurrent episodes of inflammation. At the time of implant trialing, it is important to achieve some hyperextension (of approximately 10 degrees). If you have difficulty with extension, the patient is at risk of an extension lag, which we find is more frustrating to patients than limited flexion.

Volar osteophytes are not uncommon, especially in more severe arthritis, and these can limit flexion and/or result in deviation of the finger as it flexes. It is important to remove them and confirm, when trialing, that they are not impacting joint motion and gliding. A side-cutting burr can be very helpful in these cases as it helps prepare the canals for broaching, especially in patients with sclerotic or hard bone. When indicated, I prefer impaction bone grafting over cementing into the canals and using the bone from the resected metacarpal head. Impaction grafting can help improve fit and alignment of the components.

When considering the soft tissues, the ligaments can be reinforced, tightened, or repaired by placing holes drilled with a 0.045 k-wire or a 2 mm drill in the dorsal radial aspect of the distal metacarpal or through the footprint of the origin of the collateral ligament within the metacarpal head sulcus. This repair can be achieved with absorbable or nonabsorbable sutures including a 3–0 mersilene, 3–0 fiberwire, 2–0 ticron, or 3–0 vicryl, depending on the tissue quality, sizes, and degree of laxity. It is important to have the sutures in place before placement of the final components, and secure the sutures following placement of the implant. If the implant fit is poor at the time of trialing, either more bone resection or placement of larger implants may be needed. In addition, silicone implants can serve as a bailout if stability cannot be achieved with the modular joints.

Special consideration is necessary when treating the index finger. Due to the loads across its MCP joint due to lateral pinch, proper assessment before and after surgery is important at the index finger. Instability at this joint can be very challenging. Care should be taken in preoperative assessment of these digits and intraoperative stability following implant placement. Radial collateral ligament reinforcement is often utilized in my experience, and my threshold for immobilizing the MCP joint for longer periods of time and in slight radial deviation is lower.

Finally, and not least, appropriate hand therapy is essential for a good outcome. The postoperative regimen has evolved over the years and ultimately has been simplified at our institution. Depending on intraoperative stability, the hand is immobilized with the MCP in extension, allowing for IP motion. After 1–4 weeks, depending on the diagnosis and intraoperative findings, the patient graduates to a removable orthosis that also holds the MCP joint in extension and allows for IP motion. A short arc type of protocol is begun, which progressively increases active MCP motion 10–15 degrees weekly until 75–80 degrees is reached. Patients with inflammatory arthritis require a heightened awareness of coronal plane alignment. At 3 months postoperative, the patient may begin strengthening exercises.

Because of the functional limitations associated with arthrodesis, arthroplasty is an important treatment for MCP joint arthritis in patients with both inflammatory and noninflammatory arthritis. Silicone remains the gold standard and the primary treatment for patients with RA. Newer implants, including pyrocarbon and metal-on-plastic designs, with more favorable material properties, have the potential to become the preferred option for noninflammatory arthritis. In our practice, they have already become the first choice for patients with osteoarthritis. Future advances and study will further define the role of this surgery and best treatment options.

## References


1. Swanson AB. Flexible implant resection arthroplasty. Hand. 1972;4(2):119–34.
2. Swanson AB. Silicone rubber implants for replacement of arthritis or destroyed joints in the hand. Surg Clin North Am. 1968;48(5):1113–27.
3. Swanson AB. Flexible implant arthroplasty for arthritic finger joints: rationale, technique, and results of treatment. J Bone Joint Surg Am. 1972;54(3):435–55.
4. Escott BG, et al. NeuFlex and Swanson metacarpophalangeal implants for rheumatoid arthritis: prospective randomized, controlled clinical trial. J Hand Surg Am. 2010;35(1):44–51.
5. Goldner JL, et al. Metacarpophalangeal joint arthroplasty with silicone-Dacron prostheses (Niebauer type): six and a half years' experience. J Hand Surg Am. 1977;2(3):200–11.
6. McArthur PA, Milner RH. A prospective randomized comparison of Sutter and Swanson silastic spacers. J Hand Surg (Br). 1998;23(5):574–7.
7. Moller K, et al. Avanta versus Swanson silicone implants in the MCP joint--a prospective, randomized comparison of 30 patients followed for 2 years. J Hand Surg Br. 2005;30(1):8–13.
8. Swanson AB. *Finger joint replacement by silicone rubber implants and the concept of implant fixation by encapsulation*. Ann Rheum Dis. 1969;28(Suppl 5):47–55.
9. Murakata LA, Rangwala AF. Silicone lymphadenopathy with concomitant malignant lymphoma. J Rheumatol. 1989;16(11):1480–3.
10. Smith RJ, Atkinson RE, Jupiter JB. Silicone synovitis of the wrist. J Hand Surg Am. 1985;10(1):47–60.
11. Haubold AD. On the durability of pyrolytic carbon in vivo. Med Prog Technol. 1994;20(3–4):201–8.
12. Kawalec JS, et al. Evaluation of fibrocartilage regeneration and bone response at full-thickness cartilage defects in articulation with pyrolytic carbon or cobalt-chromium alloy hemiarthroplasties. J Biomed Mater Res. 1998;41(4):534–40.
13. Beckenbaugh RD. Pyrolytic Carbon Implants. In: Simmen, editor. Hand Arthroplasties. London: Martin Dunitz; 2000. p. 323–7.
14. Garret J, et al. Pyrolytic carbon humeral head in hemi-shoulder arthroplasty: preliminary results at 2-year follow-up. JSES Open Access. 2019;3(1):37–42.
15. Houdek MT, et al. Metacarpophalangeal joint arthroplasty in the setting of trauma. J Hand Surg Am. 2015;40(12):2416–20.
16. Kim K, Gong HS, Baek GH. Pyrolytic carbon hemiarthroplasty for avascular necrosis of the metacarpal head: a case report. J Hand Surg Asian Pac Vol. 2018;23(1):140–3.
17. Pettersson K, Amilon A, Rizzo M. Pyrolytic carbon hemiarthroplasty in the management of proximal interphalangeal joint arthritis. J Hand Surg Am. 2015;40(3):462–8.
18. Santos FL, et al. APSI scaphoid hemiarthroplasty - long-term results. Rev Bras Ortop. 2018;53(5):582–8.
19. Vitale MA, et al. Pyrolytic carbon arthroplasty versus suspensionplasty for trapezial-metacarpal arthritis. J Wrist Surg. 2017;6(2):134–43.
20. Bigorre N, et al. Intermediate term evaluation of the Eclypse distal radio-ulnar prosthesis for rheumatoid arthritis. A report of five cases. Orthop Traumatol Surg Res. 2016;102(3):345–9.
21. Chung KC, et al. A multicenter clinical trial in rheumatoid arthritis comparing silicone metacarpophalangeal joint arthroplasty with medical treatment. J Hand Surg Am. 2009;34(5):815–23.
22. Beckenbaugh RD, et al. Review and analysis of silicone-rubber metacarpophalangeal implants. J Bone Joint Surg Am. 1976;58(4):483–7.
23. Chung KC, et al. A prospective study comparing outcomes after reconstruction in rheumatoid arthritis patients with severe ulnar drift deformities. Plast Reconstr Surg. 2009;123(6):1769–77.
24. Chung KC, Kotsis SV. Outcomes of hand surgery in the patient with rheumatoid arthritis. Curr Opin Rheumatol. 2010;22(3):336–41.
25. Chung KC, et al. Outcomes of silicone arthroplasty for rheumatoid metacarpophalangeal joints stratified by fingers. J Hand Surg Am. 2009;34(9):1647–52.
26. Delaney R, Trail IA, Nuttall D. A comparative study of outcome between the Neuflex and Swanson metacarpophalangeal joint replacements. J Hand Surg Br. 2005;30(1):3–7.
27. Kirschenbaum D, et al. Arthroplasty of the metacarpophalangeal joints with use of silicone-rubber implants in patients who have rheumatoid arthritis. Long-term results. J Bone Joint Surg Am. 1993;75(1):3–12.
28. Schmidt K, et al. Ten-year follow-up of silicone arthroplasty of the metacarpophalangeal joints in rheumatoid hands. Scand J Plast Reconstr Surg Hand Surg. 1999;33(4):433–8.
29. Waljee JF, Chung KC. Objective functional outcomes and patient satisfaction after silicone metacarpophalangeal arthroplasty for rheumatoid arthritis. J Hand Surg Am. 2012;37(1):47–54.
30. Goldfarb CA, Stern PJ. Metacarpophalangeal joint arthroplasty in rheumatoid arthritis. A long-term assessment. J Bone Joint Surg Am. 2003;85-A(10):1869–78.

31. Trail IA, et al. Seventeen-year survivorship analysis of silastic metacarpophalangeal joint replacement. J Bone Joint Surg Br. 2004;86(7):1002–6.
32. Boe C, Wagner E, Rizzo M. Long-term outcomes of silicone metacarpophalangeal arthroplasty: a longitudinal analysis of 325 cases. J Hand Surg Eur Vol. 2018;43(10):1076–82.
33. Claxton MR, Wagner ER, Rizzo M. Long-term outcomes of MCP surface replacement arthroplasty in patients With rheumatoid arthritis. Hand (N Y). 2020:1558944720926631.
34. Kopylov P, Tagil M. Ascension MCP metacarpophalangeal non-constrained pyrolytic carbon prosthesis in rheumatoid arthritis. J Hand Surg (Br). 2005;30B:61.
35. Parker WL, et al. Preliminary results of nonconstrained pyrolytic carbon arthroplasty for metacarpophalangeal joint arthritis. J Hand Surg Am. 2007;32(10):1496–505.
36. Syed MA, Smith A, Benjamin-Laing H. Pyrocarbon implant fracture after metacarpophalangeal joint arthroplasty: an unusual cause for early revision. J Hand Surg Eur Vol. 2010;35(6):505–6.
37. Dickson DR, et al. Pyrocarbon metacarpophalangeal joint arthroplasty in noninflammatory arthritis: minimum 5-year follow-up. J Hand Surg Am. 2015;40(10):1956–62.
38. Simpson-White RW, Chojnowski AJ. Pyrocarbon metacarpophalangeal joint replacement in primary osteoarthritis. J Hand Surg Eur Vol. 2014;39(6):575–81.
39. Wall LB, Stern PJ. Clinical and radiographic outcomes of metacarpophalangeal joint pyrolytic carbon arthroplasty for osteoarthritis. J Hand Surg Am. 2013;38(3):537–43.
40. Nunez VA, Citron ND. Short-term results of the ascension pyrolytic carbon metacarpophalangeal joint replacement arthroplasty for osteoarthritis. Chir Main. 2005;24(3–4):161–4.
41. Cook SD, et al. Long-term follow-up of pyrolytic carbon metacarpophalangeal implants. J Bone Joint Surg Am. 1999;81(5):635–48.
42. de Aragon JSM, et al. Early outcomes of pyrolytic carbon hemiarthroplasty for the treatment of trapezial-metacarpal arthritis. J Hand Surg Am. 2009;34(2):205–12.

# 18 Revision/Failed Metacarpophalangeal Joint Arthroplasty

Mohammed S. Hussain, Phillip R. Ross, and Peter J. Stern

## Introduction

Management of end-stage inflammatory arthritis of the metacarpophalangeal (MCP) joint has evolved over time. Similar to large joints, inflammatory disease can progress to stiff, malaligned, painful joints that limit daily function [1]. Left untreated, ulnar drift and inability to fully extend the fingers at the MCPJ can lead to substantial disability with weak and dysfunctional grasp [2]. The MCP joint can also be affected by primary osteoarthritis, albeit at a lower rate than the interphalangeal joints [3].

Primary MCP joint arthroplasty is indicated when the joint is malaligned, articular cartilage has been destroyed, and soft tissue support is inadequate for joint stability. The goal of arthroplasty is to correct deformity, restore function, and relieve pain [4]. Early attempts at arthroplasty were met with failure secondary to instability and implant design flaws [5]. Improved outcomes were obtained with introduction of silicone implants with the goal of creating a mobile joint, internal fibrous mold, and joint spacer. Introduced in the 1960s, silicone implants serve as a spacer which achieve stability by fibrous encapsulation combined with surgical soft tissue rebalancing [6]. Unfortunately, soft tissues are frequently in poor condition which can contribute to recurrent MCP joint deformity and poor hand function. Reliance on the soft tissue envelope for encapsulation makes revision silicone arthroplasty a less reliable surgery than the index procedure. Accordingly, revision procedures for failed MCPJ arthroplasty represent a treatment dilemma in patient selection and overall outcome.

M. S. Hussain · P. R. Ross · P. J. Stern (✉)
University of Cincinnati, Department of Orthopaedic Surgery, Cincinnati, OH, USA
e-mail: hussaimd@ucmail.uc.edu; rosspp@ucmail.uc.edu; sternpj@ucmail.uc.edu

## Arthroplasty Background

Revision procedures for MCPJ arthritis must take into consideration the specific initial implant, condition of the surrounding soft tissues, and surgical indications for the index arthroplasty. The two major forms of MCPJ replacement, silicone and pyrocarbon implants, differ in their action in treating arthritic changes and will be discussed separately.

### Silicone Arthroplasty

Silicone functions via fibrous encapsulation, balancing healing with formation of scar tissue (fibrous encapsulation) and maintaining function by earlier, controlled range of motion [7]. After an initial period of encapsulation, the integrity of the implant becomes less important as the fibrous capsule around the implant. Fibrous encapsula-


G. J. W. King, M. Rizzo (eds.), *Arthroplasty of the Upper Extremity*,
https://doi.org/10.1007/978-3-030-68880-6_18

tion along with soft tissue rebalancing (including extensor tendon centralization) creates a stable, mobile, pain-free joint.

Rheumatoid arthritis (RA) causes destructive joint synovitis leading to articular cartilage destruction, dislocation, flexion deformity, and ulnar deviation of the digits with decreased grip strength. Silicone implants have shown promise in treating these conditions which are often accompanied by severe deformity [8, 9]. Although modern medical therapy has decreased the severity and incidence of rheumatoid disease, silicone MCP arthroplasties have been a longstanding option for correction of deformity, pain relief, and improved function [10, 11]. Outcome scores are higher in patients treated with a combination of silicone arthroplasty and medical management compared to medical management alone [2]. Correction of ulnar drift using silicone implants, especially with the small and ring finger, can improve power grip and overall hand function [11]. In addition, silicone MCPJ arthroplasty in RA helps improve the flexed posture of the MCPJ and thereby changes the arc of motion from a flexed to a more extended and functionally useful arc [11]. But this may also result in a decrease in flexion [4].

Variations on the original Swanson silicone implant may also be utilized in both primary and revision scenarios. Hinged designs that include anatomic bend have shown promise in maintaining range of motion and improving occupational function scores while reducing pistoning and decreasing risk for revision surgery [3, 8, 12]. These implants have a more palmar center of rotation with collars to prevent pistoning of the implant [13]. Patients treated with these implants have shown increased flexion [8]. However, these designs are also vulnerable to implant fracture and recurrent deformity [12]. These alternative silicone implants perform similarly to the original Swanson design [14].

### Pyrocarbon Arthroplasty

In contrast, pyrocarbon implants function through a different mechanism. Thermochemical decomposition of a hydrocarbon gas creates an implant with a resultant elastic modulus similar to the bone, thus decreasing the bone stress transfer [15]. It is a non-constrained implant designed to resurface the MCPJ and preserve the collateral ligaments thereby helping to maintain joint integrity. These implants, therefore, may be a more viable option for higher-demand patients such as those with osteoarthritis [16]. Pyrocarbon implants serve as an alternative to silicone implants for patients with less deformity and structurally intact collateral ligaments [1]. Adequate soft tissue tension is needed to prevent dislocation; however, excessive tension can result in stiffness, squeaking, and aseptic loosening [9]. Despite these potential complications, pyrocarbon implants can provide a stable joint in a younger patient population.

## Epidemiology

The incidence of revision surgery for MCPJ arthroplasty has been reported in different case series and studies of both silicone and pyrocarbon implants [17] (Table 18.1). Use of silicone implants in the treatment of primary MCP joint osteoarthritis has shown good long-term results, displaying 97% survivorship at an average follow-up of 8.3 years [18]. A similar series demonstrated decreased survival of 88% at 7 years with a decrease to 68% when all implant fractures were taken into consideration [13]. The longest reported series in rheumatoid arthritis patients, consisting of 381 patients with 1336 implants, had survivorship of 80% at 10 years and 63% at 17 years post-surgery [19]. Failure was defined in the setting of revision surgery or fracture of the implant. Revision occurred in 2.9% of implants.

Pyrocarbon implants have also been utilized to replace failed silicone implants with one series of 12 conversions among 61 consecutive patients with 142 arthroplasties [16]. However, within this cohort, surgery for silicone revision led to a higher rate of major complications including subluxation, dislocation, and soft tissue rebalancing compared to primary arthroplasty at an average of 27 months follow-up. In another series of 21

**Table 18.1** Reported revision rates after silicone or pyrocarbon arthroplasty of the MCPJ

| | Arthroplasty no. (patient) | Implant | Follow-up mean | Revision rate (%) |
|---|---|---|---|---|
| Morrell et al. [18] | 40(35) | Silicone | 8.3 years | 2.5 |
| Stern et al. [10] | 208(36) | Silicone | 14 years | 7 |
| Simpson-white et al. [15] | 18(10) | Pyrocarbon | 58.6 months | 5.6 |
| Neral et al. [29] | 38(30) | Silicone | 56 months | 11 |
| Kimani et al. [13] | 66(237) | Silicone | 7 years | 12 |
| Rettig et al. [31] | 13(12) | Silicone | 40 months | 7.7 |
| Trail et al. [19] | 1336(381) | Silicone | 17 years | 5.7 |
| Beckenbaugh et al. [21] | 530(119) | Silicone | 2.5 years | 2.4 |
| Derkash et al. [32] | 89(16) | Silicone | 11.5 | 12 |
| Cook et al. [33] | 71(26) | Pyrolytic | 11.7 | 12 |

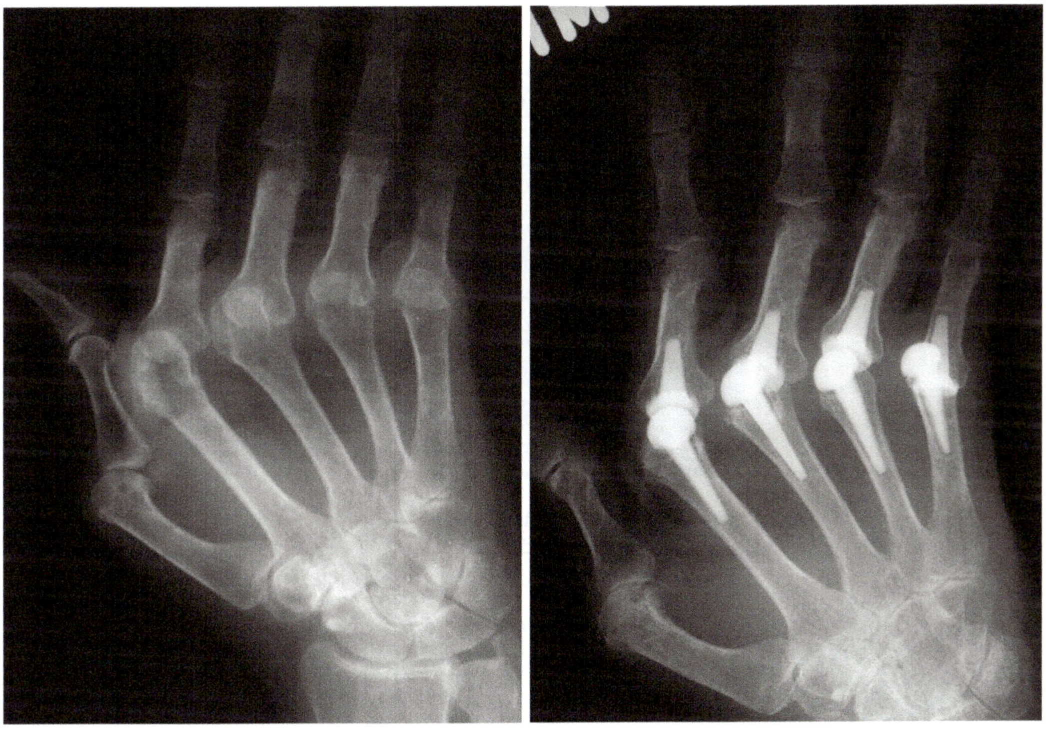

**Fig. 18.1** Preoperative and postoperative radiographs demonstrating recurrence of ulnar deformity and dislocation of the small finger MCPJ

pyrolytic implants, 3 suffered from major complications including extensor tendon rupture, implant dislocation, and chronic pain leading to ray amputation. All patients with major complications had a history of prior surgery to the MCPJ [20] (Fig. 18.1).

## Revision Arthroplasty

No formal guidelines exist regarding indications for revision MCPJ arthroplasty. Measures related to range of motion and implant integrity on radiographic imaging may not correlate with patients' satisfaction with their index procedure. If implant fracture occurs after the initial arthroplasty, the implant can still serve as a spacer within its pseudocapsule. In such cases, revision is often unnecessary.

In rheumatoid patients, isolated decrease in flexion/extension arc has been shown to occur over long-term follow-up with a minimum of 10 years [10]. In this series, patients also had recurrence of ulnar drift and a 63% percent rate of broken implants (Fig. 18.2). However, only 7% underwent revision with lack of implant integrity being the most common reason. In another report of 530 arthroplasties with a mean follow-up of 2.5 years, 26% of implants fractured with 11.3% rate of recurrent deformity [21]. Revision for recurrent deformity secondary to pain and dysfunction can also occur late, with one case undergoing revision 30 years after the index arthroplasty [17]. Silicone implants can cause particulate synovitis and foreign body reaction resulting in bony erosion and loss of bone stock (Fig. 18.3). Fortunately, this complication occurs with less frequency than seen with carpal implant arthroplasty due to decreased compression load across the MCP joint [5].

As previously seen from other studies, implant fracture does not always correlate with the need

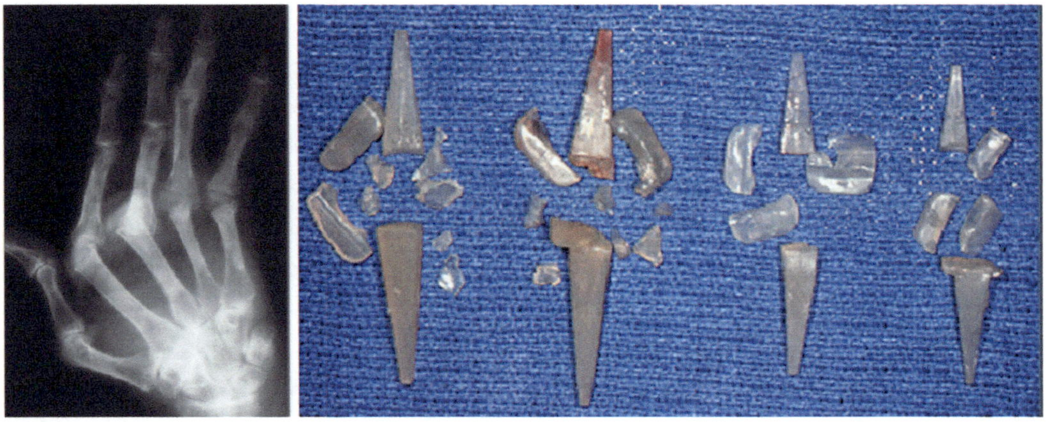

**Fig. 18.2** Recurrent deformity after silicone arthroplasty of the MCPJ in a patient with rheumatoid arthritis. Intraoperatively each implant was noted to be fractured and comminuted

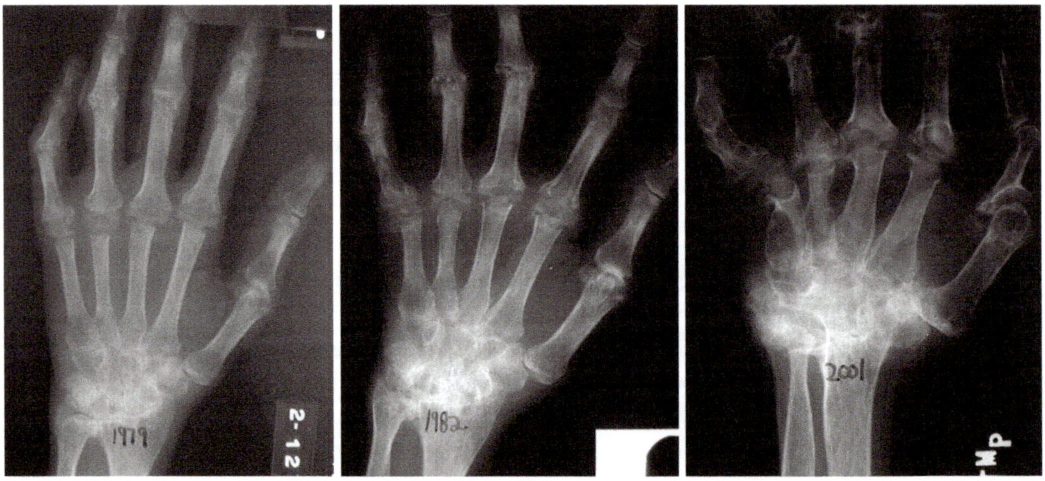


**Fig. 18.3** Subsidence and progressive osteolysis after silicone arthroplasty

for revision. One series of 40 silicone implants for primary MCPJ osteoarthritis demonstrated 5 implant fractures; however, none required revision [18]. In general though, implant fracture appears to correlate with the patient developing symptomatic recurrence of their deformity [17]. Certain factors protect against the need for revision of silicone implants. These include less preoperative deformity prior to surgery, meticulous soft tissue rebalancing at the time of surgery, and concurrent wrist realignment [19].

Intraoperative fractures of the proximal phalanx base and metacarpal shaft at the time of primary arthroplasty can usually be treated with cerclage wires and heal without additional manipulation of the original implant [15]. Over-reaming of the canal, malposition, stress shielding, and tight cortical fit have been identified as causes for this complication.

Infection, although not a common complication, has been reported between 3% and 4% in digital upper extremity implants. Diabetes, rheumatoid arthritis, and increasing ASA class have been identified as risk factors. Coating of the implant with plasma proteins that interact with bacteria can lead to the formation of a biofilm causing chronic infection [22]. Patients may lack overt signs of infection and have insidious onset of pain and swelling with implant loosening. However, erythema, rubor, swelling, and decreased range of motion may be present (Fig. 18.4).

Metallic implants may lead to metallosis and resultant soft tissue destruction. Implants, such as

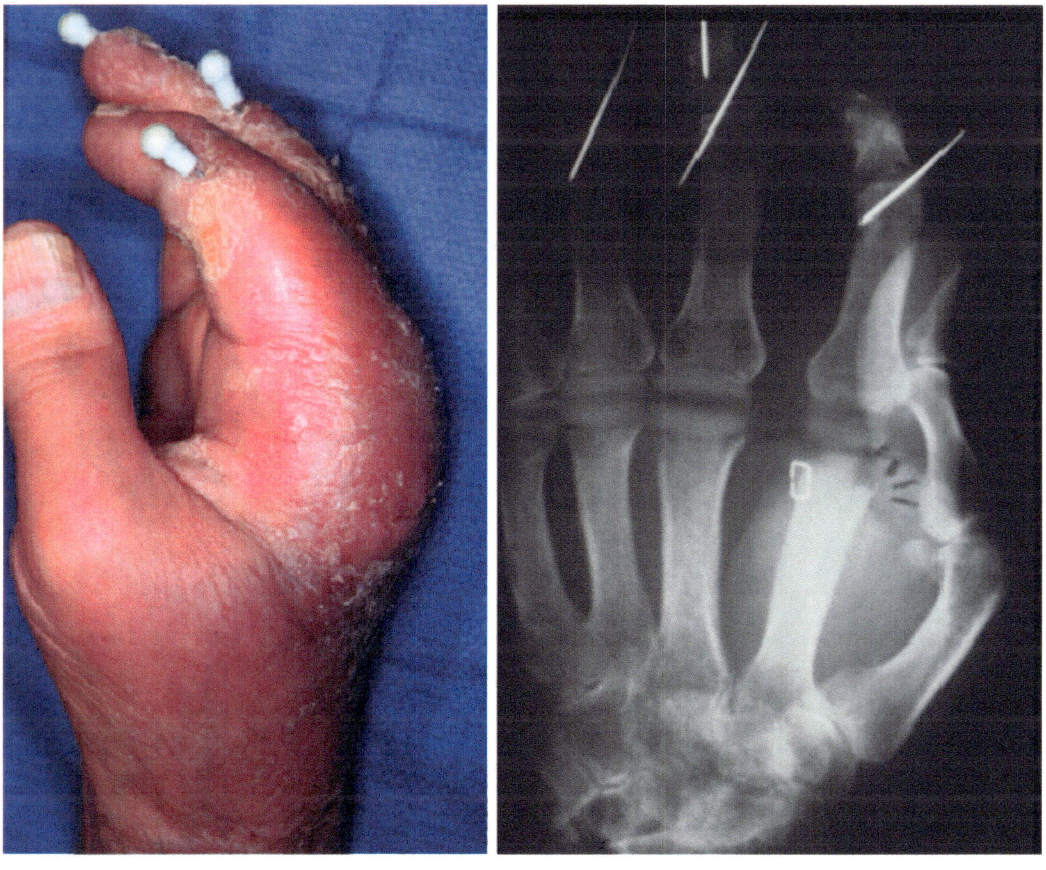

Fig. 18.4 Clinical presentation of infection following MCPJ silicone joint arthroplasty of the index finger. Note osteolysis of the radial side of the metacarpal head

vitallium, used in the early history of arthroplasty produced metal debris and did not gain widespread use [23]. Subsequently, grommets, or metallic sleeves inserted proximal and distal to the collar of a silicone implant have also been found to produce metallosis. Grommets were thought to protect silicone implants from fracture and fragmentation [24]. Malrotation and displacement of grommets can occur. In some instances, over a longer follow-up period, this can lead to recurrent deformity and metallosis necessitating revision [25] (Fig. 18.5).

## Patient Exam and Radiographic Imaging Prior to Revision Arthroplasty

Before embarking on revision MCPJ arthroplasty, a careful description of the patient's complaints and duration from the index procedure must be elicited. In patients with RA, ascertaining a medication history, including current disease-modifying antirheumatic drugs (DMARDs) and biologics, is essential. Similar to patients undergoing a primary arthroplasty, examination for patients considering revision includes assessment of the dermal integrity and

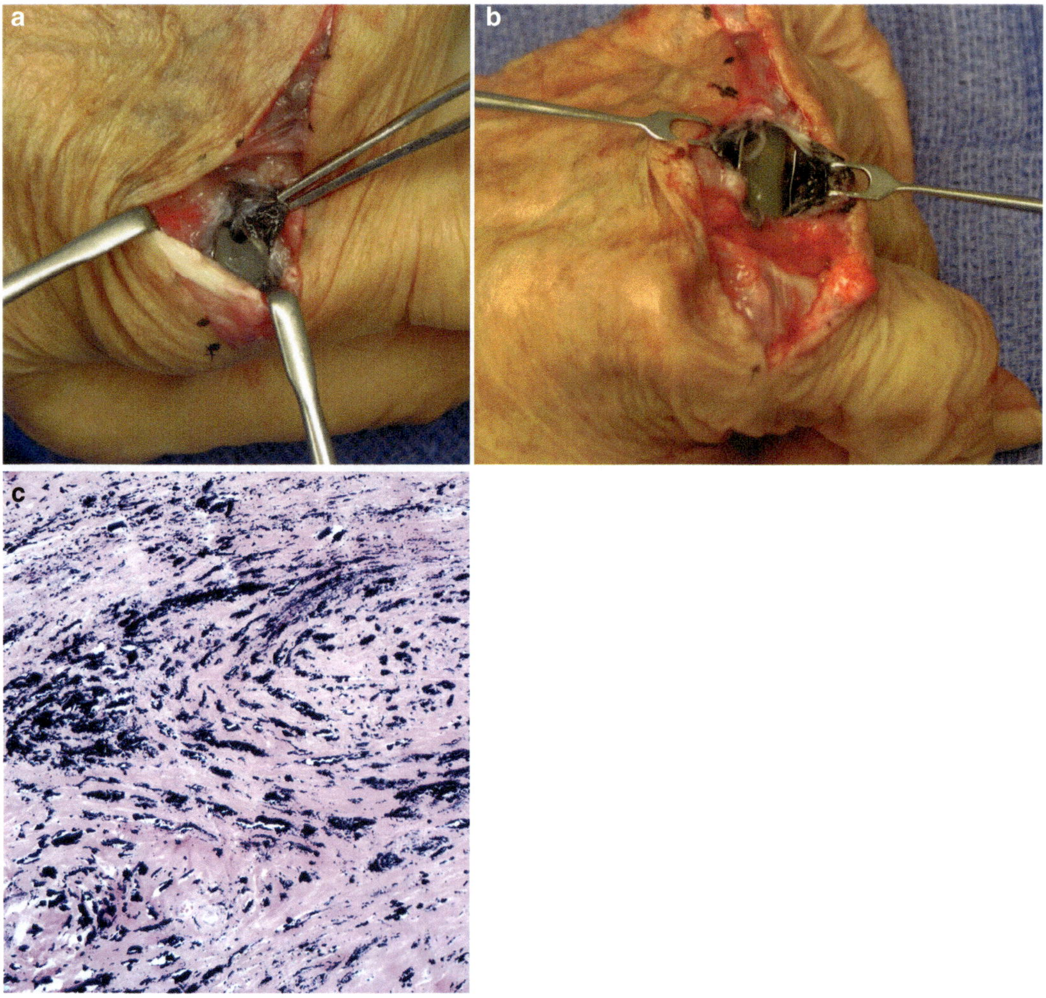

**Fig. 18.5** (**a**–**c**) Interoperative imaging of revision to the middle finger MCPJ with grommets. Soft tissue destruction and metallosis were noted (**a**, **b**). Extensive metallic particle deposition in the pseudosynovial tissue. H&E × 200 (**c**)

neurovascular status. Clinical and radiographic examination for deformity (ulnar drift and palmar subluxation of the proximal phalanx) as well as baseline measures of motion with grip and pinch strength measurements should be obtained. Extensor tendon integrity and any subluxation or imbalance should be noted. Active infection and poor soft tissue coverage are contraindications to revision arthroplasty [9]. Radiographs are mandatory to assess bone stock and implant integrity. Fractured silicone implants may be visualized, and correlation should be made with patient symptoms [10]. In some cases, implant integrity is inferred by indirect measures including subluxation of the MCPJ or bony subsidence. Ulnar deviation of greater than 45°, greater than 50% translation at the MCPJ, and proximal-distal overlap of the metacarpal and proximal phalanx can be used as surrogate markers for implant fracture [19]. Sclerosis around silicone implants may indicate decreased motion at the MCPJ [9]. Periprosthetic cyst formation can also occur around silicone implants [16].

In assessing infection, radiographs frequently show soft tissue swelling and progressive osteolysis. Cortical destruction is seen with osteomyelitis [26]. In contrast to large joint arthroplasty, systemic manifestations of periprosthetic infection may be lacking. Of patients with hand infections leading to operative debridement, one fourth demonstrate no rise in C-reactive protein (CRP) with only half of patients exhibiting an elevated erythrocyte sedimentation rate (ESR) [27]. Cytokines such as IL-6 may become more useful in the future for diagnosing indolent infections, but current clinical use is limited [22].

## Treatment

Although worsening pain, recurrent ulnar drift, and limitation of motion can be seen in asymptomatic patients, persistent symptoms associated with these measures may be an indication for revision. Similar to index arthroplasty procedures, success of revision MCPJ revision depends on the integrity of the remaining soft tissue and ligamentous stabilizers [28]. Challenges include insufficient bone stock, recurrent deformity, and soft tissue (collateral ligament and extensor tendon) insufficiency.

In cases of implant fracture with recurrence of the initial deformity, we approach the joint(s) through the prior incision. Most implant fractures occur at the distal stem junction [19]. After debriding and removing the silicone pieces, a synovial biopsy will often show foreign body reaction, refractile silicone particles, and giant cells, all consistent with particulate synovitis [6]. An assessment of the remaining bone stock is completed. Chronic subluxation of the MCPJ can cause bone loss. The proximal phalanx and metacarpal are curetted to remove an ever-present reactive jacket (cocoon) containing silicone microparticles followed by *minimal* reaming. This is needed to remove residual silicone particles and for fit of the revision implant.

After the revision silicone implant is placed, the pseudocapsule is closed, and the extensor tendon is centralized. The authors have consistently found attenuation of the extensor tendon over the MCPJ and recommend anchoring it with drill holes to the base of the proximal phalanx. The digit is then taken through a passive range of motion to ensure the extensor apparatus is centralized. Reinsertion of the radial collateral ligament although rarely possible ensures further restraint against recurrent ulnar drift.

Infection is a rare complication that can lead to considerable morbidity. Reports of infection with small joint arthroplasties are reported at less than 1% [21, 26]. Time to presentation can be variable from several days to weeks. Inciting organisms are most commonly *Staphylococcus aureus* but can include *Pseudomonas* and *Streptococcus*. Systemic sepsis is often absent with indolent infections presenting with warmth, swelling, and painful range of motion.

In revising implants in the setting of infection, either debridement with retention of implants or one-stage or two-stage revision procedure can be pursued. If concern for recurrent infection after retention or reimplantation of the prosthesis exists, removal of the implant with a resection arthroplasty is an option [26]. MCPJ joints treated in this manner may lead to a stiff pain-free joint.

In the setting of acute infection (within 6–12 weeks), isolated debridement may be sufficient [9]. However, in treating chronic infection with damage to the adjacent soft tissues and osteolysis, staged treatment may be necessary if resection arthroplasty is not performed. An antibiotic spacer can be fashioned around a Kirschner wire with re-implantation at a later date. A prolonged course of antibiotics may be necessary prior to reimplantation. Administering antibiotics targeting gram-positive organisms such as *Staphylococcus* manages the most common microorganisms associated with hand infections [27]. Gram-negative organisms may be present in immunocompromised populations requiring broader coverage. Discussion with infectious disease and rheumatology colleagues regarding the possibility of cessation of DMARDs, when possible, may also be helpful in treatment of infection. Poor bone stock precludes using arthrodesis in the setting of infection and rheumatoid arthritis [26].

The postoperative protocol following revision is similar to primary arthroplasty.

Arthrodesis can address situations where there is inadequate soft tissue envelope, lack of bone stock, or severe, recurrent deformity [6]. MCP joint fusion, however, may be difficult to achieve and may lead to worse function due to loss of range of motion in both the coronal and sagittal planes [9, 29]. Arthrodesis for failed small joint arthroplasty has been used successfully with concomitant distal radius bone graft. Mikolyzk and Stern report a technique involving use of cerclage wiring with a Steinmann pin used as an intramedullary implant [30] (Fig. 18.6). Although they used this technique in revision PIPJ arthroplasties, it can be used successfully for MCPJ fusion. In their series, all joints went on to fusion and achieved a painless, aligned joint.

## Prognosis

Few long-term studies exist on the long-term outcomes of revision MCP joint arthroplasty. Wagner studied 128 revisions performed in 64 patients done with either silicone or pyrocarbon [11]. The most common reason for revision was dislocation. Secondary causes included silicone synovitis, infection, and implant loosening. This patient population was noted to still have improvements in pain and range of motion postoperatively. Nearly 1/5 of patients required additional revision leading to an 81% 5-year survival

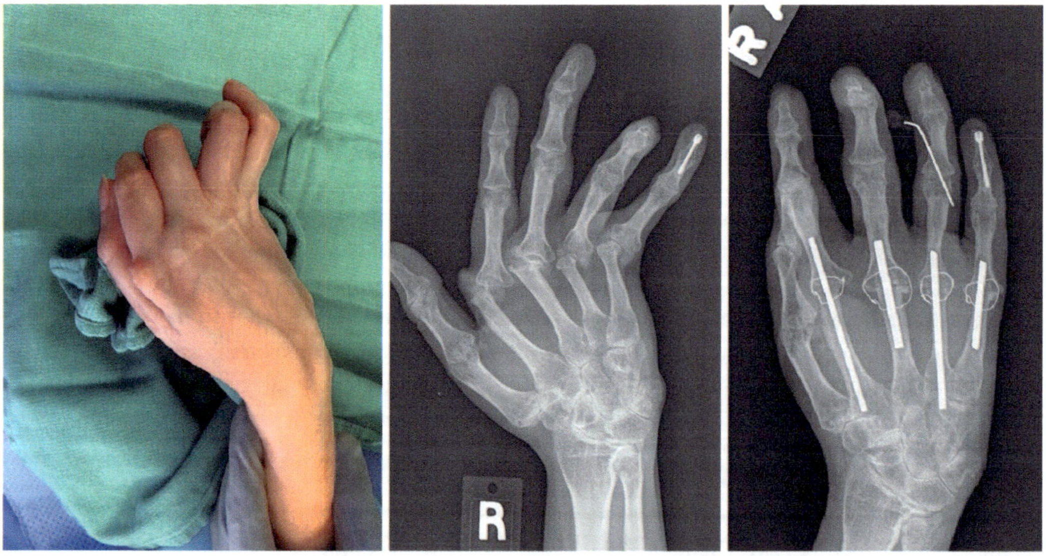


**Fig. 18.6** Recurrent deformity following initial silicone arthroplasty. Salvage procedure was undertaken via MCPJ arthrodesis using intramedullary Steinmann pins and cerclage wires

after first revision. Worse outcomes were associated with implant dislocations, and history of preoperative MCPJ instability increased risk for implant failure. Overall 10-year survival after revision was noted at 78%. Diabetes and smoking were associated with increased failure.

In another series of 20 hands in 16 rheumatoid arthritis patients undergoing revision, 76% of the original implants were noted to be fractured. Other reasons for proceeding with revision included recurrent deformity, pain, flexor digitorum profundus rupture, and loss of dexterity. After a minimum 1-year follow-up after revision, 15 implants fractured, 12 patients were satisfied, and five patients stated they would not have the procedure again. Incomplete correction of ulnar deviation correlated with dissatisfaction with revision arthroplasty. Similar motion was noted before and after revision. Overall, most patients who underwent revision for pain relief were satisfied with their surgery [6].

## Summary

Treatment of failed MCP arthroplasty is challenging, and outcomes are generally inferior to the index surgery. The indications for revision include pain, recurrent deformity, functional loss, implant failure, and infection. The most common revision option is silicone arthroplasty, with a few series that utilized non-constrained pyrocarbon implants. Arthrodesis and resection arthroplasty are options for joints that cannot support arthroplasty and carry a more guarded prognosis and result in generally less functional outcome when compared to revision arthroplasty.

## References

1. Rizzo M. Metacarpophalangeal joint arthritis. J Hand Surg Am. 2011;36(2):345–53.
2. Chung KC, Burns PB, Wilgis EFS, et al. A multicenter clinical trial in rheumatoid arthritis comparing silicone metacarpophalangeal joint arthroplasty with medical treatment. J Hand Surg Am. 2009;34(5):815–23.
3. Namdari S, Weiss A-PC. Anatomically neutral silicone small joint arthroplasty for osteoarthritis. J Hand Surg Am. 2009;34(2):292–300.
4. Bogoch ER, Escott BG, Judd MGP. Insufficient flexion of the metacarpophalangeal joint of the little finger following Swanson silicone arthroplasty for rheumatoid arthritis. Hand. 2008;3(1):24–9.
5. Adkinson JM, Chung KC. Advances in small joint arthroplasty of the hand. Plast Reconstr Surg. 2014;134(6):1260–8.
6. Burgess SD, Kono M, Stern PJ. Results of revision metacarpophalangeal joint surgery in rheumatoid patients following previous silicone arthroplasty. J Hand Surg Am. 2007;32(10):1506–12.
7. Swanson AB, Leonard JB, de Groot Swanson G. Implant resection arthroplasty of the finger joints. Hand Clin. 1986;2(1):107–17.
8. Delaney R, Trail IA, Nuttall D. A comparative study of outcome between the Neuflex and Swanson metacarpophalangeal joint replacements. J Hand Surg Br. 2005;30(1):3–7.
9. Drake ML, Segalman KA. Complications of small joint arthroplasty. Hand Clin. 2010;26(2):205–12.
10. Goldfarb CA, Stern PJ. Metacarpophalangeal joint arthroplasty in rheumatoid arthritis. A long-term assessment. J Bone Joint Surg Am. 2003;85(10):1869–78.
11. Chung KC, Kotsis SV, Wilgis EFS, et al. Outcomes of silicone arthroplasty for rheumatoid metacarpophalangeal joints stratified by fingers. J Hand Surg Am. 2009;34(9):1647–52.
12. Pettersson K, Wagnsjö P, Hulin E. NeuFlex compared with Sutter prostheses: a blind, prospective, randomised comparison of Silastic metacarpophalangeal joint prostheses. Scand J Plast Reconstr Surg Hand Surg. 2006;40(5):284–90.
13. Kimani BM, Trail IA, Hearnden A, Delaney R, Nuttall D. Survivorship of the Neuflex silicone implant in MCP joint replacement. J Hand Surg Eur Vol. 2009;34(1):25–8.
14. Parkkila T, Belt EA, Hakala M, Kautiainen H, Leppilahti J. Comparison of Swanson and Sutter metacarpophalangeal arthroplasties in patients with rheumatoid arthritis: a prospective and randomized trial. J Hand Surg Am. 2005;30(6):1276–81.
15. Simpson-White RW, Chojnowski AJ. Pyrocarbon metacarpophalangeal joint replacement in primary osteoarthritis. J Hand Surg Eur Vol. 2014;39(6):575–81.
16. Parker WL, Rizzo M, Moran SL, Hormel KB, Beckenbaugh RD. Preliminary results of nonconstrained pyrolytic carbon arthroplasty for metacarpophalangeal joint arthritis. J Hand Surg Am. 2007;32(10):1496–505.
17. Arai K, Ishikawa H, Murai T, Fujisawa J, Endo N. Revision metacarpophalangeal joint replacement 30 years after primary swanson flexible silicone implant arthroplasty in a rheumatoid patient: a case report. Hand Surg. 2009;14(1):25–9.
18. Morrell NT, Weiss A-PC. Silicone metacarpophalangeal arthroplasty for osteoarthritis: long-term results. J Hand Surg Am. 2018;43(3):229–33.
19. Trail IA, Martin JA, Nuttall D, Stanley JK. Seventeen-year survivorship analysis of Silastic metacarpopha-

langeal joint replacement. J Bone Joint Surg Br. 2004;86(7):1002–6.
20. Parker W, Moran SL, Hormel KB, Rizzo M, Beckenbaugh RD. Nonrheumatoid metacarpophalangeal joint arthritis. Unconstrained pyrolytic carbon implants: indications, technique, and outcomes. Hand Clin. 2006;22(2):183–93.
21. Beckenbaugh RD, Dobyns JH, Linscheid RL, Bryan RS. Review and analysis of silicone-rubber metacarpophalangeal implants. J Bone Joint Surg Am. 1976;58(4):483–7.
22. Edwards C, Sheppard NN. Prevention, diagnosis, and treatment of implant infection in the distal upper extremity. J Hand Surg Am. 2018;43(1):68–74.
23. Burman MS. Vitallium cup arthroplasty of metacarpophalangeal and interphalangeal joints of fingers. Bull Hosp Joint Dis. 1940;1:79–89.
24. Schmidt K, Willburger R, Ossowski A, Miehlke RK. The effect of the additional use of grommets in silicone implant arthroplasty of the metacarpophalangeal joints. J Hand Surg Br. 1999;24(5):561–4.
25. Choudhry IK, Wilson JM, Stern PJ. Metallosis following silicone metacarpophalangeal joint arthroplasties with grommets: case report. Hand. 2012;7(2):207–9.
26. Millender LH, Nalebuff EA, Hawkins RB, Ennis R. Infection after silicone prosthetic arthroplasty in the hand. J Bone Joint Surg Am. 1975;57(6):825–9.
27. Houshian S, Seyedipour S, Wedderkopp N. Epidemiology of bacterial hand infections. Int J Infect Dis. 2006;10(4):315–9.
28. Wagner ER, Houdek MT, Packard B, Moran SL, Rizzo M. Revision metacarpophalangeal arthroplasty: a longitudinal study of 128 cases. J Am Acad Orthop Surg. 2019;27(6):211–8.
29. Neral MK, Pittner DE, Spiess AM, Imbriglia JE. Silicone arthroplasty for nonrheumatic metacarpophalangeal joint arthritis. J Hand Surg Am. 2013;38(12):2412–8.
30. Mikolyzk DK, Stern PJ. Steinmann pin arthrodesis for salvage of failed small joint arthroplasty. J Hand Surg Am. 2011;36(8):1383–7.
31. Rettig LA, Luca L, Murphy MS. Silicone implant arthroplasty in patients with idiopathic osteoarthritis of the metacarpophalangeal joint. J Hand Surg Am. 2005;30(4):667–72.
32. Derkash RS, Niebauer JJ Jr, Lane CS. Long-term follow-up of metacarpal phalangeal arthroplasty with silicone Dacron prostheses. J Hand Surg Am. 1986;11(4):553–8.
33. Cook SD, Beckenbaugh RD, Redondo J, Popich LS, Klawitter JJ, Linscheid RL. Long-term follow-up of pyrolytic carbon metacarpophalangeal implants. J Bone Joint Surg Am. 1999;81(5):635–48.

# Part VII

# Proximal Interphalangeal Joint Arthroplasty

# Design Considerations for Proximal Interphalangeal Joint Arthroplasty

19

Yoshitaka Minamikawa

## Introduction

Silicone implants introduced by Swanson once enjoyed widespread popularity but declined because of disadvantages of the silicone implants that included tissue reactions such as wear-induced osteolysis, implant destruction/subsidence, cyst formation, recurrent malalignment, and pathologic fractures in association with microparticulate synovitis [1, 2]. There was enthusiasm for developing a new generation of the finger joints after the problems with silicone. None of the efforts received attention internationally except for the surface finger implant by Linscheid [3, 4]. Physiological configuration of that implant preserving soft tissue attachment with good stability had a worldwide expectation to overcome previous complications of finger implant arthroplasty. There were several issues raised from the studies, with considerable complications including motion loss and implant loosening [4]. Although studies with long-term follow-up of Swanson's PIP arthroplasty have demonstrated problems including implant fracture, subsidence, loosening, decreased motion, deformity, and high overall complications, silicone implants have remained the standard for PIP joint arthroplasty. There is limited choice for finger implants, with the only worldwide available implants being the pyrocarbon and different silicone implants more recently developed from various companies and heavily marketed.

Although finger deformities caused by rheumatoid arthritis are decreasing after the introduction of biologic pharmaceuticals, the demands of rheumatoid patient with deformities are increasing as well as cases of osteoarthritis. The need for true total finger implants has become much greater than ever [5]. Flatt and Fischer in 1969 suggested criteria for development of finger implants: restoration of functional range of motion, adequate stability, provision of a mechanical advantage equivalent to normal, firm seating with resistance to rotational stress, provision for easy implantation, and accommodation to finger/joint size [6]. Linscheid advocated, in addition to these, biologic compatibility, adequate material wear and strength characteristics, and allowance for soft tissue reconstruction. He also emphasized difficult points in his experience: small size of joints, their presence within kinematic chains, their complex soft tissue investments, and relations to adjacent rays [7]. Increasing knowledge of anatomy and biomechanical behavior of the finger joint and development of implant material and instruments have changed approaches to developing newer finger implants. Being small was considered as a disadvantage for finger implant arthroplasty; however, it can be perceived as an advantage in some points: screw-type

Y. Minamikawa (✉)
Minamikawa Orthopaedic Surgery/Numba Hand Center, Naniwaku, Osaka, Japan
e-mail: minamikawa@nambahandcenter.com



G. J. W. King, M. Rizzo (eds.), *Arthroplasty of the Upper Extremity*,
https://doi.org/10.1007/978-3-030-68880-6_19

osseointegration can be introduced for the phalanx; size of bone graft can be smaller, if required; and ligament reconstruction or augmentation can be achieved with use of local soft tissue or bone anchor sutures and even other materials available in the market. Early motion exercises can be started with minimum load to stem and bone interface compared to large joints. In this chapter, the author focuses on the historical aspect of implant arthroplasty for the PIP joint, finding reasons for failure and connecting them to future success. If finger implants require intrinsic stability how much should finger implants be responsible. Hand surgeons should choose an implant adequate for each case and, we believe, must be responsible for soft tissue reconstruction.

## Historical Overview

First total finger prosthesis of a metal hinged type was performed by Brannon and Klein in 1959 [8] (Fig. 19.1a). This ridged implant was used in both MCP and PIP joints but had high rates of loosening. Flatt modified the single stem with more flexible and longer twin stems for better fixation (Fig. 19.1b) and extensively used them for rheumatoid patients; however, both erosion and loosening or prosthetic breakage were major problems [9, 10]. With these early failures of metal hinged joints, there were only two approaches for finger implants, plastic one-piece spacers and metal-plastic constrained implants

a b

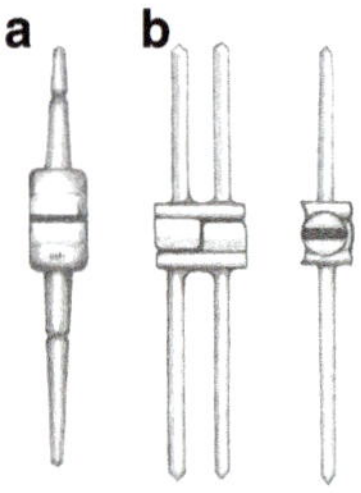

**Fig. 19.1** Metal hinged implant. (**a**) First total finger prosthesis of a metal hinged type performed by Brannon and Klein in 1959. The implant was manufactured from titanium and consisted of non-cemented proximal and distal stems articulating through a hinge stabilized by a screw. (**b**) Flatt modified the single stem with more flexible and longer twin stems for better fixation

mimicking (successful) hip components. Swanson [11] and Niebauer [12] developed silicone implants almost simultaneously but different in design and mechanical concept (Fig. 19.2). Swanson's implant allowed pistoning motion of the stem within the intramedullary cavities and used a thicker C-shaped center that held the bone ends apart and provided some intrinsic extension [13]. Niebauer introduced a Dacron-covered silicone hinge; the Dacron was to provide eventual fixation via incorporation by the tissues of the medullary canal. Niebauer's stem fixation idea was successful but resulted in producing a high implant fracture rate [14]. Cutter-Niebauer design has evolved into Sutter and Avanta prostheses [14, 15], with rectangular stems for more rotational stability, less motion at the stem-bone interface, and larger joint spacer ("shoulder") to lessen wear/subsidence (Fig. 19.2). With the success of implant arthroplasties in large joints, investors were stimulated to create similar design for fingers. Many second-generation hinged prostheses followed (Fig. 19.3), but all failed to create durable improvements in finger motion and acceptable complication rates [3, 7]. Breakage, erosion, loosening, and recurrent finger deformity were the main issues. Most researchers learned from these failures and moved to less constrained mechanisms. Competitive investigation and development of advanced implants continued; non- and minimally constrained surface implants have become standard choices for large joints, except for revision or special cases. Linscheid [16] and Beckenbaugh [17] started to use surface implants for both MP and PIP joints in the early 1970s; however, these non-constrained designs did not prevent dislocation, especially with the MP joint. There was tendency to develop a finger implant for both MP and PIP joints in the early years, but the anatomical shape and biomechanical behavior of the joints are different. Artificial congruity and semi-constrained mechanism are required for the MP joint. Linscheid et al. [18] reported favorable clinical results on 65 PIPs with an average follow-up of 4.5 years. This implant was with a more physiologic articulation, and stability was achieved via minimal bone resection to retain the

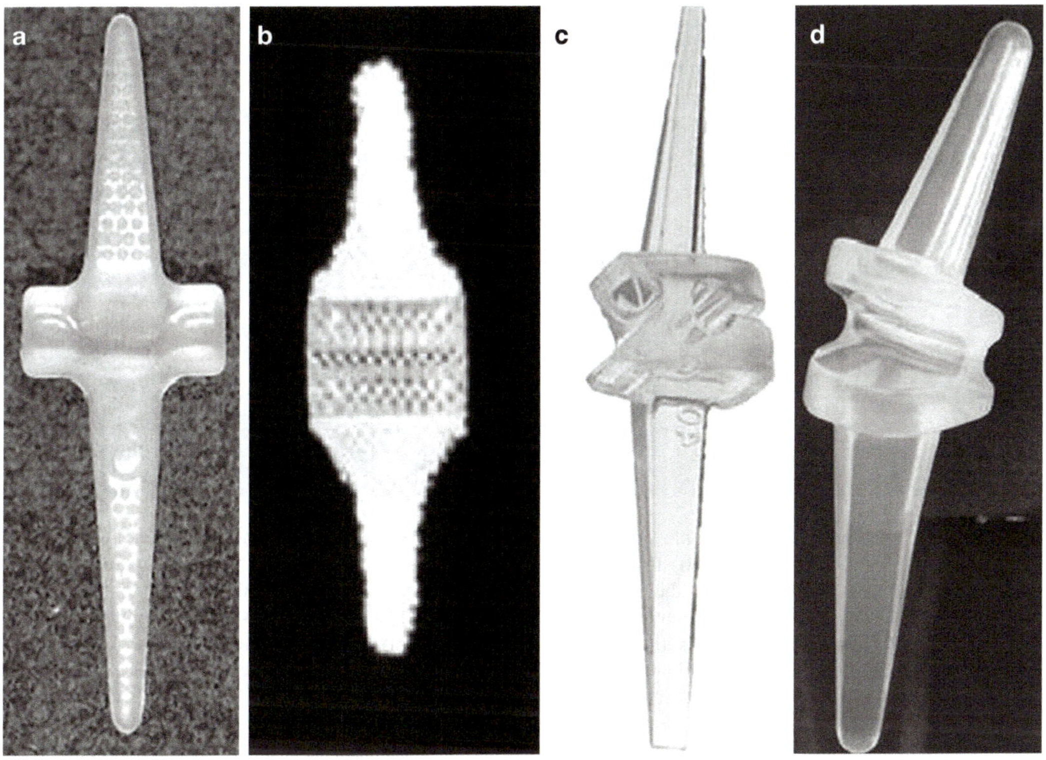


**Fig. 19.2** Silicone implant. (**a**) Swanson: one-piece silicone spacer introduced by Alfred Swanson in the early 1960s. (**b**) Niebauer: Dacron-covered thin-hinge silicone implant for stem fixation. (Reprinted with permission from Linscheid [7]). (**c**) Avanta: a thin-hinge silicone device with rectangular cross-sectioned stems for rotatory stability and flat hub facets for bony abutment. (**d**) NewFlex: 30° flexion pre-bend and a hinged designed to mimic the normal center of rotation of the MCPJ and to decrease stress on the material and improve functional range of motion (ROM), also minimizing abrasion and wear/debris formation. (Courtesy of Dr. Arnold Peter Weiss)

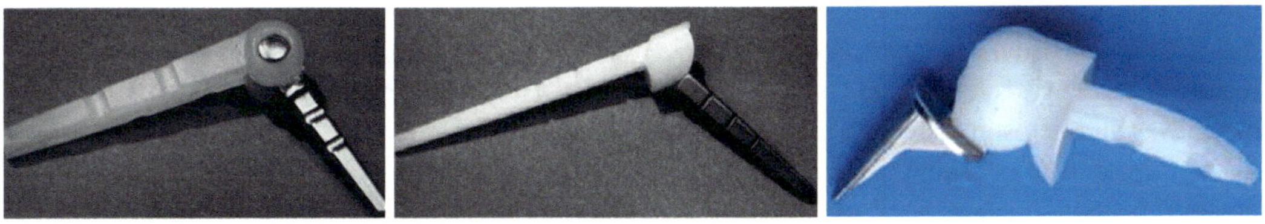

**Fig. 19.3** Metal-plastic constrained implant. (**a**) St. George-Buchholz: earlier model of so-called "second-generation" finger joint prosthesis, proximal stem composed of polyethylene which articulates metal distal stem proximally. Fixed center of rotation without and with radial and ulnar motion in later model. (**b**) Schultz: Semi-constrained cemented implant with a ball and socket articulation had changing center of rotation by incorporating a slot in articulation of the polyethylene component, which allowed distal metal articulation to glide as the joint was rotated. (**c**) In 1964, Steffee designed the first model for the thumb MCP. The distal metal component snap-locked into the proximal component, allowing pure hinged flexion and extension. In model II, adding two modifications, volar offset of center of rotation to increase the extensor moment arm and a longer distal stem to counter the tendency to tilt forward. (Reprinted with permission from Linscheid [7])

collateral ligaments (Fig. 19.4a). However, due to later failures of stem fixation, Linscheid changed from cement to press-fit "PIP SRA" (Stryker Inc., Kalamazoo, MI, USA) (Fig. 19.4b). Nonetheless, these cement-less implants had more loosening and a higher revision rate [19, 20]. In the 25th anniversary presentation of the *Journal of Hand Surgery* (American volume), 2000, Linscheid

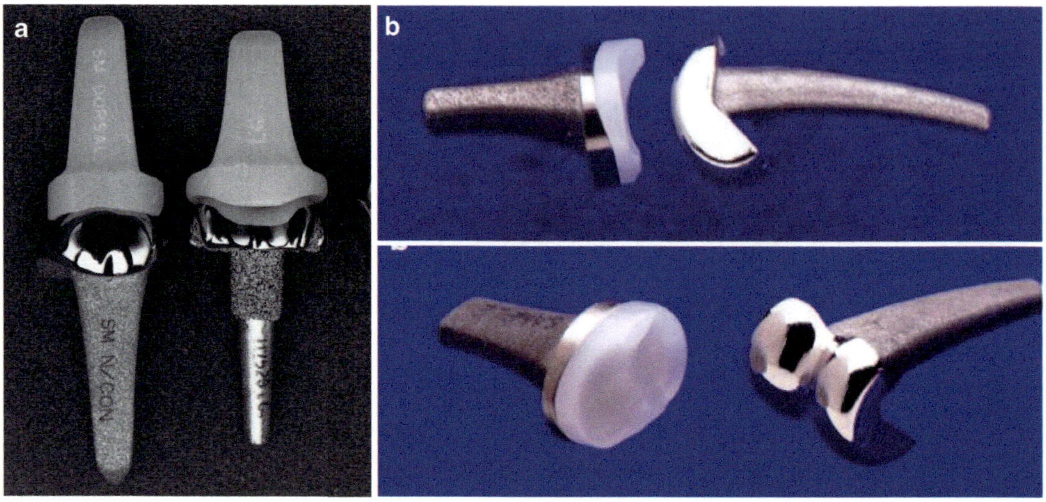


**Fig. 19.4** Surface replacement arthroplasty. (**a**) Early model of surface replacement for MP (left) and PIP (right) developed by Linscheid and Dobyns in the early 1970s. The SR MCP is a semi-constrained implant designed for minimal resection of the bone and preservation of the collateral ligaments. Manufactured from cobalt-chrome and polyethylene, the implant is intended to be implanted with bone cement (Avanta Orthopedics, San Diego, CA). The proximal components are cobalt-chrome, and the distal components are ultrahigh-molecular-weight polyethylene. Stems are to be adapted for either cement or noncement fixation. (Reprinted with permission from Linscheid [7]). (**b**) After various modifications, this implant is translated to the PIP-SRA (Small Bone Innovations, Inc., Morrisville, PA) and now at Stryker (Stryker, Mahwah, USA). Press-fit osseointegration designed stems with titanium coating. (Reprinted with permission from Jennings and Livingstone [19])

wrote "Implant Arthroplasty of the Hand: Retrospective and Prospective Considerations," the most comprehensive manuscript of finger implant arthroplasty ever produced [7]. His lifetime experience with many hand surgeons from the Mayo group had made others believe his original PIP SRA was close to the goal [20–24]. There was an interesting paper in that same year by a former Mayo fellow, Bodell, who had invented his own implant. He said, "As we move into the next millennium, it is more than sentimental to consider reflecting on the advances of… of the 20th century… to get a better sense of where we might be going and what the implications of our achievements might be, it is important to understand where we were, and how we got to where we are presently." [21] Many studies and reviews of finger implant arthroplasty followed until this moment in 2020. Most manuscripts concluded "despite substantial improvements in prosthetic joint design, outcomes have been relatively unchanged over the years" [3, 5, 19, 20, 24–26]. However, some innovative approaches that combined surface PIP implant with press-fit and consequent osteointegration have appeared from Europe in a last decade [27–29].

## Stability and Physiological Joint Motion

Stability of a joint, defined as the resistance to subluxation under physiological stresses, is normally the combined result of osteoarticular contours, dynamic support of the investing musculotendinous units, static viscoelastic constraint of the capsuloligamentous structures, and possibly the differential in atmospheric pressure between the integument and joint space [7]. There are similarities of motion and joint congruity between the knee and the PIP joint, where required motion is flexion and extension with lateral stability. It is a reasonable approach to start, in theory, with hinged implants as the first trial of finger implant arthroplasty. It has become increasingly clear that while motion at the PIP joint approximates that of a uniaxial hinge, its functional environment produces significant rotational moments demanding greater degrees of freedom as provided by the normal joint anatomy [30]. In 1990, Pellegrini compared implant arthroplasty of the PIP joint using Swanson silicone implants, biometric cemented arthroplasty (constrained), and arthrodesis and concluded the place, if any, for cemented interphalangeal arthroplasty in the hand remained in question [31]. Arthrodesis of the PIP joint for the most radial finger is recommended as the only procedure to restore key pinch strength to a level exceeding that of the contralateral hand [31]. Most textbooks and papers thereafter agreed. The author (Minamikawa) investigated motion and stability of the normal PIP joint in fresh cadaver specimens. There was 9 degrees of supination during flexion of the index, and the bicondylar joint surface congruity provide lateral stability mainly with collateral ligament tension, but other soft tissues, accessory collateral ligaments, lateral band, and flexor and extensor tendon also played important roles with muscular load [32]. Linscheid's first prosthesis with cement fixation assumption was that an unconstrained surface replacement would provide a physiological articulation if performed with minimal resection and preservation of collateral ligaments [22]. Surface PIP arthroplasty received reasonable to excellent results compared to other implants [3, 19, 20, 22]. Ashworth [33] reported silicone PIP implant prosthesis survivorship was 81%, whereas the survivorship of the SR PIP was 89% [22]. Limitations of silicone PIP joints include its lack of resistance to valgus loading (at the index and long fingers) during pinch. It was generally believed that an SR PIP that preserves the collateral ligaments would achieve greater PIP stability [4, 7]. In order to clarify this, Minamikawa et al. compared the lateral stability of the PIP joint after surface and silicone implants in cadavers. Because SRA was designed to replicate anatomic joint surface, its kinematic behavior should be similar to that of a normal joint with soft tissues preserved and concluded lateral stability with SRA was significantly greater than the silicone implant [23].

## Material of the Implant

### Silicone

The hinged silicone implant is effectively designed as a spacer and relies on the formation of scar ("pseudo capsule") around the prosthesis and ligament balance to maintain stability [13]. Swanson reported 424 PIP implant arthroplasty from 812 joints operated between 1966 and 1981 in which implant fractures were found in 22 (5.19%) joints with a mean follow-up period of 5.14 (1–16) years [34]. Although anticipated implant fracture rate of the silicone PIP joint and survivorship up to 10 years were relatively low, there were fewer reports of longitudinal study of PIPs compared to MCP implants. On the other hand, silicone MCP joint arthroplasty showed implant fracture rate as high as 63% [35] and 81% [36]. The most recent study of 325 Swanson's silicone MP arthroplasties, with a mean follow-up of 7.2 years (2–18) showed the 5-, 10- and 15-year survival rates free from revision were 98%, 95%, and 95%, respectively. The 5-, 10- and 15-year survival rates free from radiographic implant fracture were 93%, 58%, and 35%, respectively. The 5-, 10- and 15-year survival rates free from coronal plane deformity greater than 10° were 81%, 37%, and 17%, respectively [37]. Fracture and progressive recurrence of deformity are expectations rather than exceptions, and they concluded that silicone implants do not protect from progression of coronal plane deformity and have a high fracture rate [37]. Decrease of postoperative range of motion and implant subsidence were common complications with silicone. Silicone microparticulate inflammation around the stem is continuous until ankylosis of the joint or extraction of the implant; therefore, decreased motion associated with bone destruction is the rule not the exception [2]. In 1985, metal grommets were added at the stem-hub interface of Swanson implants to attempt to counteract bone erosion and implant fracture, although no significant improvements in outcomes were reported [38, 39]. The NeuFlex (Depuy, Warsaw, USA) MCPJ silicone implants came to the market in 1999 trying to improve upon Swanson's implants, reduce complications, and improve results. This implant has a 30° flexion pre-bend and a hinged design to mimic the normal center of rotation of the MCPJ, decrease stress on the material, and improve functional range of motion (ROM), also minimizing abrasion and wear/debris formation [40, 41]. Nevertheless, despite lateral instability and progressive radiological changes after silicone PIP arthroplasty, patients' satisfaction remained high, and revision additional surgery is still often not required [24, 25].

## Pyrocarbon

Pyrocarbon is a synthetic material developed in 1950, whose tribological properties and biocompatibility, particularly with blood, led to widening of its application for mechanical heart valves [42]. In 1979, the first pyrocarbon MCP joint implant was developed by Beckenbaugh as an alternative to silicone [17]. The pyrocarbon implant currently in use is an unconstrained anatomical implant with two components press-fit into the intramedullary canals [43] (Fig. 19.5). Cook et al. reported a large follow-up of pyrolytic carbon (PC) MCP implants in 53 patients for a mean follow-up of 7.2 years which revealed 94% osseointegration and 80% survivorship without adverse remodeling or bone resorption [44]. The material elasticity is remarkably like cortical bone, therefore minimizing the phenomenon of stress shielding. High compression strength and better fatigue strength appeared to show this as the best implant material [43]. The principles of interposition arthroplasty and hemiarthroplasty using pyrocarbon were developed by Pequignot and Allieu [45]. These were applied to arthroplasty of the hand and wrist, then the elbow, and more recently the foot and shoulder [45–47]. However, pyrolytic carbon implant arthroplasty for the PIP joint is relatively new and was initially introduced in Europe in 2000. It was approved for use in the United States in 2002 [48]. Daecke et al. compared PC PIP with silicone PIP joints and found PC PIP dislocations in 17% and subsidence in 33%, whereas neither of these complications occurred in the silicone arthroplasties, and secondary surgeries were performed in 39% of pyrocarbon versus 11% of silicone arthroplasties [48]. Another systematic comparison study by Chan showed not only higher complications in the pyrocarbon group, but also some studies indicated worse results in quality of life after pyrocarbon implant [49]. Furthermore, pyrocarbon PIP total joint was radiographically analyzed in 152 human cadaver fingers. Implant malposition was observed in 67% of phalanges [50]. Early results are encouraging, primarily with patient satisfaction and pain relief, but are based on low numbers. The main concerns are progressive loss of range due to implant settling, dislocation, unexplained but

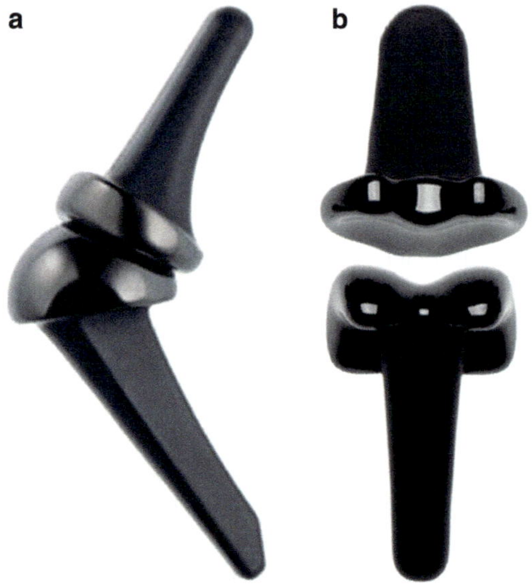

**Fig. 19.5** Pyrocarbon implant. (**a**) Pyrocarbon MP: pyrocarbon MCP joint implant was developed by Beckenbaugh in 1979. The Ascension® pyrocarbon metacarpophalangeal (MCP) implant was the first pyrocarbon implant used in orthopedics. Press-fit non cement fixation with anatomical joint configuration. (**b**) Pyrocarbon PIP: Anatomically designed pyrocarbon PIP joint was initially introduced in Europe in 2000 and was approved for use in the United States in 2002. (Reprinted with permission from Bellemere [43])

notable squeaking, and poor osteointegration with the appearance of a radiolucent line at the bone-implant interface [51]. Because of high complication rates, some authors have abandoned the PC PIP [52, 53].

## Metal-Plastic

The "Vitallium cap arthroplasty for fingers" was reported in 1940 [54]. Thereafter, implants used rigid hinge mechanisms of stainless steel and later titanium by Brannon. The problem of bone resorption and migration, sinking, and loosening of these prostheses was a focal point of the article in 1959 [8]. Titanium readily integrates with the bone and has a modulus of elasticity near that of cortical bone and facilitates load sharing at the bone-implant interface; however, it does not function well as an articulating surface. In the 1970s, metal and plastic designs became popular with efforts to mimic the success of the large joint arthroplasty experience. To date, large joint hip and knee arthroplasties are one of the most successful and well-established procedures frequently using cobalt-chromium (CoCr) and ultrahigh-molecular-weight polyethylene (UHMWPE) articulation. Linscheid and Dobyns were the first to develop surface replacement arthroplasty (SRA) utilizing this articulation with bone cement fixation and later without bone cement.

## Stem Fixation and Newer Design

Implant stability is achieved through preservation of soft tissue structures, implant-bone interface integration, and inherent implant design. Preservation of previously described surrounding soft tissue structures decreases the forces on the implant. Currently, implant-bone stability is achieved most effectively with an intramedullary stem design which provides a large surface area for contact, dispersing forces that may otherwise lead to implant loosening. An ideal stem should match the contour of the intramedullary canal and quickly incorporate into the bone [7]. Optimal fixation of finger implants remains controversial. Bone cement (polymethyl methacrylate) was used for various small implants for a long time; however, there were technical problems and cost-effectiveness. "Modern Cementing Technique Knee (MCT Knee)" addresses loosening with the objective to provide long-term implant stability in knee arthroplasty, based on scientific data from evidence-based techniques documented in the Swedish Hip Arthroplasty Register [55, 56]. Bone Bed Preparation: Cleanse all cement-receiving bone surfaces thoroughly using high pressure pulse-lavage of the entire resected surfaces in order to ensure solid cement fixation; apply bone cement first to the implant, as early as possible in the sticky phase; use a cement gun with an adequate nozzle to minimize the risk of air and blood entrapment and achieve enough pressurization, striving for penetration of 3–4 mm to help ensure optimal fixation and stress distribution. For finger implants, a disposable syringe can be used for cleaning and then injecting bone cement, curettage of intramedullary canal, and firm pressure after cementing, and alignment may be confirmed by fluoroscopy. These meticulous procedures for multiple sets of bone cement require considerable cost. Another option for firm stem fixation is press-fit osseointegration originally proposed for hip arthroplasty. Initial implant rigidity is achieved via a *press-fit*, with rigid contact between the implant stem and the load-bearing cortical bone. The stem is designed so that it is slightly larger than the femoral canal that was prepared through sequential broaching [57]. How about for finger arthroplasty? According to Linscheid, all SRA implants were cemented for several reasons: variation in endosteal configuration, porous ingrowth material cannot be easily applied to UHMWPE, and alignment using cement is easier [7]. After reports of radiological loosening, Linscheid changed to press-fit without cement: similar cobalt-chrome proximal head with titanium-coated stem and distal metal-backed polyethylene-titanium component [19] (Fig. 19.4b). Several studies reported comparisons that the cemented implant was superior to the press-fit implant [19, 20]. Cortical bone thickness of the phalanx is far smaller than that of the femur, and application of the press-fit mechanism is difficult. Remembering hitting the stem for THA with a heavy hammer, press-fit fixation for finger joints seems like an illusion to perform. Nevertheless, recent study of press-fit surface-type PIP implant showed excellent short time results (Fig. 19.6). Both the MatOrtho PIP (Mole Business Park, Leatherhead, UK) [27] and TACTYS PIP (Stryker-Memometal, Bruz, France) [28] with minimum of 2 years and the CapFlex-PIP (KLS Martin Group, Tuttlingen, Germany) [29] at 1 year follow-up showed no implant loosening or subsidence. Different ideas of stem fixation were proposed earlier, but they did not have any follow-up study afterward [7] (Fig. 19.7). The use of osseointegration screw to

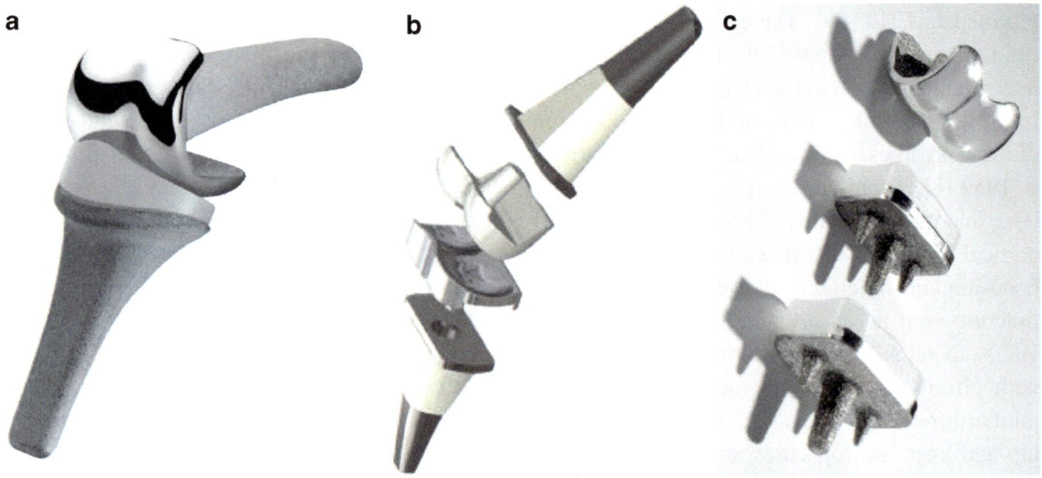

Fig. 19.6 New approach with surface articulation and press-fit fixation. (**a**) MatOrtho PIP: The implant is a cement-less cobalt-chromium metal-on-polyethylene mobile-bearing surface replacement arthroplasty. The polyethylene-bearing insert is factory pre-assembled onto the middle phalanx component to permit final rotational alignment on joint reduction for improved range of motion and implant longevity. (Reprinted with permission from Flannery [27]). (**b**) TACTYS: TACTYS PIP consists of four parts: cobalt-chrome head and UHMWPE socket with anatomical surface articular configuration and anatomical press-fit titanium stems with hydroxyapatite coating. (Reprinted with permission from Athlani et al. [28]). (**c**) Gap Flex-PIP: The CapFlex-PIP implant is a modular gliding surface PIP joint prosthesis consisting of two components. The proximal component is a bicondylar cap of cobalt-chrome alloy, and the distal component has an articular surface of ultrahigh-molecular-weight polyethylene. Both components have a titanium pore base with short pins for cement-free osteointegration. (Reprinted with permission from Schindele et al. [29])

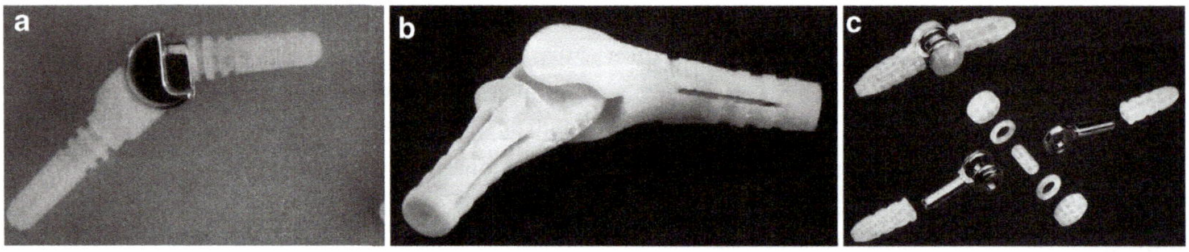

Fig. 19.7 New idea for stem fixation. (**a**) DJOA3: The DJOA3 implant (Landos, Chaumont, France) designed by Condamine for MCP and PIP joints uses elastic fixation of ellipsis-shaped polyethylene stems wedged into the intramedullary canals. (**b**) Mathy's: prostheses fabricated of polyacetyl resin proximal components and polyester distal components, which snap-lock together with a twisting maneuver. An interesting feature is the screw-expandable stems for intramedullary fixation. (**c**) DIGITOS: A modular, constrained PIP prosthesis was designed for unstable joints with impaired collateral ligaments. The metal stems inserting polyethylene sleeve permit sliding and rotate motion to reduce stress to stem and bone interface. DIGITOS (OSTEO A.G., Selzach, Switzerland). (Reprinted with permission from Linscheid [7])

achieve long-standing fixation of metal implants to the bone was first described by Brånemark et al. [58]. Finger implant arthroplasty using osteointegration technique was introduced by Lundborg and Hagert for the MP joint [59]. Titanium screw fixture (Institute for Applied Biotechnology, Göteborg, Sweden), used for edentulous patients, was placed in the phalangeal canal as a first stage, and after waiting for osteointegration to the screw, silicone-made joint mechanism (ATOS Medical, Hörby, Sweden) was placed a few weeks later (Fig. 19.8). Osseointegrated PIP joint as a one-stage surgery was also performed by the same group, who reported their 10-years' follow-up [60]. Although silicone spacers fractured in 68%, 94% osseointegration of the PC stems were observed. The joint mechanism needed further improvement, having achieved permanent fixation of the fixture to the bone structure [61, 62].

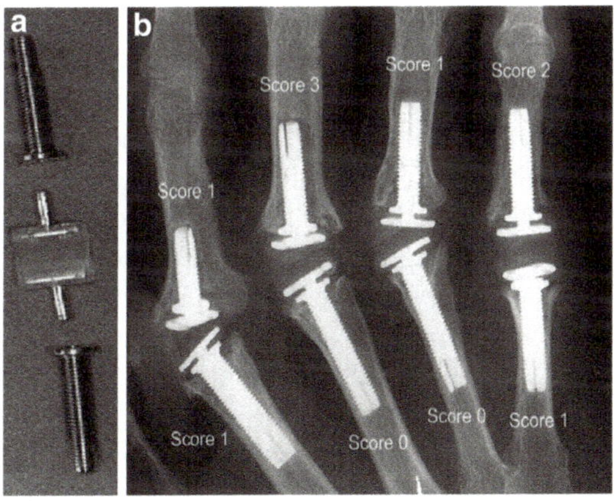


**Fig. 19.8** Osseointegration screw fixation. (**a**) The osteointegration technique for finger arthroplasty was introduced by Hagert and Brånemark for MP joint in 1986. Surgery was done in two stages, titanium screw fixture is placed in bone marrow cavities, and few weeks later, a flexible constrained silicone spacer was connected to the titanium fixtures. Lundborg later successfully used this technique in the PIP joint as a one-stage surgery. (**b**) Based on these measurements, the osseointegration of each fixture was assigned a score from 0 to 3. 0, Minimal or no change; 1, slight bone resorption under the joint connection, extending along less than half of the implant length; 2, moderate bone resorption with a narrow resorption zone extending more than half of the implant length or a wide irregular resorption zone extending at least half of the implant length; 3, obvious implant loosening, either with a wide irregular resorption zone extending around the implant or without implant subsidence or any implant subsidence of more than 1 mm on comparable radiographs with or without a narrow re- sorption zone around it. (Reprinted with permission from Möller et al. [62])

## New Design Concepts

Dissatisfaction with the performance of the available finger implants has motivated numerous investigative groups to design new implants utilizing sophisticated techniques and materials. Silastic™ and other silicone implants remain in wide use with proven clinical success, relatively low cost, and high patient satisfaction. The ideal solution for small joint arthroplasty is minimal bone resection preserving soft tissue attachments around the joint and keeping the tension of the soft tissues. Most PIP implants offer four sizes, and some use a special spacer tool to determine bone resection, with final confirmation in setting the trial implant component. To overcome this difficult but most important issue, different heights of polyethylene sockets in CapFlex-PIP [29] and modular heads and sockets with different size selections in TACTYS-PIP [28] were introduced. The CapFlex-PIP implant is a modular gliding surface PIP joint prosthesis consisting of two components. The proximal component is a bicondylar cap of cobalt-chrome alloy, and the distal component has an articular surface of UHMWPE. Both components have a titanium pore base for cement-free osteointegration. The varying height of the polyethylene articular surfaces (2.1 mm, 3.0 mm, and 4.4 mm) allows for modular adaption of joint stability based on the intraoperative findings to provide ideal collateral ligament tension (Fig. 19.6c). TACTYS PIP consists of four parts: cobalt-chrome head and UHMWPE socket with anatomical surface articular configuration and anatomical press-fit titanium stems with hydroxyapatite coating. There are four sizes (XS, S, M, L) for proximal and three sizes (S,M,L) for distal stems. Each stem fits two different size joint components (S,M,L), and the distal socket has three different heights in each size (Fig. 19.6b). MatOrtho PIP is also a precisely designed anatomical press-fit stem with hydroxyapatite coating. There are five sizes of proximal parts. The system allows the middle component to be downsized when required. The anatomically designed articular components preserve collateral ligaments, and the mobile system in distal component provides rotational stability. The polyethylene-bearing insert is factory preassembled onto the middle phalanx component (Fig. 19.6a). Compared to previous finger implants, MatOrtho PIP joint seemed the most expensive implant to make. Flannery reported a minimum of 2-year follow-up using the MatOrtho PIP replacement. One hundred implants were followed up in an average of 47 (24–77) months, and no evidence of implant loosening or subsidence was found [27].

**Self Locking Finger Joint** The Self Locking Finger Joint (SLFJ, Teijin Nakashima medical, Okayama, Japan) implant was developed for MP and PIP joints and has been used in Japan since 1999. The SLFJ implant is a cement-less articular surface replacement implant with joint anchor fixation and an intramedullary locking system of expandable legs to offer stable fixation. In addition, the implant surface anchor via a tapered screw allows the surgeon to adjust the functional height of the implant to obtain an appropriate tension of the collateral ligaments during the surgery. Tension of the collateral ligament can be further adjusted with a trial head and socket, both with limited (one size) modularity. Testing motion and stability during surgery is a great advantage of using this implant. The SLFJ prosthesis has six components: joint anchors shot-blasted titanium alloy (Ti-6AI-4V alloy). Locking screws: titanium alloy (Ti-6AI-4V alloy). Joint head: cobalt-chrome alloy (Co-Cr-Mo alloy). Joint socket: UHMWPE (ultrahigh-molecular-weight polyethylene) (Fig. 19.9a, b).

**Joint Anchor (JA)** The joint anchor consists of a tapered body with self-tapping screw with two long legs. It is designed such that 1 pitch (360°) of rotation inserts the JA 0.8 mm into the intramedullary canal. The JA is made of titanium, and its two legs are relatively thin to allow some elasticity; they are spread/secured in the canal by advancement of a locking screw within the body (Fig. 19.10a). The joint anchor is screwed into the intramedullary canal without bone cement, and therefore, the position of the joint anchor can be determined during the surgery. Because the joint components and joint anchor are connected through a square recess, the joint anchor can be positioned by every 90 degrees. The tension of the collateral ligaments is adjusted by 0.2 mm, which is 1/4 of the pitch (0.8 mm) of the screw of the JA (Fig. 19.10b). The anchor surface toward the bone is finished in rough (shot-blasted) to facilitate osteointegration. The JA is set completely within

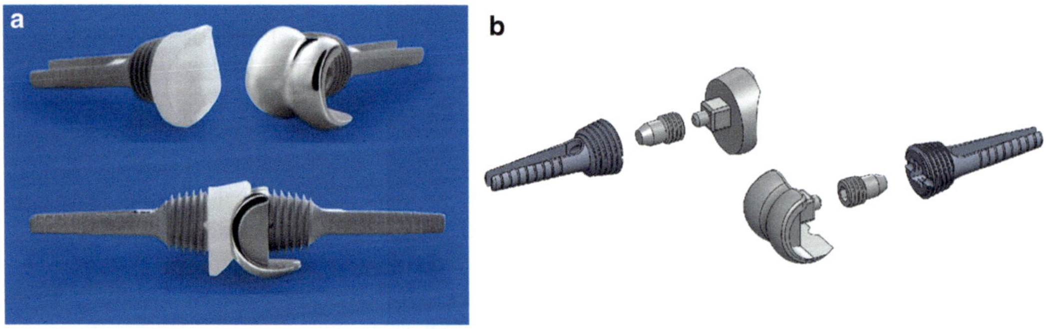


Fig. 19.9 The Self Locking Finger Joint (SLFJ) implant for proximal interphalangeal joints. (**a**) Overview of the implant. Surface replacement-type implant with bicondyle anatomical joint congruity. (**b**) The SLFJ implant has six components. Joint anchors: shot-blasted titanium alloy (Ti-6AI-4V alloy). Locking screws: titanium alloy (Ti-6AI-4V alloy) . Joint head: cobalt-chrome alloy (Co-Cr-Mo alloy). Joint socket: UHMWPE (ultrahigh-molecular-weight polyethylene)

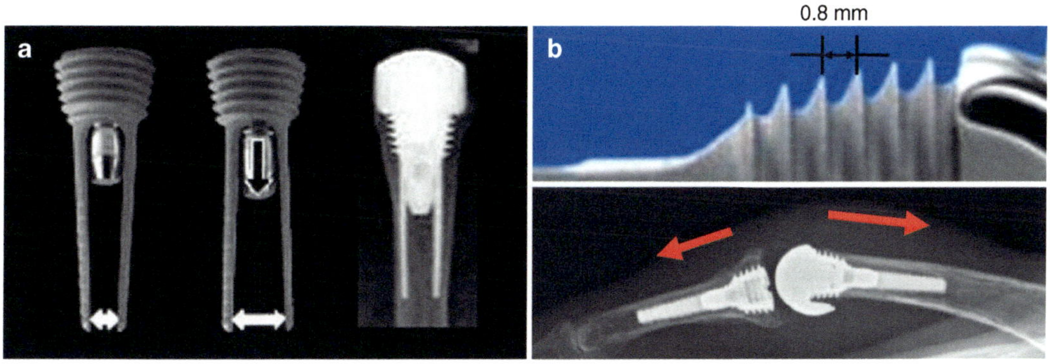


Fig. 19.10 Mechanism of the joint anchor. (**a**) Tapered screw and expandable legs: Tightening of the locking screw component will spread two legs of joint anchor inside the intramedullary canal. (**b**) Adjustable collateral tension: The joint anchor has tapered self-tapping screw. It is designed that 1 pitch (360°) of rotation inserts the joint anchor 0.8 mm into the intramedullary canal. Therefore, position of the joint anchor is 0.2 mm deeper by every 90 degrees to adjust collateral tension

the intramedullary canal after bone preparation (with a tapered reamer) after minimal resection of the head of basal phalanx and without surface resection of the middle phalanx. Soft tissue attachments are completely preserved with the SLFJ.

## Joint Component

There are two separate joint components, a cobalt-chrome joint head proximally and an UHMWPE socket distally. The square recess of the JA and square projection of the head/socket component are designed to connect these components in proper alignment (Fig. 19.9a, b). There are four sizes for the joint anchor and four sizes for the joint surface configurations. The intramedullary canal is often narrow in young rheumatoid cases or cases of OA or trauma, thus necessitating a smaller JA selection. For this reason, each joint component comes with a projection one size smaller to fit a smaller size JA. Therefore seven different heads and sockets are provided.

### Head

The proximal component is a metallic CoCr alloy with a symmetric shallow bicondylar (anatomic) configuration for the articular surface. In order to preserve as much bony support in the lateral wall as possible, the stock material behind the thin convex surface has been removed (recessed). The joint anchor has been designed to fit a few millimeters deep from the original head resection level which is distal to attachment of the collateral ligaments (Fig. 19.11). Since there are lateral wall recesses (of the head) for the collateral ligaments even if the joint anchor needs to be set in a deeper position, the collateral ligament always will be preserved for stability (Fig. 19.12).

### Socket

The distal component is fabricated from UHMWPE with the articular surface congruent with the surface of the proximal component. The shape of the cross-sectional attachment is round and matches the widest body of the joint anchor. The space between the bottom of the socket surface to attachment surface of the socket is 1 mm; therefore, the distal joint anchor is recommended to be positioned about 2 mm deeper than the original joint surface. Surface of the middle phalanx is prepared with a socket surface reamer which allows fitting of the selected socket (Fig. 19.13).

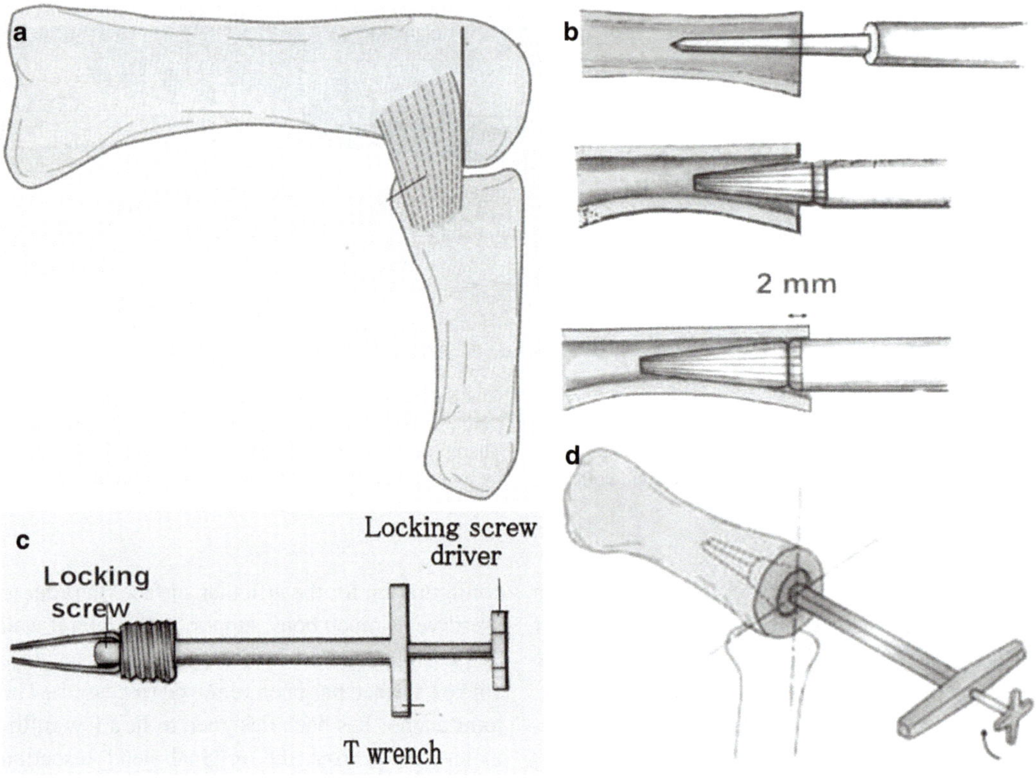


**Fig. 19.11** Surgical procedure: proximal phalanx. (**a**) Resection of the head at 1–2 mm distal to the attachment of the collateral ligaments. (**b**) Preparation of proximal canal: starter awl, tapered reamer from smaller size to larger size, until the reamer reaches the inner wall of the cortex. (**c**) Setting the joint anchor using T wrench driver. Joint anchor is placed about 2mm deeper than cutting edge. (**d**) In aligning rotational position, the handle of the T wrench should be stopped at (either) perpendicular or parallel to flexion-extension plane (axial), and the locking screw is advanced to spread the intramedullary legs

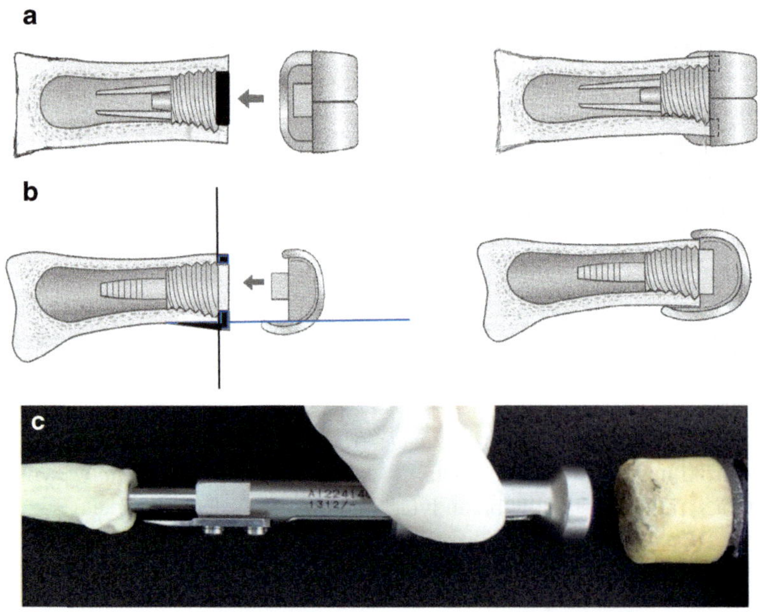


**Fig. 19.12** Surgical procedures: head setting. (**a**) Resection of dorsal and palmer cortex: In order to set the trial head component, the dorsal and palmer edges of the cortex need to be removed at the edge of the joint anchor, while lateral walls on both sides are preserved for the collaterals' attachments. (**b**) Resection palmer part of the head also needs to be removed to fit the volar part of the head. (**c**) Palmer cutting chisel is set on foam bone model to show precise cutting of the palmer bone

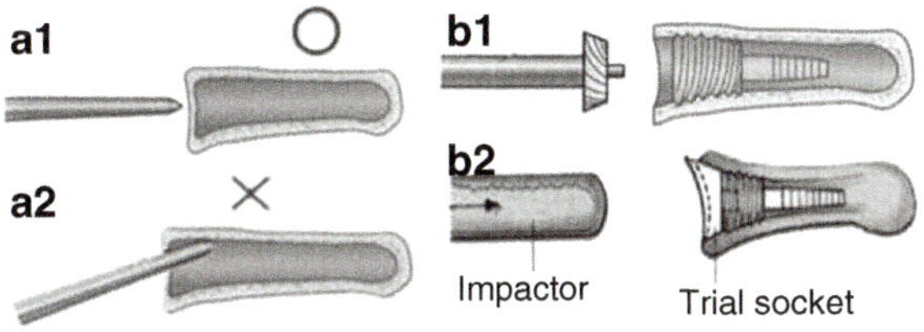


**Fig. 19.13** Surgical procedures: middle phalanx. (**a**) Preparation of middle phalanx: The starter awl is carefully inserted from the center of the joint surface toward the center of the cavity, first burring cartilage; use of x-ray images at this stage is desirable as, without resection of joint surface, this direction is sometimes inaccurate and could risk poor implant alignment. (**b**) Use the socket reamer to shape-fit the exact size of the distal socket. Trial socket is fit with impactor

## Surgical Procedures

Although the SLFJ can be implanted from either a dorsal or palmar approach, the following description will be via the dorsal approach. Preoperatively, the surgeon should estimate the size of the joint components using the provided template and the patient's x-rays. After the head of the basal phalanx is exposed, identify the collateral ligaments with the PIP joint in flexion, and resection of the head is done perpendicular to the long axis distal to the collateral ligaments using a small bone saw. This initial cutting line is not important if it does not disturb the collateral attachments (Fig. 19.11a). The starter awl is inserted into the canal at the center, or a little dorsal, going deep enough so that the awl is guided into the center of intramedullary cavity. You may check x-ray images at this point to confirm the exact location and then begin inserting the tapered reamers from small to largest size practical, until the reamer reaches the inner wall of the cortex. There is a notch at the proximal end of the tapered reamers where the actual size of the anchor should be positioned. Since initial head resection was minimal, the joint anchor needs to be 2–3 mm deeper (proximal to) the cutting line (Fig. 19.11b). In aligning the rotational position, the handle of the T wrench can be stopped at (either) perpendicular or parallel to flexion-extension plane (axis), and the locking screw is advanced to spread the intramedullary legs (Fig. 19.11d). In order to set the trial head component, the dorsal and palmer edges of the cortex need to be removed at the edge of the joint anchor, while lateral walls on both sides are preserved with the collaterals' attachments (Fig. 19.12a). Palmar cutting chisel is fitted to the square hole, and the palmar side of the head is precisely cut (Fig. 19.12b, c). Then the trial head of the same size with the JA (or one larger size) can be fitted into the joint anchor square slot. At this point, reduction of the joint without a distal implant should be possible to assess tension of the collateral ligaments. If the tension is too tight and it is difficult to reduce the joint, or motion is limited, depth of distal joint anchor or proximal can be made deeper to reduce the tension. Bone resection is not needed for the distal surface; therefore, first burr the cartilage if possible; otherwise the starter awl is vulnerable to placement in the wrong direction (Fig. 19.13a). The starter awl is carefully inserted from the center of the joint surface toward the center of the intramedullary canal. Use of x-ray images at this stage is desirable as, without resection of joint surface, this direction is sometimes inaccurate and could risk poor implant alignment. Tapered reamer is used in the same manner with proximal position of the JA adjusted according to the tested motion after proximal head setting. Check the rotational alignment in the same manner as for the proximal implant, and then use the socket reamer to shape-fit for the exact size of the distal socket (Fig. 19.13b). Trial insetting of the socket and then reinsertion of the trial head are done to reduce the joint to test motion and ligament stability.

## Development of SLFJ and Current Status with Case Examples

The author started development based on the combination of anatomical surface joint replacement secured by osseointegration. Joint components were designed to mimic Linscheid's original SRA [4, 7]. Connecting the joint component with a separate anchor (stem) mechanism became obvious when considering longitudinal screw-type osseointegration [59, 60]. The proximal tapered body with deep self-tapping screw was designed to counteract axially loaded sinking pressure. Length and width of the legs were determined to require elasticity to fit the internal surface of the canal. Leg pressure against the bone without protrusion was found to be characteristic of plastic deformation of the titanium material. After trial implantation with cadaver specimens, clinical use was approved in 1999. Most cases in the first 5 years were MP joints in patients with rheumatoid arthritis. With experience in clinical use, selection of the size of the joint anchor was found to be the most important for stable fixation. Implant breakage and loosening were found in cases with use of much smaller size of the joint anchor. Modifications of the implant were made in 2006 for joint anchor strengthening at the transition part between proximal body to legs and to change the shiny surface of the joint anchor by shot-blasting a rough surface to facilitate osteointegration. The head was changed from titanium to CoCr. The longitudinal shape of the head for the PIP joint was altered so that resection of the phalangeal head became minimal. After the modifications, breakage of the joint anchor and loosening were seldom observed. CE mark was approved in 2007, and distribution was started in Hong Kong, Singapore, and China. The author presented a preliminary report, "Cement-less Surface Finger Implant Arthroplasty" in a poster session at the 62nd annual meeting of the American Society for Surgery of the Hand, last September 2007, at Seattle, Washington. There were 98 joints in 34 rheumatoid patients (72 finger MP and 12 PIP plus 14thumb MP joints) with an average follow-up of 5.5 years (range, 4–6.5 years). Only three joints showed marked loosening. Breakage of the joint anchor was found in 7 MP and 2 PIP joints. Half of the joint anchor were found securely fixed to the bone. These cases all used the first model of SLFJ. Komatsu et al. reported 26 PIP joint arthroplasties using the SLFJ implant in 17 patients with primary or posttraumatic osteoarthritis. Their mean follow-up was 44 months (range, 24–76 months). The average active PIP joint arc of motion improved from 36° before surgery to 44° after surgery. Overall patient satisfaction was 94%. Ninety percent of implants showed osteointegration and no radiographic signs of migration or loosening [63]. From the records of the manufacturer (Teijin Nakashima Med. Co. Okayama, Japan), a total of 3890 joints (2127 PIP and 1632 finger MP plus 131 thumb MP) in 2552 patients were operated between 1999 and 2019 in 457 institutions in Japan and other Asian countries. A multicenter study of SLFJ survivorship is currently being conducted by our group. Because of widespread use over the past 10 years, osseointegration of the SLFJ is believed to occur, and now questions have even been raised about how to extract one when necessary. It is difficult to remove the JA: we suggest removal of the locking screw first, and then the body of the JA is cut and broken using strong wire cutter. In this process, the proximal bone needs to be removed to expose the JA; once the body and legs are separated, the legs are relatively easy to detach and remove. There were no strong osseointegration to the rough surface of the JA; however, two-point attachment, proximal tapered screw, and distal legs make the extraction difficult. Bone resorption is rarely observed in long-term cases. A unique mechanism of the JA is weak (elastic) attachment of the legs which distributes more load to the proximal screw. "Stress shielding effects" in hip joints occur when there is strong osseointegration in the distal stem and decreased load onto the proximal bone that causes bone absorption proximally. Longer-term follow-up, on patients over 10 years (cases 1–4), has shown less occurrence of bone resorption. Previous beliefs of contraindications for PIP arthroplasty need reevaluation. Unstable joints can be stabilized with augmentation of the collateral ligament, with tendon or other soft tissue grafting (cases 2–5). Bone deficits can be treated with bone graft. Remodeling around the stem and cortex was observed without implant loosening (cases 3–5).

Specific needs must be considered in selecting indications (e.g., cases 4 and 5). It is tempting to say that only arthrodesis is indicated for radial digits; however, we have found that arthrodesis should be reserved as the last option. Severely dislocated contracted joints can be treated with staged surgery, first using an external fixator and soft tissue reconstruction. Poor functional results may be attributed to the implant itself such as with implant breakage or loosening. Decreased motion and poor outcomes are often dependent of surgical approach and postsurgical therapy [20, 26, 64–66]. The role for total joint replacement is just as its name, to exchange a damaged part of the joint for a component. If pain and disability are due to local inflammation without joint destruction, anti-inflammatory medicine or local steroid injection is indicated. Pathology of traumatic arthrosis or degenerative conditions depend on severity and start with damage to a joint surface and are the best (easy) candidates for implant arthroplasty. Excellent results can be expected with any implant because only new parts are needed; therefore, surface implant is best for long-term durability (Case 1, Fig. 19.14). Deformed, rheumatoid, or unstable joints have two pathological problems: joint destruction and soft tissue damage. First, a new joint is needed, but ligament/tissue reconstruction should also be added to the treatment. Similarly, joint destruction with bone deficit should be considered as two pathological problems: joint destruction and bony problems like fracture and mal- or nonunion. Secure fixation of the JA with bone graft have been performed in many patients: for massive bone deficit; the key for success is to use a large bone graft to re-create the phalangeal bone before reaming (Cases 4 and 5, Figs. 19.17 and 19.18); for bone absorption or small bone loss, pack the cancellous bone before implant insertion (Cases 2 and 3, Figs. 19.15 and 19.16). Unstable joints with soft tissue loss, even also with deformity and bone loss, are not an absolute contraindication to implanting this joint.

## Summary

The author believes finger implant arthroplasty is the best chance for relief of severe pain and severe deformity with ADL (activities of daily living) disturbance if some motion is to be retained. Surface implant arthroplasty with strong, stable stem fixation is the ideal combination for long-term reconstruction. Silicone implants are easily performed with low technical demands; we believe they should be restricted to cases that give priority to short-term results over long-term expectation. There are several issues for a new implant to be distributed worldwide, and obtaining permission from each country is difficult and often not cost-effective. Use in "other parts of the world" may sometimes be influenced by language limitations; results of outcomes of numerous past Japanese implants have never been published in English [67–70]; some implant was written about only in French

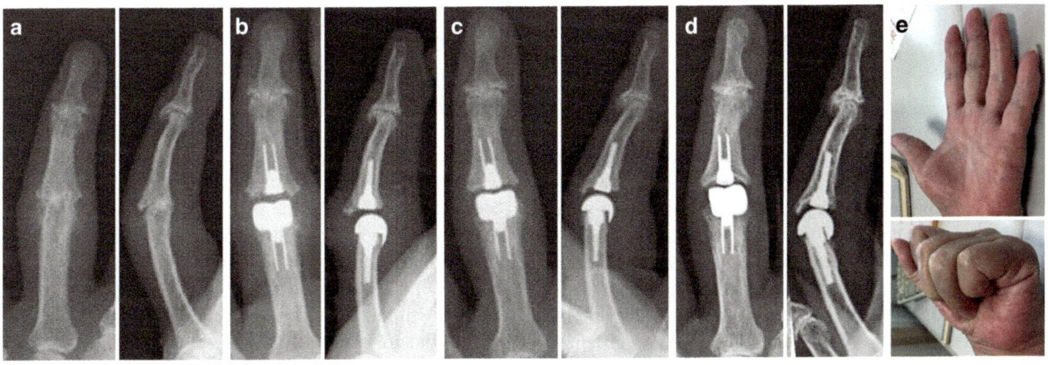


**Fig. 19.14** Case 1: 55-year-old female with painful osteoarthritis of the PIP joint in the left middle finger (**a**). Implant arthroplasty using SLFJ was performed through palmer approach. Postsurgical x-ray (**b**) 3 years (**c**) and 12 years (**d**) post-op show exact same position of the implant and very minimum bone atrophy due to stress shielding effect. Motion at last follow-up of 12 years showed extension loss of 5 and nearly full flexion(**e**) (Courtesy of the case from Dr. Y. Hamada, Kansai Medical University, Osaka Japan)

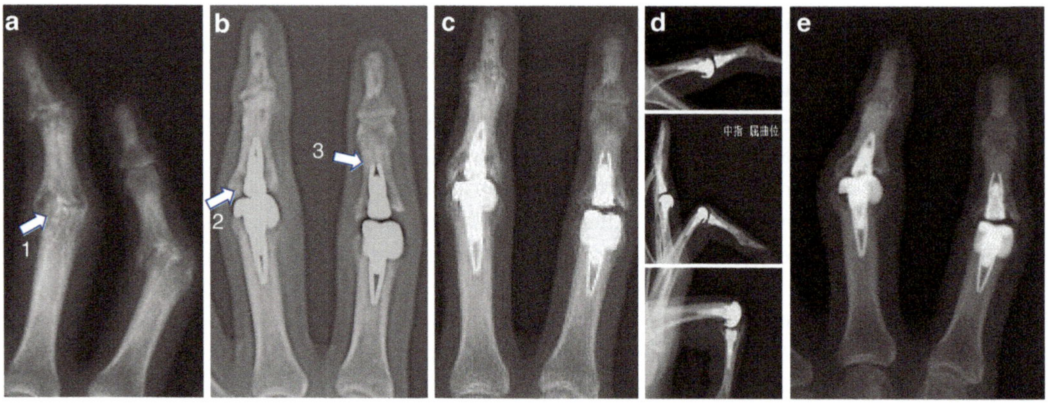


**Fig. 19.15** Case 2: 31-year-old female with rheumatoid arthritis showed ulnarly deviated PIP joint with nearly full range of motion in left index and middle fingers (**a** pre-op, **b** post-op, **c** post-op 8 years, **d** post-op 8 years lateral view, **e** post-op 15 years). Although ulnar deviation was prominent, range of the motion was not restricted without severe pain, and no surgical intervention was never recommended. Progressive deformity without ADL disturbances in young female strongly requested arthroplasty. There was bone loss at ulnar side of proximal part of middle phalanx (**a**, arrow 1). Implant arthroplasty of the PIP joint was performed through palmer approach. Bone graft was added in the middle phalanx using resected head of the basal phalanx (**b**, arrow 2), and augmentation of the radial collateral ligament was performed. Since the cortex of the middle phalanx was thick, and the cavity was so narrow, the legs JA needed to cut in short (**b**, arrow 3). JA remained the same position in every x-ray. Range of motion from the chart at 2 years for index and middle were 0–70 and 0–80, respectively, and were even better at 8 years when measured by lateral x-ray: index 0–80, middle 0–100. Anticipated bone absorption seen at 8 years (**c**) did not change afterward until 15 years follow-up (**e**). (Courtesy of Dr. T. Hojo, Kyoto Prefectural University of Medicine for providing follow-up x-ray)

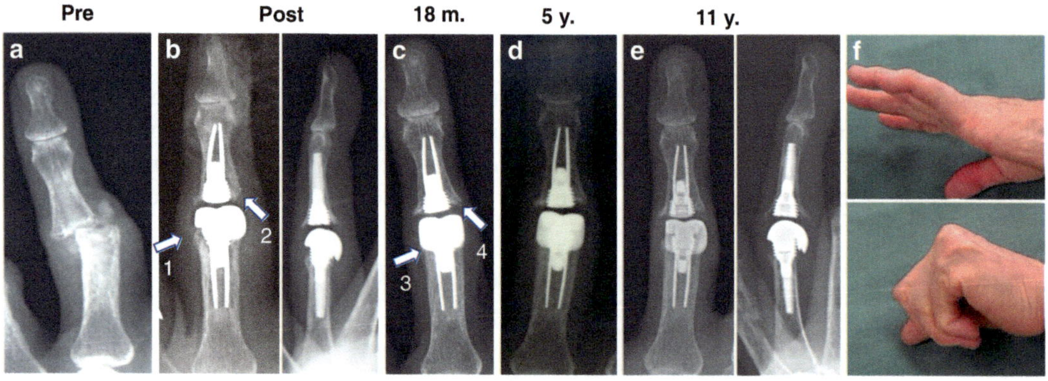


**Fig. 19.16** Case 3: 48-year-old female with rheumatoid arthritis presented painful unstable PIP joint in the left middle finger. She had history of Swanson silicone implant arthroplasty 2 years prior to consultation (**a** pre-op XP, **b** post-op **c** post-op 18 months, **d** post-op 5 years, **e** post-op 11 years, **f** post-op 11 years motion). X-ray in the initial visit clearly indicated fracture of the implant and ulnar instability. At revision arthroplasty with Chamay dorsal approach, no marked bone loss was observed. Cancellous bone graft from the iliac crest was performed with careful implant alignment. Radial collateral ligament was augmented. Post-op. X-ray showed grafted bone at radial side of middle phalanx (**b** arrow 1) and ulnar side of basal phalanx (**b** arrow 2). X-rays at post-op 18 months showed remodeling of grafted bone without any sign of loosening (**c**, arrow 3,4). Position of the JA did not change until recent follow-up of 11 years. There was minimum bone absorption in ulnar side of the middle phalanx in AP view, but lateral view showed the joint anchor is in good position within cortex (**e**). Range of motion preserved 15–75° at 11 years (**f**)

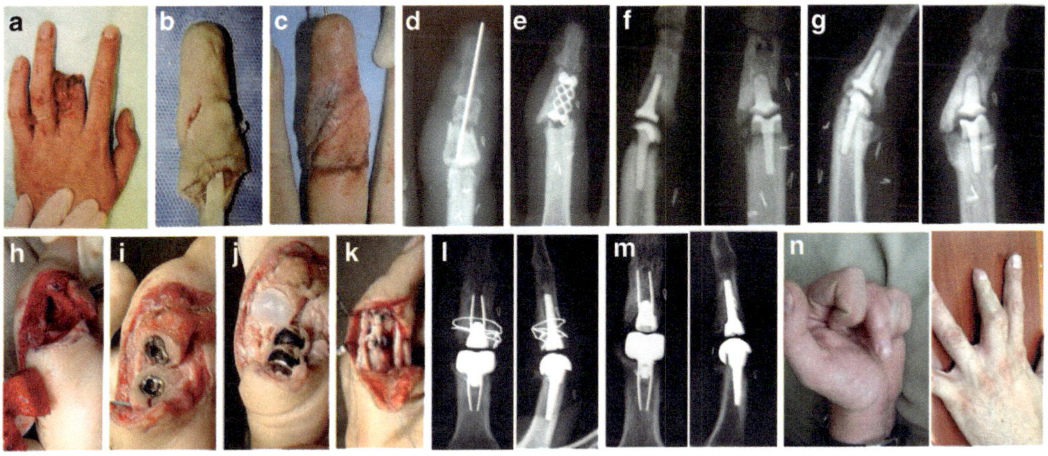


**Fig. 19.17** Case 4: 37-year-old male Hong Kong professional pilot had injury of his left middle finger during motor car rally competition in an overseas country in May 2005. His middle finger sustained an avulsion amputation at the level of middle phalanx with open dislocation of PIPJ. Microsurgical replantation with axial K wire fixation and skin graft was successful at Malaysia (**a**–**d**). However, it was complicated by nonunion of the middle phalanx. Revision plating and bone graft was performed in August 2005. The fracture healed, but there was progressive DIPJ fusion and PIPJ destruction, likely due to septic cause (**e**). Infection was treated vigorously, and finally a PIPJ arthroplasty with pyrocarbon implant was performed in August 2006 (**f**). All the treatments were given overseas. He returned to Hong Kong and resumed his duty initially. However, he noted a progressive radial deviation deformity of the middle finger with weakness and pain, which interfered his pilot work: x-ray showed aseptic loosening and implant displacement, associated with marked bone loss at the base of radial side of the middle phalanx post arthroplasty (**g**). A block of iliac bone graft was performed with periosteum attached (**h**). Revision arthroplasty was performed as advised by Minamikawa. Firm cortico-cancellous bone grafting was performed with wiring first, followed by reaming of the canal (**i**, **j**). Radial collateral ligament was reconstructed using periosteum of the grafted bone and later added with palmaris longus tendon graft (K). Stability of the joint was restored with good motion during surgery and post-op x-ray (**l**). Grafted bone was well incorporated, useful PIP ROM recovered (20°–80°), and deformity fully corrected at 1 year 4 months post revision arthroplasty. He was able to return to his work as a professional airline pilot which required independent left-hand finger motion to hold and control the thrust levers. Removal of the wire and extensor tenolysis were performed at 3 years post arthroplasty. The finger alignment and stability were good, and patient was happy with the outcome with no pain. X-ray post-op 7 years showed good alignment and bony integration of the implant, despite apparent resorption of the bone graft (M). The ROM of PIPJ at final follow-up 7 years post-arthroplasty was 40°–90°(N) (this case was presented at ASSH meeting at Las Vegas, 2019. Courtesy of P.C. Ho. Prince of Wales Hospital Hong Kong)

[71]. Adding special mechanisms and preparing different sizes and/or inserts for modular adaptability increase costs. All surrounding issues other than pure value of new implant itself make it much difficult for the manufacturer to be involved in an already small market. The author strongly believes the direction which Linscheid showed in the early 1970s [7, 16] is still valid, and short-term results have proved robust and secure fixation of the stems with osseointegration [27–29, 63]. Durable and anatomic total PIP implants are truly what everybody has wanted and should be ready for an international market.

## Case Examples

- Case 1: SLFJ PIP implant arthroplasty of the middle finger with osteoarthritis in a 55-year-old female (Fig. 19.14)
- Case 2: SLFJ PIP implant arthroplasty for unstable index and middle finger with rheumatoid arthritis in a 31-year-old female (Fig. 19.15)
- Case 3: Revision PIP implant arthroplasty using SLFJ for fractured silicone implant of the middle finger with rheumatoid arthritis in a 48-year-old female (Fig. 19.16)

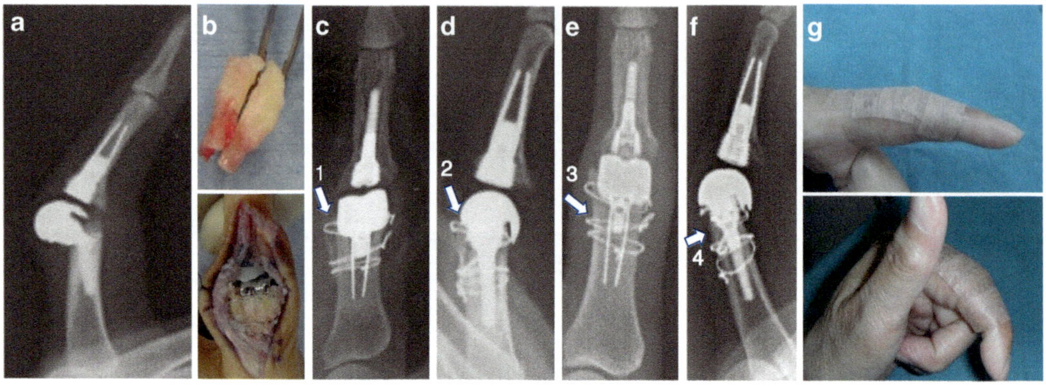


**Fig. 19.18** Case 5: 62-year-old female with rheumatoid arthritis presented painful unstable PIP joint in the left index finger. She had revision arthroplasty using SLFJ after 10 years' history of cemented surface implant at another hospital. Two years after revision surgery, she was referred for a third operation. X-ray showed fracture of the JA and displaced dorsal dislocated head (**a**). Dysfunction of the extensor apparatus was highly suspected, and removal of the joint component and arthrodesis were proposed. Patient, however, insisted another revision surgery. Because of the disease nature, her third metatarsal head was eroded and available for bone graft. Very challenging surgery was performed, and dislocated head with proximal JA was easily removed between damaged extensor and lateral band. Distal JA was completely attached to the middle phalanx, and proximal legs of the JA required small chisel to detach from the cortex. Metatarsal head was harvested from the affected third toe and divided in half (**b**) and was grafted to basal phalanx to maintain the length of phalanx. Two metal wires were used to cover the distal part of the basal phalanx completely from lateral side (**b**, **c**). Postsurgical x-ray showed metal wire indicating contour of grafted bone (**c**, **d** arrow 1,2). Extensor apparatus was repaired as much as possible. After surgery, the patient confessed she was a world famous professional Biwa (Japanese traditional stringed instrument) player. Although recovered arc was limited to 30 gegrees, she has returned (**g**), she has returned to performance after 6 months post-surgery and continued teaching and music performance. X-ray 9 years post second revision surgery showed good remodeling of grafted bone (**e**, **f**. arrow 3,4) without loosening

- Case 4: Revision PIP implant arthroplasty using SLFJ from pyrocarbon in a post replanted middle finger in a 45-year-old male (Fig. 19.17)
- Case 5: Revision PIP implant arthroplasty for failed SLFJ in the index finger with rheumatoid arthritis in a 60-year-old female (Fig. 19.18)

**Acknowledgments** The author thanks Dr. Clayton A. Peimer, Adjunct Clinical Professor of Orthopaedic Surgery, Alpert School of Medicine, Brown University, Providence, RI, for his comments that greatly improved the manuscript.

## References

1. Peimer CA, Taleisnik J, Sherwin FS. Pathologic fractures: complication of microparticle induced synovitis. J Hand Surg Am. 1991;16A:835–43.
2. Minamikawa Y, Peimer CA, Ogawa Howard C, Sherwin FS. In vivo experimental analysis of silicone implants on bone and soft tissue. J Hand Surg Am. 1994;19:575–83.
3. Adkinson JM, Chung KC. Advances in small joint arthroplasty of the hand. Plast Reconstr Surg. 2014;134(6):1260–8.
4. Linscheid RL, Dobyns JH. Total joint arthroplasty: the hand. Mayo Clin Proc. 1979;54:516–26.
5. Herren DB. Current European Practice in the treatment of proximal interphalangeal joint arthritis. Hand Clin. 2017;33(3):489–500.
6. Flatt AE, Fisher GW. Biomechanical factor in the replacement of rheumatoid finger joint. Ann Rheum Dis. 1969;28:36–41. (suppl).
7. Linscheid RL. Implant arthroplasty of the hand: retrospective and prospective considerations. J Hand Surg Am. 19 J. Hand Surg. Am. 2000;25:796–816.
8. Brannon EW, Klein G. Experiences with a finger-joint prosthesis. J Bone Joint Surg Am. 1959;41:87–102.
9. Flatt AE. Restoration of rheumatoid finger-joint function: interim report of trial of prosthetic replacement. J Bone Joint Surg. 1961;43A:753–74.
10. Flatt AE, Ellison MR. Restoration of rheumatoid finger joint function. 3. A follow-up note after fourteen years of experience with a metallic-hinge prosthesis. J Bone Joint Surg. 1972;54A:1317–22.
11. Swanson AB. Silicone rubber implants for replacement of arthritis or destroyed joints in the hand. Surg Clin North Am. 1968;48:1113–27.

12. Niebauer JJ, Shaw JL, Doren WW. Silicone-Dacron hinge prosthesis design, evaluation, and application. Ann Rheum Dis. 1969;28(suppl):56–8.
13. Swanson AB. Finger joint replacement by silicone rubber implants and the concept of implant fixation by encapsulation. Ann Rheum Dis. 1969;28(5):47–55.
14. Bass RL, Stern PJ, Nairus JG. High implant fracture incidence with Sutter silicone metacarpophalangeal joint arthroplasty. J Hand Surg [Am]. 1996;21(5):813–8.
15. Möller K, Sollerman C. Avanta versus Swanson silicone implants in the MCP joint—a prospective, randomized comparison of 30 patients followed for 2 years. J Hand Surg Br. 2005;30:8–13.
16. Linscheid RL, Dobyns JH. Total joint arthroplasty: the hand. Mayo Clin Proc. 1979;54:516–26.
17. Beckenbaugh RD. Preliminary experience with a non-cemented no constrained total joint arthroplasty for the metacarpophalangeal joints. Orthopedics. 1983;6:962–5.
18. Linscheid RL, Murray PM, Vidal MA, Beckenbaugh RD. Development of a surface replacement arthroplasty for proximal interphalangeal joints. J Hand Surg Am. 1997;22:286–98, 5–7.
19. Jennings CD, Livingstone DP. Surface replacement arthroplasty of the proximal interphalangeal joint using the PIP-SRA implant: results, complications, and revisions. J Hand Surg Am. 2008;33:1565. e1–1565.e11.
20. Johnstone BR, Fitzgerald M, Smith KR, Currie LJ. Cemented versus uncemented surface replacement arthroplasty of the proximal interphalangeal joint with a mean 5-year follow-up. J Hand Surg Am. 2008;33:726–32.
21. Bodell LS, Champagne LP. Small joint arthroplasty: the journey is not yet complete. Orthopedics Today. 2000.
22. Murray PM, Linscheid RL, Cooney WP, Baker V, Heckman MG. Long-term outcome of proximal interphalangeal joint surface replacement arthroplasty. J Bone Joint Surg Am. 2012;94:1120–8.
23. Minamikawa Y, Imaeda T, Amadio PC, Linscheid RL, Cooney WP, An K-N. Lateral stability of proximal interphalangeal joint replacement. J Hand Surg Am. 1994;19A:1050–4.
24. Srnec JJ, Wagner ER, Rizzo M. Implant arthroplasty for proximal interphalangeal, metacarpophalangeal, and trapeziometacarpal joint degeneration. J Hand Surg Am. 2017;42:817–825.4.
25. Takigawa S, et al. Long-term assessment of Swanson implant arthroplasty in the proximal interphalangeal joint of the hand. J Hand Surg Am. 2004;29:785–95.
26. Duncan SFM, Smith AA, Renfree KJ, Dunbar RM, Merritt MV. Results of the volar approach in proximal interphalangeal joint arthroplasty. J Hand Surg Asian-Pac Vol. 2018;23:26–32.
27. Flannery O, Harley O, Badge R, et al. MatOrtho proximal interphalangeal joint arthroplasty: minimum 2-year follow-up. J Hand Surg Eur Vol. 2016;41:910–6.
28. Athlani L, Gaisne E, Bellemère P. Arthroplastie de l'articulation interphalangienne proximale par prothèse TACTYS: résultats préliminaires avec un recul minimum de 2 ans. Hand Surgery and Rehabilitation. 2016;35:168–78.
29. Schindele SF, Hensler S, Audige L, et al. A modular surface gliding implant (CapFlex-PIP) for proximal interphalangeal joint osteoarthritis: a prospective case series. J Hand Surg Am. 2015;40:334–40.
30. Kuczynski K. The proximal interphalangeal joint. Anatomy and causes of stiffness in the fingers. J Bone Joint Surg Br. 1968;50(3):656–63.
31. Pellegrini VD, Burton RI. Osteoarthritis of the proximal interphalangeal joint of the hand: arthroplasty or fusion? J Hand Surg Am. 1990;15:194–209.
32. Minamikawa Y, Horii E, Amadio PC, Cooney WP, Linscheid RL, An K-N. Stability and constraint of the proximal interphalangeal joint. J Hand Surg Am. 1993;18A:198–204.
33. Ashworth CR, Hansraj KK, Todd AO, Dukhram KM, Ebramzadeh E, Boucree JB, et al. Swanson proximal inter-phalangeal joint arthroplasty in patients with rheumatoid arthritis. Clin Orthop. 1997;342:34–7.
34. Swanson AB, Maupin BK, Gajjar NV, et al. Flexible implant arthroplasty in the proximal interphalangeal joint of the hand. J Hand Surg Am. 1985;10A:796–805.
35. Goldfarb CA, Stern PJ. Metacarpophalangeal joint arthroplasty in rheumatoid arthritis. A long-term assessment. J Bone Joint Surg Am. 2003;85-A(10):1869–78.
36. Kay AG, Ljeffs JV, Scott JT. Experience with Silastic prosthesis in the rheumatoid hand: a five years follow up. Ann Rheum Dis. 1978;37:255–8.
37. Boe C, Wagner E, Rizzo M. Long-term outcomes of silicone metacarpophalangeal arthroplasty: a longitudinal analysis of 325 cases. J Hand Surg Eur Vol. 2018;10:1076–82.
38. Swanson AB, de Groot SG, Ishikawa H. Use of grommets for flexible implant resection arthroplasty of the metacarpophalangeal joint. Clin Orthop Relat Res. 1997 Sep;342:22–33.
39. Schmidt K, Witt K, Ossowski A, Miehlke RK. Therapy of rheumatoid destruction of the middle finger metacarpophalangeal joint with a Swanson silastic implant stabilized resection arthroplasty: comparative study of long and intermediate term results with and without implantation of titanium grommets. Z Rheumatol. 1997;56(5):287–97.
40. Erdogan A, Weiss APC. Metakarpophalangeale Arthroplastik mit der NeuFlex-Silastikprothese. Orthopade. 2003;32:789–93.
41. Delaney ER, Trail IA, Nuttall D. A comparative study of outcome between the Neuflex and Swanson metacarpophalangeal joint replacements. J Hand Surg Br. 2005;30:3–7.
42. Chaudhary R, Garg J, Krishnamoorthy P, Shah N, et al. On-X valve: the next generation aortic valve. Cardiol Rev. 2017;25:77–83.
43. Bellemere P. Pyrocarbon implants for the hand and wrist. Hand Surg Rehabil. 2018;37-3:129–54.

44. Cook SD, Beckenbaugh RD, Redondo J, Popich LS, Klawitter JJ, Linscheid RL. Long-term follow-up of pyrolytic carbon metacarpophalangeal implants. J Bone Joint Surg Am. 1999;81(5):635–48.
45. Gauci MO, Winter M, Dumontier C, Bronsard N, Allieu Y. Clinical and radiologic outcomes of Pyrocarbon radial head prosthesis: midterm results. J Shoulder Elb Surg. 2016;25:98–104.
46. Apard T, Casin C, Moubarak E, Bizot P. A novel pyrolytic carbon implant for hallux rigidus: a cadaveric study. Foot Ankle Surg. 2011;17:182–5.
47. Garret J, Godeneche A, Boileau P, Molé D, Etzner M, et al. Pyrocarbon interposition shoulder arthroplasty: preliminary results from a prospective multicenter study at 2 years of follow-up. J Shoulder Elb Surg. 2017;26:1143–51.
48. Daecke W, Kaszap B, Martini AK, Hagena FW, Rieck B, Jung M. A prospective, randomized comparison of 3 types of proximal interphalangeal joint arthroplasty. J Hand Surg Am. 2012;37(9):1770–9.
49. Chan K, Ayeni O, McKnight L, et al. Pyrocarbon versus silicone proximal interphalangeal joint arthroplasty: a systematic review. Plast Reconstr Surg. 2013;131(1):114–24.
50. Hohendorff B, Zhang W, Burkhart KJ, Müller LP, Ries C. Insertion of the Ascension Pyrocarbon PIP total joint in 152 human cadaver fingers: analysis of implant positions and malposition. Arch Orthop Trauma Surg. 2015;135(2):283–90.
51. Hassler M. Other coming only used biomechanical coatings: pyrolytic carbon coating. In: Driver M, editor. Coatings fr biomedical applications. 1st ed. Cambridge, UK: Woodhead Publishing Limited; 2014. p. 75–105.
52. Sweets TM, Stern PJ. Pyrolytic carbon resurfacing arthroplasty for osteoarthritis of the proximal interphalangeal joint of the finger. J Bone Joint Surg Am. 2011;93:1417–25.
53. Herren DB, Schindele S, Goldhahn J, et al. Problematic bone fixation with Pyrocarbon implants in proximal interphalangeal joint replacement: short-term results. J Hand Surg Br. 2006;31:643–51.
54. Burman MS. Vitallium cup arthroplasty of metacarpophalangeal and interphalangeal joints of fingers. Bull Hosp Joint Dis. 1940;1:79–89.
55. Malchau H, et al. Prognosis of total hip replacement. The National Hip Arthroplasty Register. 1996:9–11.
56. Malchau H, et al. The Swedish total hip replacement register. J Bone Joint Surg. 2002;84A:2–20.
57. Parcells B. Stem: Press-fit in Hip & Knee book. 4 Jan 2017. Hipandkneebook.com.
58. Brånemark P-I, Hansson BO, Adell R, et al. Osseointegrated implants in the treatment of the edentulous jaw: experience from a 10-year period. Scand J Plast Reconstr Surg Hand Surg. 1977;16(suppl 16):1–132.
59. Hagert C-G, Brånemark P-I, Albrektsson T, Strid K-G, Irstam L. Metacarpophalangeal joint replacement with osseointegrated endoprostheses. Scand J Plast Reconstr Surg. 1986;20:207–18.
60. Lundborg G, BraÊnemark PI. Osseointegrated proximal interphalangeal joint prosthesis with a peplaceable flexible joint spacer- long term results. Scand J Plast Reconstr Hand Surg. 2000;34:345–53.
61. Möller K, Sollerman C, Geijer M, Brånemark PI. Early results with osseointegrated proximal interphalangeal joint prostheses. J Hand Surg Am. 1999;24(2):267–74.
62. Möller K, Geijer M, Sollerman C, Lundborg G. Radiographic evaluation of osseointegration and loosening of titanium implants in the MCP and PIP joints. J Hand Surg Am. 2004;29(1):32–8.
63. Komatsu I, Arishima Y, Shibahashi H, Yamaguchi T, Minamikawa Y. Outcomes of surface replacement proximal interphalangeal joint arthroplasty using the self locking finger joint implant: minimum two years follow-up. Hand (N Y). 2018;13(6):637–45.
64. Bouacida S, Lazerges C, Coulet B, Chammas M. Proximal interphalangeal joint arthroplasty with Neuflex implant: relevance of the volar approach and early rehabilitation. Chir Main. 2014;33:350–5.
65. Yamamoto M, Malay S, Fujihara Y, Zhong L, Chung K. A systemic review of different implants and approaches for proximal interphalangeal joint arthroplasty. Plast Reconstr Surg. 2017;139:1139–51.
66. Schneider LH. Proximal interphalangeal joint arthroplasty: the volar approach. Semin Arthroplast. 1999;2:139–47.
67. Ishizuki M, Saito N, Wakabayashi Y, Shirota M, Ozawa H. Newly developed artificial joint of the finger joint. J Jpn Soc Surg Hand. 1998;15:188–91.
68. Masada K. New finger implant. Jpn J Rheumatol. 1998;20:497–503.
69. Nakamura K, Masada K, et al. Short-term results after metacarpophalangeal joint arthroplasty with MES finger prosthesis in rheumatoid arthritis: a multicenter study. J Jpn Soc Surg Hand. 2006;23:983–7.
70. Sekiguchi M, Suguro T, Manome T, Ohikata Y, Yamamoto K. Development of total joint (FINE total finger joint system) and clinical application based on new concept. J Jpn Soc Surg Hand. 2005;22:666–70.
71. Condamine JL, Benoit JY, Comtet JJ, Aubriot JH. Proposed digital arthroplasty: critical study of the preliminary results. Ann Chir Main. 1988;7:282–97.

# 20 Primary Proximal Interphalangeal Joint Arthroplasty

Ian A. Trail

## Introduction

Replacement of the proximal interphalangeal joint (PIP jt) has followed that of the metacarpophalangeal joint (MCP jt); however, only recently has it become the focus of increasing interest. The reason for this has been the relative success of arthrodesis or fusion in a functional position. Certainly in the presence of a normal MCP joint, PIP fusion between 30° and 50° of flexion can work well providing the patient with a pain free, stable and strong grip. However, if the MCP/DIP (distal interphalangeal) joints are themselves diseased, then fusion of the PIP joints may result in increased stiffness of the whole finger and consequently reduced function. Plainly, in these circumstances, some form of athroplasty would be advantageous. Indeed, even if these joints are relatively normal, many patients prefer the retention of some movement over none at all. This was first recognised by Carroll and Taber in an article in 1954, when they reported the results of 30 patients treated by resection arthroplasty of the PIP joint without the interposition of any other material [1]. In selected patients, they were able to demonstrate encouraging results. Pellegrini and Burton in a publication in 1990 retrospectively reviewed a number of patients who had undergone various procedures on the proximal interphalangeal joint [2]. The majority of these patients were suffering with some form of erosive osteoarthritis, and the operations undertaken were an arthroplasty using either a flexible silicone interposition or a cemented Biomeric arthroplasty or an arthrodesis. All the cemented Biomeric implants failed at an average of 2.25 years after operation. Arthrodesis of the proximal interphalangeal joint in the radial digits provided the greatest improvement in lateral pinch strength, whilst flexible silicone interpositional arthroplasty in the ulna digits provided an average flexion arc of 56° with satisfactory pain relief. Although none required revision, radiographic evidence of bone erosion around the silicone implant was seen in 35% of cases at 2 years. As a result, the authors were unable to make a recommendation as to which procedure was the most optimal.

Whilst the retention of some movement has obvious advantages, there are also attendant risks. Indeed, these risks are not only present at the time of surgery but also subsequently as the years go by. Patients with arthroplasties in situ need access to continuing care, whilst patients with an arthrodesis when solid can often be discharged. The complications of PIP arthroplasty as with all implants include dislocation, infection and loosening. At this time, however, particularly for the newer "two-part" implants which are in their infancy, the exact incidence and subsequent

I. A. Trail (✉)
Wrightington Hospital, Wigan, Lancashire, UK
e-mail: upperlimb@wrightington.org.uk


G. J. W. King, M. Rizzo (eds.), *Arthroplasty of the Upper Extremity*,
https://doi.org/10.1007/978-3-030-68880-6_20

management of these complications are poorly understood.

The history of arthroplasty of the PIP joint is undoubtedly short. In 1961, Adrian Flatt undertook trials with a metallic prosthetic replacement for the interphalangeal joints [3]. Whilst this prosthesis offered the advantage of inherent stability and an adequate range of motion, migration and erosion of the stems through the medullary canals and cortices became commonplace. This implant design is no longer available.

As with all arthroplasties of the hand and wrist, however, Al Swanson has contributed significantly to our understanding of PIP joint arthroplasty [4]. His Silastic hinged-type implant was first introduced in 1973 as an extension of the successful MCP joint Silastic interposition arthroplasty. At the same time, Neibauer (1969) introduced his version incorporating a Dacron core [5].

Further to this and as at the MCP joint other designs have subsequently been introduced. These include the Sutter (Stryker, Kalamazoo, MI, USA) and Neuflex (DePuy, Warsaw, IN, USA), the latter having a preformed angle of 15° which is said to mimic the normal resting position.

Alternatives in patients with osteoarthritis or following fracture have included excision of the articular surfaces with some form of interposition of soft tissue – the best known of these being the "volar plate" arthroplasty. Durham-Smith and McCarten from Australia reported their results in 1992 [6]. A series of 71 cases performed over 5 years were undertaken for fracture/subluxation of the joint. Sixty-two (87%) of the patients achieved a stable pain-free joint with movement from 5° to 95° within 2 months. Complications were uncommon with a high patient satisfaction rate (94%). Longer-term results of this procedure were reported by Dionysian and Eaton in May 2000 [7]. They examined 17 patients after an average of 11½ years following this procedure for fracture dislocation of the proximal interphalangeal joint. The operation was generally undertaken in a younger age group ranging from 17 to 61 years. Overall, there was satisfactory pain relief and a good active range of motion above 85°. They did note however that patients who underwent the operation earlier, that is, soon after the injury, seemed to do better. They concluded by suggesting that volar plate arthroplasty continues to be of benefit on a long-term basis. Similar results were reported by Burton et al., from Rochester, New York, in November 2002, although in this series the indication was osteoarthritis [8].

Small joint reconstruction using a perichondrial graft was first described by Johansson and Engkvist in 1981 [9]. They reported the results of perichondrial arthroplasty in 50 joints mostly at the metacarpophalangeal and proximal interphalangeal joints of the hand. At that time, the operative technique was described together with post-operative management. In the 36 joints reviewed at more than 1 year, good or excellent results were reported in 75%. A more updated study was reported by Seradge et al. from Oklahoma City in 1984 [10]. They reported a retrospective review of 36 of these procedures, 20 of which had been undertaken at the proximal interphalangeal joint, with a minimum follow-up of 3 years. The overall results showed 55% to be good and 15% fair with 30% having been revised. All procedures undertaken for post-sepsis arthritis had failed. In addition, a concomitant tendon repair was another factor associated with a high failure rate. Finally, patients over 40 seemed to have better results. In 1992, Hasegawa and Yamano from Japan reported better results using sections from the costo-osteochondral junction including an osseous portion rather than costal cartilage alone [11]. In 1995, Katsaros reported another small series with encouraging results [12].

Finally, this section would not be complete without reference to the classic articles by Harrison from the UK in 1971 and Lipscomb from the USA in 1967 [13, 14]. Harrison categorised the type of surgery applicable to the rheumatoid proximal interphalangeal joint into either symptomatic, reparative or reconstructive. Symptomatic surgery was for either acute synovitis, proliferative synovitis or fibrinous synovitis and essentially took the form of a synovectomy. The operation is well described in this article. For reparative, Harrison meant the correction of either a flexion or extension deficit, in this case a Boutonniere or "Swan Neck" deformity. Again, the surgical treatment is described. Finally, for reconstruction, he recommended either arthrodesis or arthroplasty. Lipscomb also gave a detailed description of the technique of synovectomy of the interphalangeal joint of the finger as well as the metacarpophalangeal joint of the thumb.

## Surgical Technique and Rehabilitation

As stated previously, arthroplasty of the proximal interphalangeal (PIP) joint is at a watershed and is yet to be accepted by the majority of hand surgeons. Faced with the options however of using these implants in what could already be a stiff finger, the retention of any movement seems logical. The indications for arthrodesis or arthroplasty are almost identical in that both give excellent pain relief and improvement in strength and function. Plainly, arthroplasty should allow the retention of some movement, where an arthrodesis will not. Our experience has been that patients far prefer arthroplasty despite the need for continuing care and the potential of increased complications. At this time, the only absolute contraindication at our institution would be in younger patients with an active lifestyle, in a manual worker, if there is significant bone loss or gross instability or in the presence of concomitant infection.

As with all implant surgery in the hand, it is crucial at the time of insertion that strict asepsis is observed. Whilst it is not the author's practice to wear "body exhaust suits", surgery is undertaken in a clean "laminar air" operating theatre with antibiotic cover. With regard to anaesthesia if more than one implant is being inserted, the author would normally advise the patient to have a general anaesthetic. If one finger is being operated upon, then local or regional anaesthesia is possible. The patient should be warned however that the operation can take up to 1 hour, and as such they would need to tolerate both the tourniquet and the operating room environment for that period.

With regard to the surgical approach itself, a number of techniques have been described based principally on the direction of the approach to the joint, i.e. palmar, lateral or dorsal. The palmar approach was popularised by Schneider from the USA in 1991 in an attempt to overcome the prolonged splinting required after the dorsal approach [15], the latter being required to protect the extensor tendon reconstruction. Via the volar approach, the whole flexor tendon sheath together with the palmar plate is mobilized from the middle phalanx after incision of the accessory collateral ligaments (Fig. 20.1). The dorsal components of the collateral ligaments are preserved. After repair, the joint is stable and suitable for early mobilization. Lin et al. (1995) from the USA reported their results of 69 proximal interphalangeal joint silicone arthroplasties in 36 patients inserted by this technique [16]. The average follow-up was 3.4 years. At review, they reported an improvement of the extensor deficit although the overall total active motion did not improve significantly from the pre-operative values. In addition, coronal plane deformities were not successfully corrected although pain relief was obtained in the majority of patients; five implants ultimately fractured.

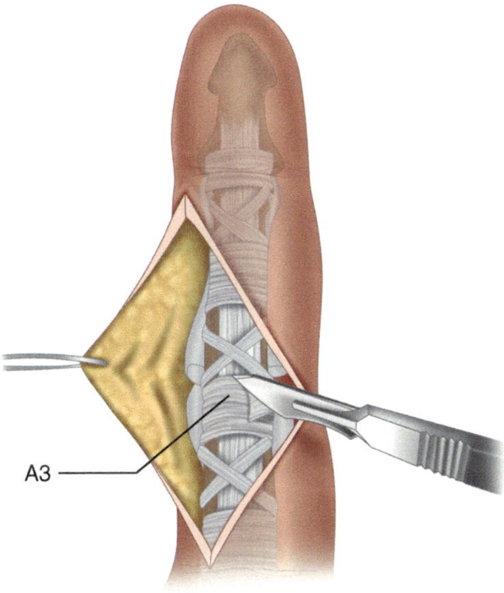


**Fig. 20.1** Volar approach to PIP joint

The lateral approach uses a midline ulnar incision centred on the midpoint of the PIP joint. The neurovascular bundle is identified and retracted in a volar direction. The retinaculum ligament is incised and the extensor tendon mobilized and retracted dorsally. The collateral ligament is then detached from the bone although generally left attached to the volar plate (Fig. 20.2). This allows the joint to be opened up "like a book." For closure, the volar plate and particularly the collateral ligament have to be repaired/reattached. The collateral ligament is reattached to its origin on the condyle of the proximal phalanx.

Undoubtedly, however, the dorsal approach has been the most widely used and is currently the approach of choice at Wrightington. The skin incision is oblique avoiding a direct longitudinal incision over the proximal interphalangeal joint (Fig. 20.3). The extensor tendon then has to be incised and retracted. This can be done either by fashioning a distally based flap in a Chevron fashion (Fig. 20.4) or by incising the tendon longitudinally dissecting the central slip off the base

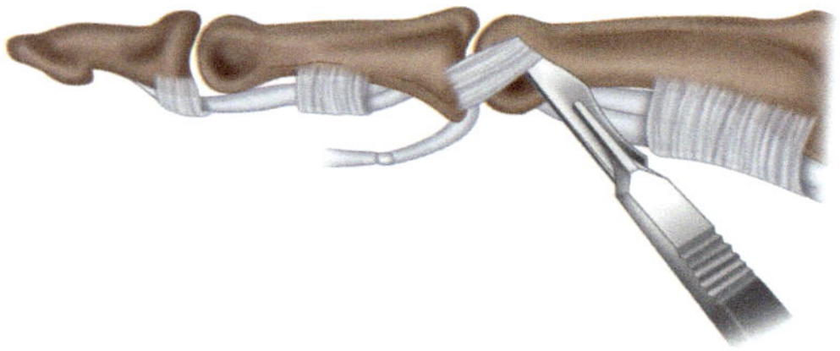

Fig. 20.2 Lateral approach to PIP joint

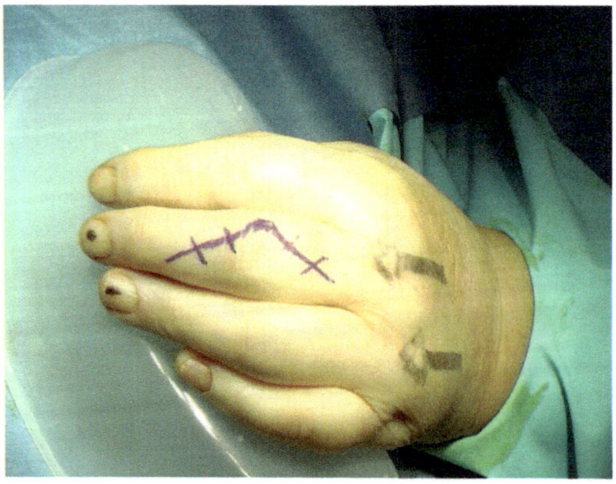

Fig. 20.3 Dorsal approach to PIP joint – skin incision

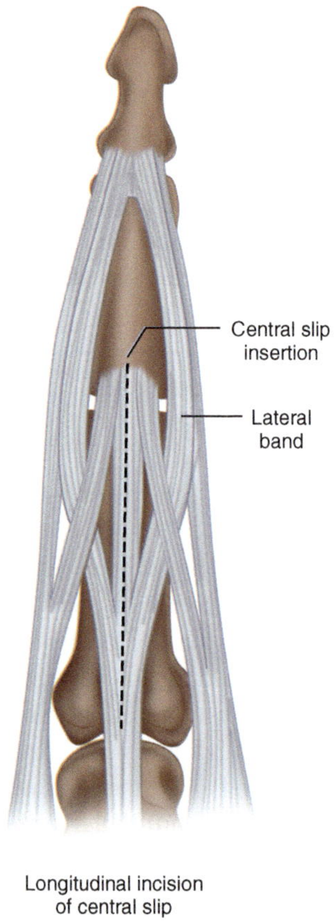


Fig. 20.4 Chevron-shaped extensor tendon flap

of the middle phalanx (Fig. 20.5). At this time, having used both approaches, the author favours the latter. More specifically, there appears to be less post-operative extension lag with this technique. It should be noted however that reconstruction of the extensor tendon is of paramount importance whichever approach is used. If the tendon is split longitudinally, the two components are re-anchored to the base of the middle phalanx by a suture passed through the bone (Fig. 20.6). This is supplemented by additional 4-0 absorbable sutures to co-apt the tendon. Usually during this approach, the dorsal quarter of the collateral ligaments has to be released to allow complete access. In addition and from time to time, a volar plate release has to be undertaken to either improve access or correct deformity. Generally, however, with this approach, an excellent view of the joint surfaces can be obtained allowing accurate resection and preparation with

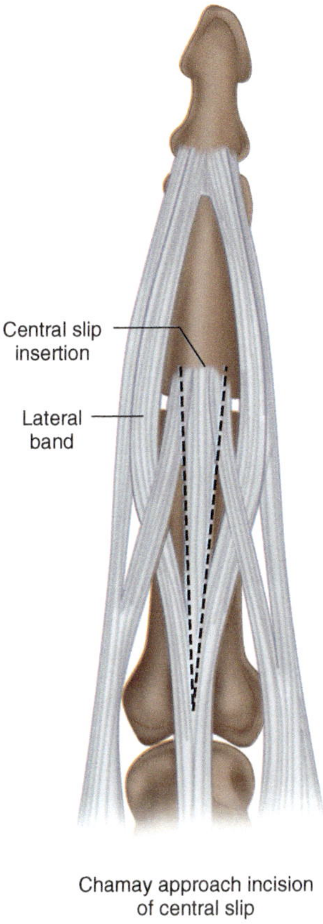


**Fig. 20.5** Release of central slip

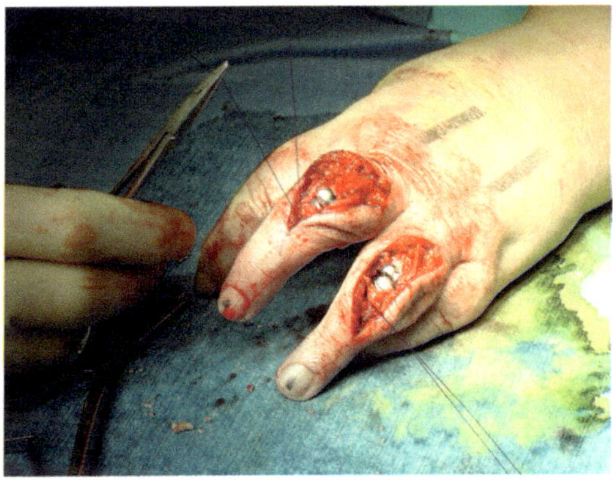

**Fig. 20.6** Reattachment of extensor tendon

better alignment of the implant. For more details on this, the reader is referred to the relevant manufacturer's instructions.

For Silastic implants however, again, it is worth emphasising the importance of the care that should be taken with any soft tissue releases and subsequent rebalancing. For the collateral ligaments, whilst generally it is the author's opinion that these should be preserved at all costs in severe deformity or stiffness, a release may be required. These cases require sharp and delicate dissection. The fibres at the origin of the collateral ligament should be preserved by releasing the collateral ligament in continuity with a sleeve of periosteal tissue. With regard to bone preparation for the Swanson implant, bevelled ends are said to be of benefit. More specifically, cuts are angled from dorsal to volar in a distal to proximal direction. This is said to facilitate flexion. For all implants, it is also important to remove any sharp bone edges or osteophytes as this may lead to abrasion of the implant. Thereafter any synovial tissue should be removed and a soft tissue release on the volar aspect of the joint undertaken if necessary. This will be required specifically if there was a pre-operative flexion contracture. At the end of all this, it is important that the release is such that with the implant in situ, there is no buckling or pinching of the device if a Silastic device is used or undue tightness if a two-piece implant is used. Sizing of the implant also requires good judgement, since the proper implant should fit snugly in the joint and be wide enough to abut both bone ends in the midsection. With regard to any repair, this is better undertaken by suturing structures directly onto the bone. To facilitate this and prior to insertion of the implant, small holes should be made and sutures passed. This will allow sound repair of collateral ligaments or the extensor mechanism. Plainly, it is important that these structures are sutured back to their correct anatomical position. For patients with a Boutonnieres deformity, a central slip advancement or lateral band reattachment to the middle phalanx should be undertaken to prevent recurrence of the contracture. In the author's opinion, it is also useful to perform a tenolysis of the long flexor tendons through a separate volar incision in the palm, particularly if there was some question about tendon excursion prior to surgery.

Finally, an alternative method of approaching the extensor expansion was described by Fahmy et al. in 2001 [17]. Essentially, they separated the lateral bands of the extensor expansion from the central slip, the tendons being retracted as necessary. On closure, the lateral bands are sutured back to the central slip. Plainly whilst this has the advantage following early active mobilization, visualisation of the proximal interphalangeal joint is more limited.

## Post-operative Management

As with all specialised surgery to the hand and wrist, the involvement of a hand therapist is strongly recommended particularly someone with experience in managing these difficult procedures. The objectives of this type of surgery are to obtain a pain-free stable joint with a functional arc of movement of approximately 60° or more. At the time of surgery, it is to be hoped that a sound soft tissue repair has been undertaken, and as a consequence, the joint is stable. Generally, after the application of a dressing, a volar slab including the forearm, wrist and the fingertips is applied. Whilst the wrist is held in neutral, the metacarpophalangeal and proximal interphalangeal joints are immobilized in slight flexion. It is of crucial importance however that the arm is elevated post-operatively to reduce swelling and that patients receive adequate analgesia during this period. At the same time, it is our routine practice to give three doses of antibiotics, the first being given on induction prior to surgery and subsequent two doses intravenously at 6 and 12 hours, respectively.

If at the conclusion of surgery the surgeon is of the view that the joint is stable and suitable for early mobilization, on day 2, the dressings can be reduced, wound inspection undertaken and early mobilization begun. Essentially this option also depends on whether single or multiple fingers have been operated upon. Whichever is the case, however, it is important that the patient is given a resting splint to be worn between periods of mobilization and most importantly at night. The splint itself holds the wrist and MCP joints in neutral yet blocks PIP extension at between 20° and 30° (Fig. 20.7). The patient is then encouraged to undertake active PIP joint flexion for between 10 and 20 repetitions per hour. It is important that whilst this is undertaken, the MCP joint remains static. If the patient had a pre-operative Boutonniere deformity, a dynamic extension splint may also be added to the resting splint maintaining the proximal interphalangeal joint in full extension. If a collateral ligament has been repaired as in the lateral approach, this should be protected by a radial outrigger or by "buddy" strapping during mobilization. This method of mobilization continues for 3–4 weeks. From that time, if flexion is poor, then further splint modifications can be instigated. These include positioning the proximal interphalangeal joints in flexion at night and the addition of flexion assist splints during the day (Fig. 20.8). If however an extension lag is the problem, then

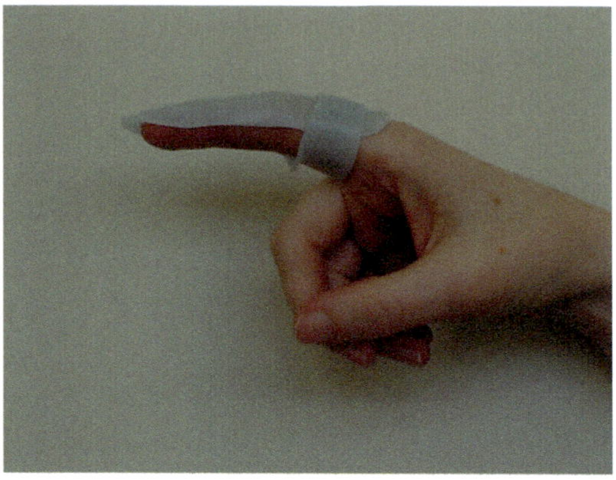

**Fig. 20.7** Extension blocking splint

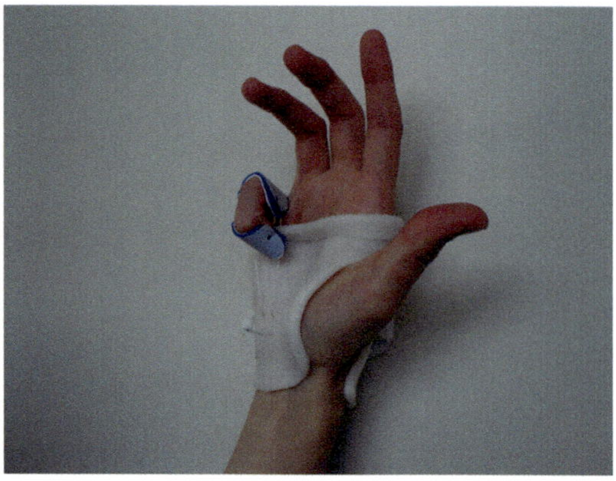

**Fig. 20.8** Flexion assist splint

extension assist splints could be introduced along with a splint to hold the PIP joints in full extension at night. During all this time, the patient is discouraged from undertaking activities of daily living, which could produce deformity of the joint, particularly power or pinch grip. At 6 weeks, protective splints are discontinued, although extension/flexion assist splints can be continued if necessary. A resting night splint is worn for a minimum of 3 months. At that time, a gradual reintroduction to normal function is begun although heavy manual work is avoided.

Finally, if at the time of surgery it is felt that joint is not stable enough to allow early active mobilization, a "delayed mobilization" programme can be instituted. Essentially this involves the patient wearing a resting splint for 3 weeks prior to mobilization. At that time, the programme described above is commenced.

## Evaluation

Outcome is related to many factors, particularly the pre-operative status of the finger, any previous surgery as well as the extent of the surgical intervention or any soft tissue reconstruction. For most surgeons working in this field, 20° of extension lag or less with 60° of flexion, that is, movement from 20° to 60°, no angulation and no pain would be regarded as a good result. All of the above with movements from 0° to 75° would be regarded as an excellent result.

Given the close proximity of other joints in the hand particularly the metacarpophalangeal joint, it is plainly difficult to evaluate the outcome of surgery to the proximal interphalangeal joint in isolation. As much all that has been written in the "Evaluation" section of the metacarpophalangeal joint chapter also applies to the proximal interphalangeal joint. This is particularly so with regard to both local and global scoring systems. At this time, whilst little has been written, certainly, it would not be inappropriate to use either the DASH or the SF36 as a single evaluation tool after this surgery.

Generally, however, as with all such systems, any evaluation should also incorporate some measure of pain relief, movement, stability and strength and finally change in function. The former is simply assessed by a visual analogue score which has the added advantage of being able to be administered by post. Movement conversely has obviously to be measured by a clinician as does strength and stability. Function however, again, can be evaluated at a distance by postal questionnaire. The ideal system for measuring function is a series of validated questions based on activities of daily living. The patient responds by indicating their ability to undertake these particular tasks again on a visual analogue score. There are a number of these available for the hand generally, but none for the PIP jt specifically. As a consequence, whilst to date the outcome of PIP joint arthroplasty has been roughly assessed in this fashion, the author is unaware of any explicit scoring or points system.

In 1979, Linscheid et al. from the Mayo Clinic, reporting their results of PIP joint arthroplasty, felt that motion of 60° or more in the usual arc of flexion with the correction of any previous existing deformity to less than 10°, minimal pain and a minimal inhibition of distal interphalangeal joint motion constituted a good result [18]. Motion of 30° or more again in a useful arc with a flexion deformity of less than 60°, an improvement of pre-existing deformity and mild discomfort were signs of a satisfactory result, while motion of 30° or less with the persistence of a swan neck or flexion deformity greater than 60°, persisting pain and recurrence of angulation were an unsatisfactory result. Finally pronounced loss of joint movement, recurrent or worsening deviation, a flexion or extension contracture and significant pain with removal of the implant or revision were signs of a poor outcome.

In 1994, Adamson et al. from Los Angeles in the USA concluded that a good result was a painless PIP joint that had a functional range of motion, a fair result was a painless joint with position or motion outside the functional range and a poor result was a painful joint with a position or motion outside of the functional range [19]. They felt that the functional range of movement of the proximal interphalangeal joint was between 35° and 85° of flexion. They also reported a radiological assessment although this does not appear to have been formalised. Indeed again from the literature whilst various radiological features have been noted, no systematic evaluation has yet been described. With regard to these various x-ray appearances, these include osteophyte or new bone formation which tends to be associated with joint stiffness. In addition, cysts or cortical erosions can be seen which are generally held to be indicators of either loosening or recurrent synovitis. Sclerotic lines around either a portion or an entire implant are also not uncommonly seen. These have been described around Silastic implants, but also the newer pyrocarbon devices. Their significance at this time, however, remains unclear, but presumably represents new bone formation. Finally, movement of the implant as seen on sequential x-rays is said to be a process known as "settling." By this, it is meant that the implants subside into the bone over a period of time. Unfortunately, on occasion, this can lead to a reduction in the peri-articular space with concomitant loss of movement.

Finally, in 1995, Iselin undertook a detailed evaluation of a number of patients who had undergone Swanson Silastic implants [20]. Their evaluation included active range of motion as measured by a goniometer, an evaluation of strength by way of a pinch metre and Jamar dynamometer, an evaluation of lateral stability and alignment, an assessment of pain and finally a radiographic review. For instability, they felt that between 10° and 15° of lateral deviation was probably of little consequence. With regard to the x-ray analysis, either bone resorption or new bone formation was seen around a small number of implants. Finally, he also reported patient satisfaction, that is, a patient evaluation of the outcome. As a result of all this, they classified their outcome into three groups:

- *Group I (good)*
  The arthroplasty met its essential goals: pain-free active flexion greater than 50°, good joint stability and alignment and very good functional results with minimal loss of strength.
- *Group II (fair)*
  Active flexion less than 50°, good stability and alignment and a good functional result.
- *Group III (poor)*
  Presence of one or more of the following: either stiffness, pain, instability or malalignment. These joints were usually further treated by revision or arthrodesis.

In the author's opinion, there is no doubt that at least where the latest designs of PIP arthroplasty are being evaluated, detailed examination is crucial. It is also important for surgeons newly undertaking these operations that an accurate outcome audit is put in place. Whilst all the modalities of evaluation described above are relevant, particularly pain relief and improvement in function, it does appear that much store is set on active movement of the proximal interphalangeal joint. It is for this reason the author would suggest that a good result would be active movement from 30° to 60°, with no angulation and pain. Excellent results would again have no angulation or pain with a greater range of motion. Anything less than this should be classified as an unsatisfactory or poor result.

## Results

### Silastic Interposition Arthroplasty

The initial results of Silastic interposition arthroplasty or implant resection arthroplasty, as it was first described by Swanson, were reported in 1973 [4] (Fig. 20.9). In this article, the philosophy, surgical technique, post-operative management and initial results are described. Swanson even detailed the concomitant treatment of swan neck and boutonniere deformities. With regard to results, the outcome of 222 PIP joint replacements in 118 hands followed up for between 1 and 6 years was reported. Predominantly these were in patients with rheumatoid arthritis. The average range of motion was from 4° extension lag through to 67° of flexion. Significant improvement was also seen in patients with a preoperative boutonniere or swan neck deformity. Complications only occurred in 2.2% with fractures in five cases (2%), subluxation in one (0.4%) and infection in one other (0.4%).

Updated results in 1985 reported 812 PIP implants; again there was a significant improvement in most cases with an active range of motion of greater than 40° [21]. In addition, the majority of patients (98.3%) reported significant pain relief, and radiologically a favourable bone response was observed. In a few cases, however, bone overgrowth was seen. A complication rate of 5.2% was noted, principally again fracture of the implant, the explanation for this being that this was with the original silicone rather than the latest composition available today. Recurrent "swan necking" was seen in 21% of cases and ulna deviation in 3.7%. Infection was again uncommon as was dislocation, the overall revision rate being 10.9%.

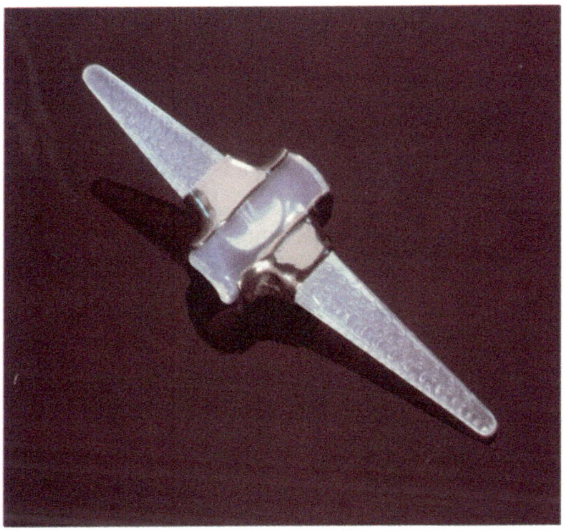

**Fig. 20.9** Swanson Silastic PIP joint replacement

Since then there have been numerous reports from various units throughout the world on this particular implant; these are detailed in Table 20.1. Essentially, in patients with inflammatory arthritis, which is probably the predominant indication, most patients achieve satisfactory pain relief. Generally, however, there is little improvement in movement from pre-operative values. In addition, in patients with a pre-operative swan neck or bou-

**Table 20.1** Results of Swanson Silastic PIP joint arthroplasty

| Author | No. of implants | Indication | ROM/results | Complications |
|---|---|---|---|---|
| Iselin 1975 [22] | 45 | Post trauma | 9–48° | 9 Failures (infection 1, stiffness 7) |
| Iselin 1984 [23] | 120 | Post trauma | 66% Good 16% fair 18% poor | Infection 13/22, rest stiffness |
| Iselin 1995 [20] | 238 | Post trauma (5–23 years follow-up) | 60° Movement long-term follow-up (up to 23 years) 67% good results | |
| Adamson 1994 [19] | 40 | Inflammatory arthritis (9 years follow-up) | 26° (identical to preop) Preop "swan neck" lost 18° 30/40 good to fair 10/40 poor | |
| Ashworth 1997 [24] | 138 | Inflammatory arthritis (5.8 years follow-up) | 5% Moderate/severe pain 38° movement preop 29° Postop function | 10 Implants fractured x-ray sclerosis 78% resorption 12% |
| Hage 1999 [25] | 16 | Post trauma (4 years follow-up) | 47% Movement of opposite side pinch strength 75% opposite side good pain relief function | 2 Failures 1 arthrodesis 1 amputation |
| Herren & Simmen 2000 [26] | 59 | OA/Inflammatory arthritis (>1 year) | 51° movement postop (palnar approach) | |
| Takigawa 2004 [27] | 70 | Predominantly inflammatory arthritis (6.5 years follow-up) | No change 30° Poor correction of deformity Pain relief 70% RA poorest group | X-ray cystic changes 45% 11 implant fractures 9 reviewed |
| Bales 2014 [28] | 38 | Osteoarthritis | Pain 0.4 flexion arc 50° | 21 out of 38 implants fractured 3 revisions |
| Proubasta 2014 [29] | 36 | Primary osteoarthritis | Pain 0.4 active arc of motion 72° | 2 Implants fractured no revision surgery |

tonniere deformity, there is often a recurrence in the long term. Despite this, most authors report a significant improvement in function. Complications however continue to be reported and principally involve fracture of the implant. Takigawa et al. in 2004 reported cystic changes in the shafts of the proximal and middle phalanx in 45% of cases, a particularly worrying finding indicative of silicone synovitis [27]. When the implant is used following trauma, the initial results are again favourable. Ultimately, however, the implant breaks and a higher revision rate has been reported. Finally, there are few reports of this implant being used in patients with primary osteoarthritis.

A number of articles pertinent to this implant have been published, these are discussed below.

## Sutter Design

The Sutter PIP joint arthroplasty is of an identical design to the Sutter MCP joint, although obviously with smaller dimensions (Fig. 20.10).

In 1999, Mathoulin and Gilbert from Paris reported their experience of 21 Sutter implants used for post-traumatic arthritis with an average follow-up of 2 years [30]. With these patients, there was a complete absence of pain in 18 with an active range of movement of 55° compared to 15° pre-operatively. Two implants however had fractured.

## Neuflex Design

The Neuflex PIP joint arthroplasty is again a modification of the Swanson with a 15° flexion prebend potentially mimicking the anatomically neutral position. A publication by Merle et al. (2011) reviewed 51 arthroplasties in 43 patients followed up for a mean of 36 months [31]. Movement improved from 38° pre-operatively to 63° post-operatively. Added to that, functional scores improved although in five cases (10%) further surgery was required. One particular issue with the lateral approach was continuing instability.

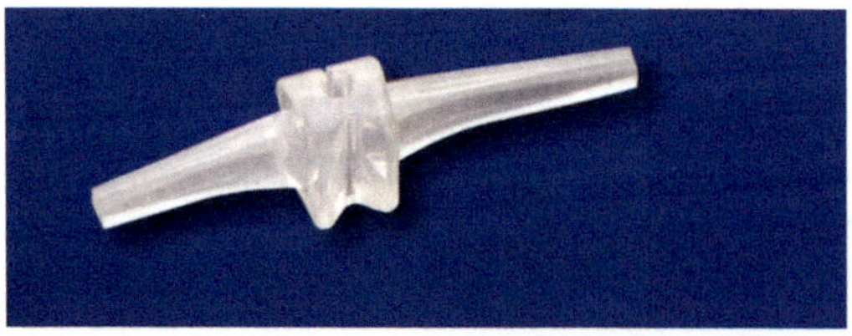

**Fig. 20.10** Silastic Sutter PIP joint arthroplasty

## Osseointegrated Implants

The first report on osseointegrated implants was from Moller et al. from Gotenberg, Sweden, in 1999 [32]. They reported the results of 32 implants in 12 patients suffering predominantly with rheumatoid arthritis. This implant has two screw-type titanium fixation devices, which are linked by a flexible silicone spacer. Iliac crest bone graft was used as a supplement in most cases. The follow-up was however short, being 27 months; movements averaged from 11° through to 67° with an average of 56° active movement. Of the 22 implants, 41 of the 44 titanium implants were osseointegrated radiologically. Unfortunately, in 4 of the 22 implants, there were fractures of the Silastic spacers, with deformity in 27%. Despite that, patient satisfaction was high, although it was felt that some modification of the Silastic spacer would be advisable.

Lundborg and Branemark in 2000 reported their results of 25 of the same implants in 19 patients [33]. The indications for surgery here were predominantly posttraumatic arthritis and primary osteoarthritis. At follow-up, at an average of 8.5 years, 47 of the 50 titanium fixtures were osseointegrated. Unfortunately, the Silastic spacers had again fractured in 68% and had to be replaced in a number. The active range of motion was 41°.

A further updated radiological evaluation, published in 2004, of 27 proximal interphalangeal and 212 metacarpophalangeal joints in 86 patients, again predominantly suffering with rheumatoid arthritis, revealed osseointegration in 94% of cases [34]. The authors also identified that, in a small number of cases, the proximal fixtures showed radiological signs of loosening mainly in the first 3 years after surgery. Again, they felt a more durable Silastic spacer would be advantageous.

## Surface Replacement

Following the general dissatisfaction with PIP joint replacement in the late 1970s, Linscheid and others from the Mayo Clinic developed a surface replacement prosthesis using the more conventional materials of cobalt chrome and ultra-high molecular weight polyethylene (UHMWPE). The design was essentially anatomical with stem fixation into the proximal and middle phalanges (Fig. 20.11), the stems themselves extending beyond the midpoint of the phalanges being fixed by the use of polymethylmethacrylate cement. The authors did acknowledge that for this type of implant to be successful, it required precise alignment together with soft tissue preservation or repair for optimal function.

In 1979, they reported their results of 66 implants in 47 patients over a 14-year period. The diagnosis in 37 cases was of osteoarthritis, 16 had posttraumatic arthritis, and 13 had rheumatoid arthritis. The mean follow-up was 4.1 years (1–14 years). Using their own criteria previously described, the results were quoted as good in 32, fair in 19 and poor in 15. Otherwise having tried all the surgical approaches, they concluded that the dorsal approach was superior to the others. In addition, pre-existing deformity or extreme bone/soft tissue loss often resulted in poor results.

A further publication by Johnstone (2001) from Australia reported on his results of 20 joints in 13 patients [35]. Again the predominant indications were osteoarthritis or posttraumatic arthritis. Excellent long-term results were seen in 18 of the 20 patients with the active range of motion being 73°. Johnstone also felt that an early active mobilization was the best post-operative therapy programme.

Thereafter, there is a publication by Jennings and Livingstone (2015) which reported on the results of 39 cases followed up for 9.3 years [36]. The average arc of motion had deteriorated from 64° following surgery to 56 degrees at the latest follow-up. There were, however, no significant x-ray changes, and no further revisions had been undertaken.

## Results of the Ascension Pyrocarbon PIP Joint Replacement

Pyrocarbon is a synthetic material formed by the pyrolysis of a hydrocarbon gas. This material is coated onto a high-strength graphite substrate to form the basis of an implant. In the case of the pyrocarbon PIP implant, this is similar in design to the surface replacement being unlinked, with stem fixation into the proximal and middle phalanges. Please note that polymethylmethacrylate cement is not used with this implant. There are however a set of instruments/cutting jigs which allow the implants to be inserted in a standard fashion, preserving the soft tissues, particularly the collateral ligaments and volar plate (Fig. 20.12).

The first published article of this implant was by Schulz et al. from Germany, who reported their results in 20 patients with idiopathic or post-traumatic arthritis affecting the proximal interphalangeal joint [37]. The range of follow-up was short between 0.5 and 2.5 years. The majority of patients were pleased with pain relief and had an average active range of motion of 50°. X-rays however did reveal some peri-prosthetic cyst for-

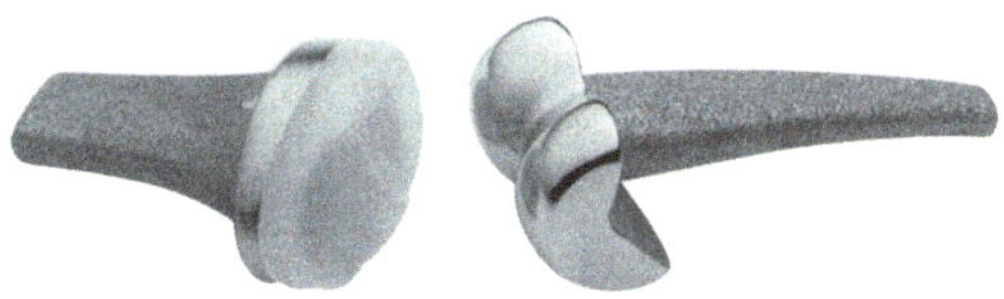

Fig. 20.11 SR unlinked PIPR joint replacement

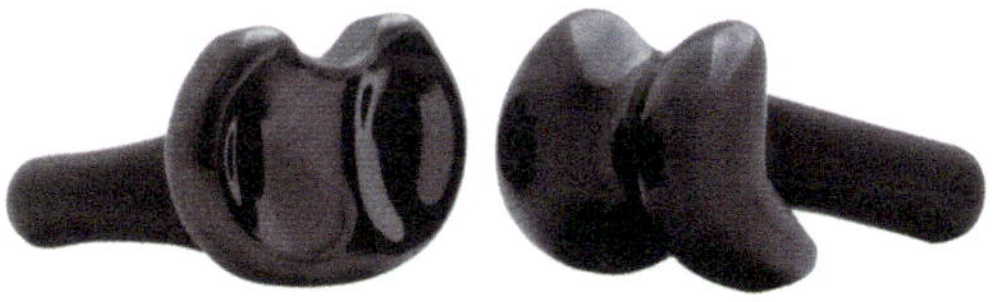

Fig. 20.12 Pyrocarbon PIP joint arthroplasty (Ascension)

**Table 20.2** Results of pyrocarbon PIP joint arthroplasty

| Author | Number of implants (follow-up) | Indications | ROM/results | Complications |
|---|---|---|---|---|
| McGuire et al. (2011) [39] | 57 (27 mo) | OA | 66° (30°)<br>88% high satisfaction | Stiffness/deformity 35%<br>Revision 9% |
| Hutt et al. (2012) [40] | 18 (6.2 years) | OA 13<br>PTOA 5 | Good pain relief<br>45° arc | 2 implant removal<br>Subsidence/migration 10/18 x-ray |
| Mashhadi et al. (2012) [41] | 24 (3 years) | OA | 46° (36°) | 9/24 (4 reoperation) |
| Tägil et al. (2014) [42] | 65 | | Good pain relief<br>54° (53°) | Revision 12%<br>Osteolysis 19 components |
| Heers et al. (2012) [43] | 13 (8.3 years) | OA | Some ongoing pain<br>58° | Significant radiolucent lines 50% |
| Reissner et al. (2014) [44] | 15 (9.7 years) | OA | Good pain relief<br>36° | High rate of migration on x-ray |
| Storey et al. (2015) [45] | 57 (7.1 years) | OA(RA) | VAS 0.3<br>0–60° mean | 3 reoperations |
| Pettersson et al. (2015) [46] | 42 (4–10 years) | OA (RA) | Pain improved<br>No improvement ROM/grip strength | 4 revisions |

mation with potential loosening of the proximal as well as the distal component in some patients. There was however no correlation between these radiological observations and clinical outcome. However, in three cases, the prosthesis had to be revised to an arthrodesis. In conclusion, the authors felt that further investigation was needed to improve the radiological results in the long term, particularly with regard to osseointegration.

At Wrightington, our initial results were presented at the British Hand Society meeting in 2003 [38]. Here the results of 32 joints in 21 patients were submitted. Again, the follow-up was short, and the majority of patients had either osteoarthritis, a post-traumatic problem or rheumatoid arthritis. All implants were put in through a dorsal approach using the appropriate instruments. A number of complications were noted, subluxation in two patients, stiffness in another two who required further surgical intervention and finally a superficial infection in one. Movement improved significantly, particularly in patients with osteoarthritis who prior to surgery had only 30° active movement, compared to 55° at the latest follow-up. Patients with posttraumatic arthritis improved similarly although those with rheumatoid less so. Overall, the vast majority of patients were satisfied, and there was no radiological evidence of loosening.

Thereafter, there are a number of articles published on the outcome of this implant. These are consolidated in Table 20.2. Effectively these show good clinical results with a modest reoperation rate, the most potentially worrying issue being a high rate of subsidence/migration on later x-rays.

## Other Proximal Interphalangeal Joint Implant Designs

Prior to the introduction of their pure surface replacement, Linscheid and others, from the Mayo Clinic, experimented with a constrained uniaxial linked implant in this situation. Again the implant was cemented and the two components linked by a polyethylene bushing. In a report in 1979, again mainly in patients with osteoarthritis, they found unsatisfactory or poor results in 47 of 67 implants followed up for 15 months, the principal problem being loosening of the components. It is my understanding that this implant is no longer available.

Dryer et al., from the University of Iowa, in 1984, reported their results with the Flatt implant amongst others in patients with rheumatoid arthritis [47]. Again, this is a linked-type implant, fixation being by two metal prongs into both the proximal and middle phalanx (Fig. 20.13). At an average 6.2-year follow-up, movements for the Flatt prosthesis ranged from 28° through to 45° with 15° of active movement. Further follow-up indicated that this movement gradually decreased over time. Radiographically cortical perforation by the prosthesis was common. Despite this, patient satisfaction was high although again I believe this implant is no longer available commercially.

In 1997, Condamine and others, from France, reported their results with the so-called digital joint arthroplasty (DJOA) implant used exclusively in patients with osteoarthritis between 1985 and 1994 [48], with the proximal interphalangeal joint being replaced in 19 cases. Range of motion at follow-up was only slightly improved by arthroplasty, measuring 50°, with some improvement in extension. The majority of patients however reported satisfactory pain relief. Radiologically there were late signs of periarticular ossification. At that time, the implant was being redesigned.

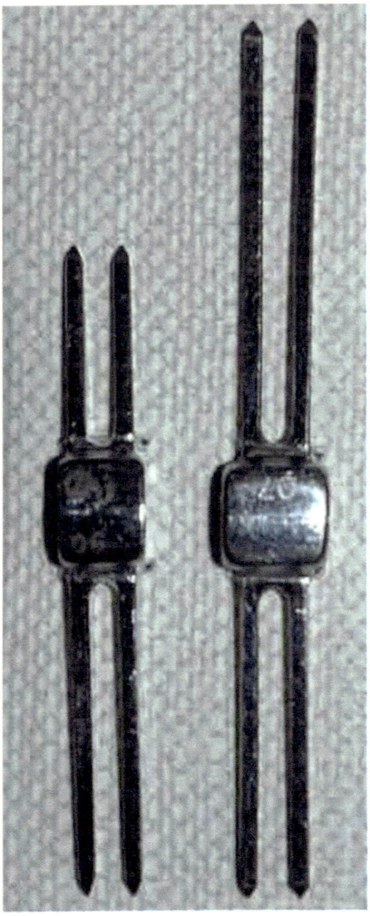

**Fig. 20.13** Flatt PIP joint arthroplasty

Subsequently in 2000, Mentzel from Ulm in Germany reported their experience with the DIGITOS-prosthesis [49]. This is a cemented, modular, hinged prosthesis, which was used in seven patients with osteoarthritis of the proximal interphalangeal joint. At follow-up of 2 years, the functional results were found to be good. Movement improved from 51.5° pre-operatively to 60.5° at 3 months after surgery, decreasing to 53° at 1 year and 49.5° by the end of the second year. Radiologically no implant was loose, and all patients were pain-free. These patients continue to be monitored carefully.

The preliminary results of the LPM prosthesis were presented at the British Society of Surgery of the Hand Autumn Meeting in 2005. Twenty-one implants had been inserted in 15 patients over a 1-year period. The average arc of movement was 50°, improving from 28° pre-operatively. The patients with osteoarthritis gained and maintained the largest improvement with those undertaken for trauma and rheumatoid arthritis less so. In this study, there were no post-operative complications, although a number of surgeons in the audience indicated that they had experienced problems including osteolysis with early to mid-term failure of the proximal component of the prosthesis. Subsequently more of these problems have been reported to the "Audit Committee" of the British Hand Society, and as a consequence, the implant has now been withdrawn.

In 2015, Schindele et al. reported the results of the CapFlex-PIP [50]. They reported ten patients in cases of osteoarthritis followed up for 12 months. They reported improved motion from 42° to 51° although this was not statistically significant. Pain,

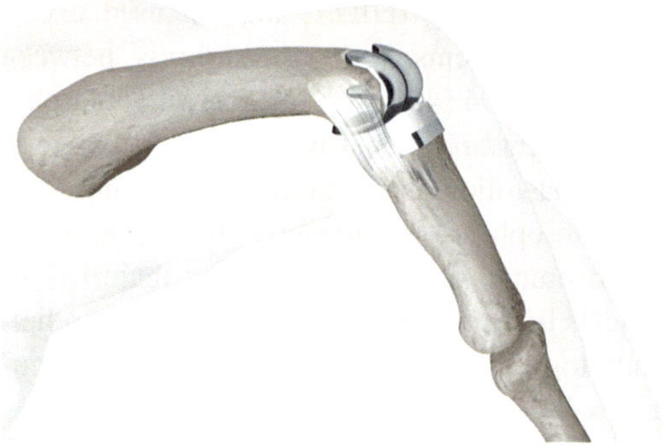

Fig. 20.14 CapFlex-PIP joint arthroplasty

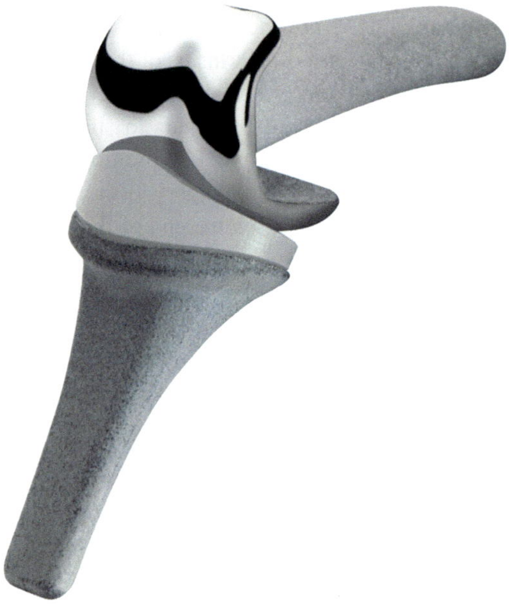

Fig. 20.15 PIPR arthroplasty (MatOrtho)

however, was reduced and functional scores improved. Two patients underwent tenolysis and tended to improve motion (Fig. 20.14).

Finally, in 2016, Flannery et al. reported the results of the MatOrtho proximal interphalangeal joint arthroplasty with a minimum 2-year follow-up [51]. This anatomical implant is based on work published by Lawrence et al. (2004) on the morphological appearance and measurements of the proximal interphalangeal joint [52]. The proximal phalanx component is made of cobalt chrome and the middle phalanx of high-density polyethylene which is mobile bearing. Both components are stemmed with hydroxyapatite coating. The implant is not linked (Fig. 20.15).

Of the original article, there were 100 implants followed up between 2 and 6.5 years. Implant survival was 85% from 4 years onwards. There were, however, 13 revisions in the first year for stiffness, instability and component disassembly. It was noted, however, that patients who had a stiff or deformed PIP joint prior to surgery did not do as well.

A more recent paper by Fowler et al. (submitted) reports the results of this implant inserted through a lateral approach rather than a dorsal [53]. It does appear that inserting this implant through a lateral approach results in significant improvement in post-operative range of motion.

## Complications and Their Management

As with all implants, the potential range of complications is large. For the Silastic replacements however, a review of literature would indicate an overall revision rate of less than 10%. The principal complication with this type of implant is fracture of the silicone (Fig. 20.16); indeed, a similar problem has been noted with the linkage part of the titanium osseointegrated-type implant. Initial published series have reported between 5% and 10% incidence of this complication. Undoubtedly, however, the longer the follow-up, the more likely it is that this complication will occur. Having said that, this does not necessarily mean that revision surgery will be required, revision only being undertaken if there is significant pain and deformity. In the author's experience, revision for this complication would take the form of either revision to another Silastic implant, arthrodesis or an excision arthroplasty.

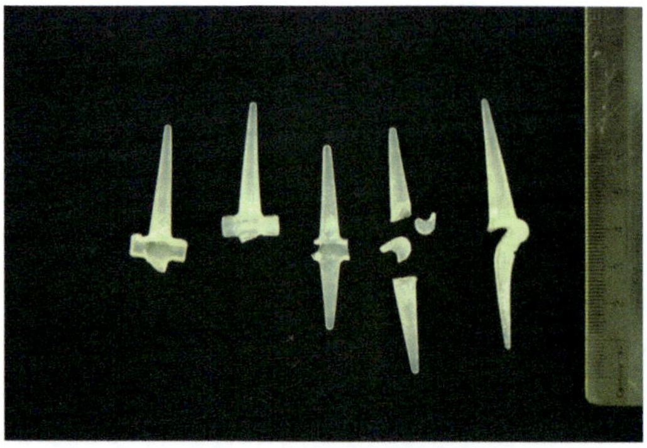

Fig. 20.16 Fracture of the silicone implant

Other complications include infection, which is obviously a complication of significant concern. Generally this is treated initially by removal of the implant, curettage and the administration of long-term antibiotics, with secondarily either leaving the joint as an excision arthroplasty, fusion or the secondary reinsertion of a further implant, either unlinked or linked (silastic). The authors' experience with this complication is fortunately small, and of the three cases seen, all have been treated by excision arthroplasty. This has resulted in a complete resolution of the infection in all cases, although the patients have been left with some instability of the proximal interphalangeal joint. Fortunately, however, some movement has been retained with a complete absence of pain. As a consequence, the patients were generally reluctant to undergo a secondary procedure. I am however aware of a patient, under a colleagues care, who did undergo the successful reinsertion of a Silastic spacer, which helped stabilize the joint. Fortunately, it did not result in a recurrence of the infection.

The third most worrying complication is dislocation or instability. Obviously, this is far more common in patients with unlinked implants and can result in deformity and loss of movement. Interestingly enough however, they often remain pain-free. With regard to management, it is the authors' opinion that for a surface replacement, the prevention of any recurrent deformity is of paramount importance. If the patient presents initially with a significant boutonniere or swan neck deformity or indeed radial or ulnar angulation, it is probably inadvisable to consider this type of implant. A better primary procedure would be either an arthrodesis or a linked-type implant. Whilst soft tissue realignment in combination with a surface replacement is feasible, the results are at best unpredictable. Secondly but of equal importance is that if at the time of surgery the surgeon is concerned that the new joint may not be stable, then he would recommend immobilization for a period of 3 weeks prior to beginning therapy. The position of immobilization would be with the PIP joint held at somewhere between 10° and 20° of flexion. Despite this, and if instability does develop, then revision can be undertaken. Again, the implant can be removed and replaced or the joint fused. However and perhaps ideally, any revision should be augmented by a soft tissue stabilization. Whilst this results in a somewhat diminished range of motion, the patient can be left with a pain-free joint, in a good functional position, with some movement. This situation is better than an arthrodesis.

Usage of some of the earlier types of linked implant with their high rates of loosening has resulted in an increase in expertise in the management of loose components. Generally, loosening of an implant will ultimately become symptomatic and result in its removal followed by either fusion, the insertion of another implant linked (Silastic) or unlinked with or without a soft tissue reconstruction. The insertion of a Silastic implant with soft tissue reconstruction has been particularly successful in the authors' experience. More specifically, the operation is often easy to perform as removal of the primary implant leaves spaces in the phalanges, which readily accept a Silastic hinged-type implant. Again whilst the spacer will stabilize the joint and result in good pain relief, movements can be limited. At this time, the author has information on two cases of pyrocarbon implants, which have been revised for loosening. The first was revised with larger components, that is, with a thicker stem, with the additional insertion of bone graft and so far has remained stable. The second was revised to a fusion again requiring the insertion of a bone graft. At this time, whilst the arthrodesis is incomplete, the patient's finger is pain-free and in a good functional position.

Another complication is bone overgrowth and stiffness. Swanson reported this in approximately 5% of his cases following Silastic replacement, although other authors have reported a higher incidence. This tends to be seen more in patients with osteoarthritis rather than rheumatoid arthritis. Interestingly enough, whilst this complication does lead to reduced movement, the patient is left with little pain, stability and satisfactory function. As a consequence of this, many patients are reluctant to undergo revision surgery. However if revision is undertaken, effectively this includes refashioning of the bony cuts, the reinsertion of often larger components and a further soft tissue release.

Whilst loosening can also occur with a Silastic implant, this complication is undoubtedly uncommon and occurs much less frequently than fracture of the stem. Radiologically however, cysts can sometimes be seen surrounding Silastic implants. These are felt predominantly to be due to silicone synovitis, which is a giant cell reaction to small fragments of silicone. A number of authors have reported this radiological finding, although surprisingly only a few have described undertaking any revision surgery. Certainly, the author has never had to perform any procedure for this complication at the PIP level. One would assume however that treatment would involve removal of the silicone implant, curettage, bone grafting and fusion as appropriate.

Finally, given the potential for complications, it should again be noted that in virtually all the series reviewed, the incidence of revision surgery is less than 10%. Even then, in patients who develop complications, there are a number of surgical options which can ultimately lead to a pain-free, stable and functional joint.

## References


1. Carroll RE, Taber TH. Digital arthroplasty of the proximal interphalangeal joint. J Bone Joint Surg. 1954;36A(5):912–20.
2. Pellegrini VD, Burton RI. Osteoarthritis of the proximal interphalangeal joint of the hand: arthroplasty or fusion? J Hand Surg. 1990;15A:194–209.
3. Flatt AE, Powers WR. Rheumatoid hand. Physical therapy following insertion of Flatt prosthesis. Phys Ther Rev. 1961;41:709–13.
4. Swanson AB. Implant resection arthroplasty of the proximal interphalangeal joint. Orthop Clin North Am. 1973;4(4):1007–29.
5. Neibauer JJ, Shaw JL, Doren WW. Silicone-dacron hinge prosthesis. Design, evaluation and application. Ann Rheum Dis. 1969;28(5:Suppl):56–8.
6. Durham-Smith G, McCarten GM. Volar plate arthroplasty for closed proximal interphalangeal joint injuries. J Hand Surg (Br). 1992;17B:422–8.
7. Dionysian E, Eaton RG. The long-term outcome of volar plate arthroplasty of the proximal interphalangeal joint. J Hand Surg. 2000;25A:429–37.
8. Burton RI, Campolattaro RM, Ronchetti PJ. Volar plate arthroplasty for osteoarthritis of the proximal interphalangeal joint: a preliminary report. J Hand Surg. 2002;27A:1065–72.
9. Johansson SH, Engkvist O. Small joint reconstruction by perichondrial arthroplasty. Clin Plast Surg. 1981;8(1):107–14.
10. Seradge H, Kutz JA, Kleinert HE, Lister GD, Wolff TW, Atasoy E. Perichondrial resurfacing arthroplasty in the hand. J Hand Surg. 1984;9A(6):880–6.
11. Hasegawa T, Yamano Y. Arthroplasty of the proximal interphalangeal joint using costal cartilage grafts. J Hand Surg (Br). 1992;17B:583–5.
12. Katsaros J, Milner R, Marshall NJ. Perichondrial arthroplasty incorporating costal cartilage. J Hand Surg [Br]. 1995;20B(2):137–42.
13. Harrison SH. The proximal interphalangeal joint in rheumatoid arthritis. Hand. 1971;3(2):125–30.
14. Lipscomb PR. Synovectomy of the distal two joints of the thumb and fingers in rheumatoid arthritis. J Bone Joint Surg. 1967;49A(6):1135–9.
15. Schneider LH. Proximal interphalangeal joint arthroplasty: the volar approach. Semin Arthroplasty. 1991;2(2):139–47.
16. Lin HH, Wyrick JD, Stern PJ. Proximal interphalangeal joint silicone replacement arthroplasty: clinical results using an anterior approach. J Hand Surg. 1995;20A:123–32.
17. Fahmy NR, Lavender A, Brew C. A conservative approach for proximal interphalangeal joint arthroplasty. J Hand Surg (Br). 2001;26B:235–7.
18. Linscheid RL, Dobyns JH, Beckenbaugh RD, Cooney WP. Proximal interphalangeal joint arthroplasty with a total joint design. Mayo Clin Proc. 1979;54:227–40.
19. Adamson GJ, Gellman H, Brumfield RH, Kuschner SH, Lawler JW. Flexible implant resection arthroplasty of the proximal interphalangeal joint in patients with systemic inflammatory arthritis. J Hand Surg. 1994;19A:378–84.
20. Iselin F, Conti E. Long-term results of proximal interphalangeal joint resection arthroplasties with a silicone implant. J Hand Surg. 1995;20A(3:Part 2):95–7.
21. Swanson AB, Maupin BK, Gajjar NV, de Groot Swanson G. Flexible implant arthroplasty in the proximal interphalangeal joint of the hand. J Hand Surg. 1985;10A:796–805.
22. Iselin F. Arthroplasty of the proximal interphalangeal joint after trauma. Hand. 1975;7(1):41–2.
23. Iselin F, Pradet G. Resection arthroplasty with Swanson's implant for posttraumatic stiffness of proximal interphalangeal joints. Bull Hosp Jt Dis Orthop Inst. 1984;44(2):233–47.
24. Ashworth CR, Hansraj KK, Todd AO, Dukhram KM, Ebramzadeh E, Boucree JB, Hansraj MS. Swanson proximal interphalangeal joint arthroplasty in patients with rheumatoid arthritis. Clin Orthop Relat Res. 1997;342:34–7.
25. Hage JJ, Yoe EPD, Zevering JP, de Groot PJM. Proximal interphalangeal joint silicone arthroplasty for posttraumatic arthritis. J Hand Surg. 1999;24A:73–7.

26. Herren DB, Simmen BR. Palmar approach in flexible implant arthroplasty of the proximal interphalangeal joint. Clin Orthop Relat Res. 2000;371:131–5.
27. Takigawa S, Meletiou S, Sauerbier M, Cooney WP. Long-term assessment of Swanson implant arthroplasty in the proximal interphalangeal joint of the hand. J Hand Surg. 2004;29A:785–95.
28. Bales JG, Wall LB, Stern PJ. Long-term results of Swanson silicone arthroplasty for proximal interphalangeal joint osteoarthritis. J Hand Surg. 2014;39A(3):455–61.
29. Proubasta IR, Lamas CG, Natera L, Millan A. Silicone proximal interphalangeal joint arthroplasty for primary osteoarthritis using a volar approach. J Hand Surg. 2014;39A(6):1075–81.
30. Mathoulin C, Gilbert A. Arthroplasty of the proximal interphalangeal joint using the Sutter implant for traumatic joint destruction. J Hand Surg. 1999;24B(5):565–9.
31. Merle M, Villani F, Lallemand B, Vaienti L. Proximal interphalangeal joint arthroplasty with silicone implants (NeuFlex) by a lateral approach: a series of 51 cases. J Hand Surg. 2011;37E(1):50–5.
32. Möller K, Sollerman C, Geijer M, Brånemark PI. Early results with osseointegrated proximal interphalangeal joint prostheses. J Hand Surg. 1999;24A:267–74.
33. Lundborg G, Brånemark PI. Osseointegrated proximal interphalangeal joint prostheses with a replacable flexible joint spacer-long term results. Scand J Plast Reconstr Surg Hand Surg. 2000;34:345–53.
34. Möller K, Sollerman C, Lundborg G. Radiographic evaluation of osseointegration and loosening of titanium implants in the MCP and PIP joints. J Hand Surg. 2004;29A:32–8.
35. Johnstone BR. Proximal interphalangeal joint surface replacement arthroplasty. Hand Surg. 2001;6(1):1–11.
36. Jennings CD, Livingstone DP. Surface replacement arthroplasty of the proximal interphalangeal joint using the SR PIP implant: long-term results. J Hand Surg. 2015;40A(3):469–73.
37. Schulz M, Müller-Zimmermann, Behrend M, Krimmer H. Frühe Ergebnisse der Fingermittelgelenkendoprothetik mit der Pyrocarbonprothese (Ascension) bei idiopathischen und posttraumatischen Arthrosen. Handchir Mikrochir Plast Chir. 2005;37:26–34.
38. Watts AC, Hearnden AJ, Trail IA, Hayton MJ, Nuttall D, Stanley JK. Pyrocarbon proximal interphalangeal joint arthroplasty: minimum 2 year follow-up. J Hand Surg. 2012;37A:882–8.
39. McGuire DT, White CD, Carter SL, Solomons MW. Pyrocarbon proximal interphalangeal joint arthroplasty: outcomes of a cohort study. J Hand Surg. 2011;37E(6):490–6.
40. Hutt JRB, Gilleard O, Hacker A, Citron N. Medium-term outcomes of pyrocarbon arthroplasty of the proximal interphalangeal joint. J Hand Surg. 2012;37E(6):497–500.
41. Mashhadi SA, Chandrasekharan L, Pickford MA. Pyrolytic carbon arthroplasty for the proximal interphalangeal joint: results after minimum 3 years of follow-up. J Hand Surg. 2012;37E(6):501–5.
42. Tägil M, Geijer M, Abramo A, Kopylov P. Ten years' experience with a pyrocarbon prosthesis replacing the proximal interphalangeal joint. A prospective clinical and radiographic follow-up. J Hand Surg. 2014;39E(6):587–95.
43. Heers G, Springorum HR, Baier C, Götz J, Grifka J, Renkawitz T. Proximal interphalangeal joint replacement with an unconstrained pyrocarbon prosthesis (Ascension): a long-term follow-up. J Hand Surg. 2012;38E(6):680–5.
44. Reissner L, Schindele S, Hensler S, Marks M, Herren DB. Ten year follow-up of pyrocarbon implants for proximal interphalangeal joint replacement. J Hand Surg. 2014;39E(6):582–6.
45. Storey PA, Goddard M, Clegg C, Birks ME, Bostock SH. Pyrocarbon proximal interphalangeal joint arthroplasty: a medium to long term follow-up of a single surgeon series. J Hand Surg. 2015;40E(9):952–6.
46. Pettersson K, Amilon A, Rizzo M. Pyrolytic carbon hemiarthroplasty in the management of proximal interphalangeal joint arthritis. J Hand Surg. 2015;40A(3):462–8.
47. Dryer RF, Blair WF, Shurr DG, Buckwalter JA. Proximal interphalangeal joint arthroplasty. Clin Orthop Relat Res. 1984;185:187–94.
48. Condamine JL, Fourquet M, Matcucci L, Pichereau D. L'arthrose primitive métacarpo- phalangienne et interphalangienne proximale à la main. Ann Chir Main. 1997;16(1):66–78.
49. Mentzel M, Hoss H, Ebinger T, Halder A, Kinzl L, Wachter NJ. DIGITOS- Fingermittelgelenkprothesen-Zweijahresergebnisse. Handchir Mikrochir Plast Chir. 2000;32:347–52.
50. Schindele SF, Hensler S, Audigé L, Marks M, Herren DB. A modular surface gliding implant (CapFlex-PIP) for proximal interphalangeal joint osteoarthritis: a prospective case series. J Hand Surg Am. 2015;40(2):334–40.
51. Flannery O, Harley O, Badge R, Birch A, Nuttall D, Trail IA. MatOrtho proximal interphalangeal joint arthroplasty: minimum 2 year follow up. J Hand Surg. 2016;41E(9):910–6.
52. Lawrence T, Trail IA, Noble J. Morphological measurements of the proximal interphalangeal joint. J Hand Surg. 2004;29B:244–9.
53. Fowler A, Arshad S, Talwalkar S, Trail IA. MatOrtho proximal interphalangeal joint arthroplasty via lateral approach: minimum 2-year follow-up. Asian Pac J Hand Surg. 2020, Submitted.

# Revision/Failed Proximal Interphalangeal Joint Arthroplasty

21

Daniel B. Herren and Stephan F. Schindele

## Introduction

Proximal interphalangeal joint (PIP) arthroplasty is an effective method to treat advanced degenerative, inflammatory, or post-traumatic changes of the PIP joint. Arthroplasty is performed significantly more often at the PIP than metacarpophalangeal (MCP) or distal interphalangeal (DIP) joints. It has been shown that PIP joint mobility is of important functional value within the scope of the entire hand and depending on its position [1, 2]. On the ulnar rays, in particular, mobility has great functional importance, since it is only possible to grasp small objects while maintaining mobility of this joint. On the radial side of the hand, especially at the index finger, stability is crucial for a strong pinch with the thumb and a firm grip. However, a stiff index finger is often a functional obstacle [3]. Therefore, PIP joint arthroplasty has become the predominant treatment option for painful PIP disorders. Yet the complication rate of PIP arthroplasty is significant and lies between 8% and 58% [4–15]. The variability of these rates is due to several factors. Firstly, a general definition for complications is lacking. According to the International Organization for Standardization, complications are defined as "any untoward medical occurrence, unintended disease or injury, or untoward clinical signs (including abnormal laboratory findings) whether or not related to the investigational medical device" [16]. This very broad definition tends to combine different post-treatment conditions, which creates difficulties in detecting the relevant postoperative problems of each patient.

Another aspect includes the varying ways in which interventions are labeled as a cause of complications. Any additional surgical intervention that is intended to improve the result of the primary intervention is referred to as a *revision operation* after a primary joint replacement. *Reoperations*, on the other hand, are defined as "all interventions that are based on a soft tissue-related cause and do not affect the primary implant." *Revision arthroplasty* is any intervention that is carried out due to an implant-related cause and is associated with a replacement of the implant or individual components. Aversano and Calfee reported soft tissue-related revision rates between 6% and 58% depending on the intervention and significantly lower rates of 8–26% for the revision of an implant itself and replacement [4].

From a clinical point of view, it is therefore meaningful to classify the complications of PIP joint replacement based on either the clinical/radiological findings or reason for revision.

D. B. Herren (✉) · S. F. Schindele
Department of Hand Surgery, Schulthess Klinik, Zurich, Switzerland
e-mail: daniel.herren@kws.ch; stephan.schindele@kws.ch


G. J. W. King, M. Rizzo (eds.), *Arthroplasty of the Upper Extremity*,
https://doi.org/10.1007/978-3-030-68880-6_21

A more detailed and practical way of categorizing PIP arthroplasty revision surgery is driven by classifying the cause of revision (Table 21.1).

This classification offers the possibility to discuss the options of revision in a more detailed and somewhat more systematic manner.

The reason for any patient undergoing another intervention can be summarized under the term of dysfunction, which includes pain, joint stiffness, joint instability, and joint deformity (Table 21.2).

It is interesting to compare the complications of small joint arthroplasty to those of other joint replacement surgeries. Labek et al. published the revision rates for the hip, knee, ankle, and elbow. For these big joints, soft tissue-induced revision surgery was quite low, and most revision procedures involved a change of one or more components. During a 10-year period, the cumulative results from worldwide joint registry datasets revealed a revision rate for primary hip and knee replacement that increased to 12%, whereas the revision rate for ankle and elbow replacement reached to 20% within a 6-year period [17].

**Table 21.1** Classification of possible complications in PIP arthroplasty

| |
|---|
| General complications: |
| Wound healing complications |
| Infection |
| CRPS |
| Soft tissue-related complications: |
| Tendon adhesions |
| Ossifications: |
| Around tendons |
| Joint capsule |
| Tendon imbalance |
| Swan neck deformity |
| Boutonniere deformity |
| Implant-related complications: |
| Joint dislocation |
| Implant loosening |
| Implant migration |
| Joint deformation |
| Joint instability |
| Joint stiffness |

**Table 21.2** Indications for revision surgery after PIP arthroplasty

| Reasons for revisions after PIP arthroplasty |
|---|
| Pain |
| Stiffness |
| Instability |
| Joint deformation |
| Implant failure |

## Complications in PIP Arthroplasty

Yamamoto and Chung conducted a meta-analysis on complications following primary PIP arthroplasty with different implants [18]. The revision rate for silicone implants was 6–11% overall. They also compared various approaches (volar, lateral, dorsal) and found that the lowest number of revisions was seen for the volar approach, whereas the lateral and dorsal approach had slightly higher revision rates of 10–11%. In contrast, the revision rate for surface replacement with first-generation implants was much higher and ranged from 18% to 37%. For surface replacement devices, a sub-analysis also revealed a difference between volar and dorsal approaches. For the latter, a high number of primary PIP surface replacements ($n = 907$) with a mean follow-up of 51 months was associated with an 18% revision rate. On the other hand, the number of implants ($n = 27$) was very low in the volar approach group, and the revision rate was 37%. Although the series are very different in terms of the interventions included, it seems that the volar approach for surface replacing implants is more demanding and might be associated with a significant learning curve. The volar placement of surface replacing components is more difficult, since the anatomical orientation is different and implant alignment is difficult to control. In terms of implant placement, silicone arthroplasty is more remitting and offers a certain degree of self-alignment due to its material properties.

A literature review of 70 articles summarizing the reasons for implant related revision included a total of 15,556 Swanson original silicone arthroplasties for all different finger joints [19]. Overall, the prevalence of complications after silicone implants was very low. The highest rate of complications comprised unspecific bone changes such as bone cysts, calcification, and bone resorption. Implant fractures were reported in only 2%. Systemic problems due to silicone particle wear (including synovitis or even lymphadenopathy) were anecdotally reported with a prevalence of around 0.6%. The reasons for revision surgery included PIP joint implant fracture in 21 of 52 reported cases. Continued pain was the primary reason for a re-intervention in 17% (9/52) of patients followed by synovitis and infections in 10% (5/52) and 8% (4/52), respectively.

A more recent retrospective study examined the results after silicone revision arthroplasty [8], where the outcome of silicone implant revision procedures in 27 cases was presented. The main reason for revision was pain (35%) and stiffness (26%). The revision procedure was best indicated in stiff joints with or without pain. Range of motion increased to a satisfactory level for most patients, and pain improved substantially. However, joint instability and axis deviation could not be sufficiently corrected, and overall patient satisfaction post-revision was inadequate.

Another recent study analyzed the results after PIP revision arthroplasty with silicone interposition arthroplasty and surface replacement using pyrocarbon implants and metal on polyethylene (PE) implants in 75 cases [20].

Although the majority of primary arthroplasties were performed with a silicone implant, these (84%) were changed to a surface replacement in order to enhance stability. The 10-year survival rate after revision was 70%. However, 25% of all revised replacements needed an additional procedure. The working group concluded that revision of a failed PIP arthroplasty remains a challenge. Overall, distorted anatomy and scar formation are less favorable outcomes of revision surgery compared to primary surgery. The salvage procedure involving the exchange of a two-component implant to a silicone arthroplasty seems a viable option. Yet instability remains an unsolved problem leading to the worst outcome of all reasons to undertake revision surgery.

In summary, all studies on PIP revision arthroplasty present a similar picture: Revision of failed or problematic PIP arthroplasty is challenging and often leads to unsatisfactory results. It appears that the only good reason for revision is residual pain, while stiffness and especially instability result in unpredictable and poor postoperative results.

## Indications for Revision PIP Arthroplasty

As previously outlined, the reasons for revision arthroplasty when primary implants fail are different and depend on the cause and symptoms but also on the implant type. Silicone implants act as a spacer only and do not replicate joint biomechanics. With its monoblock characteristic, silicone implants offer a certain primary stability in the different joint axes. Secondary stability relies on the scarring around the implant during the healing process. Together with preexisting ligamentous structures, final joint stability is mainly reached at 3–6 months after surgery. However, ongoing distorting forces to the implant may only be tolerated over a certain time, especially in joints with significant preexisting deformation and/or significant deviation forces acting on the joint (e.g., pinching thumb to index), joint instability with or without implant fracture may occur.

Since an intensive biological reaction to silicone is common, subsequent strong capsule formation can have an even greater impact over the primary stability offered by the implant. Thus, silicone implant breakage does not lead to a revision intervention due to instability. Since the implant stem has no firm connection to the bone, the silicone stems create an endomedullary reaction over time, which can be seen on radiographs as a fine sclerotic line between the implant and surrounding bone [21, 22]. In revision cases, it appears as a fine endomedullary synovial layer. This reaction is provoked by the so-called pistoning effect, a movement of the implant in the bones during flexion and extension.

The non-binding character of the implant facilitates its replacement and makes it technically easy.

Silicone implant fracture rates at the PIP joint are reported to be up to 50% [4, 7, 8, 20, 23–25].

This does not automatically mean a revision is necessary. Implant fractures often remain undetected, and it is not always obvious to detect silicone implant fractures on standard radiographs. However, the fibrous capsule usually preserves joint function, even when the implant is not intact.

Silicone implant fracture and abrasion lead to a synovial reaction [26–30]. Erosive osteolysis can be seen on radiographs, and remarkable bone defects may occur. The severity of this inflammatory reaction depends on the particle size and is more often seen with silicone wrist implants than finger arthroplasties. As a reason for PIP arthroplasty revision, silicone synovitis seems to be rare, although there is very little data to support this observation.

Fixation of two-component implants, often quoted as "surface replacement devices," follows the same principles used for other joint replacement surgeries. These devices are secured to the bone either through a press-fit cementless fixation or application of a classic bone cement with polymethyl methacrylate (PMMA). The use of cement has the advantage of immediate primary stability, while the osteointegrative binding usually takes 6–8 weeks for definitive implant fixation. In a comparative study, Johnstone et al. [31] analyzed the results of cemented versus uncemented SR-PIP implants (Stryker, Kalamazoo, MI, USA) with a mean follow-up time of 5 years and found no significant differences in pain scores or range of motion. There were more joint failures in the uncemented group with 26% (five fingers) compared to 8% (two fingers) in the cemented group, but this difference was not significant. A closer look at the results showed that soft tissue-related revisions were significantly higher in the cemented with 37% (nine fingers) versus uncemented group with no soft tissue revisions. The authors stated that this was related to the indication of surgery with more cases of post-traumatic joint destruction in the cemented group.

Despite the benefit of better primary fixation, the application of two-component implants with cement has substantial disadvantages. The revision of a cemented implant is associated with more difficulties. Well-fixed implant components that need to be removed leave rather large defects in the endomedullary bone. At times, a phalanx osteotomy may need to be applied, in a similar manner to that described for the removal of well-fixed femur components of the hip, in order to remove the implant. In addition, bone cement causes biological bone damage through its exothermic reaction during application. This impedes fixation of a revision implant, and even secondary cementation is of lesser quality. Due to these problems, many surgeons avoid cementing finger implants.

Osteointegration, on the other hand, is provided by materials that allow bone integration. Finger implants made of titanium with or without a hydroxyapatite coating are good examples of an osteointegrative device. Titanium has proven its capacity for solid bone fixation in the widespread use of dental implants. Other osteointegrative materials include ceramics and pyrocarbon, although both materials have revealed their challenges in implant fixation. Based on the reported high rates of loosening and implant migration [15, 32–37], it appears that neither ceramic nor pyrocarbon is suited for osteointegration, and osteoapposition, at best, is to be expected. Daecke et al. [38] found all titanium implants with solid osteointegration, both mechanically and histologically, while none of the implanted pyrocarbon arthroplasties showed secure bone fixation in an in vivo rabbit model. Schindele et al. [39] found that a rough titanium surface is able to achieve solid binding with the bone; an explanted surface replacement implant had a level of bone-implant contact (BIC) greater than 40%, a value well within the range characteristic of dental implants and higher than the BIC reported for surface replacement at the shoulder. Another indication for revision is implant malalignment. This naturally poses less of a problem in flexible silicone implant arthroplasty. However, for two-component implants that aim to mimic the biomechanics of the joint, positioning of the components is crucial for function. The PIP joint is a hinged joint in which the condyles are asymmetrical and vary from finger to finger [40]. It is therefore crucial to always consider the anatomical situation in order to restore as much of the normal joint kinematics as possible [41].

It is the primary goal of implant arthroplasty to restore normal joint function, and the concept of surface replacement has the potential to achieve this for a PIP joint [42]. The principal motion lies in the sagittal plane, but with a small amount of motion also in the coronal and axial planes. Lateral stability is provided by the condyles and the collateral ligament complex, including parts of the volar plate. With the pull of tendons in flexion/extension, implant components are pressed together, and lateral stability is provided through congruity of the implant and, thus, the constraint of the prosthesis. With this design concept, lateral stability can be almost restored to normal [43].

Malalignment can occur in the different planes, but not all equally affect functionality. For proper joint function, restoration of the joint center of rotation should be re-established. Factors that influence the center of rotation include the prosthetic design, especially the offset of articulation with the stem and placement of the implant within the bone [44]. There are biomechanical considerations that need to be taken into account for ideal prosthetic placement, but in vivo studies are lacking. According to various reports on implant failure and personal experience, implant arthroplasty malalignment must be analyzed for the different planes. Some imprecision seems to be better tolerated than others (Fig. 21.1).

Less problematic is the misplacement of the proximal implant in the sagittal plane (arrow A). As long as the proximal implant permits the achievable range of motion of the joint, placement in either a more volar or more dorsal fashion has very little clinical effect on joint function. However, by shifting the center of rotation either dorsal or volar, the moment arm of the flexor and extensor tendons can, at least theoretically, be altered [45]. Lateral misplacement (arrow B) might have an effect on lateral stability, since it changes the tension to the collateral ligament complex. In clinical terms, postoperative scarring of the capsule adapts somewhat to this type of implant misplacement.

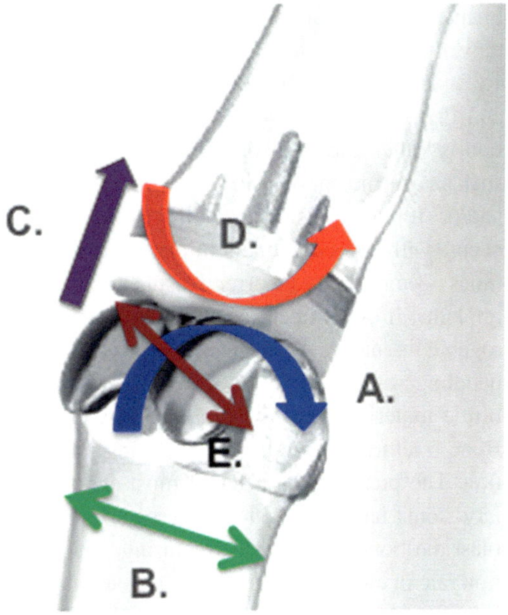


**Fig. 21.1** Different planes of implant malalignment at the PIP joint. (**a**) Sagittal plane; (**b**) Lateral; (**c**) Distal; (**d**) Axial plane; (**e**) Coronal plane

Overstuffing or overtensioning of the joint presents a more problematic situation (arrow C). Distalization of the center of rotation might be tempting in cases of severe joint defects with bone shortening. However, the soft tissue, namely, the ligaments, adapt during the process of deformation, and a tight joint replacement creates pain and difficulties, especially with extension. Correct implant placement needs to include tension-free extension on the OR table without the tendency for hyperextension. If it is difficult to extend the joint, it is overstuffed, and either a different implant needs to be chosen or the bone cuts should be corrected.

Another problem involves malpositioning in the axial plane (arrow D) with axial rotation of the implant and coronal plane asymmetry (arrow E). Both implantation errors lead to inadequate tracking of joint motion, whereby the soft tissue can hardly provide any compensation in this situation. It is important to check the tenodesis movement of the finger on the OR table after implantation and tendon reposition. The deformity becomes obvious in flexion. It is difficult to correct inadequate implant tracking during rehabilitation, and ligaments can hardly compensate the wrong movement planes. Joint dislocation accounts for 1.6% of all complications, associated with MCP and PIP arthroplasty [46]. The cause of dislocation is either due to incorrect implant placement such as insufficient primary or secondary stability and/or trauma. Dislocation almost exclusively occurs with two-component implants but is sometimes seen with incorrectly placed silicone implants. Implant fractures are rare and often iatrogenic in nature because of incorrect implant handling, especially of those made with more brittle materials such as ceramic or pyrocarbon. Bone fractures are mainly seen during implantation. The press-fit character of most endomedullary stems has the potential to create forces that blast the bone and lead to fracturing. The infection rate in elective hand surgery is generally low. However, infection related to PIP arthroplasty is an issue and is responsible [46] for 3.6% of all associated complications. Early detected superficial wound infections can often be handled conservatively with antibiotics, whereas deeper and more extensive infections require revision surgery with debridement and often implant removal. In severe cases, finger amputations have also been described [5, 19, 20, 47].

## Reoperations After Primary Implant Arthroplasty at the PIP Joint

As previously outlined, *reoperations* are defined as all interventions that are based on a soft tissue-related cause and do not affect the primary implant.

This includes tendon adhesions, ossifications, and correction of tendon imbalance.

### Tendon Adhesions/Ossifications

Joint stiffness is multifactorial, but tendon adhesions are always, at least, a concomitant reason for unsatisfactory joint mobility. Adhesions may occur together with ossifications, either along the tendons or around the joint capsule. If an implant is correctly placed and no obvious reason is detected to change the implant, arthrotenolysis might be indicated. The dorsal approach, which needs to be performed through the tendons to reach the joint, has the greater potential of provoking tendon scarring. Bodmer et al. [48] compared three different approaches with the same PIP implant and found that the Chamay approach with a V-shaped extensor tendon flap led to the largest number of reoperations due to tendon scarring.

The volar approach tends to scar the volar plate and thus provokes an extensor lag.

Technically, tendon adhesions are approached through their original surgical access point. Notable scarring around the tendon and an excessive capsular reaction around the implant is often seen, which needs to be released. The collateral ligaments play an important role in stiffness, and according to the orthopedic teaching of joint release, the scarring and capsular reaction need to be sequentially cut from inside out. After each step of release, the joint mobility needs to be controlled. Ideally, the intervention is done with a local anesthesia or the WALANT technique. This allows intraoperative control of the tendons and joint release. In addition, patients can actually observe how much mobility gain can be reached during surgery.

The results of these interventions are mixed and depend highly on the patient's motivation toward postoperative mobilization. On average, however, the benefit of this intervention was found to satisfy the majority of patients [8].

### Tendon Imbalance

The cause of tendon imbalance after PIP joint arthroplasty is often not apparent. Swan neck or boutonniere deformities can be seen with all approaches and often appear with a remarkable delay after the primary intervention. Joint tightness seems to play an important role. Loose joints tend to deform in hyperextension and assume a swan neck position, while too tight joints have the tendency to adopt a boutonniere deformity. In addition, soft tissue scarring or central slip insufficiency might be present.

It is therefore important before planning a revision intervention to evaluate the possible contribution of the implant itself to the tendon imbalance.

The reconstruction of the deformity follows the usual techniques described for this condition. For swan neck deformities, we prefer to perform a FDS hemi-sling tenodesis. One sling of the FDS is released about 1.5–2.0 cm proximal to the PIP joint. This sling is then sutured to the tendon sheet of the contralateral side at the level of the PIP with the joint in slight flexion. An extension block splint allows immediate mobilization with restrictions on extension for 6 weeks.

The correction of a boutonniere deformity is more challenging, and its indication should be discussed critically. The usual techniques for boutonniere correction may be applied, including central slip reconstruction and lateral band reconstruction with release of the transverse retinacular ligament. An experienced therapist needs to be involved during rehabilitation, and flexion loss should be avoided.

## Collateral Ligament Insufficiency

Collateral ligament insufficiency, unrelated to the type of implant, is mainly seen in trauma cases after arthroplasty joint replacement.

For this condition, a formal collateral ligament reconstruction, almost always with a free tendon graft, can be undertaken. However, it is crucial to accompany this intervention with an individually tailored rehabilitation program. Despite the postoperative therapy, the joints still tend to become stiff again.

In cases of severe instability and joint dislocation, salvage to joint fusion is often the best solution [39].

## Solutions for Failed PIP Arthroplasty

In principle, there are four different possibilities to revise a problematic PIP arthroplasty. The choice depends mainly on the reason for revision and the patient's needs, including which finger is affected. It is obvious that the soft tissue situation is also crucial in the decision-making process, and additional soft tissue procedures are often required in revision arthroplasty. Figure 21.2

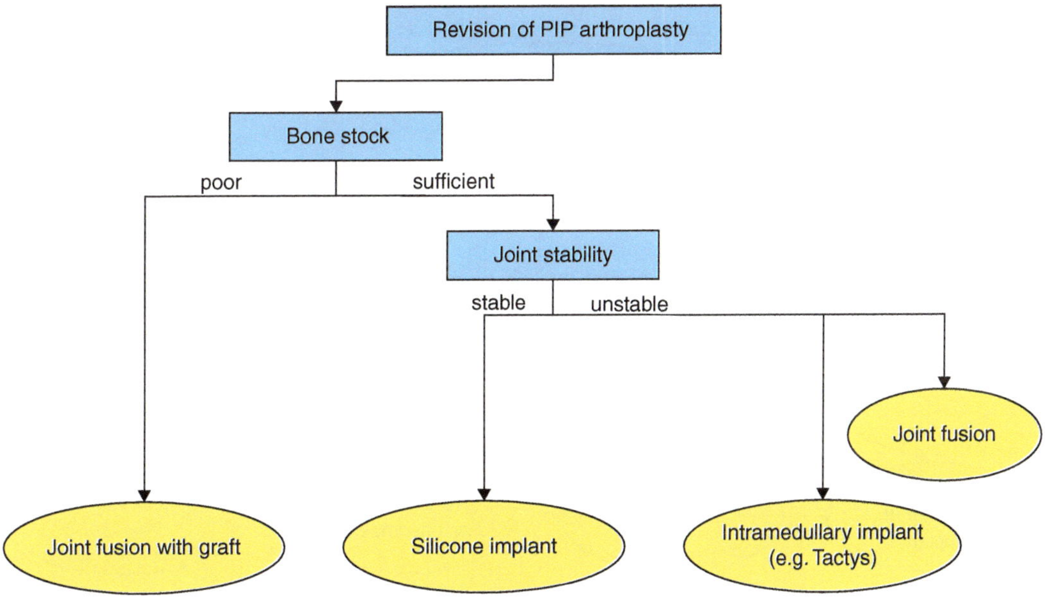


**Fig. 21.2** Simplified indication scheme for PIP arthroplasty revision

shows a simplified indication scheme for revisions taking into consideration the bone situation and the joint instability (Fig. 21.2).

In revision implant arthroplasty, the primary implant or parts of it are removed and replaced with a new implant. The same prosthesis type with a different shape or size or a completely new implant can be applied. The reason for revision dictates the main direction taken by the surgeon in choosing the type of intervention that will be undertaken. The local bone and soft tissue condition refines the final choice of surgical procedure. For example, an unstable silicone implant can either be revised with a joint fusion or a conversion to a more constrained two-component implant arthroplasty, depending on the degree of instability and local joint condition. Together with the patient, an individual solution needs to be defined. It must also be taken into consideration that every new intervention at the PIP joint contributes to an even bigger risk of additional scarring with resultant stiffness and/or pain.

*Two-component implants* can be easily adapted to the revision requirements because of their modular design and exchangeable parts (Fig. 21.3). In particular, unstable situations can be resolved if one or more components can be changed in a way that more tension in the joint can be achieved. However, overstuffing, also in revision situations, is inadvisable and leads to poor clinical results.

In situations of predominant stiffness, either a soft tissue procedure alone or joint fusion is often advisable. If joint motion needs to be preserved, the change to a silicone spacer may offer a good solution together with a meticulous soft tissue release and balancing. The silicone implant has the advantage of being flexible enough to create less tension in a joint because of its material properties.

Revision of failed *silicone implants* (Fig. 21.4) considers slightly different options, since the amount of bone resection is more extensive, and with any surgical solution, this must be taken into consideration. In addition, the quality of the endomedullary bone is limited due to the interaction with the silicone stem. As previously described, a local synovial reaction to the implant material can occur. This is an issue also associated with implant changes to fusion procedures. Since only endomedullary fixed revision implants are possible, it must be guaranteed that the bone is able to host a new implant. Uncemented revisions, in particular, need decent endomedullary bone stock quality. Arthrodesis also requires viable bone to enable bone healing, even in the presence of a bone graft.

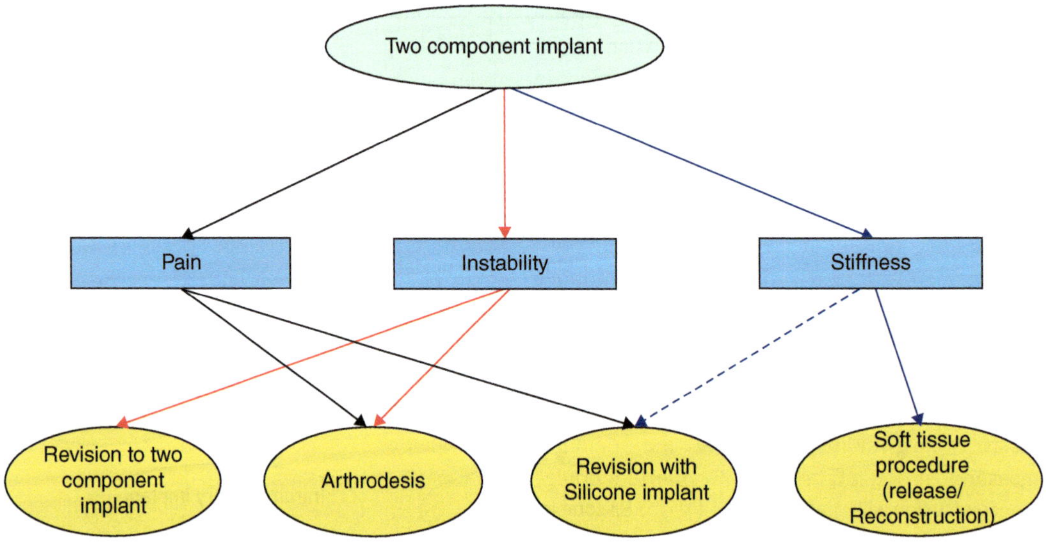


**Fig. 21.3** Decision tree for revision options in two-component implants

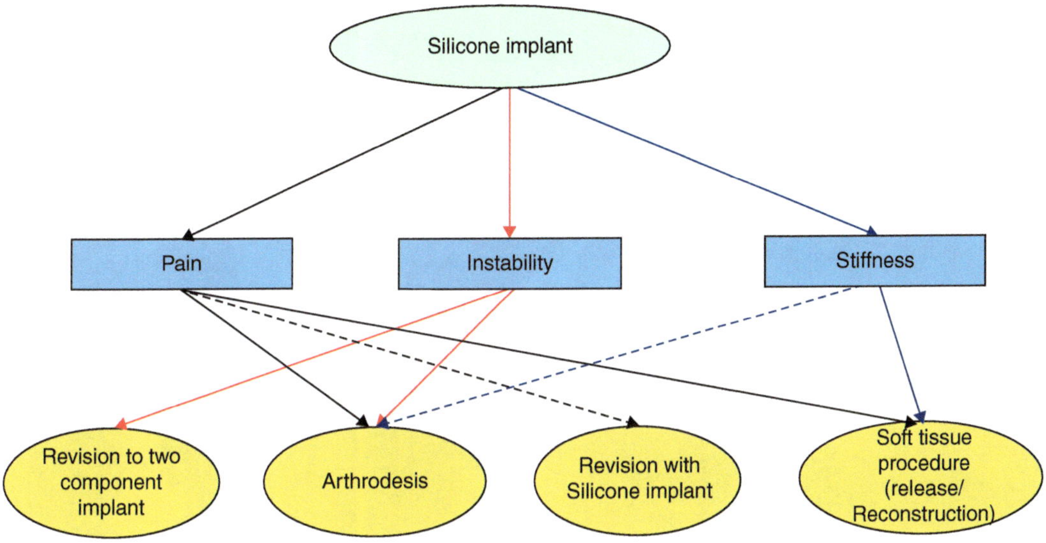


**Fig. 21.4** Decision tree for revision options in silicone implants

We have gained more and more experience in converting an unstable situation after a silicone arthroplasty with a two-component implant. For example, the TACTYS prosthesis (Stryker, Kalamazoo, MI, USA), due to its extensive modular design, offers a large range of different sized implant components that can be applied to even the largest of bone defects. Figure 21.5 demonstrates the conversion of an unstable broken silicone implant to a TACTYS arthroplasty (Fig. 21.5). Through its more constrained characteristics, this implant has the potential to correct the deformity and provide more intrinsic stability to the joint. The broad endomedullary stem allows secure primary fixation without the use of cement.

To exchange a silicone implant with another one only makes sense if the primary implant is broken and causes problems such as bone impingement. Secondary resection of the bone and replacement of the implant with a new spacer are possible. In cases of instability or deformity, it is virtually impossible to improve the situation with an implant change to another silicone prosthesis, even if additional soft tissue stabilization measures are undertaken [8]. The concept of resection-interposition arthroplasty with a volar plate, for example, is reported only for treating traumatic or post-traumatic conditions. Depending on the existing condition and the soft tissue configuration, this technique has an inherent danger of producing an unstable joint situation, especially in the radial digits.

Joint fusion is often a reliable solution to revise a difficult residual situation after primary implantation [4]. If a joint that needs a reoperation is already stiff, the decision for fusion is easy. In cases of severe instability with some functional mobility, the decision to convert the situation into a fusion is more difficult and needs to be evaluated with the patient. The two main challenges in joint fusion after arthroplasty are bone healing and positioning of the arthrodesis.

As already outlined, any type of implant arthroplasty leaves a significant bone defect and alters the local biological situation and bone healing potential. The worst situation occurs after a cemented arthroplasty where, besides the bone defect that tends to be relatively large, the endomedullary bone is partially replaced by bone cement. Together with exothermic bone damage, the biological situation to ensure bone healing for fusion is extremely unfavorable. This situation arises in a similar manner with Silastic implants. At the interface with the implant, the bone has a synovial layer, which needs to be removed before viable bone is present. In addition, a significant bone defect is created at the entrance of the

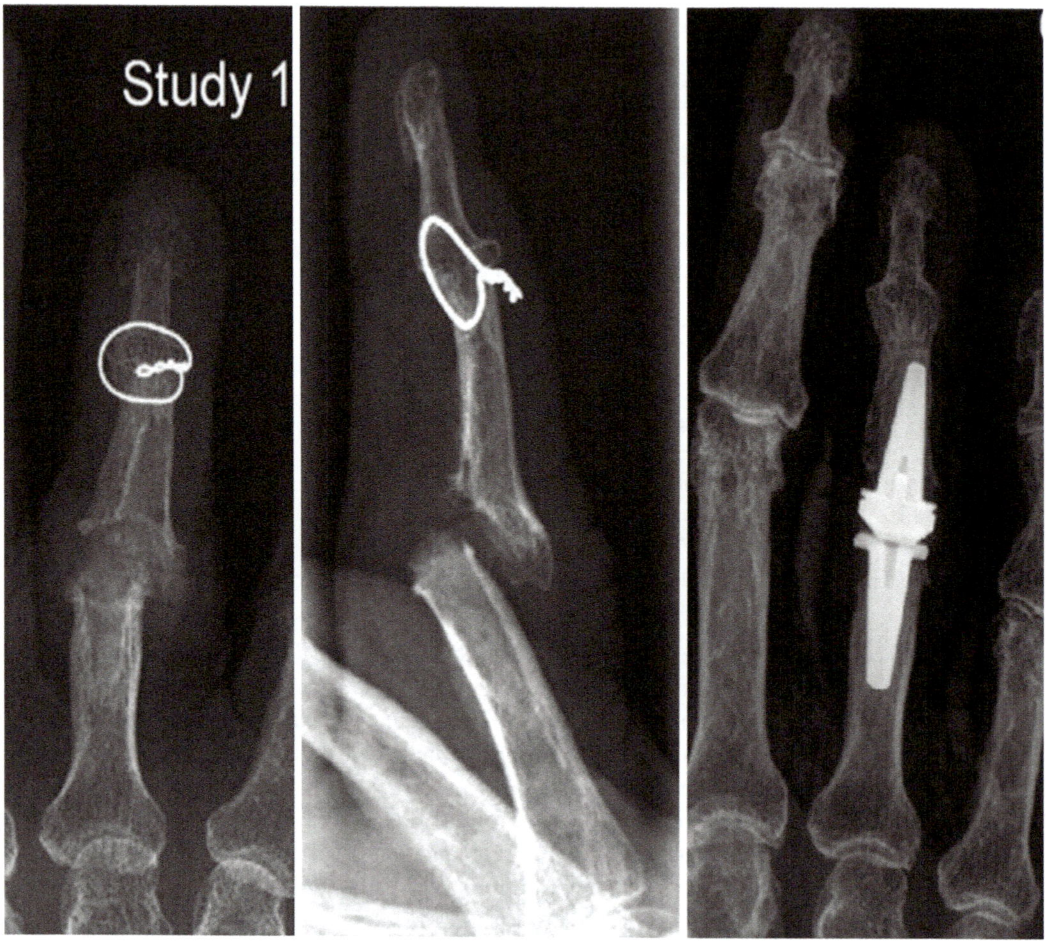


**Fig. 21.5** Example of a failed silicone implant with fracture of the implant and instability in all planes. The implant was revised with a modular two-component arthroplasty (Tactys; Stryker, Kalamazoo, MI USA)

implant into the bone due to the rather voluminous shape of the stems. Therefore, the bone surface that is needed for joint fusion is limited.

For any type of implant, a bone graft is needed to bridge the defect and maintain the general length of the treated finger. Homologous grafts, autologous grafts, or a mixture of the two can be used. We prefer bone grafts from the radius, and if several fingers are affected, bone grafts from the iliac bone crest might be needed. The volar side of the radius provides a more solid graft, and the scar is less visible. The cancellous bone can be used to fill the endomedullary cavity so as to provide some healthy bone for healing and additional primary stability. The structural graft bridges the defect. Mechanically, it is important to place the hard solid side of the graft volar and secure the bone with some sort of tension band fixation involving either a plate or K-wires combined with a tension band wire.

After removal of the implant, the local situation is unstable, and it is technically challenging to fix the joint in the desired position. Either the graft is placed between the bone ends or temporarily fixed with a wire. Figure 21.6 illustrates a case of fixed but still painful boutonnière deformity on the index and middle finger with subsequent implant removal and PIP fusion on the index finger with a graft and direct fixation in the middle

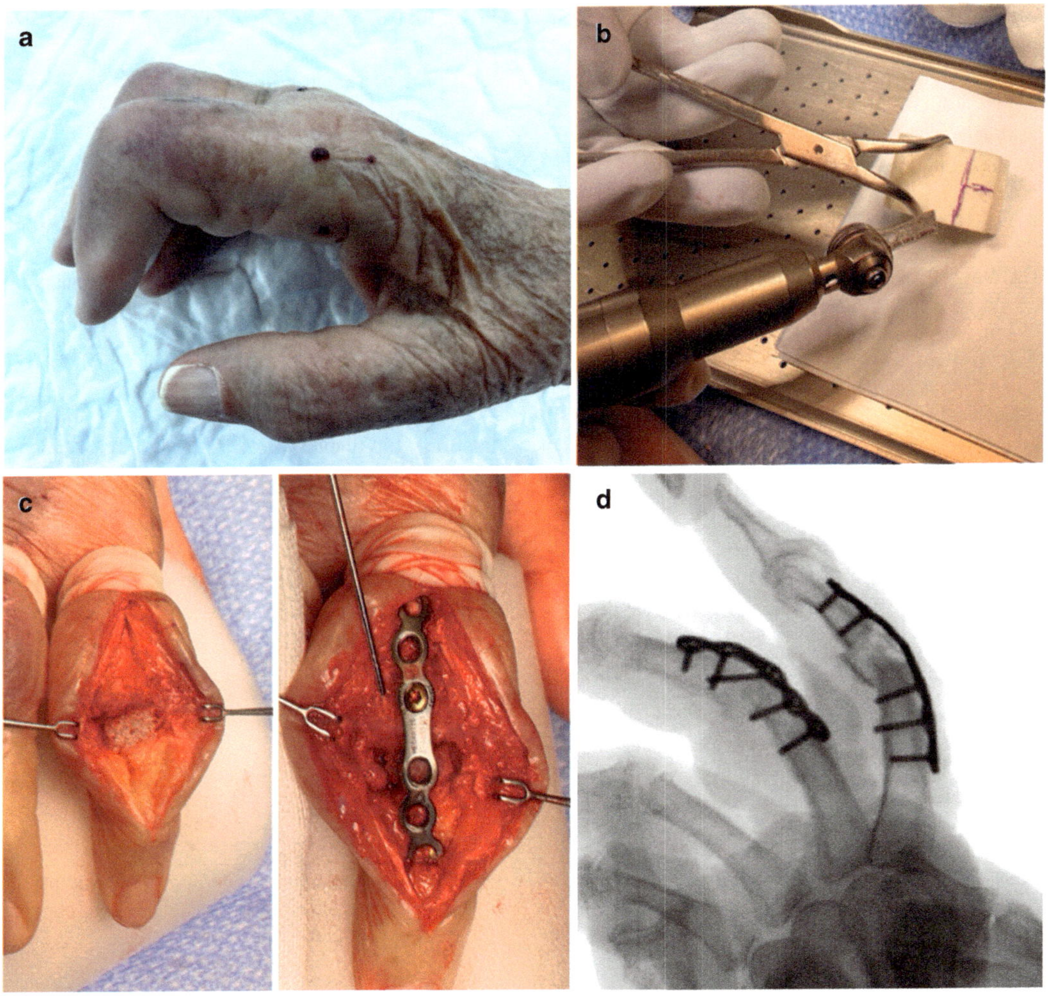

Fig. 21.6 Revision case in a patient with fixed but painful Boutonniere deformity after PIP arthroplasty. (**a**) Clinical picture with the index and middle finger in flexed deformity. (**b**) Intraoperative preparation of a homologous cortical-cancellous bone graft to bridge the defect in the index finger. (**c**) Bone graft in situ with preliminary K-wire fixation and plate adaption. (**d**) Intraoperative x-ray control with a bridge graft in the index finger and direct fixation of the middle finger PIP joint. The cortical side of the graft is faced to the volar side to offer compression stability

finger (Fig. 21.6). Alternately, the graft can be fixed to the plate first and then placed together on the bone ends. There are special plates available with a proximal horizontal hole, which allows definitive positioning of the arthrodesis in situ. The most critical factor is rotation. It is absolutely necessary to check the three-dimensional position of the finger in flexion, especially in relation to the neighboring fingers. Even minimal rotational deformity may be functionally disabling. The fusion angle depends on the position of the finger in relation to the hand and the other PIP joints. The ulnar fingers, especially the small finger, need more flexion than the index finger during pinching with the thumb.

Healing might be prolonged, especially when homologous bone grafts are used, and protection splints often need to be worn up to 3 months after surgery.

**Table 21.3** Synopsis of the different problems leading to revision surgery after PIP arthroplasty and their possible solutions

| | Cause | Therapeutical options | Salvage |
|---|---|---|---|
| *General complications:* | | | |
| Wound healing problems | Biological | Revision | |
| Infection | Biological | Revision debridement<br>Antibiotics | Amputation |
| CRPS | Dystrophic reaction | Therapy<br>Medication<br>Vitamin C | Amputation |
| *Soft tissue-driven complications:* | | | |
| Tendon adhesions | Biological<br>Inadequate therapy /noncompliance<br>Pain | Therapy<br>Tenolysis | |
| Ossifications:<br>Around tendons<br>Joint capsule | Biological<br>Surgical technique | Often nothing<br>Steroid injection<br>Removal ossification /±arthro-/tenolysis | |
| Tendon rupture/ insufficiency | Preexisting imbalances/-insufficiency<br>Tendon scarring<br>Surgical technique | Tendon reconstruction<br>Tendon transfer | Joint fusion |
| Tendon imbalances/-insufficiency:<br>Swan neck deformity<br>Boutonniere deformity | Tendon imbalances/-insufficiency:<br>Swan neck deformity<br>Boutonniere deformity | Tendon rebalancing<br>Implant characteristics | Joint fusion |
| Joint instability | Implant tensioning<br>Ligament insufficiency<br>Implant characteristics (Silicone) | Implant revision<br>Ligament reconstruction<br>Implant change (two component implant) | Joint fusion |
| *Implant-driven complications:* | | | |
| Joint instability/ dislocation | Implant tensioning<br>Ligament insufficiency<br>Adequate trauma | Implant revision<br>± Ligament reconstruction<br>Revision according to the damage | Joint fusion |
| Implant loosening | Biological<br>Insufficient primary fixation<br>Implant wear | Implant revision ±bone grafting<br>Implant change (Silicone) | Joint fusion |
| Joint deformation | Implant mal-position<br>Lateral deviation<br>Antero-posterior subluxation | Implant revision/-change<br>Ligament insufficiency | Joint fusion |
| Joint stiffness | Scarring Tendon Joint capsule Inadequate therapy/noncompliance Pain implant overstuffing | Therapy arthro-/tenolysis implant revision/change | Joint fusion |

Finger amputation as a salvage intervention must be discussed in cases of multiple revisions and unsolvable problems including infection or significant soft tissue deficiency.

Table 21.3 gives an overview of the different problems leading to a revision intervention after PIP arthroplasty and its possible solutions (Table 21.3).

## References


1. Ranney D. The hand as a concept: digital differences and their importance. Clin Anat. 1995;8(4):281–7. PubMed PMID: 7552966. Epub 1995/01/01. eng.
2. Evans DM. The PIP joint. Clin Rheum Dis. 1984;10(3):631–56. PubMed PMID: 6532646. Epub 1984/12/01. eng.
3. White WL. Why I hate the index finger. Hand (N Y). 2010;5(4):461–5. PubMed PMID: 22131935. Pubmed Central PMCID: PMC2997957. Epub 2011/12/02. eng.
4. Aversano FJ, Calfee RP. Salvaging a failed proximal interphalangeal joint implant. Hand Clin. 2018;34(2):217–27. PubMed PMID: 29625641. Epub 2018/04/08. eng.
5. Bravo CJ, Rizzo M, Hormel KB, Beckenbaugh RD. Pyrolytic carbon proximal interphalangeal joint arthroplasty: results with minimum two-year follow-up evaluation. J Hand Surg Am. 2007;32(1):1–11. PubMed PMID: 17218170. Epub 2007/01/16. eng.
6. Daecke W, Kaszap B, Martini AK, Hagena FW, Rieck B, Jung M. A prospective, randomized comparison of 3 types of proximal interphalangeal joint arthroplasty. J Hand Surg Am. 2012;37(9):1770–9. e1-3. PubMed PMID: 22916864. Epub 2012/08/25. eng.
7. Herren D. The proximal interphalangeal joint: arthritis and deformity. EFORT Open Rev. 2019;4(6):254–62. PubMed PMID: 31312517. Pubmed Central PMCID: PMC6598614. Epub 2019/07/18. eng.
8. Herren DB, Keuchel T, Marks M, Schindele S. Revision arthroplasty for failed silicone proximal interphalangeal joint arthroplasty: indications and 8-year results. J Hand Surg Am. 2014;39(3):462–6. PubMed PMID: 24503230. Epub 2014/02/08. eng.
9. Komatsu I, Arishima Y, Shibahashi H, Yamaguchi T, Minamikawa Y. Outcomes of surface replacement proximal interphalangeal joint arthroplasty using the self locking finger joint implant: minimum two years follow-up. Hand (N Y). 2018;13(6):637–45. PubMed PMID: 28918664. Pubmed Central PMCID: PMC6300185. Epub 2017/09/19. eng.
10. Naghshineh N, Goyal K, Giugale JM, Neral MK, Ferreira JV, Buterbaugh GA, et al. Proximal interphalangeal joint silicone arthroplasty for osteoarthritis: midterm outcomes. Hand (N Y). 2018:1558944718769427. PubMed PMID: 29619888. Pubmed Central PMCID: PMC6759980. Epub 2018/04/06. eng.
11. Pritsch T, Rizzo M. Reoperations following proximal interphalangeal joint nonconstrained arthroplasties. J Hand Surg Am. 2011;36(9):1460–6. PubMed PMID: 21803509. Epub 2011/08/02. eng.
12. Schindele SF, Hensler S, Audige L, Marks M, Herren DB. A modular surface gliding implant (CapFlex-PIP) for proximal interphalangeal joint osteoarthritis: a prospective case series. J Hand Surg Am. 2015;40(2):334–40. PubMed PMID: 25510157. Epub 2014/12/17. eng.
13. Vitale MA, Fruth KM, Rizzo M, Moran SL, Kakar S. Prosthetic arthroplasty versus arthrodesis for osteoarthritis and posttraumatic arthritis of the index finger proximal Interphalangeal joint. J Hand Surg Am. 2015;40(10):1937–48. PubMed PMID: 26188383. Epub 2015/07/21. eng.
14. Watts AC, Hearnden AJ, Trail IA, Hayton MJ, Nuttall D, Stanley JK. Pyrocarbon proximal interphalangeal joint arthroplasty: minimum two-year follow-up. J Hand Surg Am. 2012;37(5):882–8. PubMed PMID: 22541153. Epub 2012/05/01. eng.
15. Sweets TM, Stern PJ. Pyrolytic carbon resurfacing arthroplasty for osteoarthritis of the proximal interphalangeal joint of the finger. J Bone Joint Surg Am. 2011;93(15):1417–25. PubMed PMID: 21915547. Epub 2011/09/15. eng.
16. 14155:2011: SII. Clinical investigation of medical devices for human subjects - Good clinical practice. International Organization for Standardization. Available from: http://www.iso.org/standard/45557.html.
17. Labek G, Thaler M, Janda W, Agreiter M, Stockl B. Revision rates after total joint replacement: cumulative results from worldwide joint register datasets. J Bone Joint Surg. 2011;93(3):293–7. PubMed PMID: 21357948. Epub 2011/03/02. eng.
18. Yamamoto M, Chung KC. Joint fusion and arthroplasty in the hand. Clin Plast Surg. 2019;46(3):479–88. PubMed PMID: 31103091. Epub 2019/05/20. eng.
19. Foliart DE. Swanson silicone finger joint implants: a review of the literature regarding long-term complications. J Hand Surg Am. 1995;20(3):445–9. PubMed PMID: 7642924. Epub 1995/05/01. eng.
20. Wagner ER, Luo TD, Houdek MT, Kor DJ, Moran SL, Rizzo M. Revision proximal interphalangeal arthroplasty: An outcome analysis of 75 consecutive cases. J Hand Surg Am. 2015;40(10):1949–55 e1. PubMed PMID: 26163921. Epub 2015/07/15. eng.
21. Iselin F, Pradet G. Resection arthroplasty with Swanson's implant for posttraumatic stiffness of proximal interphalangeal joints. Bull Hosp Jt Dis Orthop Inst. 1984;44(2):233–47. PubMed PMID: 6099170. Epub 1984/01/01. eng.
22. Swanson AB, de Groot Swanson G. Flexible implant resection arthroplasty of the proximal interphalangeal joint. Hand Clin. 1994;10(2):261–6. PubMed PMID: 8040204. Epub 1994/05/01. eng.
23. Wagner ER, Robinson WA, Houdek MT, Moran SL, Rizzo M. Proximal interphalangeal joint arthroplasty in young patients. J Am Acad Orthop Surg. 2019;27(12):444–50. PubMed PMID: 31170098. Epub 2019/06/07. eng.
24. Bales JG, Wall LB, Stern PJ. Long-term results of Swanson silicone arthroplasty for proximal interphalangeal joint osteoarthritis. J Hand Surg Am. 2014;39(3):455–61. PubMed PMID: 24559624. Epub 2014/02/25. eng.
25. Takigawa S, Meletiou S, Sauerbier M, Cooney WP. Long-term assessment of Swanson implant

arthroplasty in the proximal interphalangeal joint of the hand. J Hand Surg Am. 2004;29(5):785–95. PubMed PMID: 15465226. Epub 2004/10/07. eng.

26. Pugliese D, Bush D, Harrington T. Silicone synovitis: longer term outcome data and review of the literature. J Clin Rheumatol. 2009;15(1):8–11. PubMed PMID: 19125138. Epub 2009/01/07. eng.
27. Lanzetta M, Herbert TJ, Conolly WB. Silicone synovitis. A perspective. J Hand Surg Br. 1994;19(4):479–84. PubMed PMID: 7964100. Epub 1994/08/01. eng.
28. Peimer CA, Medige J, Eckert BS, Wright JR, Howard CS. Reactive synovitis after silicone arthroplasty. J Hand Surg Am. 1986;11(5):624–38. PubMed PMID: 3531304. Epub 1986/09/01. eng.
29. Atkinson RE, Smith RJ. Silicone synovitis following silicone implant arthroplasty. Hand Clin. 1986;2(2):291–9. PubMed PMID: 3517015. Epub 1986/05/01. eng.
30. Nalbandian RM. Synovitis and lymphadenopathy in silicone arthroplasty implants. J Bone Joint Surg Am. 1983;65(2):280–1. PubMed PMID: 6337166. Epub 1983/02/01. eng.
31. Johnstone BR, Fitzgerald M, Smith KR, Currie LJ. Cemented versus uncemented surface replacement arthroplasty of the proximal interphalangeal joint with a mean 5-year follow-up. J Hand Surg Am. 2008;33(5):726–32. PubMed PMID: 18590856. Epub 2008/07/02. eng.
32. Tägil M, Geijer M, Abramo A, Kopylov P. Ten years' experience with a pyrocarbon prosthesis replacing the proximal interphalangeal joint. A prospective clinical and radiographic follow-up. J Hand Surg Eur Vol. 2014;39(6):587–95. PubMed PMID: 23461909. Epub 2013/03/07. eng.
33. Reissner L, Schindele S, Hensler S, Marks M, Herren DB. Ten year follow-up of pyrocarbon implants for proximal interphalangeal joint replacement. J Hand Surg Eur Vol. 2014;39(6):582–6. PubMed PMID: 24459251. Epub 2014/01/25. eng.
34. Herren DB, Schindele S, Goldhahn J, Simmen BR. Problematic bone fixation with pyrocarbon implants in proximal interphalangeal joint replacement: short-term results. J Hand Surg Br. 2006;31(6):643–51. PubMed PMID: 17046119. Epub 2006/10/19. eng.
35. Wesemann A, Flügel M, Mamarvar M. [Moje prosthesis for the proximal interphalangeal joint]. Handchirurgie, Mikrochirurgie, plastische Chirurgie: Organ der Deutschsprachigen Arbeitsgemeinschaft fur Handchirurgie: Organ der Deutschsprachigen Arbeitsgemeinschaft fur Mikrochirurgie der Peripheren Nerven und Gefasse. 2008;40(3):189–96. PubMed PMID: 18551388. Epub 2008/06/14. Moje-Prothese im proximalen Interphalangealgelenk. ger.
36. Hansen TB, Vainorius D. High loosening rate of the Moje Acamo prosthesis for treating osteoarthritis of the trapeziometacarpal joint. J Hand Surg Eur Vol. 2008;33(5):571–4. PubMed PMID: 18694921. Epub 2008/08/13. eng.
37. Field J. Two to five year follow-up of the LPM ceramic coated proximal interphalangeal joint arthroplasty. J Hand Surg Eur Vol. 2008;33(1):38–44. PubMed PMID: 18332018. Epub 2008/03/12. eng.
38. Daecke W, Veyel K, Wieloch P, Jung M, Lorenz H, Martini AK. Osseointegration and mechanical stability of pyrocarbon and titanium hand implants in a load-bearing in vivo model for small joint arthroplasty. J Hand Surg Am. 2006;31(1):90–7. PubMed PMID: 16443111. Epub 2006/01/31. eng.
39. Schindele SF, Sprecher CM, Milz S, Hensler S. Osteointegration of a modular metal-polyethylene surface gliding finger implant: a case report. Arch Orthop Trauma Surg. 2016;136(9):1331–5. PubMed PMID: 27450194. Epub 2016/07/28. eng.
40. Ash HE, Unsworth A. Proximal interphalangeal joint dimensions for the design of a surface replacement prosthesis. Proceedings of the Institution of Mechanical Engineers Part H. J Eng Med. 1996;210(2):95–108. PubMed PMID: 8688122. Epub 1996/01/01. eng.
41. Ash HE, Unsworth A. Design of a surface replacement prosthesis for the proximal interphalangeal joint. Proceedings of the Institution of Mechanical Engineers Part H. J Eng Med. 2000;214(2):151–63. PubMed PMID: 10825773. Epub 2000/05/29. eng.
42. Uchiyama S, Cooney WP 3rd, Linscheid RL, Niebur G, An KN. Kinematics of the proximal interphalangeal joint of the finger after surface replacement. J Hand Surg Am. 2000;25(2):305–12. PubMed PMID: 10722823. Epub 2000/03/21. eng.
43. Hensler S, Behm P, Wehrli M, Marks M, Ferguson SJ, Herren DB, et al. Lateral stability in healthy proximal interphalangeal joints versus surface replacement and silicone arthroplasty: results of a three-dimensional motion analysis study. Hand Surg Rehabil. 2020. PubMed PMID: 32376507. Epub 2020/05/08. eng.
44. Linscheid RL. Implant arthroplasty of the hand: retrospective and prospective considerations. J Hand Surg Am. 2000;25(5):796–816. PubMed PMID: 11040295. Epub 2000/10/21. eng.
45. Zhu AF, Rahgozar P, Chung KC. Advances in proximal interphalangeal joint arthroplasty: biomechanics and biomaterials. Hand Clin. 2018;34(2):185–94. PubMed PMID: 29625638. Pubmed Central PMCID: PMC5890942. Epub 2018/04/08. eng.
46. Billig JI, Nasser JS, Chung KC. National prevalence of complications and cost of small joint arthroplasty for hand osteoarthritis and post-traumatic arthritis. J Hand Surg Am. 2020. PubMed PMID: 31924436. Epub 2020/01/12. eng.
47. Murray PM, Linscheid RL, Cooney WP 3rd, Baker V, Heckman MG. Long-term outcomes of proximal interphalangeal joint surface replacement arthroplasty. J Bone Joint Surg Am. 2012;94(12):1120–8. PubMed PMID: 22717831. Epub 2012/06/22. eng.
48. Bodmer E, Marks M, Hensler S, Schindele S, Herren DB. Comparison of outcomes of three surgical approaches for proximal interphalangeal joint arthroplasty using a surface-replacing implant. J Hand Surg Eur Vol. 2019:1753193419891382. PubMed PMID: 31813305. Epub 2019/12/10. eng.

# Index




G. J. W. King, M. Rizzo (eds.), *Arthroplasty of the Upper Extremity*,
https://doi.org/10.1007/978-3-030-68880-6

GPSR Compliance

*The European Union's (EU) General Product Safety Regulation (GPSR) is a set of rules that requires consumer products to be safe and our obligations to ensure this.*

*If you have any concerns about our products, you can contact us on ProductSafety@springernature.com*

In case Publisher is established outside the EU, the EU authorized representative is:

Springer Nature Customer Service Center GmbH
Europaplatz 3
69115 Heidelberg, Germany

**Batch number: 10731393**

Printed by Printforce, the Netherlands